Thyroid and Parathyroid Diseases

Medical and Surgical Management

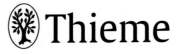 Thieme

Thyroid and Parathyroid Diseases
Medical and Surgical Management

David J. Terris
Porubsky Professor and Chairman
Department of Otolaryngology–Head and Neck Surgery
Surgical Director, MCG Thyroid Center
Medical College of Georgia
Augusta, Georgia

Christine G. Gourin
Associate Professor
Director, Clinical Research Program in Head and Neck Cancer
Department of Otolaryngology–Head and Neck Surgery
Johns Hopkins University
Baltimore, Maryland

Thieme
New York • Stuttgart

Thieme Medical Publishers, Inc.
333 Seventh Ave.
New York, NY 10001

Managing Editor: J. Owen Zurhellen
Editorial Assistant: Jacquelyn DeSanti
Consulting Medical Editor: Esther Gumpert
Vice President, Production and Electronic Publishing: Anne T. Vinnicombe
Production Editor: Kenneth L. Chumbley, Publication Services
Vice President, International Marketing and Sales: Cornelia Schulze
Chief Financial Officer: Peter van Woerden
President: Brian D. Scanlan
Medical Illustrator: Joel Herring
Compositor: Aptara, Inc.
Printer: Everbest Printing Company, Ltd.
Cover illustration drawn by Markus Voll

Library of Congress Cataloging-in-Publication Data

Thyroid and parathyroid diseases : medical and surgical management / [edited by] David J. Terris, Christine G. Gourin.
   p. ; cm.
  Includes bibliographical references and index.
  ISBN 978-1-58890-518-5 (alk. paper)
   1. Thyroid gland–Surgery. 2. Parathyroid glands–Surgery. 3. Thyroid gland–Cancer–Surgery. I. Terris, David J. II. Gourin, Christine G.
  [DNLM: 1. Thyroid Diseases–surgery. 2. Endocrine Surgical Procedures–methods. 3. Parathyroid Diseases–surgery. WK 280 T5486 2009]

  RD599.T496 2009
  617.5′39–dc22

                                                    2008017082

Important note: Medical knowledge is ever-changing. As new research and clinical experience broaden our knowledge, changes in treatment and drug therapy may be required. The authors and editors of the material herein have consulted sources believed to be reliable in their efforts to provide information that is complete and in accord with the standards accepted at the time of publication. However, in view of the possibility of human error by the authors, editors, or publisher of the work herein or changes in medical knowledge, neither the authors, editors, nor publisher, nor any other party who has been involved in the preparation of this work, warrants that the information contained herein is in every respect accurate or complete, and they are not responsible for any errors or omissions or for the results obtained from use of such information. Readers are encouraged to confirm the information contained herein with other sources. For example, readers are advised to check the product information sheet included in the package of each drug they plan to administer to be certain that the information contained in this publication is accurate and that changes have not been made in the recommended dose or in the contraindications for administration. This recommendation is of particular importance in connection with new or infrequently used drugs. Some of the product names, patents, and registered designs referred to in this book are in fact registered trademarks or proprietary names even though specific reference to this fact is not always made in the text. Therefore, the appearance of a name without designation as proprietary is not to be construed as a representation by the publisher that it is in the public domain.

Printed in China

5 4 3 2 1

ISBN: 978-1-58890-518-5

To our patients, who allowed us the privilege and honor of caring for them and learning from their experiences.

David J. Terris
Christine G. Gourin

Contents

Foreword

In recent years, diseases of the thyroid gland have drawn increased attention from the media and the public due to a steep rise in the identification of clinically occult nodular thyroid disease. This is largely attributed to increased awareness and technological advances in imaging, which often identify small intraglandular nodules in the thyroid gland, warranting the need for further workup. Discovery of such clinically occult nodules has been largely responsible for the significant rise in the identification of cancer of the thyroid gland in the United States and around the world. Such is the impact of these subclinical thyroid cancers on surgical and medical practices that they have become a major component of the clinical volume for surgeons who specialize in endocrine surgery, head and neck surgery, otolaryngology, and general surgery. Clearly, an improved understanding of the biology of these diseases and their appropriate clinical management is essential to the delivery of optimal health care to our patients.

Doctors David Terris and Christine Gourin are to be complimented for putting together this book, which reflects contemporary thinking and practice in the management of thyroid and parathyroid diseases. This is a timely publication for this topic, because the demand for a resource that provides improved understanding of these diseases is increasing. It is to be noted that nearly all of the surgical contributors to this textbook are otolaryngologists with a special interest in the field of thyroid and parathyroid surgery. This is a changing trend in clinical practice in the United States and reflects the changing pattern of specialty migration for endocrine surgery related to thyroid and parathyroid diseases. Clearly, individuals with significant interest and expertise in this subject will continue to gather experience and will become leaders in the years to come.

Thyroid cancer in particular has become an area of major interest to the media and the public. Improved understanding of its biology has drastically changed the management approach to differentiated thyroid carcinoma. The impact of prognostic factors and risk group stratification has heavily influenced the management strategies and outcomes in patients with thyroid carcinoma. Still, however, much work needs to be done on those thyroid cancers that account for the majority of deaths from this disease. Progress is likely to be made at the molecular level where newly discovered targeted therapies may play a role in the control of such aggressive cancers.

This book provides a systematic approach to understanding the pathophysiology of nonneoplastic diseases of the thyroid gland and the biological behavior of cancer of the thyroid gland. A systematic approach to the epidemiology, pathology, diagnostic workup, clinical management, and outcomes makes this a valuable resource for students, residents-in-training, and clinicians who encounter diseases and neoplasms of the thyroid and parathyroid glands in their clinical practice.

Jatin P. Shah, MD, PhD (Hon.), FACS, FRCS (Hon.),
FRACS (Hon.), FDSRCS (Hon.)
Professor of Surgery
Elliot W. Strong Chair in Head and Neck Oncology
Chief, Head and Neck Service
Memorial Sloan-Kettering Cancer Center
New York, New York

Preface

After nearly a century of performing a thyroidectomy essentially the way Theodore Kocher described, the field of thyroid and parathyroid surgery has undergone rapid change in the past few years. With the advent of high-resolution endoscopy, advanced energy sources, precise localization, and intraoperative testing and guidance, the traditional approach to thyroid and parathyroid diseases has evolved in many ways that could not even be imagined just ten years ago. The publication of a new textbook devoted to medical and surgical management of endocrine head and neck surgery is therefore timely and appropriate.

In this new book, a deliberate effort has been made to provide not only meaningful information useful to the practitioner but also high-quality figures and drawings to facilitate the understanding of innovative concepts in the field. Major thought leaders in the discipline of thyroid and parathyroid disease have generously contributed their time and expertise to this effort, and the result is a comprehensive yet lean reference that provides a fresh look at the quickly evolving concepts in thyroid and parathyroid surgery.

It is remarkable to recognize how many principles have changed since many of us were taught how to evaluate and treat patients with endocrine head and neck diseases, not so long ago, by respected giants in the field. From a minimally invasive total thyroidectomy accomplished without sutures or drains on an outpatient basis, to a directed parathyroidectomy performed under local anesthesia in which three nonpathologic parathyroid glands are allowed to remain undisturbed, patients everywhere have benefited from progress that has been made in endocrine surgery. The game has indeed changed in a significant and far-reaching way, and we have provided a suitable reference for meeting the challenges of modern thyroid and parathyroid surgery.

Acknowledgments

It is impossible to acknowledge all of the people who helped bring this project to completion. Nevertheless, it is an honor to recognize three individuals who had a profound impact on my interest and understanding of thyroid diseases and surgery: Bill Fee, Sewall Professor of Otolaryngology at Stanford, taught me to do thyroid surgery; Paolo Miccoli, Professor of Surgery at the University of Pisa, taught me the fundamentals of minimally invasive endoscopic thyroid surgery; and Ted Chin, Professor of Medicine at the Medical College of Georgia, represents a true partner in our efforts to optimally manage patients with thyroid diseases.

David J. Terris, MD, FACS
Augusta, Georgia

With gratitude to my mentors—Bob Sofferman and Jonas Johnson—surgeons, clinicians, and teachers extraordinaire.

Christine G. Gourin, MD, FACS
Baltimore, Maryland

Contributors

Adam M. Becker, MD
Resident
Department of Otolaryngology–Head and
    Neck Surgery
Medical College of Georgia
Augusta, Georgia

Brett M. Clarke, MD, MS
Resident
Department of Otolaryngology-Head and
    Neck Surgery
University of Arkansas for Medical Sciences
Little Rock, Arkansas

James I. Cohen, MD, PhD
Professor
Director, Thyroid/Parathyroid Surgery Program
Department of Otolaryngology–Head and
    Neck Surgery
Oregon Health & Science University
Portland, Oregon

Tzeela Cohen, MD
Research Fellow
Haddassah Mount Scopus Medical Center
Jerusalem, Israel

David W. Eisele, MD, FACS
Professor and Chairman
Department of Otolaryngology–Head and Neck Surgery
University of California, San Francisco
San Francisco, California

Christine G. Gourin, MD, FACS
Associate Professor
Director, Clinical Research Program in Head and Neck Cancer
Department of Otolaryngology–Head and Neck Surgery
Johns Hopkins University
Baltimore, Maryland

Jahmal A. Hairston, MD
Ear, Nose, and Throat Plastic Surgery Center
Douglasville, Georgia

Carlos M. Isales, MD
Professor
Department of Orthopaedic Surgery
Medical College of Georgia
Augusta, Georgia

Mark J. Jameson, MD, PhD
Assistant Professor
Division of Head and Neck Surgical Oncology
Department of Otolaryngology–Head and Neck Surgery
University of Virginia Health System
Charlottesville, Virginia

Jonas T. Johnson, MD, FACS
Professor and Chairman
Department of Otolaryngology
University of Pittsburgh School of Medicine
Pittsburgh, Pennsylvania

Matthew I. Kim, MD
Assistant Professor
Division of Endocrinology and Metabolism
Johns Hopkins University
Baltimore, Maryland

Michael E. Kupferman, MD
Assistant Professor
Department of Head and Neck Surgery
University of Texas
M.D. Anderson Cancer Center
Houston, Texas

Stephen Y. Lai, MD, PhD, FACS
Assistant Professor
Department of Otolaryngology
University of Pittsburgh Cancer Institute
University of Pittsburgh School of Medicine
Pittsburgh, Pennsylvania

Brian Hung-Hin Lang, MS, FRACS
Fellow
Division of Endocrine Surgery
Department of Surgery
University of Hong Kong Medical Centre
Queen Mary Hospital
Hong Kong SAR, China

Jill E. Langer, MD
Associate Professor
Department of Radiology
University of Pennsylvania School of Medicine
Philadelphia, Pennsylvania

Paul A. Levine, MD, FACS
Robert W. Cantrell Professor and Chairman
Department of Otolaryngology-Head and Neck Surgery
Chair
Division of Head and Neck Surgical Oncology
University of Virginia Health System
Charlottesville, Virginia

Chung-Yau Lo, MS, FRCS (Edin), FACS
Professor
Division of Endocrine Surgery
Department of Surgery
University of Hong Kong Medical Centre
Queen Mary Hospital
Hong Kong SAR, China

Laurie A. Loevner, MD
Professor
Departments of Radiology and Otorhinolaryngology
Codirector of Oncologic Imaging
University of Pennsylvania School of Medicine
Philadelphia, Pennsylvania

Susan Mandel, MD, MPH
Associate Professor
Associate Chief
Division of Endocrinology, Diabetes, and Metabolism
University of Pennsylvania School of Medicine
Philadelphia, Pennsylvania

Ernest L. Mazzaferri, MD
Professor
Department of Medicine
Division of Endocrinology and Metabolism
University of Florida
Gainesville, Florida

Radu Mihai, MD, PhD, FRCS
Consultant Endocrine Surgeon
Department of Surgery
John Radcliffe Hospital
Oxford, England

William H. Moretz III, MD
Resident
Department of Otolaryngology–Head and Neck Surgery
Medical College of Georgia
Augusta, Georgia

Lisa A. Orloff, MD, FACS
Professor
Department of Otolaryngology–Head and Neck Surgery
University of California, San Francisco
San Francisco, California

Kepal N. Patel, MD
Assistant Professor
Department of Endocrine Surgery
New York University School of Medicine
New York, New York

Phillip K. Pellitteri, DO, FACS
Section Head and Director of Research
Department of Otolaryngology–Head and Neck Surgery
Geisinger Health System
Danville, Pennsylvania
Clinical Professor
Department of Otolaryngology-Head and Neck Surgery
Temple University School of Medicine
Philadelphia, Pennsylvania

James Ragland, MD
Resident
Department of Otolaryngology-Head and Neck Surgery
University of Arkansas for Medical Sciences
Little Rock, Arkansas

Anatoly P. Romanchishen, MD
Professor and Chief of Endocrine Surgery
Saint Petersburg State Pediatric Medical Academy
Director of Endocrine and Surgical Oncology
Mariinsky Hosptial and Sokolv Central Hospital
Saint Petersburg, Russia

Gregory W. Randolph, MD, FACS
Associate Professor
Department of Laryngology and Otology
Harvard Medical School
Massachusetts Eye and Ear Infirmary
Boston, Massachusetts

Kathryn G. Schuff, MD
Associate Professor
Department of Medicine
Division of Endocrinology
Oregon Health & Science University
Portland, Oregon

Ashok R. Shaha, MD
Attending Surgeon, Professor of Surgery
Department of Head and Neck Service
Memorial Sloan-Kettering Cancer Center
New York, New York

Karuna Shekdar, MD
Attending Radiologist
Department of Radiology, Neuroradiology Section
The Children's Hospital of Philadelphia
Philadelphia, Pennsylvania

Maisie L. Shindo, MD, FACS
Professor
Department of Otolaryngology–Head and Neck
    Surgery
Oregon Health & Science University
Portland, Oregon

Bhuvanesh Singh, MD, PhD, FACS
Associate Attending Surgeon
Head and Neck Service
Director
Laboratory of Epithelial Cell Biology
Department of Surgery
Memorial Sloan-Kettering Cancer Center
Assistant Professor
Weil Medical College of Cornell University
Visiting Associate Physician
Rockefeller University
New York, New York

Jennifer Sipos, MD
Assistant Professor
Division of Endocrinology and Metabolism
University of Florida
Gainesville, Florida

Jason A. Smith, MD
Arkansas Otolaryngology
Little Rock, Arkansas

Robert A. Sofferman, MD, FACS
Professor
Division of Otolaryngology
University of Vermont School of Medicine
Burlington, Vermont

Brendan C. Stack Jr., MD, FACS, FACE
Professor and Vice Chairman of Adult Services
James Y. Suen, MD Chair in Otolaryngology—Head
    and Neck Surgery
Chief, Division of Head and Neck Oncology
Director of Clinical Research
Director, McGill Family Division of Clinical Research
Department of Otolaryngology–Head and Neck Surgery
University of Arkansas for Medical Sciences
Little Rock, Arkansas

David L. Steward, MD, FACS
Associate Professor
Department of Otolaryngology–Head and Neck Surgery
University of Cinncinnati College of Medicine
Cincinnati, Ohio

David J. Terris, MD, FACS
Porubsky Professor and Chairman
Department of Otolaryngology–Head and Neck Surgery
Surgical Director, MCG Thyroid Center
Medical College of Georgia
Augusta, Georgia

Ralph P. Tufano, MD, FACS
Associate Professor
Department of Otolaryngology–Head and Neck Surgery
Johns Hopkins University
Baltimore, Maryland

Randal S. Weber, MD, FACS
Professor and Chairman
Department of Head and Neck Surgery
University of Texas
M.D. Anderson Cancer Center
Houston, Texas

Anatomy and Physiology of the Thyroid Compartment

1 The History and Evolution of Techniques for Thyroid Surgery

Radu Mihai, Anatoly P. Romanchisen, and Gregory W. Randolph

Thyroidectomy has evolved through years of tortuous misunderstanding and complications to an elegant procedure of minimal morbidity, the epitome of the surgeon's art. It was primarily the pioneering work of Theodor Kocher, rewarded with the 1909 Nobel Prize, that catalyzed this evolution. This chapter reviews the evolution of thyroidectomy and offers a new classification scheme to organize thought on the current various surgical approaches available for operations on the thyroid gland.

The Normal and Enlarged Thyroid: Initial Misunderstandings

Goiters (Latin *guttur* = throat) were recognized in China as early as 2700 BC and by the Romans in the Alps in the first three centuries AD. The normal thyroid gland was not recognized until the Renaissance. In about 1500, Leonardo da Vinci drew the thyroid as a globular bilobate structure, which he regarded as two glands, filling the empty spaces in the neck. In 1543 Andreas Vesalius of Padua described two "glandulae larynges," which, he thought, lubricated the larynx. Bartholomaeus Eustachius of Rome, who also described the adrenal glands, described a single "glandulam thyroideam" (Latin for shield-shaped) with an isthmus connecting its lobes, but his work was not published until the 18th century. In 1656 Thomas Wharton of London described and named "glandula thyroidoeis." The onset of goiter in the young adult at that time led to speculation that goiter formation was associated with sexual maturity. In the late 18th century, microscopy revealed colloid-filled vesicles within the gland. Caleb Hillier Parry of Bath, England, who also described exophthalmic goiter, speculated that the thyroid provided a reservoir to prevent engorgement of the brain.[1,2]

Setons, Bootlaces, and Prison: Early Days of Thyroid Surgery

Celsus and Galen have been credited with operating on goiters in the first and second centuries, but it was not until 500 AD in Baghdad that Abdul Kasan Kelebis Abis performed the first recorded goiter excision.

Roger Frugardi, in the Italian School of Salerno, provided the first credible description of operation for goiter in approximately 1170. At that time if a large goiter failed to respond to medication, including iodine-containing marine products, two setons were inserted at right angles, with the help of a hot iron, and manipulated toward the surface twice daily until they had cut through the flesh. Another technique for those goiters that projected anteriorly involved a skin incision, grasping the tumor with a hook and then dissecting skin from the goiter. The exposed pedunculated portion of the goiter would be ligated en masse with a bootlace and removed. During such procedures the patients were tied down to tables and held firmly. In 1718 German surgeons wrote an account of thyroid surgery that differed little from that of Frugardi's.

In 1646, Wilhelm Fabricus reported the first thyroidectomy using scalpels. Unfortunately, this technical advance was associated with a poor outcome: the patient died and the surgeon was imprisoned. Pierre-Joseph Desault of Paris is the first surgeon to publish an account of a successful removal of a goiter, which he performed in 1791. He used a vertical incision, and isolated and ligated the superior and inferior thyroid arteries before cutting them and dissecting the thyroid from the trachea using the scalpel. He packed the wound, which suppurated and healed in a month. Guillaume Dupuytren followed in Desault's footsteps, and in 1808 performed the first "total thyroidectomy."

Attempts to suppress the gland by ligation of the superior thyroid artery were first made by William Blizzard in 1811. Although relatively simple due to the lateral approach, this operation fell into disuse because of minimal long-term benefit.

In the mid-19th century, William Halsted of Baltimore, in his monumental *Operative Story of Goitre,* could trace accounts of only eight thyroid operations in which a scalpel had been used between 1596 (the year of the first report) and 1800, and an additional 69 cases until 1848. In the 1850s, a variety of incisions were performed for thyroidectomy: longitudinal, oblique, Y-shaped. After a skin incision, most surgeons performed blunt dissection, and their control of bleeding was inadequate. Despite significant perioperative blood loss, bloodletting was performed for postoperative complications. Typically the wound was left open and dead spaces packed or left to fill with blood. At this time the mortality after thyroid surgery was as high as 40%. Not surprisingly, The French Academy of Medicine condemned any operative procedures on the thyroid gland, and Samuel David Gross, a prominent American surgeon, wrote in 1866: "No honest and sensible surgeon would ever engage in it!"

Through the majority of the 19th century the results of thyroid operations were so poor that most surgeons restricted their practice to very simple procedures, which could be grouped in three categories:

1. *Noncutting operations*: setons and bristles were inserted, and cysts were punctured and injected with iodine or other irritants. Deaths from hemorrhage, inflammation, or air embolus were not uncommon.
2. *Enucleation* and bootlace *ligation* of goiters.
3. *Cutting operations* with removal of thyroid tissue: These typically included ligation of thyroid arteries and division of superficial muscles and fascia.

The 19th Century Revolution: Kocher's Thyroidectomy

The 19th century marked a revolution in all fields of surgery triggered by the introduction of general anesthesia and aseptic technique. In 1849 Nikolai Pirogoff of St. Petersburg, Russia, employed ether for a thyroid operation on a 17-year-old girl whose central goiter compressed the trachea (**Fig. 1.1**). This happened only 3 years after William Morton's demonstration of ether's efficacy at Massachusetts General Hospital in 1846. Despite such progress, many surgeons at this time managed such patients without anesthesia.

One of the most distinguished surgeons of the 19th century, Albert Theodor Billroth, was involved in the new era in thyroid surgery (**Fig. 1.2**). In the early 1860s, while holding the chair of surgery in Zurich, he performed 20 thyroidectomies. Billroth, described by William Halsted as a rapid

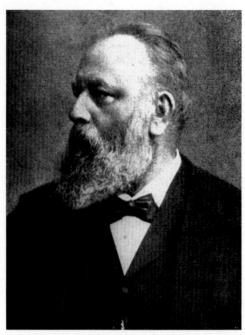

Fig. 1.2 Albert Theodor Billroth. (From Randolph GW. Surgery of the Thyroid and Parathyroid Glands. New York: Elsevier, 2003, with permission.)

thyroid operator, courageously reported his initial results, documenting a 40% mortality rate due to intraoperative hemorrhage and postoperative sepsis. After abandoning thyroid surgery for more than a decade, he started again to be attracted to this field while working in Vienna. By then antisepsis had become more established and he achieved an impressive mortality of only 8% for thyroidectomy. Billroth's technique at this time involved division of the sternocleidomastoid muscle, incision and drainage of any thyroid cysts, arterial ligation, and the use of aneurysmal needles for controlling hemorrhage. In addition to general and thyroid surgery, Billroth's other contribution impressively include the first successful laryngectomy (1873) and the first esophagectomy (1881).

Despite Billroth's pioneering work, the name that dominates the history of thyroid surgery is Theodor Kocher (**Fig. 1.3**). Kocher's appointment as chair of surgery in Bern, Switzerland, in 1872 marked the beginning of an illustrious career during which he performed over 5000 thyroidectomies. With meticulous attention to details of surgical technique, hemostasis, and antisepsis, he reported a reduction in mortality from over 12% in the 1870s to 0.2% in 1898.

Kocher's technique involved a collar incision and strap muscle preservation. It was Halsted, a visiting American surgeon attending both Billroth's and Kocher's clinics, who noted that although most of Kocher's patients after thyroidectomy developed myxedema but rarely tetany, most of Billroth's patients developed tetany but rarely myxedema. Halsted commented on Kocher's bloodless operative field, attention to detail, and removal of all thyroid tissue while preserving surrounding structures.

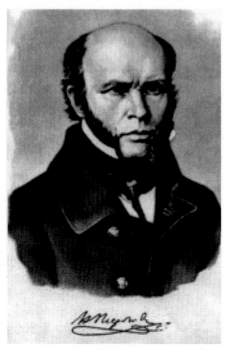

Fig. 1.1 Nikolai Pirogoff.

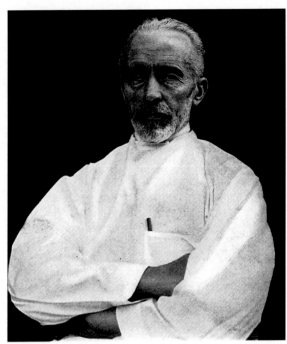

Fig. 1.3 Theodor Kocher. (From Randolph GW. Surgery of the Thyroid and Parathyroid Glands. New York: Elsevier, 2003, with permission.)

In 1909, Dr Kocher was awarded the Nobel Prize for medicine for his work on the physiology, pathology, and surgery of the thyroid gland.

The 20th Century: Maturity of Thyroid Surgery

In the late 1890s, European advances in thyroid surgery were adopted in the United States by Halsted of Baltimore, the Mayo brothers of Rochester, George Crile of Cleveland, and Frank Lahey of Boston. The well-known medical clinics that bear their names were initially financially fueled by high-volume thyroid surgery now made a safe and practical offering through the techniques of Kocher.

At the turn of the 20th century, Thomas Peel Dunhill of Melbourne began work on the treatment of thyrotoxicosis. He introduced the technique of total lobectomy with contralateral subtotal thyroidectomy, subsequently termed the Dunhill procedure. He advocated pericapsular dissection performed in a staged manner under local anesthesia and later under light general anesthesia. He achieved a mortality of only 3% while operating on severely thyrotoxic patients. In London the same operation at this time was associated with 30% mortality. Interestingly, at the time of Dunhill's presentation to the Royal Society of Medicine in London of his initial results in these patients, the society's chairman was James Berry, who described the eponymous ligament that overlies the recurrent laryngeal nerve close to its entry point into the larynx. After the First World War, Dunhill moved to London and in 1919 he published a seminal paper in the *British Journal of*

Surgery describing a detailed account of the technique of thyroidectomy, which in many aspects holds true today.[3] In the same year, Sistrunk described his radical operation for thyroglossal duct cysts, including the resection of the middle third of the hyoid bone.

Refinement of Thyroidectomy in the 21st Century: Toward a Zero Complication Rate

Outcomes

Fortunately, issues of postoperative mortality are no longer central to thyroidectomy. The technically challenging issues in thyroid surgery are dominated by postoperative hypocalcemia and voice changes. The cosmetic outcome has also become of increasing importance for a public with increasing expectations of no-risk surgery.

In today's literature, permanent hypoparathyroidism occurs in less than 2% of patients operated on by experts. Postoperative hypocalcemia and tetany were recognized as early as the mid-19th century, and the careful capsular dissection introduced by Kocher has helped to reduce its incidence. One large recent study of 5846 patients with benign and malignant thyroid disease operated on in 45 hospitals in Germany found the incidence of transient and permanent hypoparathyroidism to be 7.3% and 1.5%, respectively. On logistic regression analysis, total thyroidectomy (odds ratio [OR], 4.7), female gender (OR 1.9), Graves disease (OR 1.9), recurrent goiter (OR 1.7), and bilateral central ligation of the inferior thyroid artery (OR 1.7) constituted independent risk factors for transient hypoparathyroidism. For permanent hypoparathyroidism, total thyroidectomy (OR 11.4), bilateral central (OR 5.0) and peripheral (OR 2.0) ligation of the inferior thyroid artery, identification and preservation of none or only a single parathyroid gland (OR 4.1), and Graves disease (OR 2.4) were independent risk factors. These data reinforce the established practice of ligation of only the distal most branches of the inferior thyroid artery on the thyroid capsule rather than ligation of the main trunk of the artery.[4]

Identification of the recurrent laryngeal nerve (RLN) during thyroidectomy has been advocated for more than two decades, finally putting to rest Crile's doctrine of vulnerability, which held that a dissected nerve was an injured nerve. It is only when the RLN is identified and followed up to the entry point in the larynx that one can be reassured that the nerve has not been damaged during the procedure. Intraoperative nerve monitoring can provide additional intraoperative functional information and has application in neural identification, aids in nerve dissection, and provides prognostic information regarding postoperative function[5] and is becoming more widely adopted. An injury rate of 1 to 5% is generally quoted in expert series, but such figures appear to underestimate the rates of paralysis occurring when quality registers report on all surgeons' results and routinely examine all patients postoperatively.

The Spectrum of Thyroidectomy

We provide an overview of current techniques in thyroidectomy and comment on some advantages and disadvantages (**Table 1.1**).

Kocher's collar incision remains the hallmark of thyroidectomy. Although most surgeons take pride in a scar of minimal length, few studies report the length of the incision that is routinely used. An interesting prospective series of 200 patients from San Francisco, California, reported that the mean length of the routine incision was 5.5 cm for total thyroidectomy and 4.6 cm for lobectomy.[6] By multiple regression analysis, thyroid specimen volume and patient body mass index were independent predictors of incision length in thyroidectomy.

The boundaries and the definition of minimally invasive thyroidectomy (MIT) are not always clear-cut (**Table 1.1**).[7] Most surgeons would agree that the length of the incision is only one cosmetic parameter, and that other factors should be considered including its position in or parallel to existing neck skin creases to achieve the best cosmetic results. Subcuticular sutures, either absorbable or nonabsorbable, are used in favor of metal clips. The use of tissue glue has been promoted but has yet to become established.

The Tools of Minimally Invasive Thyroidectomy

Personal and financial factors in addition to the specific approach being used can influence surgeons' choice of equipment. Vessel control can be performed with clips, diathermy or one of the newly developed Harmonic® scalpel (Ethicon Endo-Surgery, Cincinnati, OH) or Ligasure systems (Tyco, ValleyLab, Boulder, CO). Several of these technologies have been used extensively and are considered necessary for newer minimal access approaches. We now routinely use the Harmonic scalpel at all stages during the dissection, from raising the subplatysmal flaps to sealing venous and arterial branches of up to 4 mm, including the superior thyroid artery. During dissection in the proximity of the RLN, the blades of the Harmonic scalpel are rotated so that the active blade is away from the nerve, limiting further the risk of inadvertent thermal injury to RLN. The Harmonic tip is currently too bulky to use within the ligament of Berry region of dissection where we favor fine-tip bipolar cautery or suture.

In a retrospective analysis of nearly 200 patients, operative time for total thyroidectomies performed with the Harmonic scalpel was 24 minutes shorter compared with conventional method (81 vs. 105 minutes), the mean amount of intraoperative blood loss was smaller (70 mL vs. 125 mL), there was less postoperative pain, and the costs were similar.[8] Similar data were derived from a randomized trial

Table 1.1 Classification of Thyroid Surgical Approaches

Approach*	Description	Advantages	Disadvantages
I. Standard	Kocher-type incision (neck base crease, 4 to 6 cm in length), subplatysmal flaps	Standard, proven exposure Cosmetically acceptable Suitable for any size or type lesion Monitoring applicable	Long incision
II. Small incision	Three to 4 cm, typically placed higher than standard incision, with or without strap muscle incision and subplatysmal flap	Smaller incision Monitoring applicable	Possible hypertrophic scar from skin edge retraction Less suitable for large, possibly malignant lesions, nodal resection
III. Video-assisted	A 2-cm incision overlying thyroid (i.e., high), blunt dissection, superior pole taken with video assist, then midpole and inferior pole ventrally delivered, harmonic scissors often used	Small incision Increased light and magnification Monitoring applicable Often good superior laryngeal nerve (SLN) visualization	Possible retraction keloid Precipitous ventral delivery may endanger recurrent laryngeal nerve (RLN) at ligament of Berry Patient-driven learning curve Less suitable for large, possibly malignant lesions, nodal resection
IV. Endoscopic	Central or lateral approaches, typically three puncture sites for camera and trocars, gas or retractor created working space	Small cervical incisions Increased light and magnification Monitoring applicable	Gas insufflation complications possible Less suitable for large, possibly malignant lesions, nodal resection, Substantial learning curve
V. Extracervical	Axillary or periareolar approach	No cervical scar Monitoring applicable	Extended dissection, Less suitable for large, possibly malignant lesions and nodal resection Substantial learning curve

*Any approach may be with or without general anesthesia.
Approaches II, III, and IV can be described as minimally invasive thyroid (MIT) approaches.

of 60 patients operated on using the Harmonic scalpel (HS) or the standard technique of electrocautery and ligatures: the operative time was 25 minutes shorter in the HS group (96 ± 23 vs. 121 ± 34, $p = .005$), and mean blood loss was less with HS (35 ± 27 mL vs. 54 ± 51 mL, $p = .06$).[9] An even larger prospective randomized trial of 200 patients with benign thyroid diseases confirmed a reduction of 15 to 20% in operative time when using HS. Interestingly, the global surgical charges were significantly less in the HS group (985 ± 107 Euros vs. 1148 ± 153 Euros).[10]

Some surgeons use magnifying lenses to facilitate accurate dissection in the vicinity of RLN. An extreme extrapolation of this approach has been reported by a group using a surgical microscope.[11] The rate of transient nerve palsies and the rate of transient hypocalcemia after total thyroidectomy were smaller in the group of 58 patients who had microsurgical thyroidectomy compared with a group of 40 patients undergoing standard thyroidectomy (1.7% vs. 7.5%, and 4.1% vs. 33%, respectively).

What Is Minimally Invasive Thyroid Surgery?

Some two decades after the advent of laparoscopic abdominal surgery, several enthusiasts explored the possibility of using similar equipment and techniques during thyroid surgery. The aim was to avoid the long midline cervical incision by using several 5-mm to 2-cm incisions and endoscopic instruments. In contrast with abdominal surgery, the operative space in the neck has to be actively created. This has been achieved in two ways: by a gasless technique involving blunt dissection and introduction of an endoscope through a small incision, and by insufflation of carbon dioxide (true endoscopic thyroidectomy, **Table 1.1**). What makes a procedure minimally invasive is not entirely clear, however. Key parameters in these discussions are incision length, amount of dissection, in some cases the use of local anesthesia, early discharge, and application of new technology. Certainly many patients readily prefer and seek out "minimally invasive" or "small incision" surgery, but they intrinsically assume that such options, if being offered, are as safe or safer than previous standard approaches and of clear-cut proven benefit. Further work will be needed to provide our patients with this information. We must be careful about deciding what advantages minimally invasive approaches bring to our patients but at the same time keep in mind the tremendous advances endoscopic sinus surgery and laparoscopic abdominal approaches have represented. There are benefits from skilled surgeons pushing the existing surgical envelope.

Video-Assisted Thyroidectomy

In 1998, in Pisa, Miccoli introduced the minimally invasive video-assisted thyroidectomy (MIVAT or VAT).[12] This totally gasless procedure is performed through a 15-mm central incision above the sternal notch. A 5-mm 30-degree endoscope is inserted through the skin incision. Dissection is performed under endoscopic vision using conventional and endoscopic instruments. Hemostasis is achieved using the Harmonic scalpel and small vascular clips. Surgeons from Taiwan have modified the original VAT technique by developing a self-designed Army retractor with a mosaic ring.[13]

Over 4 years some 427 patients were submitted to VAT. The technique was applied for nodules up to a maximum diameter of 3.5 cm, for small thyroid volume (under 25 cc), benign thyroid disease, or "low-risk" thyroid tumors with no evidence of nodal disease of the neck. Mean operative time was 30 minutes for lobectomy (range, 20–140 minutes) and 50 minutes for total thyroidectomy (range, 35–140 minutes). Complications were represented by permanent, recurrent nerve palsy in three patients (0.7%) and one case of definitive hypoparathyroidism (0.4%). A wound infection was reported in three cases, and there was no major bleeding that required surgical revision. A conversion to open procedure was performed in five cases (1.2%). Moreover, though not statistically proven, VAT appears to offer some advantages in terms of cosmetic results and postoperative pain.[12] VAT was subsequently studied in four tertiary-level referral centers in Italy, with leading authors Miccoli and Bellantone reporting similar results in an additional 336 patients.[14]

In another recently published series, a total of 473 VATs were attempted on 459 patients. Conversion was necessary in six cases (difficult dissection in one case, large nodule size in three, gross lymph node metastases in two). Thyroid lobectomy was successfully performed in 110 cases, total thyroidectomy in 343, and completion thyroidectomy in 14. In 66 patients with carcinoma, central neck nodes were removed through the same access. Concomitant parathyroidectomy was performed in 14 patients. Pathology showed benign disease in 277 cases, papillary cancer in 175, and medullary microcarcinoma in one. Postoperative complications included eight transient recurrent nerve palsies, 64 transient hypocalcemias, three permanent hypocalcemias, one postoperative hematoma, and two wound infections. Postoperative pain was minimal and the cosmetic result excellent. In patients with papillary cancer, no evidence of recurrent or residual disease was shown.[15]

In a randomized trial of 62 patients with single, small (<3 cm) thyroid nodules who underwent video-assisted thyroid surgery,[16] the patients' satisfaction with their scars was higher, postoperative pain in the first and second days after surgery was lower, postoperative hospital stay was lower, and there were no significant differences in complications compared with those undergoing conventional thyroidectomy.

As expected, some pushed the limits of the technique even further and managed to complete VAT using locoregional anesthesia under a superficial cervical block. During the procedure, the patients were completely awake and able to speak with members of the surgical team. Intraoperative and postoperative pain, as evaluated by a visual analogue scale, was usually negligible. No complications occurred in three thyroid lobectomies and two total thyroidectomies. All five patients were completely satisfied with the cosmetic result and the surgical outcome.[17]

The indications for VAT were subsequently extended to patients with small papillary thyroid carcinomas, and in a randomized trial it was shown that the completeness of thyroid resection was similar between patients undergoing VAT ($n = 16$) or conventional thyroidectomy ($n = 17$), with very similar postoperative iodine-131 uptake in the two groups ($5.1 \pm 4.9\%$ versus $4.6 \pm 6.7\%$).[18]

In Asia, Shimizu and Tanaka[19] developed video-assisted neck surgery as a totally gasless endoscopic surgical technique using an anterior neck-skin lifting method for thyroid and parathyroid diseases. The authors treated more than 200 cases of thyroid and parathyroid disease using this technique. The maximum tumor size was 7.4 cm in diameter. For malignant tumors, the indication for the method was limited to thyroid papillary microcarcinomas measuring less than 1 cm in diameter. Total lobectomy and prophylactic neck dissection were performed in all 10 of these cases.

Endoscopic Thyroid Surgery

Endoscopic neck surgery was first reported by Gagner's group[20] for parathyroid surgery. Significant improvements in endoscopic instrumentation (e.g., miniscopes, miniature instruments) have encouraged some surgeons to adopt these endoscopic techniques for thyroidectomy.

In the central endoscopic approach, a 5-mm incision is made slightly anterior to the sternal notch, and the cervical fascia is opened under direct vision. A subplatysmal plane is created and a purse-string suture is placed in the subcutaneous tissues of the incision to prevent gas leak during CO_2 insufflation at a pressure of 8 to 12 mm Hg. A 0-degree 5-mm scope is used to advance the dissection in front of the strap muscles to create a space in which additional trocars can be introduced: one in the midline and two along the sternocleidomastoid (SCM) border.

In Marseilles, Henry developed an endoscopic thyroidectomy based on a lateral approach similar to that used for minimally invasive parathyroidectomy. Henry developed a plane between the carotid sheath laterally and the strap muscles medially, allowing exposure for identification of the RLN and the parathyroid glands. Patients with solitary nodules smaller than 3 cm in diameter and no history of neck surgery or irradiation were offered this operation. Of the 742 thyroidectomies performed in 1 year, 38 (5.1%) were endoscopic thyroidectomies. The mean nodule size was 22 mm (range, 7–47 mm), and the mean operating time was 99 minutes (range, 64–150 minutes). In all cases, the recurrent laryngeal nerve was preserved intact. Two patients required conversion to an open thyroidectomy. The authors consider the technique safe and effective in the hands of appropriately trained surgeons.[21]

Minimal-Access Thyroid Surgery

In Sydney, Delbridge described the technique for minimal-access thyroidectomy (MAT) as an extension of the approach used for minimally invasive parathyroidectomy.[22] In short, a 2.5-cm lateral transverse incision is made directly over the nodule or over the middle of the thyroid lobe, straddling the medial margin of the SCM muscle. The subplatysmal plane is developed by finger dissection to allow mobility of the skin incision over the relevant area during the different phases of the procedure. The SCM is then retracted laterally and the space posterior to the strap muscles is opened to expose the thyroid gland. Dissection of the thyroid upper pole is achieved by retracting the upper pole laterally to open up the avascular plane, thus allowing visualization and preservation of the external branch of the superior laryngeal nerve. The superior thyroid artery or its branches are divided between metal clips. Mobilization of the lower pole is undertaken by capsular dissection, with attention being paid to the identification of the inferior parathyroid gland and recurrent laryngeal nerve.

In a group of 50 patients who underwent MAT, the mean nodule diameter was 18.5 mm. The authors feel this represents a safe and feasible surgical procedure that provides an alternative to open thyroid surgery in appropriately selected cases.

Extracervical Thyroidectomy

The desire to avoid neck scars after thyroidectomy has encouraged some authors to use incisions placed outside the cervical region, in the periareolar area,[23] in the axilla,[24] or in the subclavicular area.[25] The experience with such techniques is limited to several centers in Asia and has not been evaluated in Europe or the U.S. All these approaches involve extensive tissue dissection and as such, in our view, cannot be classified as minimally invasive thyroid surgery.

For the axillary approach, a 30-mm skin incision is made in the axilla, and 12-mm and 5-mm trocars are inserted through this incision. An additional 5-mm trocar is inserted adjacent to the incision.[26] For the anterior chest approach, a 12-mm incision is made in the skin of the anterior chest approximately 3 to 5 cm below the border of the ipsilateral clavicle. Two additional 5-mm trocars are inserted by endoscopic guidance below the ipsilateral clavicle, and CO_2 is then insufflated up to a pressure of 4 mm Hg. In extracervical gasless approaches, retraction wire devices have been employed to provide working space.

The anterior border of the SCM muscle is then separated from the sternohyoid muscle to expose the sternothyroid muscle. The thyroid gland is exposed by splitting the sternothyroid muscle. The lower pole is retracted upward and dissected from the adipose tissue to identify the recurrent laryngeal nerve. Identification of the inferior thyroid artery and careful ligation of its branches close to the gland are an excellent means of preserving the nerve and the inferior parathyroid gland. As the recurrent laryngeal nerve is exposed, the Berry ligament is exposed and incised with a 5-mm clip or slim laparoscopic coagulating shears (LCS, Johnson & Johnson Medical, Cincinnati, OH).

The cosmetic status after surgery is excellent because the small incision scar is covered by the patient's arm or a piece of clothing. The typical operative time is less than 150 minutes for the axillary approach and less than 120 minutes for the anterior approach. Large follicular tumors can be extracted by the axillary approach, whereas the anterior chest approach is advocated for removal of bilateral multinodular goiters and parathyroid lesions. Both approaches resulted in pain, swelling, and sometimes ecchymosis in the area of dissection between the skin incision and the neck in some patients, but most complaints disappeared after about 3 months, with good cosmetic results, and there was no hypesthesia or paresthesia of the neck. The present indications for pure endoscopic thyroidectomy by the axillary approach include the presence of a thyroid nodule less than 4 cm, or less than 10 mm if it is a low-risk papillary carcinoma.

Training of Future Thyroid Surgeons

Radical changes in the way surgical services are organized and delivered continue to challenge the traditional practice in many countries. Concerns have been raised in recent years about the exposure to endocrine surgery during residency programs in general surgery in the U.S. Similar concerns have been raised in the United Kingdom, and it remains doubtful whether recent changes to National Health Service (NHS) training schemes will improve the situation.

Trainees in general surgery in some programs gain minimal exposure to thyroid and parathyroid surgery, and at the end of such training programs they cannot be expected to reach the level of technical competency or have the knowledge necessary for the management of complex cases. Those who develop a subspeciality interest are subsequently encouraged to undertake a fellowship in thyroid and parathyroid surgery. In the U.K.

there is a growing desire to identify/nominate specific centers for training in thyroid/parathyroid surgery. It might be that future thyroid surgeons will embark on such fellowships at the end of either a general surgery training.

The ability to offer intense exposure to a wide spectrum of patients during a 12- to 18-month fellowship can potentially be limited by the fact that currently thyroid surgery is dispersed throughout a large number of surgeons and centers. Ideally, there is a need to concentrate the work in a small number of centers so that trainees with a declared interest could have a real opportunity to learn safe techniques for total thyroidectomy and to be exposed to a significant number of difficult cases.

It has been shown that the volume of thyroid surgery has a direct impact on the complication rates. Surgeons performing 100 or more thyroidectomies over a 6-year period had the lowest complications rates, the shortest hospital stay, and the lowest hospital charges compared with surgeons performing 30 to 100 cases or less. The high-volume surgeons had one-third fewer complications from thyroidectomy performed for benign disease and two-thirds fewer complications when operating for thyroid cancer.[27] Certainly a push toward further centralization of thyroid surgery to high volume units would be a rational response to these figures. However, it is questionable whether such units could perform all the thyroid surgery required. Currently it appears that over 80% of thyroid surgery in the U.S. is performed by the occasional thyroid surgeon.[28] A more rational plan would be to recognize the surgical educational and organizational opportunity and train a new generation of highly skilled surgeons who restrict most of their surgical work to the thyroid gland and could perform this work in their own communities.

In the wide debate about the future of thyroid surgery, the words of Theodor Billroth remain as valid as ever: "Only the man who is familiar with the art and science of the past is competent to aid in its progress in the future."

References

1. Slough CM, Johns R, Randolph GW, Lore JM, Romanchisen AP. History of thyroid and parathyroid surgery. In: Randolph GW, ed. Surgery of the Thyroid and Parathyroid Glands. Philadelphia: Saunders, 2003:3–11

2. Welbourne RB. The History of Endocrine Surgery, New York: Praeger, 1990

3. Dunhill TP. Some considerations on the operation for exophthalmic goitre. Br J Surg 1919;7:195–210

4. Thomusch O, Machens A, Sekulla C, Ukkat J, Brauckhoff M, Dralle H. The impact of surgical technique on postoperative hypoparathyroidism in bilateral thyroid surgery: a multivariate analysis of 5846 consecutive patients. Surgery 2003;133:180–185

5. Randolph GW. Surgical anatomy of the recurrent laryngeal nerve. In: Randolph GW, ed. Surgery of the Thyroid and Parathyroid Glands. Philadelphia: Saunders, 2003:300–342

6. Brunaud L, Zarnegar R, Wada N, Ituarte P, Clark OH, Duh QY. Incision length for standard thyroidectomy and parathyroidectomy: when is it minimally invasive? Arch Surg 2003;138:1140–1143

7. Terris DJ, Bonnett A, Gourin CG, Chin E. Minimally invasive thyroidectomy using the Sofferman technique. Laryngoscope 2005;115:1104–1108

8. Casadei R, Perenze B, Vescini F, Piccoli L, Zanini N, Minni F. Usefulness of the ultrasonically activated shears in total thyroidectomy. Chir Ital 2004;56:843–848

9. Cordon C, Fajardo R, Ramirez J, Herrera MF. A randomized, prospective, parallel group study comparing the Harmonic Scalpel to electrocautery in thyroidectomy. Surgery 2005;137:337–341

10. Ortega J, Sala C, Flor B, Lledo S. Efficacy and cost-effectiveness of the UltraCision harmonic scalpel in thyroid surgery: an analysis of 200 cases in a randomized trial. J Laparoendosc Adv Surg Tech A 2004;14:9–12

11. Seven H, Calis AB, Vural C, Turgut S. Microscopic thyroidectomy:

a prospective controlled trial. Eur Arch Otorhinolaryngol 2005;262:41–44

12. Miccoli P, Minuto MN, Barellini L, et al. Minimally invasive video-assisted thyroidectomy—techniques and results over 4 years of experience (1999–2002). Ann Ital Chir 2004;75:47–51

13. Chan CP, Yang LH, Chang HC, et al. An easier technique for minimally invasive video-assisted thyroidectomy. Int Surg 2003;88:109–113

14. Miccoli P, Bellantone R, Mourad M, Walz M, Raffaelli M, Berti P. Minimally invasive video-assisted thyroidectomy: multiinstitutional experience. World J Surg 2002;26:972–975

15. Lombardi CP, Raffaelli M, Princi P, De Crea C, Bellantone R. Video-assisted thyroidectomy: report on the experience of a single center in more than four hundred cases. World J Surg 2006;30:794–800

16. Bellantone R, Lombardi CP, Bossola M, et al. Video-assisted vs conventional thyroid lobectomy: a randomized trial. Arch Surg 2002;137:301–304

17. Lombardi CP, Raffaelli M, Modesti C, Boscherini M, Bellantone R. Video-assisted thyroidectomy under local anesthesia. Am J Surg 2004;187:515–518

18. Miccoli P, Elisei R, Materazzi G, et al. Minimally invasive video-assisted thyroidectomy for papillary carcinoma: a prospective study of its completeness. Surgery 2002;132:1070–1074

19. Shimizu K, Tanaka S. Asian perspective on endoscopic thyroidectomy—a review of 193 cases. Asian J Surg 2003;26:92–100

20. Naitoh T, Gagner M, Garcia-Ruiz A, Heniford BT. Endoscopic endocrine surgery in the neck. An initial report of endoscopic subtotal parathyroidectomy. Surg Endosc 1998;12:202–205

21. Palazzo FF, Sebag F, Henry JF. Endocrine surgical technique: endoscopic thyroidectomy via the lateral approach. Surg Endosc 2006;20:339–342

22. Palazzo FF, Sywak MS, Sidhu SB, Delbridge LW. Safety and feasibility of thyroid lobectomy via a lateral 2.5-cm incision with a cohort comparison of the first 50 cases: evolution of a surgical approach. Langenbecks Arch Surg 2005;390:230–235

23. Ohgami M, Ishii S, Arisawa Y, et al. Scarless endoscopic thyroidectomy: breast approach for better cosmesis. Surg Laparosc Endosc Percutan Tech 2000;10:1–4

24. Chantawibul S, Lokechareonlarp S, Pokawatana C. Total video endoscopic thyroidectomy by an axillary approach. J Laparoendosc Adv Surg Tech A 2003;13:295–299

25. Akasu H, Shimizu K, Kitagawa W, Ishii R, Tanaka S. Evaluation of an alternative, subclavicular approach to thyroidectomy. Med Sci Monit 2002;8:CS80–CS82

26. Takami HE, Ikeda Y. Minimally invasive thyroidectomy. Curr Opin Oncol 2006;18:43–47

27. McHenry CR. Patient volumes and complications in thyroid surgery. Br J Surg 2002;89:821–823

28. Saunders BD, Wainess RM, Dimick JB, Doherty GM, Upchurch GR, Gauger PG. Who performs endocrine operations in the US? Surgery 2003;134:924–931

2 Developmental and Surgical Anatomy of the Thyroid Compartment

David L. Steward and Jahmal A. Hairston

Embryology of the Thyroid Gland

The normal thyroid gland weighs approximately 10 to 20 g and is typically located anterior to the trachea, midway between the thyroid cartilage and the suprasternal notch. It is enveloped by a fibrous capsule developed from the deep cervical fascia as it divides into an anterior and posterior sheath and surrounds the gland. The thyroid consists of two lobes that lie lateral to the trachea with a central midline isthmus connecting the lobes. The lobes are typically 5.0 cm in length, and the isthmus 1.25 cm.[1] The most posterior extension of the lateral lobes (the tubercles of Zuckerkandl) maintains an important relationship to the recurrent laryngeal nerve. A pyramidal lobe is present in approximately 50% of people and is usually connected to the isthmus or one of the lobes.[1]

The thyroid gland begins its development during the fourth embryonic week. It develops embryologically from the foramen cecum, which is located at the back of the tongue between the tuberculum impar (median tongue bud) and the copula (hypobranchial eminence) (**Fig. 2.1**). The copula consists of mesoderm arising from the second pharyngeal pouch. The main central portion of the gland appears during the second and third weeks of fetal life. The thyroid primordium develops as a medial anlage from a diverticulum of the endoderm of the floor of the primitive pharynx. This thyroid diverticulum follows the primitive heart as it descends caudally, becoming a solid cord of cells that will form the follicular elements. The thyroid anlarge is connected to the base of the tongue by the thyroglossal duct. As the embryo elongates and undergoes differentiation, the diverticulum breaks in two and the proximal part retracts and disappears. The foramen cecum (located at the back of the tongue) remains, marking the origin of the primitive thyroid gland. The caudal end develops as a bilobed, encapsulated structure on either side of the midline, which descends in the neck and is connected by an isthmus in the midline.

The ultimobranchial bodies develop from the fourth pharyngeal pouch. During the fifth week of development, these cells detach from the pharyngeal wall and fuse with the posterior aspect of the main body of the thyroid as it descends into the neck. These cells differentiate into the parafollicular cells (C cells), which are the cells that secrete calcitonin.[2] The tubercles of Zuckerkandl are thickenings of the thyroid gland that represent the fusion of the ultimobranchial bodies with the medial thyroid anlage. They have importance in that it is a consistent landmark for the recurrent laryngeal nerve (RLN), which runs medial and deep to it.[3]

Anomalous Development of the Thyroid Gland

Lingual Thyroid

The lingual thyroid is relatively rare, occurring approximately in 1 in 3,000 cases of thyroid disease.[1] Although rare, it is the most common location for ectopic functioning thyroid tissue. It occurs more commonly in women than in men, and is frequently associated with a lack of a normal cervical thyroid in 70% of cases. The diagnosis is usually made in an asymptomatic patient with the incidental discovery of a mass in the back of the tongue. It can become symptomatic if it enlarges by provoking dysphagia, dysphonia, dyspnea, or a sensation of choking. Hypothyroidism is frequently present, but hyperthyroidism is rare. It has a low incidence of malignancy. The diagnosis is made with radioisotope scanning or ultrasound, and it should be suspected whenever a mass is found in the foramen cecum area of the tongue.

Thyroglossal Duct Cyst

The thyroglossal duct usually obliterates during embryonic life by the end of the fifth week of development, but it can persist as a cyst or a draining sinus tract into adulthood. A cyst or a sinus tract can develop anywhere along the course of the descent of the thyroid anlage, and occurs secondary

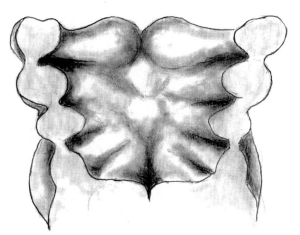

Fig. 2.1 Embryonic origin of the thyroid gland.

to persistence or incomplete obliteration of the thyroglossal duct. Anomalies of the thyroglossal duct are the most common congenital neck masses in children.[4] The lesions usually appear in the midline or just off the midline between the hyoid bone and the isthmus of the thyroid. A cyst or sinus tract may not be apparent until it becomes infected or spontaneously ruptures, usually after an upper respiratory tract infection. Historically, thyroglossal duct cysts (TGDCs) were treated with incision and drainage. Recurrence rates with this method of treatment were >50%. Currently, the standard treatment for a TGDC is the Sistrunk procedure, with recurrence rates in the 4 to 5% range. With the Sistrunk procedure, the cyst or sinus tract is meticulously dissected out along with a cuff of tissue to the base of the tongue, along with a central portion of the hyoid bone. This extensive dissection minimizes recurrence. Thyroid carcinoma can develop within a cyst, especially if the individual has received low-dose irradiation to the head and neck region in the past; thus all specimens should undergo histologic examination.

Blood Supply to the Thyroid Gland

The thyroid is an extremely vascular gland. Its main blood supply comes from the paired superior and inferior thyroid arteries. The superior thyroid artery originates either from the common carotid artery or the first or second branch of the external carotid artery. The superior thyroid arteries divide into anterior and posterior branches as they approach the gland. They then give anastomoses with their counterparts on the other side, as well as branches to the thyroid gland.

The inferior thyroid arteries contain some variability in their distribution and are absent on one side (usually the left) in approximately 0.2 to 6% of cases.[5] The inferior thyroid artery originates from the thyrocervical trunk. It divides into an upper branch and a lower branch. The upper branch goes to the posterior aspect of the gland, and the lower branch to the lower pole of the gland. There can be anastomoses with the superior thyroid artery as well as with the counterpart inferior thyroid artery across the midline.

The thyroid gland is drained by two or three large pairs of veins that anastomose within the parenchyma of the gland. The superior thyroid vein accompanies its equivalent artery and emerges from the upper pole of the thyroid. It empties into the internal jugular or common facial vein. The middle thyroid vein is present in approximately 50% of people. It typically drains into the internal jugular vein after crossing the common carotid artery anteriorly. The inferior thyroid veins emerge from the lower portion of the gland. The veins form two trunks: the left trunk drains into the left brachiocephalic vein after passing anterior to the trachea, whereas the right trunk drains into the right brachiocephalic vein after passing anterior to the brachiocephalic artery. The inferior thyroid veins may anastomose and form a plexus of veins in front of the trachea (plexus thyroideus impar).

Anomalous Vascularity of the Thyroid Gland

The vasculature to the thyroid gland may contain many variations. An aberrant inferior thyroid artery ("thyroid ima artery") may be present in 1.5 to 12.2% of people.[1] When present, it usually arises on the right side, ascending in front of the trachea. It can arise from the brachiocephalic, right common carotid, or the aortic arch. It may also arise from the internal thoracic artery, although this is rare.

Neurovasculature of the Thyroid Gland: The Recurrent and Superior Laryngeal Nerves

The relationship of the thyroid gland to the recurrent and superior laryngeal nerves is of major importance to the thyroid surgeon. Injury to these nerves can lead to dysphonia, dysphagia, and dyspnea. The vagus nerve exits the jugular foramen and descends in the neck within the carotid sheath. The cervical vagus gives off many pharyngeal branches as well as the superior laryngeal nerve. The superior laryngeal nerve divides into internal and external branches near the internal carotid artery. The internal branch of the superior laryngeal nerve provides sensation to the portion of the larynx above the vocal folds. It enters the larynx by passing through the thyrohyoid membrane. The external branch of the superior laryngeal nerve (EBSLN) provides motor innervation to the cricothyroid muscle. In the majority of cases, it lies in close proximity to the upper pole vessels and usually passes deep to the external carotid artery, where it joins the superior thyroid artery (STA). The EBSLN shows much variability, in its relation to both the STA and the inferior constrictor muscle. Studies by Cernea et al[6] and Kierner et al[7] describe the variable course of the EBSLN in relation to the STA. In this classification, type 1 EBSLN crosses the STA >1 cm cranial to the upper pole of the thyroid, type 2 crosses the STA <1 cm cranial to the upper pole of the thyroid gland, type 3 crosses the STA while covered by the upper pole of the thyroid gland, and type 4 nerves do not cross the STA at all (**Fig. 2.2**).[7] The studies of Friedman et al[8] describe the variable course of the EBSLN in relation to the inferior constrictor muscle. In these studies, the EBSLN is classified into three types. Type 1 has its entire course superficial to the inferior constrictor. Type 2 penetrates the inferior constrictor in the lower portion of the muscle approximately 1 cm proximal to the inferior constrictor-cricothyroid junction. Type 3 travels its entire course under the inferior constrictor after diving underneath its most superior fibers (**Fig. 2.3**).[8] The cricothyroid muscle raises the pitch of voice by producing a rocking motion at the joints between the thyroid and cricoid cartilages, thus increasing the tension in the vocal ligaments by pulling the front of the cricoid upward.

The recurrent laryngeal nerves are important structures in thyroid surgery, and protecting them is of paramount

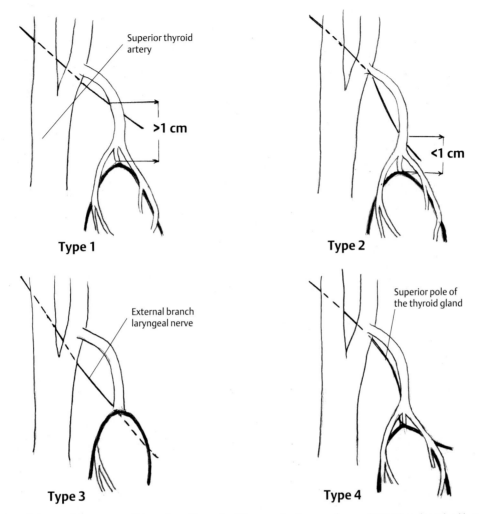

Fig. 2.2 Classification of the possible courses of the external branch of the superior laryngeal nerve (EBSLN) as described by Cernea et al.[6]

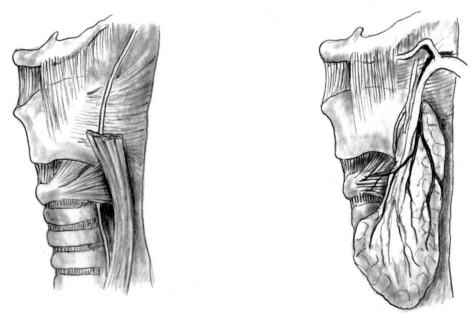

Fig. 2.3 **(A)** Type 1 variant of the course of the external branch of the superior laryngeal nerve (EBSLN courses superficial to the inferior constrictor muscle) as described by Friedman et al.[8] *(Continued on page 14)*

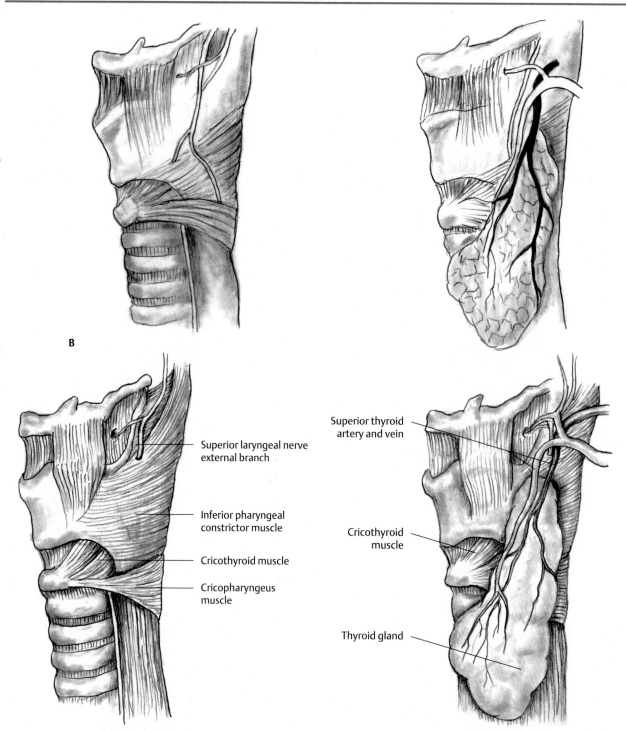

Fig. 2.3 *(Continued)* (**B**) Type 2 variant: EBSLN courses underneath the inferior constrictor muscle for part of its course. (**C**) Type 3 variant: EBSLN courses entirely deep to the inferior constrictor muscle.

importance. The RLN provides sensory, motor, and para-sympathetic innervation. These nerves innervate all of the muscles of the larynx except for the cricothyroid. More specifically, the RLN divides into an anterior and posterior branch. The posterior branch provides sensation to the vocal cords and subglottic region. The anterior branch provides motor innervation to the thyroarytenoid, the lateral and

posterior cricoarytenoid, and the transverse and oblique arytenoid. There is some variation in the course of the RLN between the left and right sides. The right recurrent laryngeal nerve descends in the neck and loops around the subclavian artery, and then ascends in the neck to innervate the larynx. The left recurrent laryngeal nerve originates from the vagus in the superior mediastinum anterior to the aortic arch. It then usually ascends in the tracheoesophageal groove to innervate the larynx, giving off branches to the trachea, esophagus, and heart.

It is important to identify the recurrent laryngeal nerve during thyroid surgery. The RLN exhibits variability in its course, and most anatomists describe these variations relative to three key landmarks: the inferior thyroid artery, the tracheoesophageal groove, and Berry ligaments. The relationship of the RLN to the inferior thyroid artery is an often-used relationship when trying to identify the nerve, despite great variability in this relationship. The arteries typically arise lateral to the nerves and then course medial to the gland. The studies of Hollinshead[9] demonstrated that on the right side, the RLN passed between the main or minor branches of the inferior thyroid artery 50% of the time, and posterior to the artery approximately 25% of the time. On the left side, the RLN passes posterior to the inferior thyroid artery 50% of the time and passes anterior to the artery in 10 to 12% of cases. The RLN's course in relation to the tracheoesophageal groove is more variable on the right side than on the left, with the left nerve being located in the tracheoesophageal (TE) groove 70% of the time, but being located in the TE groove only 59% of the time on the right side. The RLN also has a relationship with the Berry ligament and passes through it 25% or deep to it 75% of the time.[10] Despite these variations, the RLN's most consistent location is near its insertion.

The studies of Shindo et al[3] examined how to best locate the RLN surgically. Their approach was to locate the RLN distally as it approached the cricothyroid joint, identifying the nerve just below the Berry ligament. The study showed that during the initial search for the distal segment of the RLN, the dissection can be directed toward a triangle located 15 to 45 degrees from the tracheoesophageal groove, and the nerve can be expected to be found there 78% of the time.

A "nonrecurrent" recurrent laryngeal nerve can occur secondary to a vascular anomaly, but it is rare, occurring in approximately 0.63% of cases.[11] It occurs more commonly on the right side than on the left (0.04%)[11] and is associated with a retroesophageal subclavian artery. In this case, the recurrent laryngeal nerve passes directly to the larynx instead of looping around the subclavian artery. Diagnosis is made preoperatively either incidentally on chest x-ray, computed tomography (CT) scan, or barium swallow, or based on suspicion and a clinical history of impairment with swallowing.

Embryology of the Parathyroid Glands

The parathyroid glands arise from the endoderm of the third and fourth pharyngeal pouches, with the thymus also arising from the third pouch. The inferior parathyroid glands are derived from the dorsal part of the third pharyngeal pouch, whereas the thymus arises from the ventral part of third pharyngeal pouch. The superior parathyroid glands are derived from the fourth pharyngeal pouch. Because the inferior parathyroids and thymus are both derived from the same pharyngeal pouch, they ultimately migrate together. The superior parathyroids migrate with the ultimobranchial bodies.

The inferior parathyroids and thymus migrate together toward the mediastinum. They eventually separate, with the inferior parathyroids ultimately becoming localized in the majority of cases near the inferior poles of the thyroid. The thymus continues to migrate toward the mediastinum.

The superior parathyroids migrate a shorter distance than the inferior glands. This results in a relatively constant location in the neck. The superior glands migrate along with the ultimobranchial bodies, and remain in contact with the posterior part of the middle third of the thyroid lobes.

Anomalous Development of the Parathyroid Glands

The parathyroid glands can exhibit a wide variation in location secondary to migration patterns during embryogenesis. Despite this, there are certain migration characteristics that are often observed that can help to identify superior and inferior glands. The plane of the parathyroid gland in relation to the RLN is one such characteristic.[12] The superior parathyroid glands are located dorsal to the RLN and the inferior parathyroid ventral to the RLN. The superior gland migration patterns extend to the retropharyngeal, retrolaryngeal, retroesophageal, and posterior mediastinum.[13] Due to the fact that the inferior parathyroid glands migrate further than the superior glands, there is often a greater degree of variability of ectopic gland location with the inferior glands. Approximately 61% of inferior parathyroid glands are found inferior, lateral, or posterior to the lower pole of the thyroid gland.[14] The inferior parathyroid glands are also commonly found in the thyrothymic ligament or the cervical portion of the thyroid. As previously stated, the inferior glands migrate with the thymus. The descent of the thymus extends from the angle of the mandible to the pericardium, and ectopic inferior glands can lie anywhere along that path of descent, including the carotid sheath. If the inferior glands fail to separate or separation from the thymus is delayed during their descent, the inferior glands may have ectopic locations within the superior mediastinum (**Fig. 2.4**).

Parathyroid glands may be ectopically located within the thyroid gland itself. An intrathyroid ectopic location is defined as a parathyroid gland surrounded on all sides by thyroid tissue. This intrathyroid localization occurs most likely embryologically due to superior parathyroid fusion with the ultimobranchial bodies during development.

Supernumerary parathyroid glands occur secondary to accessory parathyroid fragments that result when the pharyngeal pouches separate from the pharynx. They are most often found at the level of the lower poles of the thyroid lobes or in the thymus. Supernumerary parathyroid glands may also be situated in the middle mediastinum at the level of the aortopulmonary window or lateral to the jugulocarotid axis. Such locations are most likely secondary to

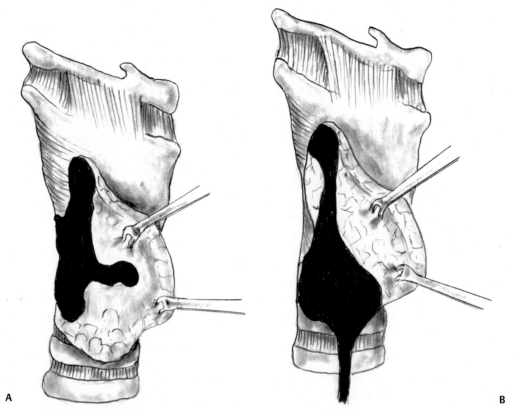

A

B

Fig. 2.4 Most common location of superior parathyroid (**A**) and inferior parathyroid (**B**) glands. Shaded areas detail the most common distribution sites of the glands.

fragmentation of the superior parathyroid rather than migration of pathologic parathyroid tissue. Intravagal parathyroid tissue has also been documented with a frequency of approximately 6%.[15,16]

Lymphatics

The lymphatic drainage of the thyroid gland travels with the venous and arterial vasculature of the gland. There is a drainage pattern for the superior, lateral, and inferior portions of the gland. The lymphatics from the superior portion of the gland and the isthmus drain into the Delphian, or prelaryngeal, lymph nodes and the jugular lymph nodes. The lymphatics from the lateral portion of the gland drain along with the middle thyroid vein. They drain into lymph node levels II to IV. The lymphatics draining the inferior portion of the gland follow the inferior thyroid veins and drain to pretracheal, paratracheal (level VI), and lower jugular (level IV) regions as well as the level VII nodes in the anterior mediastinum (**Fig. 2.5**).

The thyroid gland also has an intraglandular lymphatic network that connects the two lobes of the gland. This intraglandular network is subcapsular and significant in that it facilitates the spread of tumor within the gland.

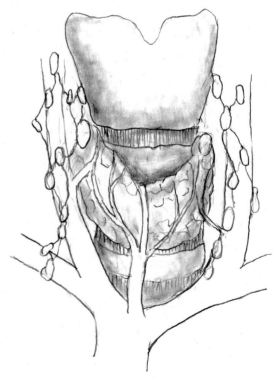

Fig. 2.5 Lymphatic network of the thyroid gland. Lymphatics parallel the venous drainage of the neck.

Embryology of the Thymus

The thymus is derived from the ventral wing of the third pharyngeal pouch and migrates into the mediastinum during development. Due to this migration, accessory thymic tissue can be found in the neck anywhere along the path of its migration (anywhere from the superior thoracic aperture to the thyroid cartilage or higher).[1] The thymus continues to grow through childhood until puberty. In adults, the gland atrophies considerably and can be difficult to locate and identify.

References

1. Hansen JT. Embryology and surgical anatomy of the lower neck and superior mediastinum. In: Falk SA, ed. Thyroid Disease. Philadelphia: Lippincott-Raven, 1990
2. Langman J, Sadler TW. Langman's Medical Embryology, 8th ed. Philadelphia: Lippincott Williams & Wilkins, 2000:504
3. Shindo ML, Wu JC, Park EE. Surgical anatomy of the recurrent laryngeal nerve revisited. Otolaryngol Head Neck Surg 2005;133:514–519
4. Choi SS. Thyroglossal duct cyst. In: Cotton RT, Myer CM III, eds. Practical Pediatric Otolaryngology. Philadelphia: Lippincott-Raven, 1999:952–954
5. Hunt PS. A reappraisal of the surgical anatomy of the thyroid and parathyroid glands. Br J Surg 1968;55:63–66
6. Cernea CR, Nishio S, Hojaij FC. Identification of the external branch of the superior laryngeal nerve (EBSLN) in large goiters. Am J Otolaryngol 1995;16:307–311
7. Kierner AC, Aigner M, Burian M. The external branch of the superior laryngeal nerve. Arch Otol Head Neck Surg 1998;124:301–303
8. Friedman M, LoSavio P, Ibrahim H. Superior laryngeal nerve identification and preservation in thyroidectomy. Arch Otolaryngol Head Neck Surg 2002;128:296–303
9. Hollinshead WH. Anatomy for Surgeons, vol 1. The Head and Neck, 2nd ed. New York: Harper & Row, 1968
10. Lore JM. Surgery of the thyroid gland. In: Tenta LT, Keyes GR, eds. Symposium on Surgery of the Thyroid and Parathyroid Glands, vol 13. Philadelphia: WB Saunders, 1980;69–83
11. Henry JF, Audiffret J, Denizot A, Plan M. The nonrecurrent inferior laryngeal nerve: review of 33 cases including two on the left side. Surgery 1988;104:977–984
12. Pyrtek L, Painter RL. An anatomic study of the relationship of the parathyroid glands to the recurrent laryngeal nerve. Surg Gynecol Obstet 1964;119:509–512
13. Randolph GW, Urken ML. Surgical management of primary hyperparathyroidism. In: Randolph GW, ed. Surgery of the Thyroid and Parathyroid Glands. Philadelphia: WB Saunders, 2003:507–528
14. Akerstrom G, Malmaeus J, Bergstrom R. Surgical anatomy of human parathyroid glands. Surgery 1984;95:14–21
15. Gilmour JR. The gross anatomy of the parathyroid glands. J Pathol Bacteriol 1938;46:133–149
16. Lack EE, Delay S, Linnoila RL. Ectopic parathyroid tissue within the vagus nerve. Arch Pathol Lab Med 1988;112:304–306

3 Physiology of the Thyroid Gland

Kathryn G. Schuff and James I. Cohen

This chapter reviews the synthesis, storage, and release of thyroid hormones; thyroid hormone delivery to the cell and action within the cell; changes in the thyroid axis in response to aging, pregnancy, medications, and nonthyroidal illness (NTI); and hypothyroidism and hyperthyroidism. Chapters 6 to 8 provide a more in-depth discussion of the pathophysiology of benign thyroid disease and medical and surgical management.

Thyroid Hormone Synthesis, Storage and Release

The thyroid hormones levothyroxine (T_4) and triiodothyronine (T_3) belong to a class of molecules referred to as thyronamines, shown in **Fig. 3.1**. They are composed of an outer

and an inner six-member ring, connected by an ether linkage. The major biologically active thyronamines are T_4 and T_3.

Thyroid Hormone Synthesis and Storage

The normal thyroid gland is composed of follicles—groups of thyroid follicular cells surrounding a central follicular lumen filled with clear, proteinaceous colloid. The thyroid follicular cells are oriented with the apical surface forming the lining of the follicular lumen and the basal surface separated from the adjacent microvascular bed by a thin basement membrane.[1] This orientation is critical to normal thyroid follicular cell function.

The process of thyroid hormone synthesis, storage, and secretion involves multiple highly coordinated steps, shown

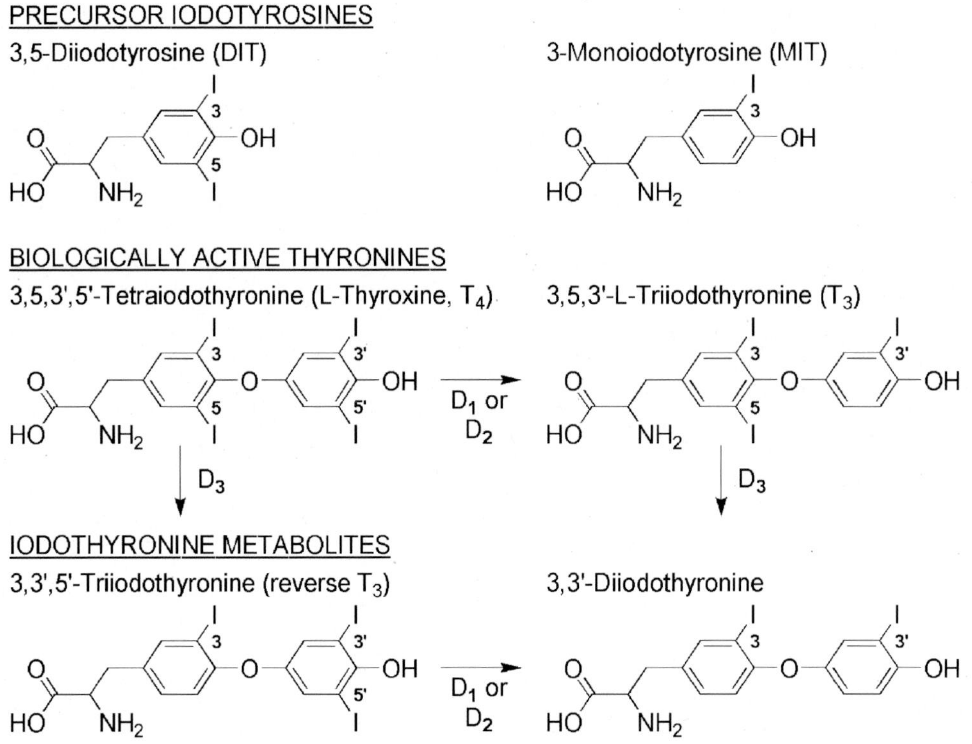

Fig. 3.1 Structure of the thyronamines. Thyroid hormones belong to the thyronamine class of molecules, composed of an outer and an inner six-member ring, connected by an ether linkage. 3,5-diiodotyrosine (DIT) and 3-monoiodotyrosine (MIT) are iodinated tyrosines that are precursors to the biologically active thyroid hormones, L-thyroxine (T_4) and triiodothyronine (T_3). Thyroxine is converted to both T_3 and reverse T_3, which are further metabolized to diiodothyronine. *Abbreviations:* DIT, diiodotyronine; MIT, monoiodotyrosine; T_4, L-thyroxine; T_3, triiodothyronine; rT_3, reverse T_3.

in detail in **Fig. 3.2**. Iodine is a crucial constituent of thyroid hormone, and the first step in thyroid hormone synthesis is active transport of iodide against a large concentration and electrical gradient from the serum into the thyroid follicular cell. This is mediated by the sodium iodide transporter (NIS) located in the basolateral membrane.[2] Intracellular iodide is transported across the apical membrane into the follicular lumen by pendrin, an iodide-chloride transporter.[3] Several other anions (pertechnetate, perchlorate, perrhenate, tetrafluoroborate, and thiocyanate) are transported or are inhibitors of iodine uptake at the NIS.[4] This forms the basis for the use of technetium-99m (^{99m}Tc) for thyroid scanning, and the perchlorate discharge test to evaluate potential organification defects.[5] Thyroglobulin, the thyroid hormone precursor protein, is transcribed within the thyroid follicular cell and transported by secretory vesicles to the apical aspect of the follicular cell.

On the luminal side of the apical membrane, thyroglobulin is then iodinated, a process referred to as organification. This is catalyzed by thyroid peroxidase (TPO) and involves iodination of specific tyrosyl residues to form monoiodotyrosine and diiodotyrosine. A coupling reaction, also catalyzed by TPO, results in conjugation of the iodinated tyrosyl residues to form T_4 or T_3 (**Fig. 3.1**). In the normal thyroid gland, T_4 is produced in preference to T_3, but T_3 is preferentially produced under conditions of iodine deficiency and some cases of hyperthyroidism.[1] Iodinated thyroglobulin is stored within the follicular lumen as colloid and serves as a large reserve of thyroid hormone.

Thyroid Hormone Release

When thyroid hormone secretion is required, stored colloid undergoes pinocytosis back into the thyroid follicular cell. The colloid droplets fuse with lysosomes, and thyroglobulin undergoes enzyme-mediated cleavage to produce T_4 and T_3, diiodotyronine and monoiodotyronine (**Fig. 3.1**). T_4 and T_3 are secreted at the basolateral membrane into venous capillary beds. Intracellular DIT and MIT are further deiodinated and metabolized, returning the iodine to the intrathyroidal pool for further thyroid hormone synthesis. DIT and MIT have historically been thought to be inactive, but recently have been proposed to have a potential role in thermogenesis and energy metabolism.[6,7]

Regulation of Thyroid Hormone Synthesis and Release

Thyroid hormone synthesis and release are highly regulated by the hypothalamic-pituitary-thyroid axis, one of the classic negative feedback loops between the pituitary and its target organs that maintain hormone levels in the physiologic range (**Fig. 3.3**). Thyroid-stimulating hormone (TSH), or thyrotropin, is secreted by the pituitary gland in pulsatile fashion with a diurnal rhythm and stimulates multiple steps in thyroid hormone synthesis and release. In turn, TSH synthesis, secretion, and bioactivity are stimulated by hypothalamic thyrotropin-releasing hormone (TRH). Thyroid hormone exerts negative feedback directly at the pituitary to inhibit TSH and indirectly at the hypothalamus to inhibit TRH. Illness inhibits TRH transcription, which is mediated by

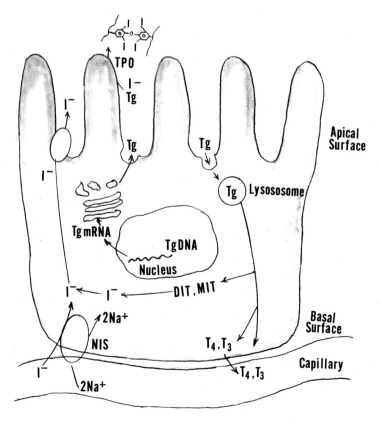

Fig. 3.2 Thyroid hormone synthesis. The thyroid follicular cell is oriented with the apical surface lining the follicular lumen and basal surface adjacent to the microvascular bed. The polar orientation is critical for iodine transport into the cytoplasm by the sodium iodide symporter and to the follicular lumen by pendrin. Thyroglobulin is transcribed, translated, and transported to the follicular lumen, where it is iodinated on specific tyrosyl residues, which are then coupled in an ether linkage to form T_4 or T_3, referred to as organification. A large pool of thyroid hormone is stored in the follicular lumen as colloid containing iodinated thyroglobulin. Stored colloid subsequently undergoes pinocytosis and fuses with lysosomes where T_4 and T_3 are cleaved from the thyroglobulin and released into the circulation. Iodine from residual DIT and MIT are recovered back into the cytoplasmic pool. *Abbreviations:* DIT, diiodotyronine; I$^-$, iodide; MIT, monoiodotyronine; mRNA, messenger ribonucleic acid; Na$^+$, sodium; NIS, sodium iodide symporter; T_3, triiodothyronine; T_4, thyroxine; Tg, thyroglobulin; TPO, thyroid peroxidase.

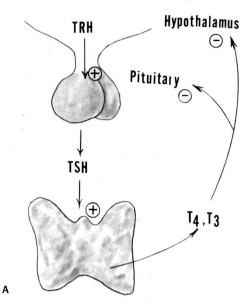

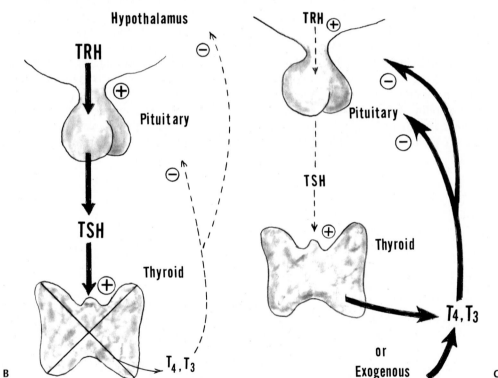

Fig. 3.3 Hypothalamic-pituitary-thyroid axis in hypothyroidism and hyperthyroidism. (**A**) Normal regulation of the hypothalamic-pituitary-thyroid axis involves a negative feedback loop. Hypothalamic TRH stimulates thyrotrophs in the pituitary gland to secrete TSH, which stimulates the thyroid gland to release T_4 and T_3. These thyroid hormones exert a negative influence on pituitary TSH secretion and hypothalamic TRH secretion. (**B**) In hypothyroidism, lack of thyroidal secretion of T_4 and T_3 reduces the negative feedback at the pituitary and hypothalamus, such that TRH secretion is increased and serum TSH levels are elevated. (**C**) In hyperthyroidism, excess T_4 and T_3 from thyroid gland overproduction (or exogenous administration) increases the amount of negative feedback, with low levels of TRH and a suppressed serum TSH level. *Abbreviations:* TRH, thyrotropin-releasing hormone; TSH, thyroid-stimulating hormone; T_3, triiodothyronine; T_4, thyroxine.

cytokines. Starvation also inhibits TRH transcription via the melanocortin system. In contrast, cold increases TRH transcription via catecholaminergic input. The three effects of TSH synthesis, secretion, and bioactivity are mediated by cytokines, the melanocortin system, and catecholaminergic input, respectively.[8] Several other minor factors regulate TSH secretion, including glucocorticoids, dopamine, and somatostatin, which inhibit TSH secretion, and vasopressin, which stimulates TSH.[9]

Thyroid-stimulating hormone is the major regulator of thyroid hormone synthesis and release. It mediates NIS tran-

scription, protein half-life and intracellular localization,[10] thyroglobulin transcription, thyroid peroxidase activity, hydrogen peroxide generation, colloid pinocytosis, and thyroid hormone release.[11] TSH binds to a seven transmembrane G-protein–coupled receptor localized at the basolateral membrane of the thyroid follicular cell.[12] The TSH receptor is coupled to multiple signaling pathways, predominantly adenylyl cyclase, but also small guanosine triphosphates, phospholipids, and phosphatidylinositide 3-kinase. In addition to thyroid hormone synthesis, the biologic actions of TSH include growth and development of the thyroid follicular cell.

Iodide is a second major regulator of thyroid hormone synthesis and secretion. It exerts TSH-independent effects on NIS transcription. Iodine deficiency upregulates NIS expression as the thyroid gland attempts to compensate; iodine excess leads to complex effects, depending on dose, time course, and underlying thyroid pathology. Acutely, iodine excess causes downregulation of NIS expression, iodide transport, and decreased thyroid hormone biosynthesis, termed the Wolff-Chaikoff effect. Escape from the Wolff-Chaikoff effect commonly occurs within days, but may be delayed or absent in patients with underlying thyroid disease. In the setting of multinodular thyroid disease, acute iodine excess results in iodine-induced hyperthyroidism, the jodbasedow effect.[13]

Thyroglobulin and a variety of cytokines (transforming growth factor-β, tumor necrosis factor-α and -β, interleukin-1, interleukin-6, and interferon-γ) inhibit NIS transcription, and some also inhibit TPO activity.[11] The clinical significance of these regulators is not clear.

Thyroid hormone synthesis and release may be manipulated pharmacologically as well. The antithyroid medications methimazole, carbimazole (which is converted to methimazole), and propylthiouracil (PTU) inhibit several steps in thyroid hormone synthesis and secretion, including iodination and coupling, endocytosis, and release of secretory granules. Perchlorate competes with iodide for transport with high affinity and can be used pharmacologically in hyperthyroidism to block thyroid hormone production. Thiocyanate and nitrate can inhibit iodide transport, with lower affinity than perchlorate.[4] However, because they are often found in the environment in higher concentrations, there may be significant alterations in thyroid function in exposed individuals. Lithium blocks iodine efflux from the thyroid follicular cell and is sometimes used as an adjunct to radioactive iodine therapy in thyroid cancer.[14]

Thyroid Hormone Activation and Metabolism

The predominant thyroid hormone secreted by the thyroid gland is T_4. T_3 is the thyroid hormone that is active at the transcriptional level. T_4 is converted to T_3 extrathyroidally by deiodination of the 5' (outer ring) iodine residue (**Fig. 3.1**) by types 1 and 2 selenodeiodinase (D1 and D2). This is the predominant source of circulating T_3, yielding 80% of circulating T_3, or approximately 25 μg. The remaining 20%, approximately 6 μg, is directly secreted by the thyroid gland.[15] T_4 activation to T_3 also occurs intracellularly in local tissues. Tissue-specific expression of the deiodinases and iodinase-specific regulation both contribute to a complex pattern of tissue-specific regulation of intracellular T_4 and T_3 concentrations, independent of serum levels. Because of the intracellular nature of this process, assessment of local production and tissue levels of T_3 is difficult and not clinically available or currently of clinical utility.

Metabolism of the active thyroid hormones to inactive compounds is mediated by the type 3 selenodeiodinase (D3). This enzyme catalyzes the 5-position (inner ring) deiodination and yields reverse T_3 (rT_3) from T_4 and diiodotyronine from T_3. D3 is highly expressed in brain, fetal tissues, the placenta, and pregnant uterus and is likely important in protecting the fetus from excess thyroid hormone during development.[15]

Selenium is an essential element for deiodinase activity. Selenium deficiency can be seen in patients on restricted protein diets, such as in phenylketonuria or the elderly, but is rarely of clinical significance with patients showing only slightly increased ratios of T_4 to T_3 and normal TSH levels.[16]

Thyroid Hormone Delivery

Thyroid Hormone Circulation

Thyroid hormones circulate highly bound to serum proteins. They bind transthyretin (TTR) and thyroxine-binding globulin (TBG) with high affinity, albumin with low affinity, and several other minor carriers including lipoproteins. Protein-bound thyroid hormone represents a large reservoir that can fluctuate with significant changes in the affinity or levels of the binding proteins. However, thyroid hormone is not biologically active until it dissociates from these proteins. This can lead to a confusing clinical picture, as total thyroid hormone levels may be abnormal due to changes in binding protein concentrations, but free hormone levels remain normal.

Importantly, although changes in thyroid hormone binding are compensated by changes in endogenous thyroid hormone production, a change in dosage may be necessary in patients on exogenous levothyroxine to maintain normal TSH and free thyroid hormone levels. **Table 3.1** lists several

Table 3.1 Conditions that Change Thyroid Binding Protein Levels or Affinities

Increased TBG, TTR, or Binding Affinity	Decreased TBG
Pregnancy	Androgens
Oral contraceptives	Corticosteroids
SERMs	Hyperthyroidism
5-fluorouracil	Proteinuria
Chronic kidney disease	Critical illness, sepsis
Hepatitis, hepatoma	Hepatic failure
Acute intermittent porphyria	Congenital absence of TBG
α_1-Antitrypsin deficiency	
Hypothyroidism	
Congenital TBG excess	
Familial dysalbuminemic hyperthyroxinemia	
Familial amyloid polyneuropathy	

Abbreviations: TBG, thyroxine-binding globulin; TTR, transthyretin; SERMs, selective estrogen receptor modulators.

clinically relevant factors that influence the concentrations and affinity of TBG and TTR.[17]

Thyroid Hormone Transport into the Cell

T_4 and T_3 are actively transported into the cell by several transporters including organic anion transporters of the Na^+/taurocholate cotransporting polypeptide (NTCP) and (Na^+-independent) organic anion transporting polypeptide (OATP) families as well as amino acid transporters of the L- and T-type such as the monocarboxylase transporter, MCT-8.

Thyroid Hormone Action

Genomic Effects

Intracellular T_3 enters the nucleus and binds to the thyroid hormone receptor (TR) as a heterodimer with the retinoid X receptor (RXR), another member of the nuclear receptor superfamily. The heterodimer binds target DNA sequences referred to as thyroid response elements (TREs) to activate or repress gene transcription. T_3 binding results in conformational changes that affect binding of coactivators and corepressors.

Nongenomic Effects

Thyroid hormone may also have nongenomic/membrane effects. Examples include effects on cell structure proteins including the actin cytoskeleton, actions on cell membrane ion channels, and mitogen-activated protein kinase (MAPK)-mediated phosphorylation of p53, $TR\beta$-1, and estrogen receptor. Cell surface receptors have been identified,[18] but the mechanism of nongenomic effects is still being evaluated.

Abnormalities of Thyroid Function

Abnormalities of thyroid function tests may reflect true abnormalities of thyroid function, either hypothyroidism or hyperthyroidism, or may reflect effects of NTI or medications on thyroid hormone blood levels. Patients may present with signs and symptoms of altered thyroid hormone levels or anatomic abnormalities such as goiter or nodules, or they may have thyroid function abnormalities discovered incidentally. In all cases, it must be determined if the thyroid function test abnormalities reflect a pathologic process. Careful correlation of the clinical assessment with measures of thyroid hormone and TSH levels is critical for appropriate management.

Assessment of Thyroid Function

In general, measurement of TSH provides the most useful information about the thyroid status of a patient. Despite TSH pulsatility and diurnal variation, TSH levels are reliable, as

Table 3.2 Situations in which the TSH Is Unreliable as a Measure of Thyroid Function

Clinical Scenario	Comment
Poor compliance with LT4	Taking several days of medication immediately prior to laboratory tests can result in a normal free T_4 but persistently elevated TSH
Delayed recovery of TSH secretion after hyperthyroidism	Can persist for many months; medications must be titrated based on free T_4 levels
Central hypothyroidism	Obligates evaluation for pituitary mass and for other pituitary hormones
TSH-secreting pituitary adenoma	Rare
Syndrome of thyroid hormone resistance	Rare mutation in $TR\beta$ causes reduced T_3 binding or altered coactivator/repressor binding; patients are clinically euthyroid with high free T_4 and "inappropriately normal" or elevated TSH levels
Heterophil antibodies	Antimouse antibody can bind the mouse-derived anti-TSH monoclonal antibody used in the TSH assay; varies by assay

Abbreviations: LT4, levothyroxine; Free T_4, free thyroxine level; TSH, thyroid-stimulating hormone; $TR\beta$, thyroid hormone receptor β isoform; T_3, triiodothyronine.

the population normal range accounts for these variations. The log-linear relationship of TSH to thyroid hormone levels is such that small changes in thyroid hormone levels, even if they remain in the population normal range, lead to significant changes in TSH in an individual patient. Additionally, in both hypothyroidism and hyperthyroidism, TSH becomes abnormal before either T_4 or T_3 levels. Further, modern TSH assays are sensitive enough to distinguish hyperthyroidism from other low TSH states such as NTI. The TSH assay is reliable, and not usually subject to significant assay interference. There are a few clinical situations (listed in **Table 3.2**) where the TSH is misleading, and correct diagnosis requires reliance on integration of the clinical assessment and free T_4 as well as the TSH levels.

Recently, consideration has been given to redefining the upper limit of the TSH normal range.[19,20] Based on data from the third National Health and Nutrition Examination Survey (NHANES III), individuals with TSH in the upper part of the normal range have higher levels of thyroid autoantibodies and may have the mildest form of subclinical hypothyroidism. Elimination of these individuals from the reference range results in contraction of the upper limit to approximately 2.5 to 3.0 mU/mL. The clinical significance of this proposed change for diagnosing new cases of hypothyroidism with TSH levels in the upper part of the current normal range (2.5–5.0 mU/mL) remains to be demonstrated. However, it is probably reasonable to titrate TSH levels of patients already on levothyroxine into this new lower range.

Measurement of T_4 and T_3 levels is more problematic. Total T_4 and T_3 measurements are technically reliable, but may be difficult to interpret due to alterations in thyroid binding proteins in euthyroid patients as listed in **Table 3.1**. Free T_4 and T_3 assays theoretically avoid this difficulty; however, there are several different assay methodologies that have assay-specific interferences and inaccuracies from binding protein changes and inhibitors. Most free T_4 assays are reliable in the absence of significant changes in binding proteins. However, levels are unpredictable when there are binding protein changes, including in pregnancy (high TBG and progressive decreases in albumin), renal failure, and any illness with decreased albumin or TBG. Although considered the "gold standard," even equilibrium dialysis can be inaccurate due to binding inhibitors. A measure of total T_4, preferably with a T_3 resin uptake and appropriate interpretation of potential binding protein changes, is probably preferable in those situations, and has been specifically recommended for pregnant women unless trimester-specific reference ranges are available.

Measurement of free T_3 is even more problematic, because free T_3 assays are not as well standardized or consistent as free T_4 assays. In addition, measurement of T_3 (total or free) is usually not helpful except in the situation of T_3 toxicosis, where the TSH is suppressed and the free T_4 is normal.

Direct measurement of thyroid binding proteins is not indicated routinely. However, it is valuable when a genetic abnormality (absence or excess) in TBG, TTR, or albumin is suspected. Abnormalities in affinity can be detected by electrophoresis after binding to radiolabeled thyroid hormone. Gene sequencing can confirm abnormal results.

A variety of different thyroid antibodies are produced in autoimmune thyroid disease. Antithyroglobulin antibodies and anti-TPO antibodies (previously termed antimicrosomal antibodies) can be measured clinically, and are seen in >90% of patients with Hashimoto thyroiditis. However, they are also seen in other thyroid diseases and in 10 to 15% of the normal population.[21] Further, they are of limited clinical utility, because they usually do not change the management of a patient with a significantly elevated TSH level. In patients with subclinical hypothyroidism, a condition where the TSH is mildly elevated but thyroid hormone levels are normal, the presence of high-level antibodies results in a higher rate of progression to overt hypothyroidism,[22] and thus may identify a group more likely to benefit from treatment. In addition, women with high levels of TPO antibodies are at higher risk of postpartum thyroiditis,[23] but there is controversy about whether this should be performed routinely in pregnant women.

Anti-TSH receptor antibodies are etiologic in Graves disease because they bind and activate the TSH receptor. They can be measured in two ways: (1) TSH-binding inhibitory immunoglobulins (TBIIs) inhibit binding of TSH to TSH receptor in vitro. (2) A bioassay measuring the ability of the antibody to stimulate cyclic adenosine monophos-

phate (cAMP) production is termed TSH receptor stimulating antibodies (TSHR-SAb). TBIIs are present in up to 99% of patients with untreated Graves disease and fall with treatment. They are also seen in lesser proportions of patients with other thyroid diseases, but in only 0.5% of normal subjects. TSHR-SAb is found in approximately 90% of patients with Graves disease. Measurement of these antibodies can occasionally be helpful in cases of hyperthyroidism where the etiology is not clear (e.g., Graves disease with nodularity, postpartum thyroiditis versus Graves disease) and can predict neonatal thyrotoxicosis when measured in the third trimester.[24] However, these assays are expensive, and usually do not add significant information to the patient's evaluation.

Thyroid-stimulating hormone receptor antibodies can also block the TSH receptor and cause thyroprivic hypothyroidism, which is characterized by atrophy of the thyroid gland.[1] They will be detected by the TBII assay, but not the TSHR-SAb.

Thyroid Hormone Changes in Physiologic and Environmental Challenges and Nonthyroidal Illness

Aging

There appears to be little change in the thyroid axis with healthy aging, although the concomitant presence of illness may lead to abnormal thyroid function tests in elderly patients. The thyroidal T_4 secretion rate falls slightly with age, but without any change in serum T_4 levels, attributed to slowed metabolism of thyroid hormone. Over the age of 80 years, there is a slight fall in serum T_3 levels and a slight decrease in TSH.[25]

Pregnancy

The physiologic changes in the thyroid axis with pregnancy are complex and clinically significant (see recent review by LeBeau and Mandel[24]). One of the most significant changes is a twofold increase in TBG, which occurs early in the first trimester and persists for the duration of the pregnancy. Additional T_4 is required to saturate thyroxine binding; transplacental passage and placental metabolism of T_4 also increase T_4 requirements. In addition, the glomerular filtration rate, and therefore renal clearance of iodide, increases. These changes stimulate maternal thyroid production. Further, because of cross-reactivity of TSH and human chorionic gonadotropin (hCG), there is direct stimulation of the thyroidal TSH receptor by hCG resulting in increased T_4 production and a small increase in thyroid gland size (though usually not a clinically detectable goiter).[26] These effects can be significant enough to cause transient hyperthyroidism, known as gestational thyrotoxicosis, particularly during twin or molar pregnancies. The thyrotoxicosis resolves spontaneously when hCG levels decline after 20 weeks' gestation.[24]

As a result of these changes, thyroid function tests in the first trimester typically show lower TSH levels due to hCG thyroidal stimulation, with 9% of euthyroid pregnant women having TSH levels <0.05 mU/L, 9% having TSH levels from 0.05 to 0.4 mU/L and a 95% upper limit of TSH normal range of 2.5 mU/L. Free T_4 levels in automated assays are variable because of assay differences, none of which has trimester-specific normal ranges established. The true free T_4 probably increases slightly; total T_4 levels increase 50%.

The most important implication of these changes is recognition of the early (by 4 to 8 weeks' gestation) and dramatic (25–47%) increase in exogenous levothyroxine requirements in hypothyroid pregnant women. On this basis, it is recommended that women increase their levothyroxine dose by approximately 30% (two extra pills/week) immediately upon learning they are pregnant, with close monitoring of TSH in the first trimester. Women with underlying autoimmune thyroid disease who are euthyroid prior to conception may have reduced thyroidal reserve and should be monitored during pregnancy, with a goal TSH of less than 2.5 mU/mL.

Nonthyroidal Illness

Acute illness, including medical illness, surgery, trauma, and caloric deprivation, causes several thyroid hormone abnormalities, termed nonthyroidal illness (NTI). These abnormalities often do not reflect any pathologic change in thyroid function, but are part of the neuroendocrine response to illness. It is hypothesized that this is an adaptive response, reflecting attempts to maintain homeostasis. These changes may be compounded by medication effects, described in the next section. Evaluation of patients with suspected NTI is complex; the clinical evaluation is difficult and laboratory evaluations are unreliable and misleading.

The most typical pattern and duration of thyroid function changes are shown in **Table 3.3** and include a decrease in serum T_3 and increase in reverse T_3 levels. The severity of illness correlates with the degree of T_3 decrement. Decreases in D1 activity due to either drugs or cytokines and increases in type 3 deiodinase (D3) activity explain these changes.[27] Free T_3 levels are preserved or may show a lesser decrement. Serum T_4 levels are either normal or slightly decreased unless the patient is critically ill; severely low T_4 levels are associated with higher mortality.[28] Free T_4 levels vary by the assay used and can be affected by several interfering substances present in the serum of ill patients. Studies using reliable methods suggest that free T_4 remains normal.[17] Serum TSH levels are usually normal, but it can be low in critical illness, although rarely totally suppressed. Proposed mechanisms for low TSH levels include drug effects, decreased TRH production, a direct effect of cytokines on pituitary thyrotrophs, and increases in pituitary D2 activity. Importantly, TSH levels may temporarily increase to above the normal range during recovery from NTI.

Nonthyroidal illness is common, occurring in up to 50% of hospitalized patients. Treatment with thyroid hormone, either T_4 or T_3, is controversial.[27,29] Most treatment studies were limited by design, and the heterogeneity and small numbers of patients. Most thyroidologists recommend against treatment, based on concern of worsening catabolism and lack of evidence for benefit.

Iodine Deficiency

Because of the critical role of iodine in thyroid hormone synthesis, iodine deficiency results in hypothyroidism, goiters, and nodules. Maternal iodine deficiency is particularly detrimental, leading to impaired fertility, increased perinatal and infant mortality, and decrements in fetal physical and mental development. Iodine deficiency is the leading and most preventable cause of mental retardation in the world. Despite efforts of the World Health Organization to assist governments in establishing and monitoring iodine supplementation programs, 36.5% of the world population, nearly 2 billion people, remain iodine deficient.[30] In the past, iodine deficiency was a significant problem in the United States, particularly in the "goiter belt" of the Great Lakes region and Pacific Northwest.[31] This has essentially been eliminated with an optional salt iodization program. The current Institute of Medicine recommends a daily iodide intake of 150 μg per day for adults and 220 μg daily for pregnant and lactating women. Recent studies show that although iodine intake is adequate for the general U.S. population, it is marginal for women of childbearing age.[32] Further, most commonly available prenatal vitamins do not contain supplemental iodine.[33]

Medications and Foods

Medications and chemicals in foods or the environment may cause several changes in thyroid function tests. Alterations are observed at every level of the thyroid axis, as detailed in **Table 3.4**. The mechanism of these effects has been

Table 3.3 Thyroid Hormone Changes in Nonthyroidal Illness

Parameter	Mild	Severe	Recovery
T_3	↓	↓↓	Rapidly normalizes
Free T_3[a]	Mild ↓	↓	Rapidly normalizes
Reverse T_3	↑	↑	
TSH	Normal	Low but usually not suppressed	Normal or ↑
T_4	Normal or mild ↓	Low	↑
Free T_4[a]	Normal or ↑ by ED, low by analogue methods	Normal	Rapidly normalizes, may be ↑

Abbreviations: T_3, triiodothyronine; TSH, thyroid-stimulating hormone; T_4, thyroxine; ED, equilibrium dialysis.
[a] Varies by method.

Table 3.4 Medications and Foods that Affect the Thyroid Axis

Medication	Clinical Presentation
Impaired thyroid hormone absorption	Increases levothyroxine requirement
Calcium carbonate	
Aluminum hydroxide	
Carafate	
Omeprazole	
Ferrous sulfate	
Bile acid sequestrants	
Ciprofloxacin	
Raloxifene	
Charcoal	
Soy infant formulas	
Increased thyroid hormone binding	Increases total T_4, normal free T_4
	Increases levothyroxine requirement
Oral estrogens and SERMs	
5-Fluorouracil	
Clofibrate	
Opiates	
Perphenazine	
Heroin	
Methadone	
Decreased thyroid hormone binding	Decreases total T_4, normal free T_4
	Decreases levothyroxine requirement
NSAIDs: acetylsalicylic acid (aspirin), salsalate, meclofenamate, fencolofenac	
Sulfonylureas	
Phenytoin	
Diazepam	
Chloral hydrate	
Glucocorticoids	
Androgens	
Furosemide	At high doses, e.g., large IV boluses
L-asparaginase	
Free fatty acids (e.g., hyperalimentation, hemodialysis or by activation of lipoprotein lipase by heparin)	Increased free T_4 due to in vitro effect on the assay
Heparin, enoxaprin	Increased free T_4 due to in vitro effect on the assay
Induce primary thyroid disease	
Cytokines: interferons, interleukin-2, GM-CSF	Induces transient or permanent immunologic-mediated goiter, hypothyroidism or hyperthyroidism
	Silent thyroiditis
	Asymptomatic thyroid autoantibody production
Amiodarone	Iodine-induced thyrotoxicosis or destructive thyroiditis
Decreased TSH secretion	Central hypothyroidism
Dopamine	
Glucocorticoids	
Somatostatin	
RXR agonists (bexarotene)	
Carbamazepine	
Opiates	
Salicylate	
Metformin	
Thyroid hormone synthesis and secretion	
Lithium	Goiter, hypothyroidism
Thionamides: propylthiouracil, methimazole, carbimazole	Used clinically to treat hyperthyroidism
	Can cause goiter, hypothyroidism
Iodine-containing medications including iodinated contrast	Transient hypothyroidism or hyperthyroidism
Amiodarone	Transient hypothyroidism or hyperthyroidism (independent of induction of primary thyroid disease, see above)

(continued on page 26)

Table 3.4 *(Continued)* **Medications and Foods that Affect the Thyroid Axis**

Medication	Clinical Presentation
Interferons, interleukin-1, TNF-α	Transient hypothyroidism
Phenylbutazone	Goiter, hypothyroidism
Goitrogens: cassava, maize, bamboo shoots, sweet potatoes, yellow turnips and Brassica seeds, cabbage, turnips, kale, kohlrabi, rutabaga, mustard	Contain thiocyanate that competes for iodine uptake or direct inhibition of T_4 synthesis
	Goiter, hypothyroidism in areas of iodine deficiency
Environmental pollutants: perchlorate, thiocyanate	Competes for iodine uptake
	Goiter, hypothyroidism in areas of iodine deficiency
Thyroid hormone metabolism	
Deiodinase inhibitors:	Decreases T_3
Propranolol	Not observed with other beta-blockers
Glucocorticoids	High dose
Propylthiouracil	Augments T_4 synthetic blockade in treatment of hyperthyroidism
Amiodarone	Increases total and free T_4, decreases T_3 (independent of induction of primary thyroid disease, see above)
Lipid soluble iodinated contrast agents: Iopanoic acid	Increases total and free T_4, decreases T_3
Sodium ipodate	
Tyropanoate	
Growth hormone	Increases T_3 production
P-450 inducers:	Decreases T_4, free T_4 with minor increase in TSH, no change in T_3
Phenytoin	Increases levothyroxine requirement
Phenobarbital	
Carbamazepine	
Nicardipine	
Rifampicin	
Rifampin	
Imanitib	Increases levothyroxine requirement
Thyroid hormone action	
RXR agonists (bexarotene)	Central hypothyroidism from TSH gene repression

Abbreviations: T_4, thyroxine; SERMs, selective estrogen receptor modulators; NSAIDs, nonsteroidal antiinflammatory drugs; IV, intravenous; GM-CSF, granulocyte-macrophage colony-stimulating factor; TNF, tumor necrosis factor; T_3, triiodothyronine, TSH, thyroid-stimulating hormone; RXR, retinoic acid receptor.

reviewed,[34–38] and will only be highlighted here. In addition, medications that have in vitro effects but have not been demonstrated to be clinically significant are not addressed here.

Clinically, the most important medication effect is impairment of absorption of exogenous levothyroxine. Some medications are direct inhibitors, and others may impair absorption by effects on gastric acidity.[39] Inhibition of absorption by soy appears to be clinically significant only in infants on soy formula.

A second clinically important effect is medications that alter thyroid hormone binding in the serum. These can change levothyroxine requirements, particularly oral contraceptives. However, in individuals without thyroid disease, medications that alter thyroid hormone binding rarely cause clinically relevant disease because of compensation of endogenous function.

A third relatively common medication effect is the induction of primary thyroid disease, probably by an effect of modulating the immune system (cytokines, particularly interferon-α) or by initiating an inflammatory process within the thyroid gland (amiodarone).

A fourth medication effect is suppression of TSH secretion, caused by agents including dopamine and glucocorticoids.

The clinical significance of these effects is controversial, because most patients who received these medications also have NTI, with overlapping effects.

Finally, some medications inhibit thyroid hormone synthesis, secretion, or deiodinase activity. Often, goiter is observed in these patients, with or without biochemical changes, and usually the biochemical changes are mild. The two most significant agents are iodine-containing agents, which can cause transient thyroid dysfunction, and lithium, which can cause goiter and hypothyroidism.

Hypothyroidism

There are several symptoms that patients suffer from related to low thyroid hormone levels, including fatigue, lethargy, sleepiness, mental impairment, depression, cold intolerance, hoarseness, dry skin, weight gain, constipation, menorrhagia, arthralgias, and paresthesias. However, the signs and symptoms are relatively nonspecific and commonly found in the general population, so any particular symptom may or may not be attributable to the thyroid dysfunction. The diagnosis of primary hypothyroidism is straightforward, relying upon detection of an elevated TSH level (**Fig. 3.3**). In subclinical hypothyroidism only the TSH is abnormal; this probably represents the mildest form of hypothyroidism.

Several pathologic processes can cause primary hypothyroidism in the adult, the most common of which is autoimmune thyroid disease. Hashimoto thyroiditis with autoimmune destruction of thyroid tissue and subsequent fibrotic replacement results in inadequate thyroid hormone production (see Chapter 6 for further details). The other acquired etiologies of hypothyroidism include postsurgical or postradiation (from iodine-131 due to previous Graves disease or external beam irradiation), and rare infiltrative diseases (amyloidosis, scleroderma). Transient hypothyroidism can be seen in postpartum thyroiditis and silent and subacute thyroiditis. Usually, the etiology is diagnosed on clinical grounds.

The etiologies of congenital hypothyroidism are several. In addition to thyroid dysgenesis, genetic defects in any of the essential steps in thyroid hormone synthesis will result in congenital hypothyroidism, including defects in iodine transport (NIS and pendrin) and organification (*DUOX2* and TPO), thyroglobulin, and the thyroid hormone cellular transporter MCT-8.[40]

Secondary or central hypothyroidism is an infrequent cause of hypothyroidism and is more challenging but very important to diagnose. It must be suspected when a patient with hypothyroid symptoms has a low or low normal free T_4 but does not have an elevated TSH. It is usually due to organic pituitary or hypothalamic disease.

Treatment of hypothyroidism is also relatively straightforward, consisting of levothyroxine replacement; routine replacement with T_4-T_3 combination therapy is not currently recommended.[41] Treatment of benign thyroid disease, including hypothyroidism, is the topic of Chapters 7 and 8.

Hyperthyroidism

Overproduction of thyroid hormone results in symptoms that vary in their manifestation based on the severity of the thyrotoxicosis and the age of the patient. Common symptoms include nervousness, increased sweating and heat intolerance, palpitations, fatigue, weight loss, dyspnea, and weakness. Young patients often tolerate significant thyrotoxicosis relatively well; the elderly frequently present with predominantly cardiovascular symptoms, depression, lethargy, and weakness, termed "apathetic hyperthyroidism." The diagnosis is made on the basis of a suppressed TSH and elevated free T_4 or T_3 level (**Fig. 3.3**); in subclinical hyperthyroidism only the TSH is abnormal, and this probably represents the mildest form of hyperthyroidism.

The most common cause of hyperthyroidism is Graves disease, an autoimmune disease resulting in production of TSH-receptor stimulating antibodies. Covered in Chapter 6, other causes include toxic nodules, toxic multinodular goiter and thyroiditic processes including subacute thyroiditis, postpartum thyroiditis, iodine and amiodarone-induced thyrotoxicosis, and, rarely, suppurative thyroiditis. Symptoms are similar among the different etiologies, except the specific symptoms related to the nonthyroidal manifestations of Graves disease (exophthalmos, inflammatory eye changes, dermopathy, and acropachy). The thyroid examination obviously varies by disease process and assists in the diagnosis. Often the diagnosis is made on the basis of the clinical presentation alone. In other cases, results of an iodine-123 thyroid scan, ultrasonography and measurement of thyroid stimulating immunoglobulins are required to ensure an accurate diagnosis.

Management of thyrotoxicosis is covered in Chapters 7 and 8. In all cases, patients exhibit significant symptomatic improvement from beta-blockade until definitive treatment tailored to the etiology of the thyrotoxicosis can be given.

References

1. Larsen PR, Davies TF, Schlumberger MJ, Hay ID. Thyroid physiology and diagnostic evaluation of patients with thyroid disorders. In: Larsen PR, Kronenberg HM, Melmed S, Polonsky KS, eds. Williams Textbook of Endocrinology. Philadelphia: WB Saunders, 2003:331–373

2. Dai G, Levy O, Carrasco N. Cloning and characterization of the thyroid iodide transporter. Nature 1996;379:458–460

3. Scott DA, Wang R, Kreman TM, Sheffield VC, Karniski LP. The Pendred syndrome gene encodes a chloride-iodide transport protein. Nat Genet 1999;21:440–443

4. Van Sande J, Massart C, Beauwens R, et al. Anion selectivity by the sodium iodide symporter. Endocrinology 2003;144:247–252

5. Hilditch TE, Horton PW, McCruden DC, Young RE, Alexander WD. Defects in intrathyroid binding of iodine and the perchlorate discharge test. Acta Endocrinol (Copenh) 1982;100:237–244

6. Silvestri E, Schiavo L, Lombardi A, Goglia F. Thyroid hormones as molecular determinants of thermogenesis. Acta Physiol Scand 2005;184:265–283

7. Goglia F. Biological effects of 3,5-diiodothyronine (T(2)). Biochemistry (Mosc) 2005;70:164–172

8. Mastorakos G, Pavlatou M. Exercise as a stress model and the interplay between the hypothalamus-pituitary-adrenal and the hypothalamus-pituitary-thyroid axes. Horm Metab Res 2005;37:577–584

9. Hollenberg AN. Regulation of thyrotropin secretion. In: Braverman LE, Utiger RD, eds. Werner & Ingbar's The Thyroid: A Fundamental and Clinical Text. Philadelphia: Lippincott Williams & Wilkins, 2005:197–213

10. Dohan O, De la Vieja A, Paroder V, et al. The sodium/iodide symporter (NIS): characterization, regulation, and medical significance. Endocr Rev 2003;24:48–77

11. Kopp P. Thyroid hormone synthesis. In: Braverman LE, Utiger RD, eds. Werner & Ingbar's The Thyroid: A Fundamental and Clinical Text. Philadelphia: Lippincott Williams & Wilkins, 2005:52–76

12. Beau I, Misrahi M, Gross B, et al. Basolateral localization and transcytosis of gonadotropin and thyrotropin receptors expressed in Madin-Darby canine kidney cells. J Biol Chem 1997;272:5241–5248

13. Nuovo JA, Wartofsky L. Adverse effects of iodide. In: Becker KL, ed. Principles and Practice of Endocrinology and Metabolism. Philadelphia: Lippincott Williams & Wilkins, 2001:360–366

14. Koong SS, Reynolds JC, Movius EG, et al. Lithium as a potential adjuvant to 131I therapy of metastatic, well differentiated thyroid carcinoma. J Clin Endocrinol Metab 1999;84:912–916

15. Bianco AC, Larsen PR. Intracellular pathways of iodothyronine metabolism. In: Braverman LE, Utiger RD, eds. Werner & Ingbar's The Thyroid: A Fundamental and Clinical Text. Philadelphia: Lippincott Williams & Wilkins, 2005:109–133

16. Beckett GJ, Arthur JR. Selenium and endocrine systems. J Endocrinol 2005;184:455–465

17. Stockigt JR. Free thyroid hormone measurement: a critical appraisal. Endocrinol Metab Clin North Am 2001;30:265–289

18. Davis PJ, Davis FB, Cody V. Membrane receptors mediating thyroid hormone action. Trends Endocrinol Metab 2005;16:429–435

19. Surks MI, Goswami G, Daniels GH. The thyrotropin reference range should remain unchanged. J Clin Endocrinol Metab 2005;90:5489–5496

20. Wartofsky L, Dickey RA. The evidence for a narrower thyrotropin reference range is compelling. J Clin Endocrinol Metab 2005;90:5483–5488

21. Hollowell JG, Staehling NW, Flanders WD, et al. Serum TSH, T(4), and thyroid antibodies in the United States population (1988 to 1994): National Health and Nutrition Examination Survey (NHANES III). J Clin Endocrinol Metab 2002;87:489–499

22. Huber G, Staub JJ, Meier C, et al. Prospective study of the spontaneous course of subclinical hypothyroidism: prognostic value of thyrotropin, thyroid reserve, and thyroid antibodies. J Clin Endocrinol Metab 2002;87:3221–3226

23. Stagnaro-Green A. Postpartum thyroiditis. Best Pract Res Clin Endocrinol Metab 2004;18:303–316

24. LeBeau SO, Mandel SJ. Thyroid disorders during pregnancy. Endocrinol Metab Clin North Am 2006;35:117–136 vii

25. Mariotti S, Barbesino G, Caturegli P, et al. Complex alteration of thyroid function in healthy centenarians. J Clin Endocrinol Metab 1993;77:1130–1134

26. Glinoer D, de Nayer P, Bourdoux P, et al. Regulation of maternal thyroid during pregnancy. J Clin Endocrinol Metab 1990;71:276–287

27. Stathatos N, Wartofsky L. The euthyroid sick syndrome: Is there a physiologic rationale for thyroid hormone treatment? J Endocrinol Invest 2003;26:1174–1179

28. Chinga-Alayo E, Villena J, Evans AT, Zimic M. Thyroid hormone levels improve the prediction of mortality among patients admitted to the intensive care unit. Intensive Care Med 2005;31:1356–1361

29. DeGroot LJ. "Non-thyroidal illness syndrome" is functional central hypothyroidism, and if severe, hormone replacement is appropriate in light of present knowledge. J Endocrinol Invest 2003;26:1163–1170

30. Andersson M, Takkouche B, Egli I, Allen HE, de Benoist B. Current global iodine status and progress over the last decade towards the elimination of iodine deficiency. Bull World Health Organ 2005;83:518–525

31. Trowbridge FL, Hand KE, Nichaman MZ. Findings relating to goiter and iodine in the Ten-State Nutrition Survey. Am J Clin Nutr 1975;28:712–716

32. Caldwell KL, Jones R, Hollowell JG. Urinary iodine concentration: United States National Health and Nutrition Examination Survey 2001–2002. Thyroid 2005;15:692–699

33. Lee SL, Roper J. Inadequate iodine supplementation in American multivitamins. Endocr Pract 2004;10(suppl 1):46

34. Berberoglu M. Drugs and thyroid interaction. Pediatr Endocrinol Rev 2003;1(suppl 2):251–256

35. Siraj ES, Gupta MK, Reddy SSK. Raloxifene causing malabsorption of levothyroxine. Arch Intern Med 2003;163:1367–1370

36. Vigersky RA, Filmore-Nassar A, Glass AR. Thyrotropin suppression by metformin. J Clin Endocrinol Metab 2006;91:225–227

37. de Groot JW, Zonnenberg BA, Plukker JT, van Der Graaf WT, Links TP. Imatinib induces hypothyroidism in patients receiving levothyroxine. Clin Pharmacol Ther 2005;78:433–438

38. Cooper JG, Harboe K, Frost SK, Skadberg O. Ciprofloxacin interacts with thyroid replacement therapy. BMJ 2005;330:1002

39. Centanni M, Gargano L, Canettieri G, et al. Thyroxine in goiter, Helicobacter pylori infection, and chronic gastritis. N Engl J Med 2006;354:1787–1795

40. Park SM, Chatterjee VK. Genetics of congenital hypothyroidism. J Med Genet 2005;42:379–389

41. Grozinsky-Glasberg S, Fraser A, Nahshoni E, Weizman A, Leibovici L. Thyroxine-triiodothyronine combination therapy versus thyroxine monotherapy for clinical hypothyroidism - Meta-analysis of randomized controlled trials. J Clin Endocrinol Metab 2006; In press

4 Physiology of the Parathyroid Glands

Carlos M. Isales

Of all the ions in the blood chemistry, calcium is one of the most tightly regulated, highlighting the critical role this ion plays in everything from intracellular signaling to muscular contraction. Thus even small deviations in calcium values outside the normal range usually signify some underlying pathology. Disorders involving hypercalcemia are more common than those involving hypocalcemia because of all the compensatory systems that respond to a drop in serum calcium. In an outpatient setting the most common cause of hypercalcemia is primary hyperparathyroidism. The diagnosis of early primary hyperparathyroidism increased dramatically with the advent of automated multiple sample blood chemistry analysis. It remains to be seen whether changes in the current way blood chemistries are ordered will negatively impact the advances in the early diagnosis of this disease. The corollary of the fact that early diagnosis is routinely made in patients with primary hyperparathyroidism is that rarely do we encounter patients as dramatic as Captain Charles Martell anymore.[1] Therefore, to be able to better diagnose and treat patients with diseases of the parathyroid gland who do not necessarily have significant clinical signs or symptoms, it is important to have a clear understanding of the factors involved in the regulation and secretion of parathyroid hormone.

History

The comparative anatomic description and naming of parathyroid glands is credited to Sandstroem in 1880[2,3] who examined the necks of humans and other mammals (dog, cat, rabbit, horse, and ox) for the glands he eventually named "glandulae parathyroidea."[4] As a medical student in the Department of Anatomy at the University of Uppsala, he examined the necks of human cadavers and identified the same organs he had observed in animals in 43 of 50 cadavers: "found on both sides of the inferior border of the thyroid an organ of the size of a small pea which judging from its exterior, did not appear to be a lymph gland, or an accessory thyroid gland and which upon histological examination showed a rather peculiar structure."[4] At that time, only two parathyroid glands were recognized to be present in humans. Interestingly, the description of parathyroid glands as distinct organs in animals had been made as far back as 1852 by Owen,[5] who identified "a small compact yellow glandular body attached to the thyroid" in the Indian rhinoceros.[2] A potential role of these organs was not clear until the French physiologist Eugene Gley demonstrated that tetany did not occur in experimental animals upon thyroidectomy if the parathyroid glands were excluded.[4] However, it was felt that the parathyroid gland's role was to remove toxins from the body (methyl guanidine) and that it was the accumulation of toxins that was precipitating the tetany.[6] It was not until almost 20 years later that MacCallum and Voegtlin[7] demonstrated that removal of the parathyroid glands was associated with hypocalcemia and that infusion of calcium prevented tetany.[6]

A connection between overproduction of parathyroid hormone and a specific disease was proposed in 1915 when the pathologist Friedrich Schlagenhaufer, based on two autopsies he was performing on patients with hyperparathyroidism, speculated that an enlarged parathyroid gland (adenoma) could result in parathyroid bone disease (osteitis fibrosa cystica).[4,6] Subsequently, in 1925 this hypothesis was put to the test when Dr. Felix Mandl successfully removed an enlarged parathyroid gland in a patient, with marked improvement in the accompanying bone disease.[6]

Around this time Fuller Albright and colleagues[8–12] at the Massachusetts General Hospital began careful metabolic studies to characterize calcium and phosphate turnover. A New England sea captain by the name of Charles Martell had developed severe parathyroid bone disease and was operated on by Dr. Edward Richardson, head of the Department of Surgery at the Massachusetts General Hospital. No abnormal parathyroid tissue was located in the neck despite repeated surgeries. Dr. Oliver Cope,[13] then a surgical resident, undertook a study of normal variations in the parathyroid glands. In 1932, Dr. Edward Churchill together with Dr. Cope, in Martell's seventh surgery, extended the incision to the chest with a sternotomy and successfully removed a parathyroid adenoma from the mediastinum.[13] Unfortunately, Martell went on to die from renal failure related to kidney stone disease from the many years of severe hyperparathyroidism.

During that time, work was also proceeding on the purification of parathyroid hormone (PTH; called "parathyrin" at that time). Hanson,[14] followed by James Collip,[15] were able to successfully make a purified extract of parathyroid hormone from bovine parathyroids. Collip, who had previously assisted in the preparation of an insulin extract with Drs. Banting and McLeod, demonstrated that administration of his extract successfully prevented the development of tetany in a patient.[16] Further characterization of the PTH molecule required more pure preparations, and this was eventually accomplished by Aurbach[17] and Rasmussen and Craig[18] in 1959.

Parathyroid Physiology

Evolutionarily, parathyroid glands are known to be present in amphibians and mammals but not fish. In view of calcium's multiple essential roles in the body, it has been hypothesized that as the organisms migrated from the ocean (with a high calcium content) to land, they required a mechanism for regulating this key ion and thus the appearance of parathyroid glands.[19] In humans, the parathyroid glands develop from the endoderm of the third and fourth pharyngeal pouches. A key transcription factor in the development of the parathyroid glands is Gcm-2.[20] This transcription factor appears to be exclusively expressed in the parathyroid glands, and in phylogenetic studies it has also been shown to be expressed in pharyngeal pouches in fish (from which the internal gill buds develop).[21] Thus Graham et al[22] speculate that the evolution of the parathyroid glands was a natural progression from the gills in fish to their present form and thus the reason for the glands' location in the neck.

Calcium Receptors

Calcium is the key regulator of PTH secretion. Until recently, it was not clear how this cation regulated PTH secretion. It is now know that there is a distinct calcium receptor that belongs to the G-protein–coupled seven transmembrane domain receptor family.[23] In addition to the chief cells in the parathyroid gland, the calcium receptor is expressed in multiple other tissues including the C cells in the thyroid, kidney, bone cells, cartilage, intestine, placenta,[24] brain, lung, and keratinocytes,[25] where it plays a key role in regulating calcium balance. Although this receptor has the highest affinity for calcium, it also binds other polyvalent cations, such as magnesium, and aromatic amino acids, such as l-phenylalanine and l-tryptophan.[26] In fact, the presence of the calcium receptor on antral G cells (which secrete gastrin), gastric parietal cells (which secrete acid), and renal cortical thick ascending limb cells (which regulate urinary calcium) may explain why ingestion of protein or amino acids results in increased gastrin, acid secretion, and urinary calcium excretion, respectively.[26] Further, discovery of a distinct calcium receptor served to clarify the pathophysiology of some inherited disorders of calcium handling, with both inactivating and activating mutations of the calcium receptor having been identified. Familial hypocalciuric hypercalcemia (FHH) is an inactivating mutation of the calcium receptor that results in elevation of serum calcium, low urinary calcium excretion, and high or high normal levels of parathyroid hormone. Autosomal dominant hypocalcemia with hypercalciuria (ADHH) results from an activating mutation of the calcium receptor.[27]

Binding of calcium to the calcium receptor results in suppression of PTH secretion. Stimulation of PTH secretion because of hypocalcemia follows a sigmoidal curve with large increases in PTH secretion occurring with only small drops in serum calcium. The parathyroid tissue expresses very high levels of the calcium receptor, and calcium binding results

in activation of phosphoinositide phospholipase C (PI-PLC) and activation of protein kinase C (PKC). In addition to this signal transduction pathway, calcium binding to its receptor also activates the phospholipase A_2 (PLA_2), phospholipase D (PLD), and mitogen-activated protein kinase (MAPK) pathways.[28,29] These calcium-receptor–regulated proliferative pathways have a major impact on parathyroid tissue proliferation. Under normal conditions there is very little proliferative activity in parathyroid tissue; however, hypocalcemia markedly stimulates parathyroid cell proliferation, as seen in patients with renal failure.[30] Calcium receptor binding in parathyroid tissue also activates the inhibitory G protein (G_i), inhibits adenylate cyclase, and lowers cyclic adenosine monophosphate (cAMP) levels.[31] Interestingly, these signal transduction pathways can also be modulated by other cations. It has long been known that hypomagnesemia inhibits PTH secretion. It has been demonstrated that this hypomagnesemic-induced inhibition of PTH secretion is secondary to an increased activation of the inositol pathway and greater inhibition of cAMP.[32]

Recently, several drugs have been developed that can either bind to and activate (calcimimetic) or inhibit (calcilytic) the calcium receptor.[33,34] Calcimimetics (such as cinacalcet), by binding to the calcium receptor, can alter PTH secretion, and have been used successfully to treat primary or secondary hyperparathyroidism and even parathyroid carcinoma.[35–37] Calcilytics, on the other hand, by interfering with calcium binding, increase PTH secretion and may be of benefit in conditions such as osteoporosis.[34]

Parathyroid Hormone Secretion

Parathyroid hormone secretion is primarily regulated by the calcium concentration via the calcium receptor as discussed above. The parathyroid gland is primed to secrete PTH tonically, and it is calcium binding that inhibits this PTH secretion. PTH is synthesized in the chief cells as a 115-amino-acid long peptide (pre-pro PTH), which is then cleaved in the endoplasmic reticulum to a peptide of 90 amino acids in length (pro-PTH), and finally six additional amino acid residues are cleaved in the Golgi to result in an 84-amino-acid peptide stored in secretory vesicles for immediate release. For more prolonged hypocalcemia (lasting greater than 1 hour), PTH degradation is markedly reduced. In addition, the form of PTH secreted can vary according to calcium levels.[38–40] For example, under normocalcemic conditions PTH is predominantly secreted from the parathyroid glands as the intact molecule (1–84) that is then processed in the liver and kidneys into several fragments thought to be biologically inert. Under hypercalcemic conditions the proportion of carboxy-terminal fragments (PTH7–84, PTH24–84, PTH28–84, PTH34–84, PTH37–84, and PTH43–84) secreted by the parathyroid gland increases and PTH 1–84 decreases. Ultimately, if hypocalcemia persists, there is proliferation and hyperplasia of the parathyroid tissue.

In addition to hypocalcemia, hyperphosphatemia also stimulates PTH secretion in vitro through a decrease in cytosolic PLA_2 activity.[41] Phosphate stimulates PTH gene expression by decreasing the degradation of the PTH transcript. It would also appear that $1,25(OH)_2D_3$ decreases PTH secretion and inhibits parathyroid gland hyperplasia.

Parathyroid Hormone Receptors

The classic actions of PTH on kidney and bone are mediated by the amino-terminal 1–34 residues of the molecule through a seven transmembrane domain G-protein–coupled receptor, PTH1R. This receptor couples to both adenylyl cyclase and PI-PLC.[42] Two previously identified PTH receptors, PTH2R and PTH3R, have turned out not to be true PTH receptors.

A second putative receptor for PTH was cloned from a rat cerebral cortex complementary DNA (cDNA) library.[43] The amino acid sequence shares 51% amino acid homology with PTH1R. This PTH2R is distributed less widely than PTH1R and is found predominantly in the brain and pancreas, with lesser expression in the placenta and testis. The PTH2R binds PTH1–34 preferentially over PTHrP1–36 and appears to activate the adenylate cyclase signal transduction pathway at relatively low concentrations of PTH (between 10^{-10} and 10^{-9} M [Molar]). This receptor does not respond to comparable doses of PTHrP, suggesting that it is a specific PTH receptor. However, PTH2R appears to have a higher affinity for the tuberoinfundibular peptide (TIP34) than for PTH.[44] Thus PTH2R may be a misnomer, because it would appear that this is not a true PTH receptor and may actually be a TIP receptor.

A third putative PTH receptor was identified in zebrafish and has homology to PTH1R.[45] However, there does not appear to be a human homologue, and it may have evolved through gene duplication. Thus, even though three putative PTH receptors have been identified (PTH1R to PTH3R), only PTH1R appears to be a true PTH receptor.

An additional putative carboxy-terminal PTH receptor, was characterized by Inomata et al.[46] Using radiolabeled C-terminal PTH fragments for binding and cross-linking studies, these investigators characterized two proteins of 90 and 40 kd in size in a rat osteosarcoma cell line (ROS 17/2.8). These putative receptors demonstrate a higher affinity for C-terminal fragments of PTH (PTH19–84, PTH39–84, PTH53–84) than for N-terminal fragments of PTH or for C-terminal fragments of PTHrP. Carboxy-terminal PTH fragments do not bind to the PTH1 receptor and do not elevate cellular cAMP levels.

Parathyroid Hormone Target Organs

Parathyroid hormone is a classic endocrine hormone in that it is secreted by the parathyroid glands and is transported in the bloodstream to act on distant target tissues, in particular bone and kidney.

Multiple studies have attempted to identify the bioactive portions of the PTH molecule. The full-length circulating form of the PTH peptide consists of 84 amino acids; however, the amino portion of the molecule 1–34 has been considered to have full biologic activity. The first three amino acids of the peptide are essential for activating adenylate cyclase. Amino acids 24 to 32 provide PTH with its amphiphilic α-helical conformation, which is important in PTH receptor binding (pth-1) and PKC activation.[47] Carboxy-terminal fragments distal to amino acids 1 to 34 (i.e., 35–84) were not considered to have any biologic activity even though this portion of the molecule is highly conserved. More recent studies have demonstrated, however, that carboxy-terminal PTH fragments do have specific cellular effects. There is at present no consensus concerning the importance of these effects in terms of either the cell biology or physiology of PTH action.

Parathyroid Hormone Actions on the Kidney

Parathyroid hormone has multiple actions in the kidney including decreasing phosphate and bicarbonate reabsorption in the proximal tubule, increasing calcium reabsorption in the distal tubule, and increasing the activity of the 1α-hydroxylase enzyme in the mitochondrial of the proximal tubule, which converts 25-hydroxyvitamin D to the more active 1,25-dihydroxyvitamin D, which in turn increases calcium absorption in the small intestine.[48] Because of these PTH actions in the kidney, the most common electrolyte abnormalities in primary hyperparathyroidism are hypercalcemia with hypophosphatemia and a hyperchloremic metabolic acidosis. About 50% of patients with primary hyperparathyroidism have a serum phosphorus less than 2.5 mg/dL, and 40% of patients have a chloride greater than 107 mEq/L.[49]

Parathyroid Hormone Actions on Bone

Parathyroid hormone has complex effects on the bone. PTH receptors are present on the bone-forming cells, osteoblasts, and in the osteoblast precursors, mesenchymal stem cells. In patients with longstanding hyperparathyroidism, there is an increase in the number of cells that break down bone, osteoclasts, but this appears to be an indirect effect mediated by release of soluble factors from the osteoblast stimulated by PTH. Osteoclast number and activity is regulated by the balance between factors that stimulate osteoclastic maturation (such as the receptor for activated nuclear factor κB [NF-κB] ligand [RANKL]) and those factors that inhibit osteoclastic development (such as osteoprotegrin [OPG], which is a soluble decoy receptor for RANKL). Both of these factors are produced by osteoblasts, and PTH favors the production of RANKL over OPG, thus increasing the number and activity of osteoclasts.[48] On the other hand, PTH increases the number of osteoblasts by decreasing osteoblast apoptosis[50,51] and increases the production of growth factors by osteoblasts like insulin-like growth factor I (IGF-I).[52,53] The anabolic effect of

PTH predominates, which is evidenced by the fact that PTH is currently used for the treatment of osteoporosis. The key difference seems to be that in primary hyperparathyroidism PTH levels are elevated in a sustained manner, whereas PTH when used for treatment of osteoporosis is administered in an intermittent fashion.

Parathyroid Hormone Actions on Nonclassic Target Organs

For many years, the exclusive target cells for PTH action were thought to be those in several segments of the proximal and distal renal tubules, and certain bone cells.[54,55] However, later work led to the discovery that there are effects of PTH on a variety of other cells, including cardiac myocytes, adrenal glomerulosa cells,[56] vascular endothelial cells,[57] and vascular smooth muscle cells.[56,58,59] It was initially thought that PTH might be a vasoconstrictor, because there is a higher incidence of essential hypertension in patients with primary hyperparathyroidism and because parathyroidectomy in spontaneously hypertensive rats (SHRs) prevents the development of hypertension. However, investigators found that if PTH was infused in vivo, it caused smooth muscle relaxation,[60] and if PTH was infused into animals or humans, there was an initial rapid (though transient) fall in blood pressure. The initial hypotensive effect is seen with amino terminal PTH fragments 1–34; it is most effective when the muscle is precontracted, and is predominantly a cAMP and not a nitric oxide (cyclic guanosine monophosphate [cGMP]) mediated relaxation. PTH has also been reported to block L-type calcium channel current in a neural cell line, suggesting an alternate possible mechanism for its ability to induce smooth muscle relaxation.[61] PTH receptors have also been shown to be present in vascular endothelial cells,[57] and PTH can modulate secretion of the potent vasoconstrictor endothelin-1. Thus some of the discrepancies in the observations of PTH effects on muscle and vasculature may relate to differences in direct PTH effects on smooth muscle versus indirect effects through endothelial cells.

The closely related peptide PTHrP also appears to be a potent vasorelaxant.[62] It is possible that the action of PTH on smooth muscle relaxation is mediated through a parathyroid hormone related peptide (PTHrP) receptor. PTHrP message and protein are known to be present in vascular smooth muscle and endothelial cells. Therefore, it has been proposed that PTHrP may be a vasodilatory paracrine factor secreted to regulate smooth muscle contraction.[63–66]

Parathyroid hormone has also been shown to potentiate angiotensin II stimulated aldosterone secretion in vitro and thus play a role in the higher incidence of high blood pressure seen in patients with primary hyperparathyroidism,[56] although high PTH concentrations were utilized in the published studies. It is possible that this PTH effect is seen only in vivo in situations of sustained elevations of PTH such as in primary hyperparathyroidism.

Conclusion

Calcium regulation is exquisitely regulated in vivo, with small changes in serum calcium leading to large changes in PTH secretion and additional changes in calcium handling by the kidney and intestine. Because of the evolutionary transition from a calcium-rich ocean environment to a calcium poor land environment, the human body contains multiple homeostatic mechanisms to protect against hypocalcemia, and thus this is a relatively rare occurrence. Hypercalcemic disorders, on the other hand, are common, and may range from benign to malignant processes involving the parathyroid glands. The present availability of agents that modify calcium binding to its receptor in the parathyroid gland (calcilytic or calcimimetic agents), parathyroid gland growth and proliferation (vitamin D analogues), or parathyroid hormone processing makes it essential that the clinician have a clear understanding of the normal physiologic regulation of PTH secretion to make more rational therapeutic decisions.

Acknowledgment

Dr. Isales's work is supported in part by funding from the National Institutes of Health (NIDDK 68020).

References

1. Spence HM. The life and death of Captain Charles Martell and kidney stone disease. J Urol 1984;132:1204–1207

2. Medvei VC. A History of Endocrinology. Hingham, MA: MTP Press, 1982

3. Sandstroem IV. Om en ny kortel hos menniskan och atskilliga Daggdjur. Upsala Lakaref. 1880;15:441–471

4. Modarai B, Sawyer A, Ellis H. The glands of Owen. J R Soc Med 2004;97:494–495

5. Owen R. On the anatomy of the Indian rhinoceros. (Rh. Unicornis L.). Trans Zool Soc 1852;4:31–58

6. Eknoyan G. A history of the parathyroid glands. Am J Kidney Dis 1995;26:801–807

7. MacCallum WG, Voegtlin C. On the relation of the parathyroid to calcium metabolism and the nature of tetany. Bull Johns Hopkins Hosp 1908;19:91–92

8. Albright F, Bauer W, Aub JC. Studies of calcium and phosphorus metabolism: VIII. The influence of the thyroid gland and the parathyroid hormone upon the total acid-base metabolism. J Clin Invest 1931;10:187–219

9. Albright F, Bauer W, Claflin D, Cockrill JR. Studies in parathyroid physiology: III. The effect of phosphate ingestion in clinical hyperparathyroidism. J Clin Invest 1932;11:411–435

10. Albright F, Bauer W, Cockrill JR, Ellsworth R. Studies on the physiology of the parathyroid glands: II. The relation of the serum calcium to the serum phosphorus at different levels of parathyroid activity. J Clin Invest 1931;9:659–677

11. Albright F, Bauer W, Ropes M, Aub JC. Studies of calcium and phosphorus metabolism: IV. The effect of the parathyroid hormone. J Clin Invest 1929;7:139–181

12. Albright F, Ellsworth R. Studies on the physiology of the parathyroid glands: I. Calcium and phosphorus studies on a case of idiopathic hypoparathyroidism. J Clin Invest 1929;7:183–201

13. Cope O. The study of hyperparathyroidism at the Massachusetts General Hospital. N Engl J Med 1966;274:1174–1182

14. Hanson AM. An elementary chemical study of the parathyroid gland in cattle. Mil Surgeon 1923;52:280–284

15. Collip JB. The extraction of parathyroid hormone which will prevent or control parathyroid tetany and which regulates the level of blood calcium. J Biol Chem 1925;63:395–438

16. Collip JB, Leitch DB. A case of tetany treated with parathyrin. Can Med Assoc J 1925;15:59–60

17. Aurbach GD. Isolation of parathyroid hormone after extraction with phenol. J Biol Chem 1959;234:3179–3181

18. Rasmussen H, Craig LC. Purification of parathyroid hormone by use of countercurrent distribution. J Am Chem Soc 1959;81:5003

19. Greep RO. Parathyroid hormone. In: vonEuler US, Heller H, eds. Comparative Endocrinology. New York: Academic Press, 1963:325–370

20. Kim J, Jones BW, Zock C, et al. Isolation and characterization of mammalian homologs of the Drosophila gene glial cells missing. Proc Natl Acad Sci U S A 1998;95:12364–12369

21. Okabe M, Graham A. The origin of the parathyroid gland. Proc Natl Acad Sci U S A 2004;101:17716–17719

22. Graham A, Okabe M, Quinlan R. The role of the endoderm in the development and evolution of the pharyngeal arches. J Anat 2005;207:479–487

23. Brown EM, Gamba G, Riccardi D, et al. Cloning and characterization of an extracellular Ca(2+)-sensing receptor from bovine parathyroid. Nature 1993;366:575–580

24. Brown EM. The extracellular Ca2+-sensing receptor: central mediator of systemic calcium homeostasis. Annu Rev Nutr 2000;20:507–533

25. Bikle DD, Ng D, Tu CL, Oda Y, Xie Z. Calcium- and vitamin D-regulated keratinocyte differentiation. Mol Cell Endocrinol 2001;177:161–171

26. Conigrave AD, Quinn SJ, Brown EM. L-amino acid sensing by the extracellular Ca2+-sensing receptor. Proc Natl Acad Sci U S A 2000;97:4814–4819

27. Thakker RV. Diseases associated with the extracellular calcium-sensing receptor. Cell Calcium 2004;35:275–282

28. Kifor O, MacLeod RJ, Diaz R, et al. Regulation of MAP kinase by calcium-sensing receptor in bovine parathyroid and CaR-transfected HEK293 cells. Am J Physiol Renal Physiol 2001;280:F291–F302

29. McGehee DS, Aldersberg M, Liu KP, Hsuing S, Heath MJ, Tamir H. Mechanism of extracellular Ca2+ receptor-stimulated hormone release from sheep thyroid parafollicular cells. J Physiol 1997;502(pt 1):31–44

30. Canadillas S, Canalejo A, Santamaria R, et al. Calcium-sensing receptor expression and parathyroid hormone secretion in hyperplastic parathyroid glands from humans. J Am Soc Nephrol 2005;16:2190–2197

31. Makita N, Sato J, Manaka K, et al. An acquired hypocalciuric hypercalcemia autoantibody induces allosteric transition among active human Ca-sensing receptor conformations. Proc Natl Acad Sci U S A 2007;104:5443–5448

32. Quitterer U, Hoffmann M, Freichel M, Lohse MJ. Paradoxical block of parathormone secretion is mediated by increased activity of G alpha subunits. J Biol Chem 2001;276:6763–6769

33. Hebert SC. Therapeutic use of calcimimetics. Annu Rev Med 2006;57:349–364

34. Steddon SJ, Cunningham J. Calcimimetics and calcilytics–fooling the calcium receptor. Lancet 2005;365:2237–2239

35. Block GA, Martin KJ, de Francisco AL, et al. Cinacalcet for secondary hyperparathyroidism in patients receiving hemodialysis. N Engl J Med 2004;350:1516–1525

36. Brown EM. Clinical lessons from the calcium-sensing receptor. Nat Clin Pract Endocrinol Metab 2007;3:122–133

37. Dong BJ. Cinacalcet: an oral calcimimetic agent for the management of hyperparathyroidism. Clin Ther 2005;27:1725–1751

38. Akerstrom G, Hellman P, Hessman O, Segersten U, Westin G. Parathyroid glands in calcium regulation and human disease. Ann N Y Acad Sci 2005;1040:53–58

39. Silver J, Levi R. Regulation of PTH synthesis and secretion relevant to the management of secondary hyperparathyroidism in chronic kidney disease. Kidney Int Suppl 2005;95:S8–S12

40. Silver J, Levi R. Cellular and molecular mechanisms of secondary hyperparathyroidism. Clin Nephrol 2005;63:119–126

41. Almaden Y, Canalejo A, Ballesteros E, Anon G, Rodriguez M. Effect of high extracellular phosphate concentration on arachidonic acid production by parathyroid tissue in vitro. J Am Soc Nephrol 2000;11:1712–1718

42. Abou-Samra AB, Juppner H, Force T, et al. Expression cloning of a common receptor for parathyroid hormone and parathyroid hormone-related peptide from rat osteoblast-like cells: a single receptor stimulates intracellular accumulation of both cAMP and inositol trisphosphates and increases intracellular free calcium. Proc Natl Acad Sci U S A 1992;89:2732–2736

43. Usdin TB, Gruber C, Bonner TI. Identification and functional expression of a receptor selectively recognizing parathyroid hormone, the PTH2 receptor. J Biol Chem 1995;270:15455–15458

44. Usdin TB, Bonner TI, Hoare SR. The parathyroid hormone 2 (PTH2) receptor. Receptors Channels 2002;8:211–218

45. Gensure RC, Ponugoti B, Gunes Y, et al. Identification and characterization of two parathyroid hormone-like molecules in zebrafish. Endocrinology 2004;145:1634–1639

46. Inomata N, Akiyama M, Kubota N, Juppner H. Characterization of a novel parathyroid hormone (PTH) receptor with specificity for the carboxy-terminal region of PTH-(1–84). Endocrinology 1995;136:4732–4740

47. Neugebauer W, Gagnon L, Whitfield J, Willick GE. Structure and protein kinase C stimulating activities of lactam analogues of human parathyroid hormone fragment. Int J Pept Protein Res 1994;43:555–562

48. Brown EM, Juppner H. Parathyroid hormone: synthesis, secretion and action. In: Favus MJ, ed. Primer on the Metabolic Bone Diseases and Disorders of Mineral Metabolism. Washington, DC: ASBMR, 2006

49. Younes NA, Shafagoj Y, Khatib F, Ababneh M. Laboratory screening for hyperparathyroidism. Clin Chim Acta 2005;353:1–12

50. Bellido T, Ali AA, Plotkin LI, et al. Proteasomal degradation of Runx2 shortens parathyroid hormone-induced anti-apoptotic signaling in osteoblasts. A putative explanation for why intermittent administration is needed for bone anabolism. J Biol Chem 2003;278:50259–50272

51. Jilka RL, Weinstein RS, Bellido T, Roberson P, Parfitt AM, Manolagas SC. Increased bone formation by prevention of osteoblast apoptosis with parathyroid hormone. J Clin Invest 1999;104:439–446

52. Canalis E, McCarthy TL, Centrella M. Growth factors and cytokines in bone cell metabolism. Annu Rev Med 1991;42:17–24

53. Zhang M, Xuan S, Bouxsein ML, et al. Osteoblast-specific knockout of the insulin-like growth factor (IGF) receptor gene reveals an essential role of IGF signaling in bone matrix mineralization. J Biol Chem 2002;277:44005–44012

54. Chase LR, Aurbach G. The effect of parathyroid hormone on the renal excretion of adenosine 3'5'-adenylic acid. Proc Natl Acad Sci U S A 1967;58:518–525

55. Chase LR, Aurbach G. The effect of parathyroid hormone on the concentration of adenosine 3'5' monophosphate in skeletal tissue in vitro. J Biol Chem 1970;245:1520–1525

56. Isales CM, Barrett PQ, Brines M, Bollag W, Rasmussen H. Parathyroid hormone modulates angiotensin II-induced aldosterone secretion from the adrenal glomerulosa cell. Endocrinology 1991;129:489–495

57. Isales CM, Sumpio B, Bollag RJ, et al. Functional parathyroid hormone receptors are present in an umbilical vein endothelial cell line. Am J Physiol Endocrinol Metab 2000;279:E654–E662

58. Mok LL, Nickols GA, Thompson JC, Cooper CW. Parathyroid hormone as a smooth muscle relaxant. Endocr Rev 1989;10:420–436

59. Rampe D, Lacerda A, Dage R, Brown A. Parathyroid hormone: an endogenous modulator of cardiac calcium channels. Am J Physiol 1991;261:H1945–H50

60. Pang PK, Yang MC, Shew R, Tenner TE. The vasorelaxant action of parathyroid hormone fragments on isolated rat tail artery. Blood Vessels 1985;22:57–64

61. Pang PK, Wang R, Wu LY, Karpinski E, Shan J, Benishin CG. Control of calcium channels in neuroblastoma cells (N1E–115). Exp Gerontol 1990;25:247–253

62. Shan J, Pang PK, Lin HC, Yang MC. Cardiovascular effects of human parathyroid hormone and parathyroid hormone-related peptide. J Cardiovasc Pharmacol 1994;23:S38–S41

63. Hongo T, Kupfer J, Enomoto H, et al. Abundant expression of Parathyroid Hormone-related Protein in primary rat aortic smooth muscle cells accompanies serum-induced proliferation. J Clin Invest 1991;88:1841–1847

64. Okano K, Wu S, Huang X, et al. Parathyroid hormone (PTH)/PTH-related protein (PTHrP) receptor and its messenger ribonucleic acid in rat aortic vascular smooth muscle cells and UMR osteoblast-like cells: cell-specific regulation by angiotensin-II and PTHrP. Endocrinology 1994;135:1093–1099

65. Pirola CJ, Wang HM, Strgacich MI, et al. Mechanical stimuli induce vascular parathyroid hormone-related protein gene expression in vivo and in vitro. Endocrinology 1994;134:2230–2236

66. Rian E, Jemtland R, Olstad OK, et al. Parathyroid hormone-related protein is produced by cultured endothelial cells: a possible role in angiogenesis. Biochem Biophys Res Commun 1994;198:740–747

5 Imaging of the Thyroid Gland

Laurie A. Loevner, Karuna Shekdar, Susan Mandel, and Jill E. Langer

The thyroid gland plays a critical role in the regulation of many metabolic functions, including cardiac rate and output, lipid catabolism, skeletal growth, as well as heat production. As a result, patients with hypothyroidism or hyperthyroidism present with a spectrum of symptoms. The evaluation of such patients requires an understanding of the hormonal functions performed by the thyroid gland. In addition, thyroid nodules are a common clinical problem and are detected by physical examination in up to 7% of the United States population. Although the majority are benign, 5 to 7% represent thyroid carcinomas.

Imaging may be useful to assess the thyroid gland. Nuclear scintigraphy reveals functional information about the thyroid gland, whereas cross-sectional imaging including ultrasound (US), computed tomography (CT), and magnetic resonance imaging (MRI) provide important adjunctive anatomic information. In addition, cross-sectional imaging provides important information about related structures in the neck, including the presence or absence of cervical and mediastinal lymphadenopathy, or extension of thyroid disease into adjacent soft tissues including the mediastinum, trachea, and carotid sheath.

This chapter reviews the anatomy and physiology of the thyroid gland; discusses developmental, autoimmune, inflammatory, metabolic, and neoplastic diseases of the thyroid; and addresses the role of radiologic imaging to evaluate each of these thyroid abnormalities.

Anatomy and Endocrinology of the Thyroid Gland

The thyroid gland is shield-shaped in the majority of patients, and consists of right and left lobes adjoined by the isthmus, although occasionally the isthmus may be absent. The thyroid isthmus is anterior to the trachea (usually overlying the first through third tracheal rings). Infrequently, it may reside anterior to the cricoid cartilage. The thyroid is anterior to the prevertebral and paraspinal musculature, and deep to the sternothyroid and sternohyoid muscles. Usually, the thyroid gland terminates above the clavicles; however, substernal extension into the superior mediastinum may occur. An accessory lobe, the pyramidal lobe, may be present in 50 to 70% of people, and usually arises from the isthmus and extends superiorly along the course of the distal thyroglossal duct.[1] It may be attached to the hyoid bone. Uncommonly, the pyramidal lobe may arise from the medial aspect of the right or left thyroid lobe. A pyramidal lobe is most commonly recognized in patients with Graves disease because it is enlarged and readily identified on nuclear scintigraphy.

The visceral fascia, part of the middle layer of the deep cervical fascia, attaches the thyroid gland to the larynx and trachea. As a result, the gland or abnormalities related to it will move with the larynx during swallowing. The thyroid gland is encapsulated, and septa from the capsule extend into the substance of the gland.

The thyroid gland has a rich vascular supply including paired superior and inferior thyroidal arteries. The right and left superior thyroidal arteries are the first branches off the respective external carotid arteries, and they travel inferiorly to the thyroid gland. The thyrocervical trunks originate from the subclavian arteries, and each gives rise to an inferior thyroidal artery. The *thyroidea ima* is an inconstant artery, which, when present, arises directly from the aortic arch and helps supply the inferior thyroid gland. Superior and middle thyroidal veins drain into the internal jugular veins, and inferior veins drain into the innominate vein. The vagus nerve and the cervical sympathetic plexus innervate the thyroid gland. Sympathetic fibers descend from the sympathetic trunk, whereas parasympathetic fibers are along the course of the vagus nerve. This autonomic innervation is felt to strongly influence perfusion to the thyroid gland.

The thyroid gland contains multiple lobules, each composed of multiple follicles. Thyroglobulin is stored within colloid in these follicles, and the follicular cells secrete thyroid hormones. Parafollicular C cells are also dispersed throughout the stroma of the gland and secrete thyrocalcitonin.

The primary function of the thyroid gland is the synthesis of hormones that regulate numerous metabolic functions. Two hormones, triiodothyronine (T_3) and thyroxine (T_4), are synthesized within the thyroid gland. They are released from the thyroid in response to a feedback mechanism with the pituitary-hypothalamic axis.

The synthesis of hormones within the thyroid is a regulated, systematic process. The first step involves trapping of iodide from the circulating plasma via active transport into the thyroid gland, where it is concentrated within follicular cells, and oxidized by thyroid peroxidase into its chemically active form. Subsequently, organification, a process in which tyrosine residues on thyroglobulin molecules are iodinated to form monoiodotyrosine (MIT) and diiodotyrosine (DIT) occurs. The coupling of MIT and DIT forms triiodotyrosine, and the coupling of two molecules of DIT forms T_4. Next, T_3

Table 5.1 Common Medications that May Decrease Thyroid Iodide Uptake

Iodine-containing contrast agents

Oral cholecystographic agents

Thyroxine (Synthroid™, Levoxyl™)

Liothyronine (Cytomel™)

Antithyroid medications [propylthiouracil (PTU), methimazole]

Amiodarone

Iodide preparations

and T_4 are released from thyroglobulin and secreted into the circulation in free and bound forms.[2] Simultaneously, deiodination of free MIT and DIT occurs for iodide salvage and recycling within the thyroid gland. Aberrant organification usually results from enzymatic defects that interfere with the oxidation of iodide or the iodination of tyrosine. Rarely, there may be failure of iodide trapping.

In the circulation, carrier proteins transport thyroid hormones. Thyroxine-binding globulin carries approximately 70% of T_3 and T_4, thyroxine binding preglobulin carries approximately 5% of T_3 and 25% of T_4, and albumin carries the remaining hormones. The active form of T_3 and T_4 is the free unbound form, representing only 0.3% of T_3 and 0.03% of T_4. T_4 is synthesized entirely within the thyroid, whereas 80% of T_3 is synthesized by peripheral conversion of T_4 in the liver and muscle.

Several medications may temporarily interfere with the intrathyroidal transport or organification of iodide including iodinated contrast materials frequently used in CT studies (**Table 5.1**). As a result these medications will alter radioactive iodine uptake measurements and hence should be discontinued prior to nuclear scintigraphy.

Clinical Manifestations of Thyroid Disease

Thyrotoxicosis is a clinical syndrome that develops when circulating levels of T_4 and T_3 are increased (thyroid-stimulating hormone [TSH] is usually suppressed). Hyperthyroidism is sustained thyroid hyperfunction with increased thyroid hormone synthesis and release. Thyrotoxicosis is manifested by a variety of symptoms including warmth and flushing, reflecting peripheral vasodilatation, increased heat loss, weight loss, myopathy, and increased appetite. Patients, especially children, may be hyperactive. Cardiac manifestations are more common in older patients and include tachycardia, palpitations, arrhythmias, and cardiomegaly.

Thyrotoxicosis associated with hyperthyroidism is most frequently seen with Graves disease, but may be seen with toxic multinodular goiter and rarely a hyperfunctioning TSH-secreting pituitary adenoma or a thyroid neoplasm.

Toxic multinodular goiter associated with hyperthyroidism (Plummer disease), commonly develops after 50 years of age and is related to a hyperfunctioning thyroid nodule.[3] Thyrotoxicosis not associated with hyperthyroidism (low radioactive iodine uptake) may be related to inflammatory thyroid disease or ectopic thyroid tissue (struma ovarii), or it may be factitious (exogenous hormone use) (**Table 5.2**).

Thyroid ophthalmopathy, more common in women, is characterized by enlargement of the bellies of the extraocular muscles with sparing of the tendinous insertions, and is most commonly seen in Graves disease. The most common patterns of extraocular involvement are enlargement of all of the muscles, or of the inferior or inferior and medial muscle complexes with relative sparing of the lateral rectus muscles (**Fig. 5.1**).[4] Isolated involvement of the lateral rectus muscle is unusual and when present should raise suspicion for a different disease process such as myositis or pseudotumor. Clinical signs and symptoms of thyroid ophthalmopathy include proptosis due to increased orbital fat and an increase in the volume of the extraocular muscles related to edema and lymphocytic infiltrates, lid retraction that may result in corneal exposure, and decreased eye motion. Exophthalmos may be unilateral or bilateral.[4] An intraorbital mass must be excluded in patients with unilateral proptosis. Extraocular muscle enlargement may cause compression of the optic nerve at the orbital apex, resulting in visual loss (**Fig. 5.1**) that may require surgical decompression if refractory to medical therapy. Late in disease, contractures, fatty infiltration, and fibrosis of the extraocular muscles may lead to abnormal eye movements.

Hypothyroidism refers to decreased thyroid hormone synthesis (serum TSH is usually high whereas T_3 and T_4 levels are low). Primary hypothyroidism may be secondary to structural or functional abnormalities of the thyroid gland, and in adults most often results from processes that destroy thyroid tissue such as autoimmune disease or iodine-131 (I-131) treatment. In children it may be related to enzyme deficiencies, defects in organification, or congenital anomalies such as a lingual thyroid or thyroid agenesis.[5] Central hypothyroidism results from decreased thyroid stimulation by TSH related to pituitary disease (secondary hypothyroidism)

Table 5.2 Evaluation of the Hyperthyroid Patient

TFTs elevated	RAIU (normal)	RAIU (low)	RAIU (high)
Graves disease	Plummer disease	Thyroiditis	Graves disease
	de Quervain	Plummer disease	
		Subacute lymphocytic	
		Struma ovarii	
		Factitious	

RAIU, 24-hour radioactive iodine uptake (normal, 10 to 30%); TFTs, thyroid function tests.

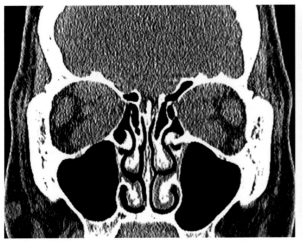
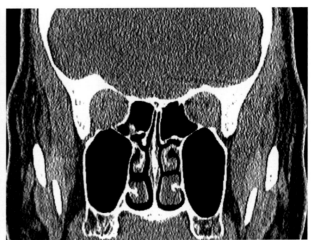

Fig. 5.1 Thyroid ophthalmopathy. **(A)** Coronal computed tomography (CT) image shows diffuse, bilateral enlargement of the extraocular muscles, most prominently the medial and inferior muscle complexes.

(B) Coronal CT image posterior to **A** shows compression of the optic nerves secondary to extraocular muscle enlargement.

or hypothalamic thyrotropin-releasing hormone deficiency (tertiary hypothyroidism). Here, serum TSH levels are inappropriately normal in the presence of low serum T_3 and T_4 concentrations. Unless readily identified and managed, hypothyroidism occurring in the prenatal period or during infancy results in cretinism. Hypothyroidism occurring in older children and adults (myxedema) has variable clinical manifestations ranging from fatigue to coma, and in part depending on the degree and duration of hypothyroidism.

Secondary manifestations of thyroid disease are frequently responsible for clinical presentation. Any condition that causes marked enlargement of the thyroid gland, most commonly multinodular goiter, but also neoplastic and inflammatory processes, may compress the adjacent esophagus and trachea causing dysphagia and respiratory distress (**Fig. 5.2**). Because the recurrent laryngeal nerve travels in the tracheoesophageal groove, thyroid lesions that extend to this area may present with vocal cord paralysis. Cervical lymphadenopathy in the presence of a thyroid mass, or direct extension of a thyroid lesion into the trachea or carotid sheath structures, is usually indicative of thyroid neoplasia.

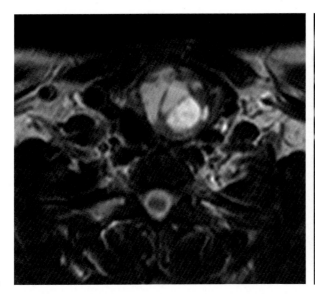
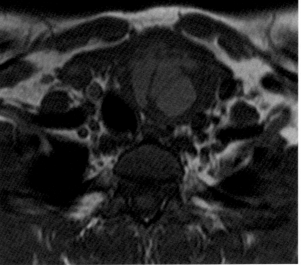

Fig. 5.2 Hyperplastic nodule within thyroid goiter in a patient who presented with wheezing. **(A)** Unenhanced axial T1-weighted magnetic resonance imaging (MRI) shows a complex mass of the inferior pole of the left lobe of the thyroid gland without intervening normal tissue that causes mass effect on the trachea, which is markedly displaced from left to right. **(B)** Corresponding T2-weighted MRI shows the complex mass pushing the trachea but without significant airway luminal narrowing.

Imaging of the Thyroid Gland

Nuclear Scintigraphy

Nuclear scintigraphy provides excellent functional information about the thyroid gland because the radionuclides used to image the gland do so by utilizing some step of hormone synthesis within the thyroid. The primary role of scintigraphy is in the evaluation of patients with abnormal thyroid function tests, particularly hyperthyroidism. Scintigraphy is able to demonstrate if the cause of hyperthyroidism is a diffuse process such as Graves disease or an autonomously functioning nodule. Scintigraphy of a focal thyroid mass in euthyroid patients may be used to determine whether a lesion is functioning (extremely low incidence of malignancy) or nonfunctioning "cold," a feature carrying a reported risk of malignancy ranging from 8 to 25%.[6–8]

Morphologic detail of the thyroid gland is obtained using technetium-99m (Tc-99m) pertechnetate, or preferably iodine 123 (I-123). Technetium-99m is trapped by the thyroid, allowing an estimate of thyroid activity as early as 5 minutes following its administration, whereas I-123 is also organified, providing a "true" assessment of diffuse or focal regions of uptake.[9] Routes of administration and doses of these radionuclides are listed in **Table 5.3**. Imaging is performed approximately 20 minutes following administration of Tc-99m pertechnetate, 4 to 24 hours after oral ingestion of I-123, and 24 to 72 hours following administration of I-131. The normal thyroid gland shows homogeneous radionuclide uptake and distribution. The isthmus may demonstrate slightly less activity than the thyroid lobes.

Table 5.3 Radionuclides Used in Imaging the Thyroid Gland

Radionuclide	Administration	Dose	Half-Life
Tc-99m	Intravenous	2–10 mCi	6.02 hours
I-123	Oral	200–400 μCi	13.6 hours
I-131 (diagnostic)	Oral	30–100 μCi	8.05 days
I-131 (whole body)*	Oral	2–5 mCi	
I-123 (whole body)*	Oral	1–2.5 mCi	
I-131 (treatment)**	Oral	100 mCi	
I-131 (treatment)***	Oral	100–200 mCi	

*Diagnostic whole-body scan following thyroidectomy to evaluate for residual thyroid tissue in the thyroid bed or to detect distant metastases; to detect ectopic thyroid tissue such as struma ovarii; in hyperthyroid patients with no demonstrable iodine uptake in the thyroid.

**Cancer treatment following thyroidectomy with the goal being to ablate residual thyroid tissue (may require hospital admission depending on dose).

***Cancer treatment with the goal being to ablate thyroid metastases (may require hospital admission depending on dose).

Iodine 123 is used for obtaining the 24-hour thyroid iodine uptake. Thyroid uptake reflects the percentage of the dose given to the patient that is accumulated within the gland, corrected for radioactive decay. Normal 24-hour uptake ranges from 10 to 30%. Several medications, iodine-containing topical solutions, and intravenous iodinated contrast agents used for imaging may temporarily interfere with the organification of iodide, altering radioactive iodine uptake measurements for as long as 6 weeks (**Table 5.1**).[10–13] The uptake of radioactive iodine may be reduced by as much as one half at 1 week following injection of iodinated agents for CT examination.[10–12] Furthermore, in over one third of patients with underlying thyroid disease, temporary changes in thyroid function may occur following injection of iodinated contrast material.[10] Therefore, if cross-sectional imaging is felt to be necessary in a patient who will also be studied with nuclear scans using iodinated radionuclides, MRI should be obtained. If the patient has a contraindication for MRI, then CT should be performed without intravenous contrast administration, and if contrast is desired, then CT should be performed following nuclear scintigraphy.

Iodine 131 is used in both the evaluation and treatment of patients with thyroid cancers that concentrate iodine. It is particularly useful in the follow-up of patients after thyroidectomy to evaluate for residual thyroid tissue in the operative bed as well as to assess for recurrent or distant metastatic disease (see Malignant Thyroid Neoplasms, later in chapter).

Increasingly, 18-fluorodeoxyglucose positron emission tomography ([18]FDG-PET) has played an important role in the follow-up of patients treated for thyroid cancer. It may be particularly useful in metastatic thyroid tumors that do not concentrate radioiodine.[14,15] It is increasingly used in the context of rising thyroglobulin levels in patients following thyroidectomy with clinically negative exams.[16] Whole-body scans are obtained to identify regions of FDG uptake. Potential pitfalls include indolent or well-differentiated thyroid tumors that take up FDG poorly, and FDG uptake that may not be related to metastatic thyroid cancer.

Ultrasonography

Sonography is the primary imaging modality for the evaluation of the thyroid disease. Compared with other imaging modalities including MRI,[17,18] sonography provides the highest resolution and therefore is best able to detect and characterize diffuse and focal thyroid abnormalities.

Real-time ultrasound (US) of the thyroid gland is usually performed with a high-resolution linear array transducer ranging from 7.5 to 12 MHz.[19] The patient is placed in the supine position and the neck is mildly hyperextended. The thyroid gland is imaged in its entirety both in transverse and longitudinal planes. The carotid arteries and jugular veins are posterior and lateral to the thyroid lobes, respectively, and provide excellent anatomic markers during the examination. The exam also includes assessment of the midline neck from

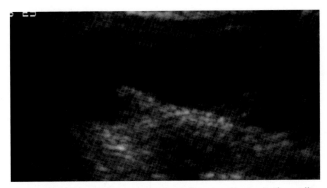

Fig. 5.3 Thyroglossal duct cyst. Sagittal ultrasound image in the midline of the neck above the hyoid bone shows a comma-shaped cystic lesion, typical of a thyroglossal duct cyst.

the sternal notch to above the hyoid bone to detect lesions such as thyroglossal duct cysts (**Fig. 5.3**). The sonographer should also image the lateral cervical lymph nodes, particularly in the setting of suspected malignancy.

The normal thyroid gland is uniformly hyperechoic relative to the strap muscles and homogeneous in background echotexture.[19,20] The surface of the thyroid is smooth and demarcated from the adjacent soft tissue structures by the overlying thin capsule. The superior and inferior thyroidal arteries and veins and their intrathyroidal branches are commonly seen by sonography.

Limitations of sonography include the high degree of operator dependency and the inability of sonography to detect retrotracheal and intrathoracic extension of an enlarged thyroid due to overlying air or bone. Ultrasound is also limited in detecting extension of thyroid malignancy into the adjacent trachea, esophagus, or other adjacent soft tissue structures of the head and neck.

Ultrasound may also be used successfully to guide fine-needle aspiration of nodular disease within the thyroid, or to guide aspiration of suspicious cervical lymph nodes in the setting of thyroid cancer (**Fig. 5.4**).[21–23]

Cross-Sectional Imaging

Computed tomography and MRI provide important adjunctive anatomic information in select clinical scenarios, especially in assessing advanced thyroid carcinomas at presentation as well as in the evaluation of recurrent thyroid cancer following thyroidectomy. These modalities may play a critical role in the detection of lymph node metastases, especially nodal metastases in areas poorly assessed by ultrasound (retropharynx and mediastinum), and are critical in evaluating the extension of thyroid disease to adjacent tissues in the neck. Specifically, invasion of the paraspinal musculature, esophagus, trachea/larynx, and jugular vein may be assessed[17] (**Fig. 5.5**). The anatomic information provided by CT and MRI can also be valuable in guiding the surgical approach.

The normal thyroid gland has a density of 80 to 100 Hounsfield units on CT due to its iodide content. The intravenous injection of iodinated contrast material usually

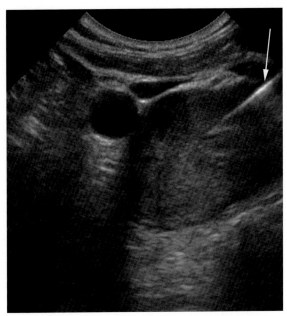

Fig. 5.4 Ultrasound-guided fine-needle aspiration (FNA). Transverse image of a dominant, solid thyroid nodule shows the needle (arrow) in the mass. Cytologic evaluation revealed a follicular neoplasm.

diffusely increases the density of the gland. Again, although iodinated contrast material may provide additional information about lesions within the gland, because the contrast contains iodine it will alter radioactive iodine uptake measurements for up to 6 weeks following the study. Therefore, in patients in whom nuclear scintigraphy is also going to be performed, contrast should not be administered. If both functional and enhanced cross-sectional anatomic studies are felt to be necessary, nuclear imaging can be performed prior to CT, or MRI with contrast material (gadolinium) may be used in conjunction with scintigraphy, as this contrast agent does not interfere with iodide uptake or organification by the thyroid.

Magnetic resonance imaging is performed with an anterior neck coil centered over the thyroid gland, which provides high-quality images with the best soft tissue resolution. Nodules as small as 4 mm may be detected.[18] Multiple pulse sequences should be obtained including unenhanced sagittal and axial T1-weighted (T1W) images, as well as axial fast spin echo T2-weighted (T2W) images with the application of fat saturation. Following the intravenous administration of gadolinium, axial T1W images with the application of fat saturation are acquired. Because lesions may be hyperintense (bright) and fat in the neck is hyperintense on T1W and T2W images, fat suppression is necessary to increase lesion conspicuity. On T1W images, the normal thyroid gland shows homogeneous signal intensity slightly greater than that of the musculature in the neck. On T2W images, the thyroid gland is hyperintense relative to the neck musculature. Following contrast administration, the normal gland enhances homogeneously.

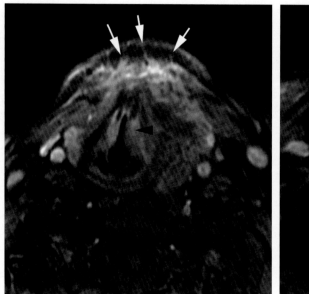 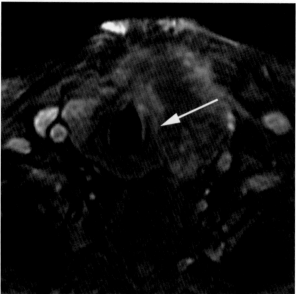

Fig. 5.5 Tall cell variant of papillary carcinoma invading the larynx. (**A**) Gadolinium-enhanced T1-weighted MRI shows a large mass of the left lobe and isthmus of the thyroid gland. Soft tissue stranding in the subcutaneous fat anterior to the gland (arrows) represents extracapsular spread of neoplasm. There is frank extension into the left hemilarynx (arrowhead) at the level of the vocal cord. (**B**) Enhanced T1-weighted MRI more inferiorly shows perichondral spread to the cricoid cartilage (arrow).

Developmental Anomalies of the Thyroid Gland

The thyroid gland develops in the first trimester of pregnancy, beginning at around the fifth week of gestation, and is completed by the tenth week of gestation. It develops from median and paired lateral anlages. The median anlage arises in the midline oropharynx at the fourth to fifth gestational week and gives rise to follicular thyroid tissue, which will ultimately secrete hormones.[24] The lateral anlages are believed to arise from the ultimobranchial bodies, which are derived from the fourth and fifth branchial pharyngeal pouches at around the fifth week of gestation. They give rise to the parafollicular C cells, which are thought to derive from the neural crest.[24] The parafollicular cells ultimately secrete calcitonin. By the tenth week in utero, the right and left lateral anlages fuse with the median anlage, resulting in the bilobed thyroid gland.[24,25]

During fetal development, the thyroid gland descends from its place of origin, the foramen cecum located at the base of the tongue, to its final adult destination in the lower neck. The thyroid is attached to the tongue base by the thyroglossal duct, which is lined by squamous epithelium. During the caudal descent of the gland, this duct elongates and subsequently degenerates.

Abnormal development or aberrant caudal descent of the thyroid gland results in a spectrum of anomalies. Arrest of descent can occur anywhere from the tongue down to the lower neck. Ectopic thyroid has rarely been reported in the submandibular and lateral neck regions,[26] and these ectopias may be misinterpreted as other disease processes. Failure of descent of the median thyroid anlage, or complete failure of descent of the thyroid, results in a lingual thyroid gland at the base of the tongue, the most common type of functioning ectopic thyroid tissue. In these cases, up to 75% of patients may have no functioning thyroid tissue in the neck.[27–29] If the tissue at the base of the tongue is not recognized as thyroid and is resected, the patient may become acutely and severely hypothyroid.[30] Nuclear imaging plays a major role in establishing the diagnosis of a lingual thyroid gland as well as in determining whether there is normal functioning thyroid tissue in the neck. On CT lingual thyroid is hyperdense due to its iodine content, and on MRI it is high in signal intensity on T1W and T2W imaging compared with the tongue musculature. Avid enhancement is seen following contrast administration.

Overdescent of the thyroid may result in ectopic thyroid in the lower neck or mediastinum. On rare occasion thyroid tissue may be found in remote locations, described within the heart as well as within ovarian teratomas (struma ovarii).[31,32] In the handful of reported cases of intracardiac thyroid tissue, all arose from the right ventricular aspect of the interventricular septum, and none was associated with abnormalities of thyroid function.[32] Intratracheal thyroid ectopia may occur, with aberrant thyroid tissue most often located at or just below the cricoid cartilage.[33] The majority of patients with this condition are female, and most present with acute or chronic respiratory distress. Intratracheal thyroid tissue may be connected to the thyroid gland by a bridge of tissue or a thin fibrous strand.[33] Any pathology that may

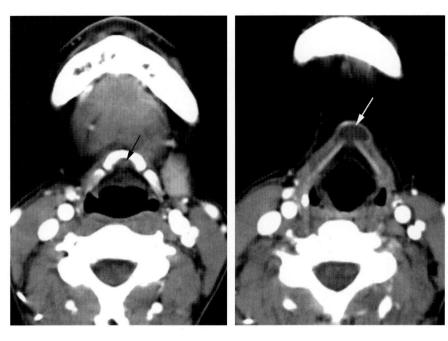

A, B

Fig. 5.6 Thyroglossal duct cyst at hyoid level. (**A**) Contrast-enhanced CT image at the level of the hyoid bone shows a small region of tissue just deep to the hyoid bone (*arrow*) typical of thyroglossal duct cysts at this level. (**B**) Enhanced CT image 3 mm inferior to **A** shows the characteristic midline cyst.

arise within normally located thyroid may also arise in ectopic tissue. Though extremely rare, carcinoma has been described in ectopic thyroid.[29,34] Scintigraphy using Tc-99m pertechnetate or I-123 should be performed when ectopic thyroid is suspected.[35]

Other developmental anomalies of the thyroid gland include agenesis or hemiagenesis of one lobe (most often the left lobe), with normal formation of the contralateral lobe and isthmus.[7,35,36]

Incomplete degeneration of the thyroglossal duct may result in a persistent fistulous tract, or in a thyroglossal duct cyst along the path of migration of the thyroid gland from the foramen cecum at the tongue base to the anterior lower neck. Thyroglossal duct cysts are anterior midline neck masses when they occur at or above the hyoid bone (**Fig. 5.6**), and tend to be paramedian in location especially when below the hyoid bone (**Fig. 5.7**). Over half of these cysts have normal thyroid follicular tissue in their walls.[37] Approximately 65% of thyroglossal duct cysts are infrahyoid in location and are encased by the thyroid strap muscles (**Fig. 5.7**). Approximately 20% of thyroglossal duct cysts are suprahyoid, occurring at the tongue base/floor of mouth, and are in the hyoid region above the strap muscles in 15% of cases.

On sonography, the classic thyroglossal duct cyst has well-defined margins and will appear as a simple anechoic lesion (**Fig. 5.3**) with thin walls. However, many thyroglossal duct cysts contain internal echoes due to debris and septations, and may have thick walls.[38,39] On cross-sectional imaging uncomplicated thyroglossal duct cysts are usually well demarcated. On CT scans they may be isodense to cerebrospinal fluid (CSF), or they may be hyperdense when there is a high protein content. On MRI, they typically have signal characteristics similar to CSF on T1W and T2W images. When the contents of the cyst are proteinaceous, cysts may be hyperintense on T1W images, and usually remain intermediate-to-hyperintense on T2W scans. Thick peripheral enhancement is unusual unless a cyst is secondarily infected or traumatized.

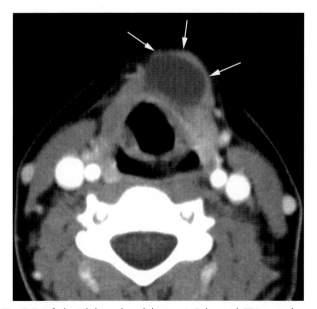

Fig. 5.7 Infrahyoid thyroglossal duct cyst. Enhanced CT image shows a left paramedian location of the cyst below the hyoid bone. Note that the cyst is completely enveloped by the strap muscles (arrows), radiologically characteristic of infrahyoid thyroglossal duct cysts.

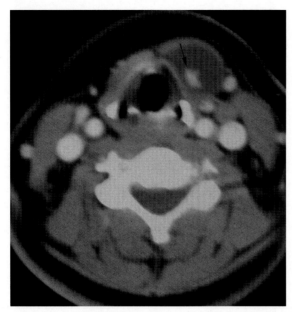

Fig. 5.8 Papillary carcinoma arising in a thyroglossal duct cyst. Enhanced CT image shows a typical infrahyoid thyroglossal duct cyst deep to the strap muscles. A solid nodule within the cyst (arrow) should always suggest the presence of papillary cancer as in this case.

When large, thyroglossal duct cysts are clinically detected as palpable midline neck masses. A pathognomonic sign is vertical motion of the mass with swallowing or tongue protrusion. Small thyroglossal duct cysts are usually clinically occult and may be recognized only if they become secondarily infected or traumatized, or if they are incidentally noted on imaging studies of the neck that are performed for unrelated reasons. Rarely, thyroglossal duct cysts may undergo malignant degeneration, usually into papillary carcinoma, and this should be suspected when a soft tissue component or nodule exists within or around the cyst (**Fig. 5.8**), or if the cyst has calcifications.[38]

Diseases of the Thyroid Gland

Autoimmune Disease and Thyroiditis

Thyroiditis, infiltration of the thyroid gland with inflammatory cells, may be seen in a diverse group of autoimmune, inflammatory, and infectious processes. Thyroiditis may be acute and self-limiting, or chronic and progressive. Several autoimmune disorders, such as Grave disease and Hashimoto thyroiditis, may affect the thyroid gland. Each differs in pathophysiology and clinical presentation. Graves disease and silent thyroiditis are usually associated with thyroid hyperfunction, whereas Hashimoto (chronic lymphocytic thyroiditis) is typically associated with hypofunction.

The diagnosis of thyroiditis is based on the clinical presentation and laboratory analysis of thyroid function. Imaging is not a critical component of the initial workup of these patients because the findings by themselves are usually not distinguishable from other thyroid pathology including goiter and neoplasia; however, imaging can be useful, especially in patient follow-up and monitoring of disease.

Graves Disease

Graves disease is the most common autoimmune disorder occurring in approximately 0.4% of the population in the United States.[2] The peak incidence is in the third to fourth decades of life with a female predominance. There is a familial predisposition. In Graves disease the thyrotropin receptor on the follicular cells is the target for thyroid autoantibodies that bind to these receptors, stimulating them as though TSH triggered the receptor. This results in constant autonomous function of the thyroid, resulting in hyperthyroidism. Serologic tests for specific autoimmune markers may be elevated, confirming the diagnosis. Marked enlargement of the thyroid gland without focal nodules, referred to as diffuse toxic goiter, results. There may be prominent enlargement of a pyramidal lobe (**Fig. 5.9**). Pathologically, in the thyroid gland there is diffuse hyperplasia of the follicular epithelial cells and depletion of colloid. Vascularity is increased. Graves disease is associated with other autoimmune diseases of the thyroid including Hashimoto thyroiditis.

Radionuclide scintigraphy may be useful in evaluating a patient with suspected Graves disease as well as in differentiating it from acute thyroiditis. In Graves disease, the thyroid gland is diffusely enlarged with intense radiotracer uptake often as high as 80% in 24 hours.

In contrast to Graves disease, where there is concordance between the clinical presentation of thyrotoxicosis and increased radionuclide uptake, in the acute phase of thyroiditis when the patient is clinically hyperthyroid the thyroid synthetic function may be so impaired that there is little observable radionuclide uptake, usually less than 10% (normal, 10–30%). The hyperthyroid phase of thyroiditis results from the leakage of stored thyroid hormone from the damaged thyroid gland into the bloodstream, not from increased hormone production. The radiotracer uptake usually returns to normal if the gland recovers and the patient reverts to a euthyroid state, and may even become transiently elevated if the patient enters the hypothyroid phase. Differentiation between Graves disease and subacute thyroiditis is important for appropriate patient management. Patients with Graves disease often require medication to treat the secondary manifestations of hyperthyroidism, radioiodine ablation of the thyroid gland, or surgery when required. Thyroiditis is treated conservatively, although beta-blockers may be useful to alleviate cardiac symptomatology.

In toxic multinodular goiter, there are areas of both increased and decreased uptake within an enlarged gland distinct from the homogeneous uptake seen in Graves disease. The overall uptake is not as avid as in Graves disease. In toxic adenoma, there is focal uptake in a single nodule. If the nodule is autonomous, there is suppression of the remaining normal glandular tissue.

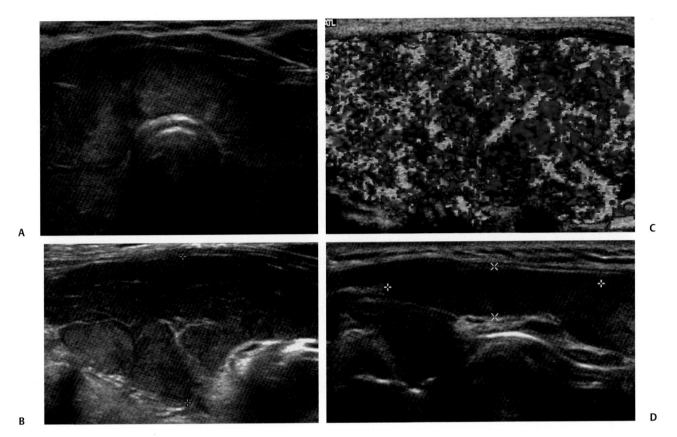

Fig. 5.9 Graves disease. (**A**) Transverse image shows that the thyroid gland is diffusely enlarged and slightly heterogeneous in echotexture. (**B**) Sagittal view shows an enlarged right lobe with exaggeration of the lobular contour. (**C**) Color Doppler sagittal images shows markedly increased vascularity of the entire lobe, a finding referred to as "thyroid inferno," characteristic of Graves disease. (**D**) A prominent pyramidal lobe is noted in the midline neck extending superiorly from the isthmus. Normally the pyramidal is very small and may not be seen by sonography.

On ultrasound, the gland is diffusely enlarged, with a smooth but lobular surface contour and may range from isoechoic to diffusely hypoechoic. The echotexture is homogeneous without discrete nodules, but patchy areas of altered echotexture may occur (**Fig. 5.9A,B**). There is a characteristic marked increase in thyroid vascularity observed on color Doppler exam called "the thyroid inferno" (**Fig. 5.9C**), the severity of which tends to parallel the patient's degree of hyperthyroidism.[40,41] On CT and MRI, findings in Graves disease are nonspecific. The enlarged thyroid demonstrates avid enhancement. The CT density is actually decreased, reflecting a decrease in iodine concentration even though there is an overall increase in iodine content in the gland. Even after treatment, density values may not return to normal.[42]

Hashimoto Thyroiditis

Hashimoto thyroiditis, also called chronic lymphocytic thyroiditis, is the prototype autoimmune thyroiditis. Pathologically, the thyroid gland is enlarged and has lymphocytic and plasma-cell infiltration, follicular cell atrophy, and interlobular fibrosis.[43] The normal follicular epithelial cells may be altered, being replaced with pink oxyphilic epithelium (Hürthle or Askanazy cells).[44] Hashimoto thyroiditis is usually associated with goiter, but in later stages the thyroid may become atrophic. The pathogenesis of Hashimoto thyroiditis involves both cellular and humoral mechanisms. Autoantibodies have been identified against thyroglobulin, thyroperoxidase, and TSH receptors. In reported cases, when TSH receptor blocking antibodies disappeared, normal thyroid function returned.[45] Chronic lymphocytic thyroiditis has also been reported to occur with increased frequency in patients with other autoimmune disorders including lupus, Graves disease, and pernicious anemia.

Hashimoto thyroiditis occurs predominantly in women, most commonly presenting in the fourth and fifth decades of life. It may also be the most common thyroiditis in children.[46] The clinical presentation is frequently that of asymptomatic hypothyroidism.[47] Antibody titers are usually elevated.

On scintigraphy, there is no typical pattern in Hashimoto thyroiditis. Uptake of radioiodine or Tc-99m pertechnetate is most commonly heterogeneous and patchy, and may be uniformly increased or mildly to severely decreased.[44,48] In children, a homogeneous distribution of tracer is more common.[46]

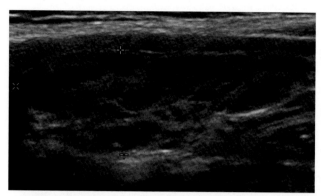

Fig. 5.10 Chronic lymphocytic thyroiditis. Sagittal view of the right lobe of the thyroid shows multiple small geographic hypoechoic patches throughout the thyroid, which pathologically correspond to regions of lymphocytic infiltration. The thyroid was slightly small in size; the patient was euthyroid.

Ultrasonography shows a spectrum of patterns in patients with chronic lymphocytic thyroiditis. The thyroid gland may be small, normal or enlarged in size depending on the duration and severity of the disease. In patients with mild or previously undetected chronic lymphocytic thyroiditis, the gland may be normal with multiple small irregular, hypoechoic areas with a surrounding echogenic rim (**Fig. 5.10**).[49] These "micronodules" pathologically correspond to focal areas of infiltration by lymphocytes and plasma cells. With more advanced lymphocytic infiltration, there is enlargement and architectural distortion of the gland, which becomes diffusely heterogeneous, but predominantly hypoechoic in appearance, approaching the echogenicity of the adjacent strap muscles (**Fig. 5.11**).[50–52] There may be numerous poorly defined hypoechoic regions separated by fibrous strands.[21] This appearance is often mistaken for a multin-

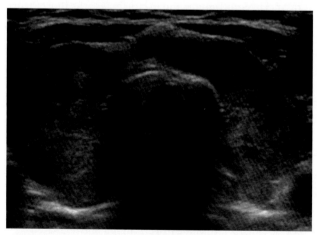

Fig. 5.11 Chronic lymphocytic thyroiditis. Transverse image of a hypothyroid patient with chronic lymphocytic thyroiditis shows diffuse enlargement of the gland with marked diffuse hypoechogenicity equal to that of the overlying strap muscles of the neck. In general, the degree of hypoechogenicity of the thyroid in patients with chronic lymphocytic thyroiditis correlates with the likelihood that the patient will be hypothyroid.

odular goiter both on sonography and physical examination. Although a diffuse process, chronic lymphocytic thyroiditis may also present as a focal palpable abnormality simulating nodular disease.[53] In end-stage disease, the thyroid gland may become severely atrophied and fibrotic, resulting in a heterogeneous or hypoechoic gland.

On CT, there is an inhomogeneous distribution of iodine. With MRI, T2W images may show areas of increased signal intensity. Linear, septated low-intensity bands thought to represent fibrosis have been described.[18] Following contrast there may be regions that enhance more than the remainder of the gland.

Ultrasound may be used to follow patients with Hashimoto thyroiditis to detect occult malignancy. Both benign and malignant nodules may occur in these patients, and although relatively rare, there is a known increased risk for non-Hodgkin lymphoma of the thyroid in this setting.[54–57] Thyroid lymphoma may produce solitary or multiple focal hypoechoic lesions or diffuse disease that may be difficult to distinguish from the underlying Hashimoto thyroiditis.[54,55] The presence of a large or infiltrating hypoechoic nodule, a nodule with microcalcifications, or the development of respiratory obstructive symptoms or cervical lymphadenopathy raises suspicion for a malignancy.[54,58]

Subacute Lymphocytic Thyroiditis

Silent painless thyroiditis and postpartum thyroiditis are two different types of subacute lymphocytic thyroiditis that are usually self-limited. When this inflammatory process occurs in the absence of pregnancy, it is termed painless thyroiditis. Antithyroid antibodies may be present and the disorders are thought to be autoimmune.

During the early phase of lymphocytic infiltration and follicular disruption with hormone release, patients usually present with thyrotoxicosis that progresses to transient hypothyroidism before returning to a euthyroid state.[59] Patients may or may not have glandular enlargement. Radioactive iodine uptake is low and the pattern on scintigraphy varies from no tracer uptake to diffuse or heterogeneous uptake.[36] Nuclear scans may return to normal in conjunction with resolution of the process.

Postpartum thyroiditis typically occurs 4 to 6 weeks following delivery. It occurs in up to 5% of postpartum women and may recur with subsequent pregnancy.[60] As with silent thyroiditis, women may present with goiter, thyrotoxicosis, and antithyroid antibodies. The process usually resolves after transient hypothyroidism; however, some patients progress to chronic lymphocytic thyroiditis.

De Quervain Thyroiditis (Subacute Granulomatous Thyroiditis)

De Quervain thyroiditis is a self-limited inflammatory process that usually occurs following a viral upper respiratory tract infection.[2,24] Among the viral infections that have been associated with subacute thyroiditis are Coxsackie and the mumps.[61] The peak incidence is in the second to fifth decades of life, occurring three times more frequently in women. Early in the inflammatory process, follicles may be replaced with neutrophils forming microabscesses. Later, macrophages and multinucleated giant cells surround the damaged follicles, stimulating a granulomatous process.[2] Viral inclusions have not been found in the inflamed gland. With healing, there is regeneration of the follicles. Clinical presentation may include painful enlargement of the thyroid gland, fever, and thyrotoxicosis with low radioactive iodine uptake. Scintigraphy shows a variable pattern that usually reverts to normal as the patient returns to a euthyroid state.[6]

Acute Suppurative Thyroiditis

Acute suppurative thyroiditis is uncommon and typically occurs due to seeding of the thyroid gland by bacterial and occasionally fungal organisms in immunocompromised or debilitated patients.[24] It may be associated with a branchial cleft abnormality. The role of imaging is to exclude a fistula (from the pyriform sinus) as an etiology of the thyroiditis.[62] On cross-sectional imaging, the affected portion of the gland (lobe or isthmus) is enlarged and heterogeneous. With disease progression, focal abscesses may develop and there may be obliteration of the adjacent soft tissues in the neck resulting from associated myositis and cellulitis.[63]

Riedel Thyroiditis

Riedel thyroiditis (struma) is a rare form of chronic thyroiditis characterized by a fibrosing reaction similar to that seen in retroperitoneal fibrosis, which destroys the thyroid and extends into the adjacent soft tissues of the neck. Within the fibrosing tissue are lymphocytic and plasma-call infiltrates and a vasculitis (phlebitis).[64] Stridor, dysphagia, and vocal cord paralysis from recurrent laryngeal nerve involvement may occur. The cause is unknown. It is more common in women and usually occurs in the fourth to seventh decades of life. On palpation, the thyroid is frequently firm, which may be confused with a malignancy.[65] One third of patients develop hypothyroidism. On ultrasound the thyroid may be hypoechoic, and on CT the involved thyroid may be hypodense compared with normal thyroid.[19,66] The characteristic MRI appearance includes decreased signal intensity on T1W and T2W images felt to correspond to fibrosis, as well as infiltration of adjacent soft tissues in the neck.[66] Riedel may be associated with mediastinal or retroperitoneal fibrosis as well as sclerosing cholangitis.

Thyroid Goiter

Goiter refers to any enlargement of the thyroid gland. Nodular goiter is characterized by excessive growth with structural or functional transformation of one or several areas within an otherwise normal thyroid gland. In the absence of autoimmune thyroid disease, thyroiditis, thyroid dysfunction, and thyroid malignancy, this condition is termed simple nodular goiter.[67] The pathogenesis of simple nodular goiter

appears to be related to environmental factors, most importantly iodine deficiency, as well as genetic factors. To compensate for inadequate thyroid hormone output, follicular epithelium undergoes compensatory hypertrophy to achieve a euthyroid state. Hypo- or hyperthyroidism may develop. Initially, the goitrous enlargement is diffuse; however, with time it usually becomes nodular. If the impediment to thyroid hormone output abates, the thyroid gland may revert to normal during the diffuse state.

Diffuse nontoxic goiter represents diffuse, nonnodular enlargement of the thyroid associated with a euthyroid state. There are two stages in its development. The first is hyperplasia (follicular cell growth) characterized by diffuse glandular enlargement and hyperemia. The second stage is colloid involution, which occurs when a euthyroid state is maintained. Endemic goiters are prevalent in iodine-deficient areas. In simple sporadic goiter, there is a female predominance and a peak incidence at puberty.[2] With time, most simple goiters progress to multinodular goiters that may remain nontoxic.

Multinodular goiter is characterized by nodularity, focal hemorrhage, focal calcifications, cyst formation, and scarring. Glandular enlargement may be asymmetric, involving one lobe more than the other, or involving the isthmus. Thyroid goiters may extend substernally and into the anterior mediastinum.

Multiple patterns may be identified with nuclear scintigraphy. Radioactive iodine or Tc-99m pertechnetate may accumulate in multiple foci throughout the gland, or less typically in only a few nodules. Some nodules may demonstrate autonomous function. In patients with thyrotoxicosis, therapeutic doses of I-131 may be required to reduce thyroid function. Although it was previously thought that a solitary cold nodule in a multinodular gland was less likely to be malignant than a solitary cold nodule in a normal gland, several studies that have used sonography or histology to determine the number of nodules have demonstrated similar rates of malignancy.[68–70] A dominant or enlarging mass within a goitrous thyroid raises concern for a malignancy and should be biopsied (**Fig. 5.12**).[71]

Sonography is often able to differentiate among the various causes of an enlarged thyroid gland. A multinodular goiter appears as an enlarged gland with multiple superimposed nodules, typically of varying sizes. These benign hyperplastic nodules most commonly contain complex cystic areas, representing pools of colloid, often mixed with areas of internal hemorrhage and necrosis (**Fig. 5.13**). Dystrophic calcification is also common in multinodular goiter and is typically multiple, large, and coarse. On CT multinodular goiter is asymmetric with multiple low-density areas reflecting regions of hemorrhage, cyst formation, or necrosis. Focal regions of hyperdensity are common, reflecting calcifications, hemorrhage, or colloid. On MRI, multinodular goiter may show a wide spectrum of appearances.[72] On T1W images, multiple foci of high signal intensity may represent cysts containing colloid or hemorrhage. On T2W images, diffuse heterogeneity may be present,[72] and nodules as small as 3 to 5 mm can

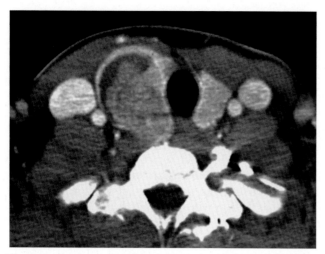

Fig. 5.12 Dominant thyroid nodule. Contrast-enhanced CT image shows a dominant 3.5-cm complex nodule of the right lobe of the thyroid gland. There is no radiologic feature of nodules isolated to the thyroid gland that can distinguish a benign from a malignant lesion. Ultrasound-guided FNA in this case revealed a benign hyperplastic nodule within a goitrous gland.

be visualized.[18] Alternatively, multiple large heterogeneous nodules may be present. Enhancement is usually inhomogeneous. Unlike CT, calcifications may be difficult to detect.

Computed tomography and MRI are the most valuable imaging modalities in assessing secondary manifestations of goiter including compression and displacement of the trachea, esophagus, and adjacent vessels (**Fig. 5.2**). Importantly, substernal and mediastinal extension are readily detected. When symptoms related to compression of the aerodigestive tract or vessels occur in elderly patients, nonsurgical candi-

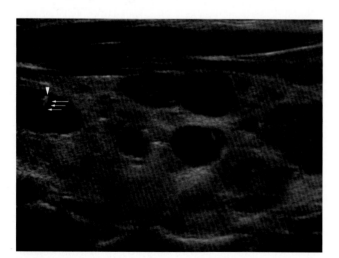

Fig. 5.13 Colloid nodules. Multiple cystic or predominantly cystic nodules are scattered throughout the thyroid. One of the nodules demonstrates a punctate focus of increased echogenicity (arrowhead) that causes reverberation artifact, appearing as multiple tightly clustered and diminishing echogenic lines (arrows) behind the nodule. Crystals in the colloid cause this sonographic artifact. In the absence of a solid component within the nodules, this artifact is a very reliable predictor of a benign colloid cyst.

dates, or those refusing surgery, therapy with I-131 may be effective in reducing thyroid volume.[73]

Evaluation of Thyroid Nodules

Nodules in the thyroid gland are common, with palpable nodules occurring in approximately 4 to 7% of the adult population in the United States.[75] Fine-needle aspiration (FNA) of all palpable nodules in euthyroid patients is the accepted standard of care for assessing the nodule for cancer. In the hands of experienced cytologists, FNA has a high accuracy rate.[76]

The likelihood that a nodule is cancer is influenced by a variety of risk factors. Malignancy is more common in patients under 20 or over 60 years of age. Findings on physical examination associated with an increased risk of malignancy include firmness of the nodule, rapid growth, fixation to adjacent structures, vocal cord paralysis, and enlarged cervical lymph nodes. A history of neck irradiation or a family history of thyroid cancer increases the risk that a thyroid nodule is malignant.[77–79]

On CT and MRI studies of the neck performed for other reasons, as many as 14.5% of patients may have detectable thyroid nodules.[69,77] Nodules are detected in up to 70% of adults undergoing sonography, increasing in frequency with advancing age, and in 50% of adults on pathologic review of the thyroid.[80–83] Over 50% of patients with a solitary nodule on physical exam have additional nodules demonstrated by sonography.[82] Most nodules are benign. The challenge lies in identifying those lesions that are malignant in the most cost-effective, noninvasive manner.

It was once thought that the number of thyroid nodules in a gland influenced the risk of malignancy. Newer studies of large groups of patients undergoing thyroid sonography and ultrasound-guided FNA have shown the overall incidence of cancer in patients with thyroid nodules to be approximately 9 to 13%, no matter how many nodules are present on sonography.[84–86] In patients with multiple nodules, the cancer rate per nodule decreases, but the decrease is approximately proportional to the number of nodules, so that the overall rate of cancer *per patient*, 10 to 13%, is the same as in patients with a solitary nodule. Although the thyroid cancers found in patients with multiple nodules are often in the dominant or largest nodule, in approximately one third of cases, the cancer is in a nondominant nodule.[87,88]

Many studies have assessed the ability of sonography to predict whether a thyroid nodule is benign or malignant.[84,85,89,90] Several sonographic features present within a nodule or cervical lymph nodes are associated with an increased risk of thyroid cancer including the presence of calcifications (**Fig. 5.14**), hypoechogenicity (**Fig. 5.15**), irregular margins, absence of a halo, purely solid, and nodular vascularity (**Figs. 5.15** and **5.16**). The feature with the highest sensitivity (70–75%) is solid composition; however, this feature has a fairly low positive predictive value (15–27% chance of being malignant). The feature with the

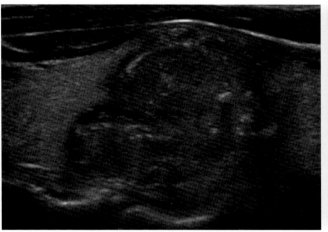 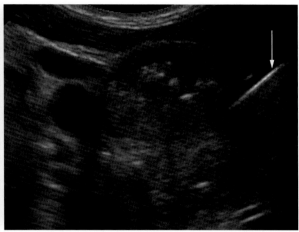

A   B

Fig. 5.14 Papillary carcinoma. (**A**) Sagittal image of this 54-year-old man with a palpable nodule demonstrates a 3-cm calcified nodule. The lesion contains some larger coarse calcifications, but also fine stippled microcalcifications seen as scattered foci of increased echogenicity. The presence of microcalcifications in a thyroid nodule carries very high specificity for papillary cancer. (**B**) Transverse view shows a 25-gauge needle (arrow) within the lesion during ultrasound-guided FNA procedure.

highest positive predictive value, ranging from 42 to 94%, is the presence of microcalcifications, defined as less than 1 mm nonshadowing echogenic foci. However, microcalcifications have a relatively low specificity, and are found in only 26 to 59% of cancers. Combining factors improves the positive predictive value of ultrasound. A predominantly solid nodule with microcalcifications has a 32% likelihood of being cancer, compared with a predominantly cystic nodule (>75% cystic) with no calcification that has a 1.0% likelihood of being cancer.[87] The presence of coarse calcification within a predominantly solid nodule also increases the risk of malignancy. Nodule size is not predictive of malignancy.[84,87,90] Although no sonographic feature has sufficient sensitivity, specificity, or positive predictive value to determine if a nodule is malignant, the sonographic features of nodules can aid in determining which nodules should undergo FNA.[87]

Patients noted to have one or more palpable nodules on physical exam usually undergo serum TSH determination. If the TSH is low, I-123 scintigraphy is helpful to determine if one or more of the nodules is autonomously "hot." If a nodule shows uniform, increased uptake compared with the remainder of the thyroid, there is an extremely low risk of malignancy. Approximately 5% of all palpable nodules are autonomous. Scintigraphy of a focal thyroid mass in euthyroid patients may be used to determine whether a lesion is functioning "hot" or nonfunctioning "cold." Cold nodules carry a reported risk of malignancy ranging from 8 to 25%.[6–8,70] However, the true risk of a hypofunctioning nodule being cancer is much less because smaller hypofunctioning nodules are often not detected by this technique.[91–93] In the case of complex solid and cystic nodules (**Figs. 5.17** and **5.18**), care must be taken to consider the functionality of only the solid component of the nodule, and not mistake the cystic component as a nonfunctioning nodule. However, because the vast majority of nodules are nonfunctioning, and the vast majority of them are benign, scintigraphy is not felt to play

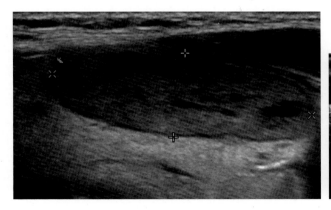 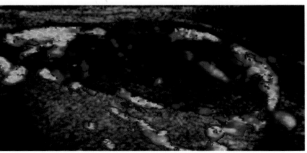

A   B

Fig. 5.15 Hypoechoic nodule. (**A**) Sagittal image of the right lobe of the thyroid gland shows a hypoechoic nodule. (**B**) The use of color Doppler is helpful in improving the diagnostic rate of FNA by allowing targeted biopsy of the solid flow-positive component, particularly in mixed cystic and solid nodules.

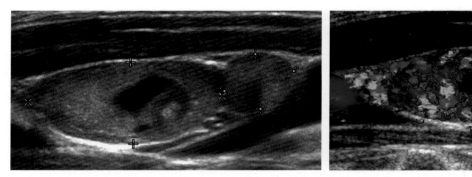

Fig. 5.16 Metastatic papillary cancer. (**A**) Sagittal image of the mid-right neck shows complex solid and cystic lymph nodes. (**B**) Corresponding color Doppler shows marked vascularity in the solid components that proved to be metastatic papillary carcinoma.

an important role in the initial evaluation of most patients with nodular thyroid disease.[79]

Fine-needle aspiration with US guidance that ensures the correct positioning of the needle within the lesion has gained wide acceptance as an accurate diagnostic method for evaluating thyroid nodules (**Figs. 5.4** and **5.14**).[20,94,95] In many cases, nodules that are palpable undergo biopsy without imaging guidance. Sonography is pursued for guidance if the patient has had a prior nondiagnostic biopsy, or if the nodule is known to be complex because sonography can guide FNA of the solid component and significantly decrease the likelihood of a nondiagnostic aspirate.[96–98] Even if the patient has had a diagnostic FNA by palpation, sonography of the gland may be indicated to search for nonpalpable coexistent nodules, which may influence management in up to 63% of patients.[82] Specimens may be obtained with 22- to 25-gauge needles. Typically, three separate passes are made to ensure the most adequate specimen possible. Interpretation requires a skilled cytopathologist. Benign nodules may be followed and malignant or suspicious nodules are usually surgically resected. In instances where FNA is nondiagnostic,

repeat aspiration in 6 to 8 weeks or surgical excision may be necessary.[95]

Neoplasms of the Thyroid Gland

Benign Adenomas

Thyroid adenomas are true benign neoplasms distinct from the adjacent thyroid tissue and encased by a fibrous capsule. They are usually solitary and nonfunctioning, commonly detected in young and middle-aged adults. Autonomously functioning adenomas smaller than 3 mm are not usually associated with hyperthyroidism.[99] Toxicity is usually seen with large lesions and advanced age. Follicular adenomas slowly increase in size, usually not exceeding 4 cm.[2] Sudden enlargement of a follicular adenoma is usually related to spontaneous hemorrhage within the lesion.[100] Spontaneous degeneration of an adenoma may occur. Most thyroid cysts represent degeneration of adenomas. The presence of carcinoma within an adenoma is exceedingly rare.[100]

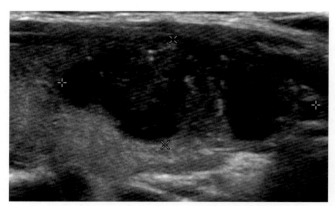

Fig. 5.17 Benign hyperplastic nodule. This nodule (outlined by electronic calipers) has both solid and cystic components. There are several punctate areas of increase echogenicity that have distal reverberation artifact. This finding is related to the presence of colloid within this nodule and allows differentiation of these echogenic foci from microcalcifications that cause shadowing.

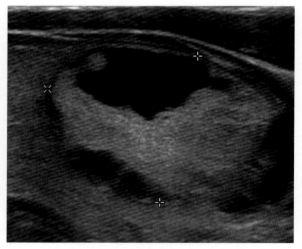

Fig. 5.18 Solid and cystic thyroid cancer. Sagittal ultrasound image shows a complex solid and cystic intrathyroidal tumor (outlined by electronic calipers).

If an adenoma is autonomous (independent of TSH), ablation with I-131 may be performed because the short-acting β-radiation will deposit preferentially in the nodule. Alternatively, the nodule may be surgically removed. In either case, the risk of postprocedural hypothyroidism is small. The previously suppressed normal thyroid tissue resumes normal function following treatment. Ethanol injection including with ultrasound guidance has been reported[76–82]; however, it has not gained wide acceptance. Ethanol injection should be considered only for sclerosis of benign cystic nodules. It is not an effective therapy to shrink benign solid nodules because it is painful, has a higher incidence of complications, and requires numerous sessions to achieve a response.[101–109]

Malignant Thyroid Neoplasms

The incidence of thyroid cancer in men and women increased up through 1975, which was thought to reflect the years in which low-dose radiation was used to treat conditions in the head and neck, particularly in children for benign diseases such as thymic enlargement and adenoidal hypertrophy.[110] There is a linear dose–response relationship between 100 and 2000 rad.[6,111] Approximately 15 to 30% of patients who received radiation in this dose range develop a thyroid nodule, and 6 to 8% develop papillary thyroid cancer. Long-term follow-up is necessary because the latent period for the development of cancer may be as long as 30 years. Thyroid carcinoma following high-dose irradiation (greater than 2000 rad) is rare, likely because radiation at these doses destroys thyroid tissue.[6] Approximately 20,000 to 30,000 new cases of thyroid carcinoma are diagnosed in the United States each year. The annual death rate is approximately 1500.[112] Of interest, the prevalence of incidental thyroid carcinomas identified at autopsy is up to 18%,[113,114] and at surgery is 10.5%.[115]

Differentiated thyroid carcinomas including papillary (60–80%) and follicular subtypes are most common and have a favorable prognosis.[6,116] Thyroid carcinomas arise from both follicular and parafollicular C cells. Malignant potential and behavior ranges from low grade (papillary carcinoma) to aggressive (anaplastic carcinoma), and is reflected by mortality rates: papillary carcinoma 8 to 11%, follicular carcinoma 24 to 33%, medullary carcinoma 50%, and anaplastic carcinoma 75 to 90%.[78] The prognosis is affected by gender, the tumor's biologic behavior, tumor size, and the tendency for hematogenous or lymphatic metastases.

The role of the radiologist in assessing patients with a known or suspected thyroid malignancy is to evaluate for findings related to local invasion, including invasion through the thyroid capsule and infiltration of adjacent tissues and structures in the neck, and to identify the presence of cervical and mediastinal lymph nodal metastases.

Papillary Carcinoma

Papillary carcinoma is a low-grade malignancy occurring most commonly in adolescent girls and young adults. It comprises up to 80% of thyroid cancers. Papillary carcinoma histologically may have a spectrum of findings and may be purely papillary, mixed papillary and follicular, or completely follicular.[117–119] The mixed papillary subtype behaves like papillary carcinoma.[117] The completely follicular variant is also included under papillary carcinomas because both biologically and clinically they behave like these tumors.[24,120] Frequently, papillary carcinoma is multifocal in the thyroid gland and is felt to represent intraglandular lymphatic spread rather than multiple synchronous tumors. However, other patterns of papillary cancer are also common including occult cancers (less than 1.5 cm), intrathyroidal encapsulated, and extrathyroidal.[121,122] At gross pathology, these tumors may have calcifications, hemorrhage, necrosis, or cysts. Histologically, papillary cancer is characterized by the presence of papillae (epithelial cells encasing a fibrovascular core), and clear nuclei.[118,119] Psammoma bodies (calcified remnants of papillae) are present in over one third of papillary cancers.

There are uncommon histologic subtypes of papillary cancer that have been noted to behave more aggressively, including tall-cell and columnar-cell variants.[123] The tall-cell variant is composed of oxyphilic (pink) cells.[123] At presentation these malignancies are frequently extrathyroidal, with vascular or laryngeal invasion and a poorer prognosis compared with other papillary carcinomas (**Fig. 5.5**).

The imaging appearance of papillary carcinoma is variable and may include a dominant nodule, multifocal nodules, or diffuse infiltration of the gland. The most common features of papillary cancer on sonography include a hypoechoic nodule with solid echotexture, microcalcifications, and intrinsic vascularity[124] (**Fig. 5.14A**).

Papillary carcinoma has the highest incidence of the thyroid malignancies for cervical lymph node metastases, seen in up to 50% of cases. Metastatic lymph nodes are frequently normal in size and may be calcified, vascular, cystic, or hemorrhagic, or they may contain colloid (**Fig. 5.16**).[125] Cystic nodes are different from the necrotic nodes frequently seen with metastatic squamous cell carcinoma that have central low density but retain a thick rind of residual lymphatic tissue. Thyroglobulin- and colloid-containing cancerous lymph nodes may be hyperintense relative to the neck muscles on unenhanced T1W MRI (**Fig. 5.19**), and may have hemorrhage-fluid levels (**Fig. 5.20**). The differing signal characteristics of complex fluid on T1W and T2W MRI is a reflection of viscosity, protein concentration, cross-linking of glycoproteins, and water content. Though the vast majority of nodal metastases from thyroid cancer occur in the lateral cervical lymph chains and less commonly in the upper mediastinum, occasionally (2%) metastases occur in retropharyngeal nodes (**Fig. 5.21**).

Hematogenous spread to the lungs, bones, and central nervous system may occur; however, this is less common (approximately 5%), especially in the absence of nodal disease. Because many papillary carcinomas concentrate radioiodine, scanning with I-131 following thyroidectomy may

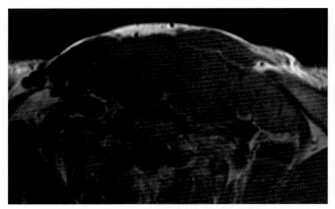

Fig. 5.19 Colloid/thyroglobulin-containing metastatic lymph nodes. Axial unenhanced T1-weighted MRI shows extensive left neck nodal disease that is hyperintense relative to cerebrospinal fluid (CSF) and muscle.

be valuable in identifying recurrent/residual thyroid disease in the operative bed of the neck as well as in detecting distant metastases. Treatment subsequently with I-131 may be performed (**Table 5.3**). The prognosis for papillary thyroid carcinoma is excellent, with a 20-year survival rate of over 90%.[118,119,121,122]

Follicular Carcinoma

True follicular carcinomas constitute 5% of all thyroid cancers. Follicular carcinomas are well-differentiated, relatively low-grade malignancies that are more common in the setting of iodine deficiency. They are slightly more aggressive than papillary carcinomas if vascular invasion is present. Pathologically, they are characterized by capsular and vascular invasion, and are usually solitary. Distant metastases to the

lung and bone related to hematogenous seeding are more common than lymph node spread; the latter is seen in less than 8 to 10% of cases.[126] The 5-year survival rate for encapsulated variants is approximately 90%; however, invasive tumors have a poorer prognosis. Though less often than papillary carcinomas, follicular cancers concentrate iodine, and I-131 imaging may be useful in the follow-up of these patients.

Hürthle-Cell Tumor

Hürthle cells are derived from follicular epithelium.[127] A Hürthle-cell neoplasm must meet specific criteria including that of an isolated thyroid mass, composed predominantly of Hürthle cells, and in the absence of inflammatory cells.[127,128] These tumors are diagnosed according to the criterion of malignancy used for follicular neoplasms of the thyroid gland. Regional nodal metastases in addition to hematogenous dissemination may occur.

Medullary Carcinoma

Medullary carcinoma is relatively uncommon and has a higher mortality rate than well-differentiated papillary and follicular malignancies. Sporadic medullary carcinomas are usually solitary lesions. They may invade adjacent tissues in the neck, spread to cervical lymph nodes,[129] and may have hematogenous seeding with distant metastases most commonly to the lungs, bones, and liver. Because of their origin from parafollicular C cells that secrete calcitonin (up to 90% of medullary carcinomas secrete calcitonin), calcitonin is an excellent hormonal marker for following these patients.[56,130]

Medullary carcinoma occurs sporadically, but may also be inherited as an autosomal dominant trait (approximately 15% of cases are familial) and comprises a component of

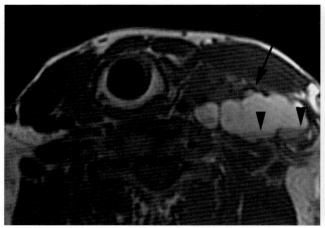
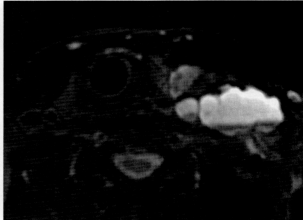

A
B

Fig. 5.20 Fluid-fluid level in complex cystic metastatic cervical lymph nodes. (**A**) Axial unenhanced T1-weighted MRI shows a complex left lateral neck nodal mass (arrow) with fluid-fluid level/meniscus (arrowheads). The nondependent fluid is hyperintense relative to CSF and muscle, and can reflect thyroglobulin (as it did in this case), colloid, or blood. (**B**) Corresponding T2W image shows the nondependent fluid remains hyperintense (bright), whereas the dependent fluid is relatively hypointense. Differing signal characteristics of complex fluid on T1- and T2-weighted MRI is a reflection of viscosity, protein concentration, cross-linking of glycoproteins, and water content.

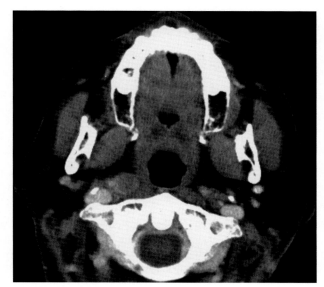

Fig. 5.21 Metastatic retropharyngeal lymph node in a 54-year-old patient with rising thyroglobulin following thyroidectomy. Clinical and ultrasound examination of the lateral necks were negative. Axial enhanced CT image shows a 1-cm pathologic right retropharyngeal lymph node. CT-guided transfacial biopsy showed papillary carcinoma.

the multiple endocrine neoplasia (MEN) syndromes, types IIA and IIB, which include medullary thyroid carcinoma and adrenal pheochromocytomas.[131,132] Hyperparathyroidism is common in MEN type IIA (Sipple syndrome) due to hyperplasia of the parathyroid glands.[131,132]

Medullary carcinomas may be encapsulated or infiltrative on gross pathology.[131,132] There is a broad spectrum of histologic and biochemical subtypes. The prognosis for medullary thyroid cancer is variable. Patients with thyroid cancer in the setting of MEN type IIB tend to have very aggressive, often fatal tumors that frequently occur at a young age, whereas those in association with MEN type IIA have more favorable outcomes.[133] Sporadic tumors may behave in an indolent manner or may be aggressive.[133] Serum levels of calcitonin and carcinoembryonic antigen, as well as immunostaining of resected tumor, may help in predicting tumor behavior.[134]

Medullary carcinoma does not concentrate radioiodine. However, radionuclides specific for neuroendocrine tissue, such as I-131 metaiodobenzylguanidine (MIBG) and the somatostatin analogue indium-111 pentetreotide have been used with some success to evaluate primary as well as metastatic medullary thyroid carcinoma.[135–138]

Anaplastic Carcinoma

Anaplastic carcinoma usually presents in older patients and is highly aggressive and rapidly fatal. Life expectancy is measured in months. It commonly occurs in patients with long-standing goiter. These cancers grow rapidly and typically compress and invade the aerodigestive tract and vessels. Lymph node metastases occur in the majority of patients and are necrotic in approximately 50% of cases.[56,139] These

neoplasms do not concentrate radioiodine. On US they are frequently hypoechoic.[19,20,129] On CT punctate calcifications and necrosis are frequently present.[139]

Rare Malignancies Affecting Thyroid Gland

Primary lymphoma of the thyroid gland is uncommon, and usually presents in elderly women with a long history of goiter. Patients with Hashimoto thyroiditis also have an increased incidence of developing thyroid lymphoma, which is usually non-Hodgkin in nature.[54,55] Imaging including MR cannot reliably distinguish lymphoma from thyroiditis in patients with Hashimoto.[1,140] Patients usually present with a rapidly enlarging thyroid mass and obstructive symptoms related to compression of the aerodigestive tract.[1,54] Thyroid lymphoma may present as multiple nodules, but more commonly (80%) presents as a solitary mass.[1,54] It is usually hypoechoic on US[19,20] and hypodense on CT.[54] Lymphoma is typically cold on iodine and technetium scintigraphy. Necrosis and calcification are uncommon.[54]

Primary squamous cell carcinoma of the thyroid gland is rare and may result from squamous metaplasia of epithelial cells. Rare sporadic cases of mucoepidermoid carcinoma may occur. These are typically seen in patients with a long history of goiter and have a poor prognosis. There are no diagnostic imaging findings to distinguish these from other neoplasms. Primary sarcomas of the thyroid gland are extremely rare, may be radiation-induced, and have a poor prognosis.

Metastatic disease to the thyroid gland is uncommon. Lung and breast carcinoma are the most common metastases found at autopsy, whereas renal carcinoma is the most common metastasis detected clinically.[141] Melanoma and colon carcinoma metastatic to the thyroid gland have also been reported.[142] Single or multiple thyroid masses may be present in the setting of metastatic disease (**Fig. 5.22**). When atypical histology of a resected thyroid mass is detected, metastatic disease should be considered. Testing to establish the presence of thyroglobulin or calcitonin, supporting the notion that the neoplasm is thyroid in origin, may be extremely useful. The absence of these markers favors metastatic disease.

Role of the Radiologist in the Evaluation of Thyroid Cancer

At Initial Clinical Presentation

The role of the radiologist in the assessment of patients presenting with differentiated thyroid cancer is twofold: (1) to determine the extent of the primary thyroid cancer, and (2) to search for regional nodal metastases. Rarely, patients at initial presentation have distant metastatic disease. If the initial clinical presentation is uncomplicated, namely an isolated asymptomatic thyroid mass detected because it is palpable or because it is incidentally noted on imaging being performed for other reasons, all that may be needed is

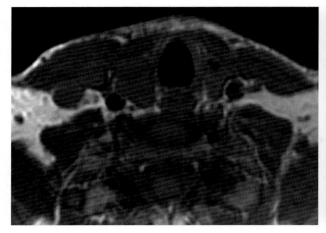
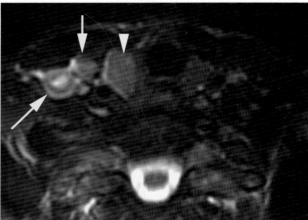

A
B

Fig. 5.22 Base of tongue cancer metastatic to thyroid gland. A 64-year-old patient treated for right base of tongue cancer had neck MRI for restaging. (**A**) Axial unenhanced T1-weighted MRI and (**B**) axial T2-weighted MRI show regional right neck metastases (arrows). Also noted is a dominant right thyroid mass (arrowhead), which was fluorodeoxyglucose (FDG) avid, and at biopsy revealed metastatic squamous cell carcinoma similar to the original base of tongue primary cancer.

thyroid ultrasound. It is not uncommon for the neck to be clinically negative despite the presence of metastatic disease in cervical lymph nodes (up to 65% of nodes harboring thyroid cancer are normal in size at pathology). In these cases and in the hands of skilled clinicians, imaging outside of ultrasound may not be necessary because nodes with microscopic cancer are readily managed with iodine radioablation following thyroidectomy. In the minority of patients with non–iodine-avid tumors, imaging may be done to plan neck dissection.

If the patient presents with a fixed, immobile thyroid mass or is symptomatic, including palpable cervical adenopathy, hoarseness, dysphagia, or respiratory symptoms, unenhanced CT or preferably MRI should be obtained. It is essential that the radiologist determine the extent of the primary tumor including the identification of the following: (1) spread outside the thyroid capsule to the soft tissues of the neck, (2) spread to the airway (larynx or trachea) (**Fig. 5.5**), (3) esophageal invasion on rare occasions, (4) vascular invasion (jugular vein), and (5) mediastinal extension (may necessitate planned combined procedure with thoracic surgery). In the setting of palpable cervical nodal disease, imaging is frequently requested by the surgeon to plan the extent of the neck dissection and to evaluate the contralateral neck and central compartment for surgical planning.

Imaging the Treated Neck with Rising Thyroglobulin

Following thyroidectomy for differentiated thyroid cancer, serum thyroglobulin is an excellent marker to detect the presence of recurrent cancer. One of the most significant dilemmas clinicians face is in detecting the site of recurrence

in patients following thyroidectomy with rising thyroglobulin and normal clinical examination (no palpable disease). Recurrent disease is frequently within lymph nodes, but less commonly may represent distant metastases to the lungs, bones, and occasionally the brain. The role of imaging in the setting of the treated neck with rising thyroglobulin is to identify nonpalpable metastases.

Imaging in recurrent disease may include ultrasound of the lateral neck with FNA as required, cross-sectional imaging (CT or MRI), I-131 whole-body scan, or PET/CT.[143–146] Ultrasound is sensitive in detecting cancer in lateral cervical lymph nodes that are normal in size, as it readily detects abnormal echogenicity and blood flow in them (**Figs. 5.14** and **5.16**), but has low accuracy in assessing the deep spaces of the head and neck (retropharyngeal nodes and mediastinum), which are the strengths of CT and MRI (**Figs. 5.21** and **5.23**). Diagnostic CT often requires iodinated contrast that may be contraindicated if I-131 whole-body scanning or radioablation is under consideration. Whole-body I-131 imaging is most accurate in detecting iodine-avid metastases, and can miss up to 50% of differentiated/dedifferentiated thyroid metastases. In patients with thyroid cancer, whole-body I-131 scanning has an overall sensitivity of approximately 50%, and specificity over 95%.[144] It may require withdrawal of thyroid hormone therapy or the administration of TSH. The advantage of MRI in detecting metastases is that there are no concerns about iodinated contrast agents. In addition, lymph nodes harboring metastatic thyroid cancer frequently have high protein content due to the presence of thyroglobulin, colloid, and occasionally blood products, making them detectable on MRI ("bright" hyperintense on unenhanced T1W imaging) even if normal in size (**Fig. 5.24**). Magnetic resonance imaging is 90 to 95% sensitive when thyroglobulin is elevated. In patients in whom

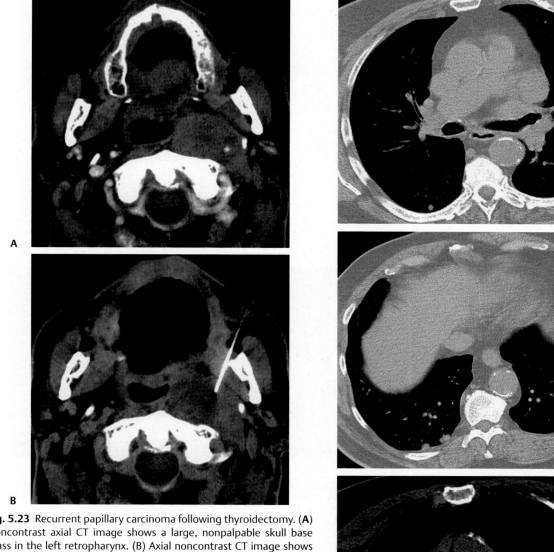

Fig. 5.23 Recurrent papillary carcinoma following thyroidectomy. (**A**) Noncontrast axial CT image shows a large, nonpalpable skull base mass in the left retropharynx. (B) Axial noncontrast CT image shows CT-guided FNA with the needle placed into the mass using a transfacial approach. Cytology showed recurrent papillary carcinoma with regions of anaplastic transformation.

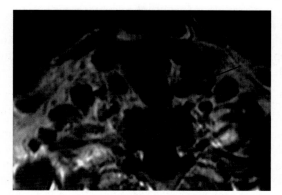

Fig. 5.24 A 47-year-old man with rising thyroglobulin following thyroidectomy. Axial unenhanced T1-weighted MRI shows a "bright" or hyperintense pathologically confirmed lymph node recurrence in the base of the left neck (arrow).

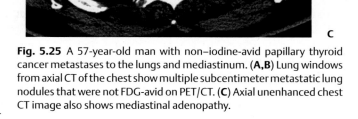

Fig. 5.25 A 57-year-old man with non–iodine-avid papillary thyroid cancer metastases to the lungs and mediastinum. (**A,B**) Lung windows from axial CT of the chest show multiple subcentimeter metastatic lung nodules that were not FDG-avid on PET/CT. (**C**) Axial unenhanced chest CT image also shows mediastinal adenopathy.

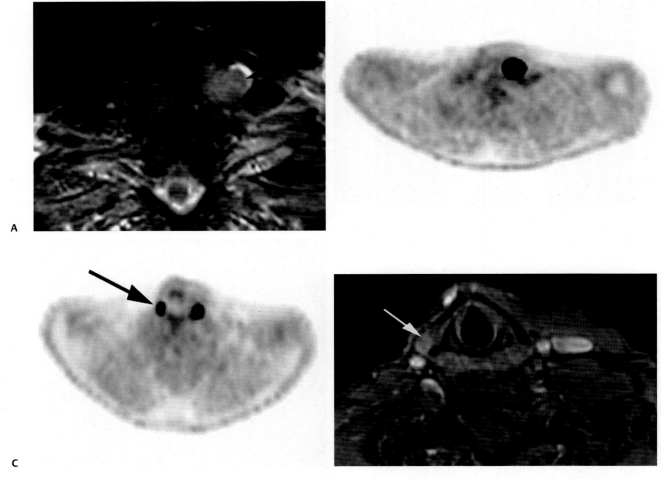

Fig. 5.26 Recurrent iodine-avid papillary thyroid cancer. (**A**) Axial T2-weighted MRI shows a metastatic node at level IV in the left neck (arrow). (**B**) Corresponding FDG-PET image shows avid FDG uptake in this mass. (**C**) FDG-PET image approximately 10 mm cephalad to image **B** shows a second focus of FDG uptake in the right neck lateral to the inferior thyroid cartilage (arrow) that also represented metastatic disease. (**D**) Axial fat-suppressed gadolinium enhanced T1-weighted MRI shows a 4-mm nodule (arrow) in the right neck corresponding to the focus seen on the PET (**C**). This was not detected prospectively on MRI.

MRI or CT identifies nodes suspected of harboring cancer, CT-guided FNA can readily be performed for histologic confirmation (**Fig. 5.23B**).

The role of PET or PET/CT in the assessment of differentiated thyroid cancer recurrence is still evolving. The uptake of FDG in general is inversely proportional to iodine uptake/differentiation.[145] Its overall sensitivity is approximately 65% (iodine avid, 50–65%; non–iodine avid, 70–85%).[143–145] Its overall specificity is greater than 95%.[145] Another limitation of PET is that cancerous nodes may not be detected on PET due to low cellularity, or because they are predominantly cystic or necrotic. In addition, even non–iodine-avid small metastases such as in the lungs may be missed due to relatively low cellularity volume (**Fig. 5.25**). Some clinicians see an additional role of PET/CT in the evaluation of recurrent papillary cancer; namely, it may provide additional information that confirms or changes the management plan, and importantly enhances patient and physician confidence in both the diagnosis of metastatic disease (**Fig. 5.26**) and the management plan.[145,147] It is also important to note that iodine-based PET agents are in development, so it will be interesting to see what the future holds.

Conclusion

Recommendations for imaging in the setting of rising thyroglobulin in patients treated for differentiated thyroid cancer with a negative clinical exam should include ultrasound of the lateral neck, I-131 scan, and MRI of the neck and upper mediastinum (or chest CT). In our practice, PET/CT is used when US, MRI, and I-131 scanning are negative or equivocal because it is in this group that the sensitivity of PET is highest.

References

1. Shibata T, Noma S, Nakano Y, et al. Primary thyroid lymphoma: MR appearance. J Comput Assist Tomogr 1991;15:629–633
2. De Lellis RA. The endocrine system. In: Cotram R, Kumar V, Robbins SL, eds. Robbins' Pathologic Basis of Disease, 4th ed. Philadelphia: WB Saunders, 1989:1214–1242
3. Plummer HS. The clinical and pathologic relationship of simple and exophthalmic goiter. Am J Med Sci 1913;146:790–803
4. Villadolid MC, Yokoyama N, Izumi M, et al. Untreated Graves disease patients without clinical ophthalmopathy demonstrate a high frequency of extra-ocular muscle (EOM) enlargement by magnetic resonance. J Clin Endocrinol Metab 1995;80:2830–2833
5. Takashima S, Nomura N, Tanaka H, et al. Congenital hypothyroidism: assessment with ultrasound. AJNR Am J Neuroradiol 1995;16:1117–1123
6. Price DC. Radioisotopic evaluation of the thyroid and parathyroids. Radiol Clin North Am 1993;31:991–1015
7. Sandler MP, Patton JA, Ossoff RH. Recent advances in thyroid imaging. Otolaryngol Clin North Am 1990;23:251–270
8. Price DC. Radioisotope evaluation of the thyroid and parathyroids. Radiol Clin North Am 1993;31:991–1015
9. Smith JR, Oates E. Radionuclide imaging of the thyroid gland; patterns, pearls and pitfalls. Clin Nucl Med 2004;29:181–193
10. Nygaard B, Nygaard T, Jensen LI, et al. Iohexol: effects on uptake of radioactive iodine in the thyroid and on thyroid function. Acad Radiol 1998;5:409–414
11. Laurie AJ, Lyons SG, Lassen EC. Contrast material iodides: potential effects on radioactive thyroid uptake. J Nucl Med 1992;33:237–238
12. Sternthal E, Lipworth L, Stanley B, Abreau C, Fang SL, Braverman LE. Suppression of thyroid radioiodine uptake by various doses of stable iodide. N Engl J Med 1980;303:1083–1088
13. Laurberg P, Boye N. Inhibitory effect of various radiographic contrast agents on secretion of thyroxine by the dog thyroid and on peripheral and thyroidal deiodination of thyroxine to triiodothyronine. J Endocrinol 1987;112:387–390
14. Feine U, Lietzenmayer R, Hanke J, Wohrle H. Fluorine-18-FDG and iodine-131 uptake in thyroid cancer. J Nucl Med 1996;37:1468–1472
15. Dietlein M, Scheidhauer K, Voth E, Theissen P, Schicha H. Fluorine-18 fluorodeoxyglucose positron emission tomography and iodine-131 whole body scintigraphy in the follow-up of differentiated thyroid cancer. Eur J Nucl Med 1997;24:1342–1348
16. Wang W, Larson SM, Fazzari M, et al. Prognostic value of [18F] fluorodeoxyglucose positron emission tomographic scanning in patients with thyroid cancer. J Clin Endocrinol Metab 2000;85:1107–1113
17. Gotway MB, Higgins CB. MR imaging of the thyroid and parathyroid glands. Magn Reson Imaging Clin North Am 2000;8:163–182
18. Gefter WB, Spritzer CE, Eisenberg B, et al. Thyroid imaging with high-field strength surface-coil MR. Radiology 1987;164:483–490
19. Hegedus L. Thyroid ultrasound. Endocrinol Metab Clin North Am 2001;30:339–360
20. Solbiati L, Volterrani L, Rizzatto G, et al. The thyroid gland with low uptake lesions: evaluation by ultrasound. Radiology 1985;155:187–191
21. Hopkins CR, Reading CC. Thyroid and parathyroid imaging. Semin Ultrasound CT MR 1995;16:279–295
22. Quinn SF, Nelson HA, Demlow TA. Thyroid biopsies: fine-needle aspiration biopsy versus spring-activated core biopsy needle in 102 patients. J Vasc Interv Radiol 1994;5:619–623
23. Sanchez RB, vanSonnenberg E, D'Agostino HB, et al. Ultrasound guided biopsy of nonpalpable and difficult to palpate thyroid masses. J Am Coll Surg 1994;178:33–37
24. LiVolsi VA. The thyroid and parathyroid. In: Sternberg SS, ed. Diagnostic Surgical Pathology, 2nd ed. New York: Raven Press 1994:523–560
25. Pintar JE, Toran-Allerand CD. Normal development of the hypothalamic-pituitary-thyroid axis. In: Braverman LE, Utiger RD, eds. Werner and Ingbar's, The Thyroid, 6th ed. Philadelphia: JB Lippincott, 1991:7–21
26. Hammond RJ, Meakin K, Davies JE. Case report: lateral thyroid ectopia — CT and MRI findings. Br J Radiol 1996;69:1178–1180
27. Morgan NJ, Emberton P, Barton RP. The importance of thyroid scanning in neck lumps–a case report of ectopic tissue in the right submandibular region. J Laryngol Otol 1995;109:674–676
28. Guneri A, Ceryan K, Igci E, et al. Lingual thyroid: the diagnostic value of magnetic resonance imaging. J Laryngol Otol 1991;105:493–495
29. Montgomery ML. Lingual thyroid: comprehensive review. West J Surg 1935;43:661–671
30. Neinas FW, Gorman CA, Devine KD, et al. Lingual thyroid. Clinical characteristics of 15 cases. Ann Intern Med 1973;79:205–210
31. Kantelip B, Lusson JR, DeRiberolles C, et al. Intracardiac ectopic thyroid. Hum Pathol 1986;17:1293–1296
32. Fujioka S, Takatsu Y, Tankawa H, Yamanaka K, Ando F. Intracardiac ectopic thyroid mass. Chest 1996;110:1366–1368
33. Brandwein M, Som P, Urken M. Benign intratracheal thyroid. Arch Otolaryngol Head Neck Surg 1998;124:1266–1269
34. Dominguez-Malagon H, Guerrero-Medrano J, Suster S. Ectopic poorly differentiated (insular) carcinoma of the thyroid. Report of a case presenting as an anterior mediastinal mass. Am J Clin Pathol 1995;104:408–412
35. Takashima S, Nomura N, Tanaka H, et al. Congenital hypothyroidism: assessment with ultrasound. AJNR Am J Neuroradiol 1995;16:1117–1123
36. Shibutani Y,Inoue D,Koshiyama H,Mori T.Thyroid hemiagenesis with subacute thyroiditis. Thyroid1995;5:133–135. New reference: Ahuja AT, Kind AD, King W,Metreweli C. Thyroglossal duct cysts: sonographic appearance inadults. AJNR Am J Neuroradiol1999;20:579–58210319964
37. Pollice L, Caneso G. Struma cordis. Arch Pathol Lab Med 1986;110:452–453
38. Hays LL, Marlow SF. Papillary carcinoma arising in a thyroglossal duct cyst. Laryngoscope 1968;78:2189–2193
39. Ahuja AT, Kind AD, King W, Metreweli C. Thyroglossal duct cysts: sonographic appearance in adults. AJNR Am J Neuroradiol 1999;20:579–582
40. Ralls PW, Mayekawa DS, Lee KP, et al. Color-flow Doppler sonography in Graves disease: "thyroid inferno. AJR Am J Roentgenol 1988;150:781–784
41. Castagnone D, Rivolta R, Rescalli S, et al. Color doppler sonography in Graves' disease: value in assessing activity of disease and predicting outcome. AJR Am J Roentgenol 1996;166:203–207
42. Kaneko T, Matsumoto N, Fukui K, et al. Clinical evaluation of thyroid CT values in various thyroid conditions. J Comput Tomogr 1979;3:1–4
43. Volpe R. The pathology of thyroiditis. Hum Pathol 1978;9:429–438
44. Wang PW, Chen HY, Li CH, et al. Tc-99m pertechnetate trapping and thyroid function in Hashimoto's thyroiditis. Clin Nucl Med 1994;19:177–180
45. Takasu N, Yamada T, Takasu M, et al. Disappearance of thyrotropin-blocking antibodies and spontaneous recovery from hypothyroidism in autoimmune thyroiditis. N Engl J Med 1992;326:513–518

46. Alos N, Huot C, Lambert R, et al. Thyroid scintigraphy in children and adolescents with Hashimoto's disease. J Pediatr 1995;127:951–953

47. Doniach D, Bottazzo GF, Russell RCG. Goitrous autoimmune thyroiditis (Hashimoto's disease). Clin Endocrinol Metab 1979;8:63–80

48. Intenzo CM, Park H, Kim SM, et al. Clinical, laboratory, and scintigraphic manifestations of subacute and chronic thyroiditis. Clin Nucl Med 1993;18:302–306

49. Yeh HC, Futterweit W, Gilbert P. Micronodulation: ultrasonographic sign of Hashimoto thyroiditis. J Ultrasound Med 1996;15:813–819

50. Takashima S, Matsuzuka F, Nagareda T, et al. Thyroid nodules associated with Hashimoto thyroiditis: assessment with US. Radiology 1992;185:125–130

51. Marcocci C, Vitti P, Cetani F, et al. Thyroid ultrasonography helps to identify patients with diffuse lymphocytic thyroiditis who are prone to develop hypothyroidism. J Clin Endocrinol Metab 1991;72:209–213

52. Set PAK, Oleszczuk-Raschke K, VonLengerke JH, Brämswig J. Sonographic features of Hashimoto thyroiditis in childhood. Clin Radiol 1996;51:167–169

53. Langer JE, Khan A, Nisenbaum HL, et al. Sonographic appearance of focal thyroiditis. AJR Am J Roentgenol 2001;176:751–754

54. Takashima S, Ikezoe J, Morimoto S, et al. Primary thyroid lymphoma: evaluation with CT. Radiology 1988;168:765–768

55. Ott RA, Calandra DB, McCall A, et al. The incidence of thyroid carcinoma in patients with Hashimoto's thyroiditis and solitary cold nodules. Surgery 1985;98:1202–1206

56. Compagno J, Oertel JE. Malignant lymphoma and other lymphoproliferative disorders of the thyroid gland: clinicopathologic study of 245 cases. Am J Clin Pathol 1980;74:1–11

57. Clark OH, Greenspan FS, Dunphy JE. Hashimoto's thyroiditis and thyroid cancer: indications for operations. Am J Surg 1980;140:65–71

58. Nordmeyer JP, Shafeh TA, Heckmann C. Thyroid sonography in autoimmune thyroiditis: a prospective study on 123 patients. Acta Endocrinol (Copenh) 1990;122:391–395

59. Mizukami Y, Michigishi T, Hashimoto T, et al. Silent thyroiditis: a histologic and immunohistochemical study. Hum Pathol 1988;19:423–431

60. Hamburger JI. The various presentations of thyroiditis: diagnostic considerations. Ann Intern Med 1986;104:219–224

61. Hay ID. Thyroiditis: a clinical update. Mayo Clin Proc 1985;60:836–843

62. Hatabu H, Kasagi K, Yamamoto K, et al. Acute suppurative thyroiditis associated with pyriform sinus fistula: sonographic findings. AJR Am J Roentgenol 1990;155:845–847

63. Kawanaka M, Sugimoto Y, Suehiro M, et al. Thyroid imaging in a typical case of acute suppurative thyroiditis with abscess formation due to infection from a persistent thyroglossal duct. Ann Nucl Med 1994;8:159–162

64. Malotte MJ, Chonkich GD, Zuppan CW. Riedel's thyroiditis. Arch Otolaryngol Head Neck Surg 1991;117:214–217

65. Fontan FJP, Carballido FC, Felipe FP, et al. Case report: Riedel thyroiditis: US, CT, and MR evaluation. J Comput Assist Tomogr 1993;17:324–325

66. Perez Fontan FJ, Cordido Carballido F, Pombo Felipe F, et al. Riedel thyroiditis: US, CT, and MR evaluation. J Comput Assist Tomogr 1993;17:324–325

67. Langer JE, Khan A, Nisenbaum HL, et al. Sonographic appearance of focal thyroiditis. AJR Am J Roentgenol 2001;176:751–754

68. Belfiore A, LaRose GL, LaPorta GA, et al. Cancer risks in patients with cold thyroid nodules: relevance of iodine intake, sex, age, and multinodularity. Am J Med 1992;93:363–369

69. Cerise EJ, Spears R, Ochsner A. Carcinoma of the thyroid and nontoxic nodular goiter. Surgery 1952;31:552–561

70. McCall A, Jarosz H, Lawrence AM, et al. The incidence of thyroid carcinoma in solitary cold nodules and in multinodular goiters. Surgery 1986;100:1128–1132

71. Shulkin BL, Shapiro B. The role of imaging tests in the diagnosis of thyroid carcinoma. Endocrinol Metab Clin North Am 1990;19:523–543

72. Noma S, Kanaoka M, Minami S, et al. Thyroid masses: MR imaging and pathologic correlation. Radiology 1988;168:759–764

73. Huysmans DA, Hermus AR, Corstens FH, et al. Large, compressive goiters treated with radioiodine. Ann Intern Med 1994;121:757–762

74. Langer JE, Khan A, Nisenbaum HL, et al. Sonographic appearance of focal thyroiditis. AJR Am J Roentgenol 2001;176:751–754

75. Dworkin HJ, Meier DA, Kaplan M. Advances in the management of patients with thyroid disease. Semin Nucl Med 1995;25:205–220

76. Gharib H, Goellner J. Fine-needle aspiration biopsy of the thyroid: an appraisal. Ann Intern Med 1993;118:282–289

77. Yousem DM, Huang T, Loevner LA, Langlotz CP. Clinical and economic impact of incidental thyroid lesions discovered by CT and MR imaging. AJNR Am J Neuroradiol 1997;18:1423–1428

78. Harvey HK. Diagnosis and management of the thyroid nodule. An overview. Otolaryngol Clin North Am 1990;23:303–337

79. Hegedus L, Bonnema SJ, Bennedbaek FN. Management of simple nodular goiter: current status and future perspectives. Endocr Rev 2003;24:102–132

80. Brander A, Viikinkoski P, Nickels J, Kivisaari L. Thyroid gland: US screening in a random adult population. Radiology 1991;181:683–687

81. Bruneton JN, Balu-Maestro C, Marcy P, Melia P, Mourou M. Very high frequency (13MHz) ultrasonographic examination of the normal neck: detection of normal lymph nodes and thyroid nodules. J Ultrasound Med 1994;13:87–90

82. Marqusee E, Benson C, Frates M, et al. Usefulness of ultrasonography in the management of nodular thyroid disease. Ann Intern Med 2000;133:696–700

83. Mortenson JD, Woolner LB, Bennett WA. Gross and microscopic findings in clinically normal thyroid glands. J Clin Endocrinol Metab 1955;15:1270–1280

84. Papini E, Guglielmi R, Bianchini A, et al. Risk of malignancy in nonpalpable thyroid nodules: predictive value of ultrasound and color Doppler features. J Clin Endocrinol Metab 2002;87:1941–1946

85. Kunreuther E, Orcutt J, Benson C, et al. Prevalence and distribution of carcinoma in the uninodular and multinodular goiter. 76th Annual Meeting of the American Thyroid Association, Vancouver, BC, 2004

86. Nam-Goong IS, Kim HY, Gong G, et al. Ultrasonography-guided fine-needle aspiration of thyroid incidentaloma: correlation with pathological findings. Clin Endocrinol (Oxf) 2004;60:21–28

87. Frates MC, Benson CB, Charboneau JW, et al. Management of thyroid nodules detected at US: Society of Radiologists in Ultrasound consensus conference statement. Radiology 2005;237:794–800

88. Tollin SR, Mery GM, Jelveh N, et al. The use of fine-needle aspiration biopsy under ultrasound guidance to assess the risk of malignancy in patients with a multinodular goiter. Thyroid 2000;10:235–241

89. Khoo ML, Asa S, Witterick I, Freeman J. Thyroid calcification and its association with thyroid carcinoma. Head Neck 2002;24:651–655

90. Kim E-K, Park C, Chung W, et al. New sonographic criteria for

recommending fine-needle aspiration biopsy of nonpalpable solid nodules of the thyroid. AJR Am J Roentgenol 2002;178:687–691

91. Knudsen N, Perrild H, Christiansen E, Rasmussen S, Dige-Petersen H, Jorgensen T. Thyroid structure and size and two-year follow-up of solitary cold thyroid nodules in an unselected population with borderline low iodine deficiency. Eur J Endocrinol 2000;142:224–230

92. Shamma FN, Abrahams JJ. Imaging in endocrine disorders. J Reprod Med 1992;37:39–45

93. Klieger PS, Wilson GA, Greenspan BS. The usefulness of the dynamic phase in pertechnetate thyroid imaging for solitary hypofunctioning nodules. Clin Nucl Med 1992;17:617–622

94. Gharib H, Goellner JR, Johnson DA. FNA cytology of the thyroid: a 12 year experience with 11,000 biopsies. Clin Lab Med 1993;13:699–709

95. Gharib H, Goellner JR. Fine needle aspiration of the thyroid: an appraisal. Ann Intern Med 1993;118:282–289

96. Carmeci C, Jeffrey RB, McDougall IR, et al. Ultrasound-guided fine-needle aspiration biopsy of thyroid masses. Thyroid 1998;8:283–289

97. Danese D, Sciacchitano S, Farsetti A, et al. Diagnostic accuracy of conventional versus sonography-guided fine-needle aspiration biopsy of thyroid nodules. Thyroid 1998;8:15–21

98. Erdogan MF, Kamel N, Aras D, et al. Value of re-aspirations in benign nodular thyroid disease. Thyroid 1998;8:1087–1090

99. Hamburger JI. Evolution of toxicity in solitary nontoxic autonomously functioning thyroid nodules. Clin Endocrinol Metab 1980;50:1089–1093

100. Ross DS. Evaluation of the thyroid nodule. J Nucl Med 1991;32:2181–2192

101. Valcavi R, Frasoldati A. Ultrasound-guided percutaneous ethanol injection therapy in thyroid cystic nodules. Endocr Pract 2004;10:269–275

102. Papini E, Pacella CM, Verde G. Percutaneous ethanol injection (PEI): what is its role in the treatment of benign thyroid nodules? Thyroid 1995;5:147–150

103. Livraghi T, Paracchi A, Ferrari C, et al. Treatment of autonomous thyroid nodules with percutaneous ethanol injection: preliminary results. Work in progress. Radiology 1990;175:827–829

104. Monzani F, Goletti O, Caraccio N, et al. Percutaneous ethanol injection treatment of autonomous thyroid adenoma: hormonal and clinical evaluation. Clin Endocrinol (Oxf) 1992;36:491–497

105. Mazzeo S, Toni MG, DeGaudio C, et al. Percutaneous injection of ethanol to treat autonomous thyroid nodules. AJR Am J Roentgenol 1993;161:871–876

106. Papini E, Panunzi C, Pacella CM, et al. Percutaneous ultrasound-guided ethanol injection: a new treatment for toxic autonomously functioning thyroid nodules? J Clin Endocrinol Metab 1993;76:411–416

107. Livraghi T, Paracchi A, Ferrari C, et al. Treatment of autonomous thyroid nodules with percutaneous ethanol injection: 4-year experience. Radiology 1994;190:529–533

108. Ozdemir H, Ilgit ET, Yucel C, et al. Treatment of autonomous thyroid nodules: safety and efficacy of sonographically guided percutaneous injection of ethanol. AJR Am J Roentgenol 1994;163:929–932

109. Solbiati L, Pra LD, Ierace T, et al. High-resolution sonography of the recurrent laryngeal nerve: anatomic and pathologic considerations. AJR Am J Roentgenol 1985;145:989–993

110. Duffy BJ, Fitzgerald PJ. Cancer of the thyroid in children: a report of 28 cases. J Clin Endocrinol Metab 1950;10:1296–1311

111. Favus MJ, Schneider AB, Stachura ME, et al. Thyroid cancer occur-ring as a late consequence of head-and-neck irradiation: evaluation of 1,056 patients. N Engl J Med 1976;294:1019–1025

112. Mazzaferri EL. Management of a solitary thyroid nodule. N Engl J Med 1993;328:553–559

113. Mazzaferri EL. Management of a solitary thyroid nodule. N Engl J Med 1993;328:553–559

114. Mazzaferri EL, de los Santos ET, Rofagha-Keyhani S. Solitary thyroid nodule: diagnosis and management. Med Clin North Am 1988;72:1177–1211

115. Pelizzo MR, Piotto A, Rubello D, et al. High prevalence of occult papillary thyroid carcinoma in a surgical series for benign thyroid disease. Tumori 1990;76:255–257

116. Sutton RT, Reading CC, Charboneau JW, et al. US-guided biopsy of neck masses in postoperative management of patients with thyroid cancer. Radiology 1988;168:769–772

117. Chen KT, Rosai J. Follicular variant of thyroid papillary carcinoma. A clinicopathologic study of 6 cases. Am J Surg Pathol 1977;1:123–130

118. Rosai J, Zampi G, Carcangiu ML. Papillary carcinoma of the thyroid. Am J Surg Pathol 1983;7:809–817

119. Carcangiu ML, Zampi G, Pupi A, Castagnoli A, Rosai J. Papillary carcinoma of the thyroid. A clinicopathologic study of 244 cases treated at the University of Florence, Italy. Cancer 1985;55:805–828

120. Chen KT, Rosai J. Follicular variant of thyroid papillary carcinoma: a clinicopathologic study of six cases. Am J Surg Pathol 1977;1:123–130

121. Vickery AL. Thyroid papillary carcinoma. Pathological and philosophical controversies. Am J Surg Pathol 1983;7:797–807

122. Hay ID. Papillary thyroid carcinoma. Endocrinol Metab Clin North Am 1990;19:545–576

123. Hawk WA, Hazard JB. The many appearances of papillary carcinoma of the thyroid. Cleve Clin Q 1976;43:207–216

124. Chan BK, Desser TS, McDougall IR, Weigel RJ, Jeffrey RB. Common and uncommon sonographic features of papillary thyroid carcinoma. J Ultrasound Med 2003;22:1083–1090

125. Som PM, Brandwein M, Lidov M, et al. The varied appearance of papillary carcinoma cervical nodal disease: CT and MR findings. AJNR Am J Neuroradiol 1994;15:1129–1138

126. Franssila KO, Ackerman LV, Brown CL, Hedinger CE. Follicular carcinoma. Semin Diagn Pathol 1985;2:101–102

127. Roediger WEW. The oxyphil and C cells of the human thyroid gland. Cancer 1975;36:1758–1770

128. Bondeson L, Bondeson AG, Ljungberg O, Tibblin S. Oxyphil tumors of the thyroid. Follow-up of 42 surgical cases. Ann Surg 1981;194:677–680

129. Gorman B, Charboneau JW, James EM, et al. Medullary thyroid carcinoma: role of high-resolution US. Radiology 1987;162:147–150

130. Melvin KEW, Miller HH, Tashjian AH. Early diagnosis of medullary carcinoma of the thyroid by means of calcitonin assay. N Engl J Med 1971;285:1115–1120

131. Steiner AL, Goodman AD, Powers SR. Study of a kindred with pheochromocytoma, medullary thyroid carcinoma, hyperparathyroidism, and Cushing's disease: multiple endocrine neoplasia type 2. Medicine 1968;47:371–409

132. Wolfe HJ, DeLellis RA. Familial medullary thyroid carcinoma and C-cell hyperplasia. Clin Endocrinol Metab 1981;10:351–365

133. Kakudo K, Carney JA, Sizemore GW. Medullary carcinoma of thyroid: biologic behavior of the sporadic and familial neoplasm. Cancer 1985;55:2818–2821

134. Busnardo B, Girelli ME, Simioni N, Nacamuilli D, Busetto E. Non-parallel patterns of calcitonin and carcinoembryonic antigen levels in the follow-up of medullary thyroid carcinoma. Cancer 1984;53:278–285

135. Dorr U, Wurstlin S, Frank-Raue K, et al. Somatostatin receptor scintigraphy and magnetic resonance imaging in recurrent medullary thyroid carcinoma: a comparative study. Horm Metab Res Suppl 1993;27:48–55

136. Lebouthillier G, Morais J, Picard M, et al. Tc-99m sestamibi and other agents in the detection of metastatic medullary carcinoma of the thyroid. Clin Nucl Med 1993;18:657–661

137. Krenning EP, Kwekkeboom DJ, Bakker WH, et al. Somatostatin receptor scintigraphy with [111-In-DTPA-D-phe]- and [I-123-tyr]-Octreotide: the Rotterdam experience with more than 1,000 patients. Eur J Nucl Med 1993;20:716–731

138. Dorr U, Sautter-Bihl ML, Heiner B. The contribution of somatostatin receptor scintigraphy to the diagnosis of recurrent medullary carcinoma of the thyroid. Semin Oncol 1994;21:42–45

139. Takashima S, Morimoto S, Ikezoe J, et al. CT evaluation of anaplastic thyroid carcinoma. AJR Am J Roentgenol 1990;154:1079–1085

140. Ohnishi T, Noguchi S, Murakami N, et al. MR imaging in patients with primary thyroid lymphoma. AJNR Am J Neuroradiol 1992; 13:1196–1198

141. Haugen BR, Nawaz S, Cohn A, et al. Secondary malignancy of the thyroid gland: a case report and review of the literature. Thyroid 1994;4:297–300vfill

142. Czech JM, Lichtor TR, Carney JA, vanHeerden JA. Neoplasms metastatic to the thyroid gland. Surg Gynecol Obstet 1982;155: 503–505

143. Dietlein M, Scheidhauer K, Voth E, Theissen P, Schicha H. Fluorine-18 fluorodeoxyglucose positron emission tomography and iodine–131 whole-body scintigraphy in the follow-up of differentiated thyroid cancer. Eur J Nucl Med 1997;24:1342–1348

144. Grunwald F, Kalicke T, Feine U, et al. Fluorine-18 fluorodeoxyglucose positron emission tomography in thyroid cancer: results of a multicentre study. Eur J Nucl Med 1999;26:1547–1552

145. Nahas Z, Goldenberg D, Fakhry C, et al. The role of positron emission tomography/computed tomography in the management of recurrent papillary thyroid carcinoma. Laryngoscope 2005;115:237–243

146. Zimmer LA, McCook B, Meltzer C, et al. Combined positron emission tomography/computed tomography imaging of recurrent thyroid cancer. Otolaryngol Head Neck Surg 2003;128:178–184

147. Frilling A, Tecklenborg K, Gorges R, et al. Preoperative diagnostic value of [18F] fluorodeoxyglucose positron emission tomography in patients with radioiodine-negative recurrent well-differentiated thyroid carcinoma. Ann Surg 2001;234:804–811

Benign Thyroid Diseases

6 Introduction to Benign Thyroid Diseases

Maisie L. Shindo

Benign thyroid diseases comprise nodular diseases and inflammatory thyroid conditions. Nodular diseases can be categorized as solitary thyroid nodules and goiters. The term *goiter,* derived from the Latin word *guttur,* meaning throat, is used to describe a pathologic enlargement of the thyroid gland. Goiters can be classified as diffuse or nodular, and toxic or nontoxic. Inflammatory thyroid conditions include autoimmune thyroiditis, subacute thyroiditis, and Riedel thyroiditis.

The prevalence of clinically evident thyroid nodules is approximately 5%, depending on age, sex, and geographic location.[1] In autopsy series the prevalence of solitary nodules is approximately 10% and of thyroid nodularity is as high as 50%.[2] In recent years imaging modalities have become more ubiquitous and more sensitive, and asymptomatic unexpected thyroid nodules are being discovered serendipitously during an unrelated procedure, which are referred to as incidentalomas. With routine use of imaging modalities such as ultrasound, computed tomography (CT), magnetic resonance imaging (MRI), and positron emission tomography (PET) scans, the incidence of thyroid incidentalomas is likely to be similar to the prevalence of nodules found on autopsy. The incidence of malignancy in a solitary nodule ranges from 10 to 40%, depending on the patient's age and sex, the characteristics of the nodule, the selective criteria for surgery, and the presence of risk factors.[3-6] In evaluating a thyroid nodule, a complete history should be elicited regarding factors that may predict the risk of malignancy such as radiation exposure, voice change, hemoptysis, and family history of thyroid malignancy.[3,5-8] Radiation exposure can be from prior head and neck irradiation for lymphoma or benign conditions (acne, thymus, enlarged adenoids, tinea capitis),[9,10] total body irradiation for bone marrow transplantation,[11,12] and exposure to fallout from the Chernobyl incident, particularly in patients under 15 years of age.[13-15]

In reviewing the patient's medical history, it is also important to be aware that nodular thyroid diseases may be associated with various hereditary syndromes, particularly when present at a younger age. Familial adenomatous polyposis is an autosomal dominant disease caused by mutation of *APC* gene, and is characterized by polyposis of the colon, epidermoid cysts of the skin, desmoid tumors of the abdominal wall, retinal pigmented epithelium, and thyroid carcinoma. A small subset of these patients presents with osteomas, referred to as Gardner syndrome. Thyroid carcinomas occur in 1 to 2% of these patients and is usually papillary carcinoma.[16,17] Cowden disease is an autosomal dominant disease characterized by tumors of the thyroid, breast, colon, endometrium, and brain, and hamartomas and tumors of the skin. The thyroid abnormalities may present in childhood as multinodular goiters, multifocal follicular adenomas, and adenomatous nodules.[17,18] Carney complex is a multiple neoplasia syndrome consisting of spotty skin pigmentation, myxomas, endocrine overactivity, and schwannomas.[19] It is also autosomal dominant. Multiple endocrine organs are affected, resulting in thyroid tumors and primary pigmented nodular adrenocortical disease, which can result in Cushing syndrome, prolactin-producing pituitary tumors, testicular tumors causing precocious puberty, and ovarian tumors.[19] Up to 75% of patients with Carney complex have multiple thyroid nodules, and some may also present with thyroid malignancy.[19] Skin manifestations include spotty pigmented skin lesions, blue nevi, and café-au-lait spots. The myxomas can involve the heart, breast, and skin.[19] Pendred syndrome is an autosomal recessive disease manifesting as a combination of goiter and congenital deafness. Goiters may be present from childhood to early adolescent years. The genetic defect with this disease has been shown to be mutation of the *PDS* gene on chromosome 7q22–31.1.[20]

In the evaluation of nodular thyroid disease, the head and neck examination should not only include the characteristics of the thyroid gland, but one should also search for lymphadenopathy and assess cranial nerve function, particularly vocal cord mobility. A thyroid nodule associated with ipsilateral vocal cord paralysis is highly suspicious for a malignancy. In the rare patient who may also have hemoptysis, flexible laryngoscopy should be performed not only to assess laryngeal pathology but also to examine the upper trachea for presence of intratracheal extension from a thyroid malignancy.

Evaluation and Management of Solitary Thyroid Nodules

The natural course of thyroid nodules is not fully understood. One long-term study showed that 23% of thyroid nodules ultimately increased in size.[21] The most important goal in the diagnostic evaluation of a thyroid nodule is to exclude malignancy. Because thyroid nodules, including the incidentalomas, are quite prevalent, the challenge for the clinician is in deciding which nodules need to be biopsied or surgically excised, and which can be observed. Thyroid sonography and a serum thyroid-stimulating hormone (TSH) level are very useful initial diagnostic tests for a solitary thyroid nodule.

Ultrasound is far superior to physical examination for detection of thyroid nodules, and is an excellent adjunct to physical examination of the thyroid.[3,22–24] Thyroid sonography provides very useful information for management that includes accurate measurement of the size of the nodule, whether the nodule is purely cystic, solid, or mixed, the presence of other nonpalpable nodules, and findings that are concerning for a malignancy, such as microcalcifications and irregular margins, intranodular hypervascularity, and marked hypoechogenicity.[24–26] Thyroid uptake scan for solitary nodules is not particularly useful, unless the TSH level is suppressed (i.e., below normal). In that case, a thyroid uptake scan can be obtained to see if the nodule is hyperfunctioning, indicative of a toxic single adenomatous nodule. Fine-needle aspiration (FNA) is a very important and useful tool in the diagnostic evaluation of solitary nodules.[5,27]

There is no uniform consensus on when a solitary nodule should be biopsied. In general, a solitary nodule requires histologic evaluation, either by FNA or surgical excision, when associated with risk factors for malignancy, which include rapid enlargement, associated lymphadenopathy, associated vocal cord paralysis, prior radiation exposure, age over 60 or under 20, and a family history of thyroid cancer in a first-degree relative. Nodules with sonographic findings suspicious for malignancy as discussed above should be biopsied.[25] The incidence of malignancy in a solitary nodule of childhood is greater than in an adult and has been reported to be as high as 50%.[9,28–30] Therefore, serious consideration should also be given to biopsy or surgical excision of thyroid nodules detected during childhood, particularly if greater than 1.5 cm and solid. Solid thyroid nodules in patients over 65 years of age have a higher risk of being malignant. Furthermore, a higher percentage of the malignancies in this age group tend to be of the more aggressive type.[4,31,32] In a recent study of 21,748 patients with thyroid nodules who underwent ultrasound-guided FNA and surgical pathologic correlation in 3629 patients, 37% of the nodules occurring in those over age 65 were found to be malignant, and up to 36% of the malignancies diagnosed were anaplastic or metastatic.[4] Therefore, aggressive pursuit of a cytologic or pathologic diagnosis is warranted in elderly patients who present with a new thyroid nodule, particularly if it is rapidly growing. Incidentalomas pose a management dilemma. Silver and Parangi[33] recommend ultrasound-guided FNA for incidentally found nodules that are greater than 1.5 cm, and observation of nodules smaller than 8 mm, with reevaluation in 6 months using ultrasound. For nodules between 8 mm and 1.5 cm, they recommend ultrasound-guided FNA if one or more worrisome ultrasound features are present.[33]

Other laboratory testing in the evaluation of a thyroid nodule are serum calcitonin and thyroglobulin levels. A serum calcitonin level should be obtained if there is a family history of medullary thyroid carcinoma, or if FNA of the nodule reveals atypical small round cells or spindle cells, which are not typical of cells derived from follicular origin. Serum thyroglobulin is not very helpful as a diagnostic tool. An elevated thyroglobulin in itself is not indicative of a thyroid malignancy, because benign conditions such as an adenomatous nodule, as well as recent FNA, can cause elevation of serum thyroglobulin. However, should the nodule turn out to be a follicular cell–derived thyroid carcinoma, an elevated preoperative level obtained prior to FNA is indicative of a thyroglobulin-secreting tumor and it can reliably be used for cancer surveillance.

Thyroid FNA cytologic findings are generally categorized as malignant, indeterminant, benign, or nondiagnostic. The indeterminate category includes those that are suspicious for malignancy, follicular neoplasm, and Hürthle cell neoplasm. A nondiagnostic FNA results from poor preservation of specimen or low cellularity obtained from the aspiration, which can occur for several reasons: small nodules, densely fibrotic or calcified nodules, cystic nodules, and operator inexperience. The diagnostic yield of FNA can be improved when performed under ultrasound guidance.[34,35] Furthermore, with ultrasound guidance, small nonpalpable nodules can be biopsied with high yield.[33] The rate of nondiagnostic aspiration can be further reduced to less than 2% when the biopsy is performed under ultrasound guidance with on-site cytologic preparation where cytotechnologists or cytopathologists can provide immediate feedback on whether or not the aspirate is sufficiently cellular.[4,36,37]

Thyroidectomy should be recommended if the FNA cytology is consistent with a malignancy or is indeterminate. The risk of malignancy in an indeterminate nodule is approximately 20%.[38–40] The decision is not as straightforward when the FNA cytology is nondiagnostic. According to the American Thyroid Association (ATA) Guidelines Task Force of 2005, surgery should be recommended if the cytologically nondiagnostic nodule is solid.[5] The patient's age and underlying medical condition also need to be factored into the decision making. In young patients with large solid nodules, particularly if they are solid or demonstrate some atypia, surgical excision for definitive diagnosis and long-term treatment is preferred over observation. In elderly patients with this scenario, if the patient has little or no anesthesia risks, surgical excision should be considered. However, in those with significant comorbidities, it would be appropriate to repeat the FNA and closely observe the nodule.[41] Cystic nodules are diagnostically challenging because aspiration of the fluid usually yields a hypocellular specimen. The risk of malignancy in cystic thyroid nodules among adults range from approximately 15 to 30%, similar to that of solid nodules, and the risk of a false-negative aspirate is high.[42–44] The recommendation formulated by the ATA is that cystic nodules that repeatedly yield nondiagnostic aspirates need surgical excision or close observation with fastidious follow-up and repeat FNA.[5] A cystic nodule containing a large solid component, particularly with microcalcifications, or with an irregular and finger-like pedunculated mass extending into the lumen, is suspicious for a cystic papillary carcinoma.[45,46] If the initial FNA of a cystic nodule with these ultrasound characteristics is nondiagnostic, either the FNA should be repeated with ultrasound guidance and on-site cytologic evaluation, or surgery should be recommended. When performing FNA on a cystic nodule, the diagnostic yield can be improved by first aspirating the fluid content and then reaspirating under ultrasound of the remaining cyst wall or solid component.[46–48] A cystic thyroid nodule associated with cystic lymphadenopathy in the paratracheal region is strongly suggestive of cystic papillary thyroid carcinoma and should be treated as such until proven otherwise. FNA of the thyroid nodule and cystic node, particularly if performed under ultrasound and cytologic guidance, should confirm the diagnosis. A cystic thyroid nodule associated with cystic lymphadenopathy in the lateral neck is more challenging to establish a diagnosis cytologically because the aspirate from the lymph node can be hypocellular or mimic lesions of nonthyroid origin, such as a branchial cleft cyst.[43,49] In that setting, the fluid from the lymph node aspiration can be sent to the lab for a thyroglobulin level; an elevated level would be diagnostic of cystic papillary carcinoma, but a normal level does not exclude malignancy. Measuring the thyroglobulin level in the fluid obtained from FNA of a cystic thyroid nodule is generally not helpful because it can also be elevated in a benign nodule. If FNA of a thyroid nodule associated with cystic cervical lymphadenopathy cannot establish a diagnosis, surgery with frozen section is warranted.

Nodular Goiters

Nodular goiters encompass several different pathologic conditions: hyperthyroidism, hypothyroidism, autoimmune thyroiditis, and malignancy. In the absence of such conditions, it constitutes an entity described as simple nodular goiter, often interchangeably termed multinodular goiter. Multinodular goiter is the most common endocrine disorder worldwide. Goiters can occur endemically and sporadically. An endemic goiter is one that occurs in a region where its prevalence in children 6 to 12 years of age is greater than 5%.[50] The best known endemic areas are located in high mountain regions, such as the Andes and Pyrenees. Sporadic goiter is one that occurs in a nonendemic region in a euthyroid individual.

Pathogenesis

The etiology of nodular goitrous enlargement is multifactorial, and can be categorized as environmental and genetic.[50,51] Iodine deficiency is the most common environmental factor contributing to formation of endemic goiters.[52] Iodine deficiency affects the organification step in thyroxine synthesis, resulting in inadequate thyroid hormone production, which leads to increased TSH production by the pituitary. TSH stimulation ultimately causes the growth of thyroid follicles and glandular enlargement. After iodine was supplemented in diet as iodized salt, the prevalence of goiters decreased significantly in many parts of the world. Al-

though iodine deficiency may also be a cause of goiters in nonendemic regions, the etiology in most cases of sporadic goiters is unclear. Various natural substances that interfere with the iodine trapping mechanism have been implicated in the development of goiters.[53] Some of these natural goitrogens, such as cyanogenic glycosides and thiocyanates, are found in vegetables; others are found in grass and weed, which are then transmitted through cows and animals that consume them. Female gender is also associated with increased risk of nodular goiter formation. Other etiologies that have been implicated in development of goiters are smoking,[50,54,55] medications,[50,56] and stress.[50,57] Rarely, iodine excess has also been advocated as a cause of goiter.

Genetics has also been implicated in the formation of nodular goiters. A gene located on chromosome 14 at the multinodular-1 (MNG-1) locus has been identified as being associated with familial nontoxic multinodular goiter.[58,59] Another locus on chromosome 14, known as GD-1, has also been mapped as a major susceptibility locus for Graves disease.[60] Capon and colleagues[61] mapped a dominant form of multinodular goiter to chromosome Xp22. In addition, pleomorphism of codon 727 of human TSH receptor has been seen with toxic goiters.[62] Immunogenic stimulation has also be speculated as a potential cause of goiter formation. Immunoglobulins that can stimulate growth of thyroid follicles in vitro have been detected in patients with both toxic and nontoxic nodular goiters[63,64]; however, their role in the development of these goiters has yet to be clearly established. Regardless of the thyrotrophic stimulating agent, be it TSH or immunoglobulin, the initial response in the thyroid is diffuse enlargement. With chronic stimulation, various areas of the gland continue to proliferate at different rates. Some areas become hypofunctional and others become hyperfunctional. The increased tissue mass is also modulated by apoptosis, resulting in death of thyrocytes and involution in some areas. The apoptosis is thought to be mediated by the Fas antigen.[65]

Patterns of Growth

The natural history of untreated euthyroid multinodular goiters can be somewhat variable.[66,67] Some continue to grow in volume, up to 20% in a year, while remaining euthyroid.[67] As growth continues, the enlarging thyroid gland can extend outside of the thyroid bed and spread inferiorly to the mediastinum or posteriorly along the sides or behind the pharynx. Chin and colleagues[68] studied the patterns of growth on CT scans in 190 patients with goiters. They reported that in 44% of the patients the goiters spread outside of the thyroid bed. Thirty-seven percent of the goiters demonstrated extension into the mediastinum, and 7% extended along or behind the pharynx. Of those that extended into the mediastinum, all extended into the anterior compartment and 7% extended into the posterior compartment.

Evaluation and Management of Nontoxic Goiters

Approaches to management of nontoxic goiters differ considerably among physicians of the same specialty or in different specialties, on different continents, and for young versus old patients. In a survey of 140 North American members of the ATA, there was a wide variation in opinions as to what should be the optimum diagnostic tests in a patient with a nontoxic multinodular goiter.[69] The most common diagnostic tests utilized by North American clinicians was serum TSH (100%), followed by FNA (74%) and thyroid ultrasound (59%). The majority of the clinicians preferred utilization of ultrasound guidance for FNA. Thyroid uptake scintigraphy and serum calcitonin levels were utilized less frequently by North American clinicians compared with European clinicians. There is also considerable disagreement among clinicians on the management of nontoxic goiters. In the same survey reported by Bonnema et al,[69] one third preferred observation, whereas approximately half used levothyroxine, despite a lack of evidence from prospective clinical trials demonstrating its value. Seventy-eight percent recommend surgery if rapid growth is observed; 69% recommend surgery for compressive symptoms. Surgery was also preferred by approximately two thirds of the clinicians if there is a history of prior head and neck radiation or a family history of thyroid malignancy. With no uniform consensus on approaches to management of nontoxic goiters, a logical approach would be to base the decision on the presence or absence of dominant nodules, and on whether or not the goiter is causing compression. The patient's age and sex, the history of rapid growth, prior head and neck irradiation exposure, and a family history of thyroid malignancy also need to be factored into the decision.

Noncompressive Goiters

In the absence of any associated risk factors for malignancy, small nontoxic goiters with small nodules can generally be observed. Observation is best done with periodic thyroid sonograms. Nodules should be biopsied when growth is observed. Dominant nodules in a multinodular goiter, particularly if they are hypofunctional, should undergo FNA. Guidelines on when to biopsy a thyroid nodule were discussed in the previous section on solitary nodules. However, guidelines on which nodules one should biopsy in a multinodular goiter are not as well defined, and opinions regarding this have varied in the past. The most recent ATA Guidelines Task Force recommendations are as follows: (1) In the presence of two or more thyroid nodules larger than 1 cm, those nodules with a suspicious sonographic appearance should be aspirated preferentially. (2) If none of the nodules has a suspicious sonographic appearance and multiple sonographically similar nodules are present, the largest nodule should be biopsied.[5]

Guidelines for recommending thyroidectomy are similar to those for a solitary nodule. The most common indications for surgical removal of a noncompressive goiter are the presence of a malignancy, suspicion for malignancy, and nondiagnostic nodule(s) on FNA. Other indications are enlarging nodules in a goiter and for cosmesis. The extent of thyroidectomy that should be performed for nontoxic multinodular goiters depends on the location, size and cytologic findings on FNA. Total thyroidectomy is the recommended treatment for most patients with thyroid malignancy.[5] If surgery is performed for an indeterminant diagnosis or for nondiagnostic reasons in a multinodular goiter, hemithyroidectomy is appropriate if the other nodules are all in the same lobe. Total thyroidectomy is indicated if the nodules are bilateral or if both lobes are markedly enlarged.

In recent years the use of ethanol injection for long-term management of cystic nodular goiters has been advocated by some as an alternative to surgical excision. With this technique, the cyst is decompressed under ultrasound guidance, and highly concentrated ethanol (i.e., 95%) is injected. Several studies have shown that volume reduction by as much as 95% can be achieved with low recurrence rates.[70–74] Some have even advocated that cysts up to a volume of 40 mL can be successfully treated.[71,72] One of the limitations of this technique is in treating cysts with high viscosity, which tend to be difficult to evacuate. For these types of cysts, Zieleznik and colleagues[75] described a two-stage ethanol injection technique where ethanol is injected into the cyst under ultrasound during the first procedure and left for 2 weeks, which helps reduce the viscosity. In the second stage, the thinner fluid is aspirated and 95% ethanol is reinjected under ultrasound.[75] The authors reported a 92% reduction in volume and no recurrence. The therapeutic use of ethanol injection for thyroid nodules remains controversial. Opinions range from those who believe that this is still an investigative technique, to those who use it selectively in patients who cannot undergo surgery, to those who use it routinely.[50,71,76,77] Although this has become a popular primary treatment modality for thyroid cysts and toxic adenomatous nodules in Europe and Asia, this procedure is generally not favored as the primary treatment of choice in the United States.

Compressive and Substernal Goiters

When nodular goiters become sufficiently large, they can cause deviation or compression of the aerodigestive tract. With further extension inferiorly, they can extend into the mediastinum and become substernal goiters. Lahey and Swinton[78] defined a substernal goiter as a "gland in which [the] greatest diameter of the intrathoracic mass by roentgenogram is well below the upper aperture of the thoracic cage made by the sternum, first rib, [and] vertebral bodies." The incidence of substernal goiter in the general population based on screening chest x-ray is 0.02 to 0.5%.[79,80] Several classification systems have been proposed for substernal goiters. Higgins[81] originally described a classification system based on the percentage of the goiter in the neck versus the thorax. He classified a goiter as intrathoracic if at least four fifths of the gland lies in the thorax. In addition, he described substernal (part or all of the gland extending below the sternum) and subclavicular (part or all of the gland extending below the clavicle) components. Another classification was developed by Cohen and Cho[82] based on the percentage of mediastinal component of the substernal goiter. Grade I is defined as up to 25% of the goiter in the chest, grade II defined as 26 to 50%, grade III is defined as 51 to 75%, and grade IV is defined as greater than 75%.

Compressive cervical and substernal goiters can grow considerably for years before causing any symptoms. When sufficiently large, they can impinge on the trachea and cause deviation or narrowing of the tracheal lumen. Many patients with tracheal narrowing are asymptomatic, but some may experience dyspnea. Patients with tracheal deviation are usually asymptomatic. Large goiters can also impinge on the esophagus and cause dysphagia. Substernal goiters can occasionally impinge on the intrathoracic great vessels and cause venous obstruction. When venous compression is severe, it can impede venous outflow from the head and neck, resulting in facial erythema when arms are raised above the head, known as the Pemberton sign. In those who are symptomatic from a substernal goiter the most common compressive manifestation is dyspnea (48–67%), followed by dysphagia (26–53%) and stridor (11–17%).[83–88]

Despite the fact that radioactive iodine has been shown to be effective in reducing the volume of goiters,[89–91] the majority of North American clinicians tend to recommend surgery over radioactive iodine for treatment of compressive and substernal goiters.[69] In the United States, thyroidectomy is the preferred treatment modality for young patients with cervical and substernal compressive goiters. The decision for thyroidectomy is not as straightforward in the elderly with such goiters because of associated comorbidities. Certainly, rapid enlargement of a goiter in an elderly patient is worrisome for a thyroid malignancy and therefore requires at least FNA, if not thyroidectomy. Observation is a reasonable approach for the asymptomatic elderly patient with a cervical or substernal compressive goiter that is known to have been present for years with very little change in size and degree of compression. Compressive goiters that are incidentally discovered on imaging studies performed for some other reason, however, pose a management dilemma in elderly patients. In this situation, if the patient is asymptomatic and radiographs demonstrate only mild to moderate tracheal deviation or narrowing (**Fig. 6.1**), observation with FNA of dominant nodule(s) is a reasonable approach. If the patient is experiencing dysphagia or shortness of breath, it is important to differentiate if their symptoms are actually due to compression by the goiter or due to some other conditions that frequently coexist in this age group, such as congestive heart failure, cricopharyngeal spasm, or esophageal dysmotility. Pulmonary functions tests with flow loops may

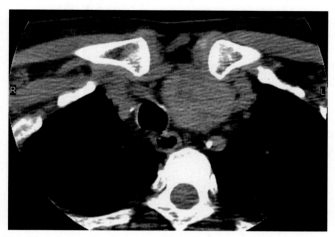

Fig. 6.1 Substernal goiter with mild tracheal narrowing and compression.

be helpful if extrathoracic obstruction is seen, but a normal flow loop does not necessarily exclude symptomatic tracheal compression. An esophagram, if it demonstrates extrinsic compression, may also provide supportive evidence that the goiter is causing dysphagia. However, a normal study does not necessarily mean that the goiter is not the cause of the dysphagia. It is also important to obtain a noncontrast CT of the neck and chest to determine the extent of tracheal compression or if the goiter is actually compressing on the esophagus to help determine if the patient would truly benefit from thyroidectomy. For routine imaging of the thyroid, intravenous contrast is unnecessary and should be avoided because the gland often is well visualized on CT. Thus, in an elderly patient with a large compressive goiter (intrathoracic or cervical) and symptoms of compression such as dysphagia, dyspnea, and facial venous congestion, in the absence of other concurrent conditions that can explain these compressive symptoms, subtotal or near-total thyroidectomy should be recommended, provided the patient's anesthesia risk is low. Otherwise, radioactive iodine can be used, which has been shown to decrease the goiter size by approximately 50%.[89–91]

Thyroidectomy for substernal goiters can be performed safely with proper preoperative planning. Review of the patient's chest CT is essential to determine the location and extent of spread in the mediastinum. Extension of the goiter into the posterior mediastinum increases the risk of recurrent laryngeal nerve injury because the nerve may course anterior to the goitrous nodule rather than posteriorly. Preoperative assessment of the extent of tracheal compression and deviation is important in the planning of initial airway management. Netterville et al[83] reported that a CT- or MRI-demonstrated tracheal deviation was seen in 77% and tracheal compression in 73% of substernal goiters. Despite the high incidence of tracheal displacement or compression, orotracheal intubation can generally be successfully achieved without difficulties, as long as the patient

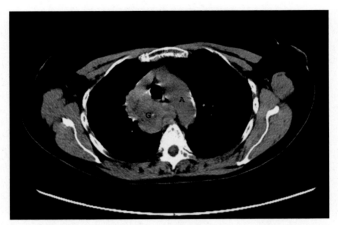

Fig. 6.2 Substernal goiter with significant extension below the aortic arch and into the posterior mediastinum. *Abbreviations:* A, aortic arch; G, substernal goiter.

Table 6.1 Causes of Thyrotoxicosis

- Hyperthyroidism
- Thyroiditis
- Thyrotoxicosis factitia
- Increased thyroxine-binding globulin (TBG) or T_4-binding prealbumin
- Medications
- Abnormal binding to albumin
- Peripheral resistance to thyroid hormone
- Endogenous antibodies to T_4
- Familial dysalbuminemia
- Thyroid-stimulating hormone (TSH) producing pituitary tumor

does not have any upper airway abnormalities that would result in difficult exposure of the vocal cords. Where one may potentially encounter difficulty is with a massive goiter that causes significant pharyngeal compression and impairs adequate visualization of the vocal cords with direct laryngoscopy. In this rare situation, awake fiberoptic intubation may be helpful. If a CT scan demonstrates a very narrow tracheal lumen (i.e., less than 1 cm diameter), it would be prudent to discuss the findings with the anesthesiologist prior to induction so that a smaller size endotracheal tube and a rigid bronchoscope are available should it be difficult to pass the endotracheal tube through the narrowest portion of the lumen. The great vessels, such as the internal jugular vein, innominate vein, carotid artery, innominate artery, and aorta, may be displaced in up to 50% of patients with substernal goiters.[83] Such information is important in planning for the potential need for sternotomy to safely remove the goiter without a major vascular complication. Most substernal goiters can be removed safely through a transcervical approach. However, those that extend well below the aortic arch or into the posterior mediastinum (**Fig. 6.2**) or encase the great vessels are best removed through a sternotomy.

Evaluation and Management of Toxic Goiters

In the evaluation of toxic goiters, it is important to differentiate between hyperthyroidism and thyrotoxicosis. Thyrotoxicosis is a condition in which circulating levels of the thyroid hormones thyroxine (T_4) and triiodothyronine (T_3) are elevated. Hyperthyroidism is a condition in which elevation of serum T_4 and T_3 levels is due to sustained overproduction and release of thyroid hormones by the thyroid gland. **Table 6.1** lists various etiologies of thyrotoxicosis. A toxic goiter is an enlarged thyroid associated with hyperthyroidism. It can manifest with overt clinical symptoms, such as anxiety, palpitations, tremor, weight loss, insomnia, and heat intolerance. Elderly patients may present with con-

gestive heart failure or atrial fibrillation. Very rarely, elderly patients with hyperthyroidism can present with apathetic thyrotoxicosis, where they appear frail, significantly wasted, depressed, and myxedematous. Loose bowel movement, which is a frequent complaint in young hyperthyroid patients, is a rare complaint in elderly patients with hyperthyroidism. Rather, those who normally have chronic constipation may note that their bowel movements are more normal. In severe, uncontrolled hyperthyroidism thyroid storm can precipitate, the manifestations of which are severe arrhythmias, hyperthermia, agitation, pulmonary edema, and cardiovascular collapse.

Surgeons who are evaluating a "hyperthyroid" patient for thyroidectomy need to review the thyroid function tests and confirm that the patient truly has hyperthyroidism and not thyrotoxicosis secondary to nonhyperthyroid causes. **Table 6.2** summarizes typical laboratory findings that are seen with some of the different causes of thyrotoxicosis. As shown in **Tables 6.1** and **6.2**, many causes of thyrotoxicosis are not due to hyperthyroidism. For example, because T_4 and T_3 are tightly bound to proteins, medications such as estrogen replacement and oral contraceptives can increase the level of

Table 6.2 Typical Laboratory Findings Seen with Different Causes of Thyrotoxicosis

Cause	Total T_4 and T_3 Levels	TSH
Clinical hyperthyroidism	Elevated	Low
Subclinical hyperthyroidism	Normal or slightly elevated	Low
Subacute thyroiditis (initial phase)	Normal or elevated	Low
Medications that increase binding proteins	Elevated	Normal
Excess intake of exogenous thyroid hormone	Slightly elevated	Low
TSH producing pituitary tumor	Elevated	Elevated

binding proteins and result in elevated total T_4 and T_3 levels; however, the free T_4 and TSH levels are actually normal, and the patient does not have hyperthyroidism. Another cause of elevated T_4 and T_3 is a TSH-secreting pituitary adenoma, an extremely rare entity, where the TSH is also elevated. Thus the diagnosis of hyperthyroidism is not made based on elevated total T_4 and T_3 levels but rather is made based on a low TSH level, and serum T_4 and T_3 levels provide information on the degree of the hyperthyroidism. A low TSH with elevated T_4 and T_3 levels is consistent with the diagnosis of hyperthyroidism. Subclinical hyperthyroidism is where the TSH level is suppressed but the T_4 and T_3 values are within normal range, and the patient rarely has any symptoms of hyperthyroidism. Two other conditions should also be considered in the differential diagnosis when the TSH is low and T_4 and T_3 are suppressed: (1) overmedication with thyroxine replacement (thyrotoxicosis factitia), which is easily diagnosed by reviewing the patient's medication history; and (2) transient thyrotoxicosis resulting from thyroiditis (see Inflammatory Thyroid Conditions, later in chapter).

Once the diagnosis of hyperthyroidism is established, the next diagnostic step is to differentiate its etiology, which is important in treatment selection and planning. The causes of hyperthyroidism are toxic adenomatous nodule, Graves disease (toxic diffuse goiter), and toxic multinodular goiter. A thyroid uptake scan is helpful in differentiating these three conditions. The scan should be obtained prior to initiating therapy with antithyroid medications, which interferes with the uptake of the radioisotope by the gland. A toxic adenomatous nodule is seen on the uptake scan as a single hot nodule, usually with very little uptake in the remainder of the gland, indicative of its suppression. Graves disease is an autoimmune disorder with hyperthyroidism resulting from sustained stimulation of the thyroid gland by immunoglobulins. The diagnosis of Graves disease can be made clinically by laboratory studies or nuclear scintigraphy. The clinical diagnosis of Graves disease can be made when at least two of the three manifestations of this disease—hyperthyroidism, ophthalmopathy, and dermopathy—are present. An elevated serum thyroid-stimulating immunoglobulin (TSI) also helps confirm the diagnosis, though it is not always elevated. A thyroid uptake scan is also helpful in establishing the diagnosis and will demonstrate diffuse increased uptake, often greater than 40% in 24 hours. The appearance of a toxic multinodular goiter on nuclear scintigraphy is heterogeneous uptake with multiple hyperfunctioning and hypofunctioning areas, and the 24-hour uptake is above the normal range but not as high as that of a Graves gland.

Untreated hyperthyroidism in the elderly can potentially result in life-threatening complications and therefore warrants prompt management. The treatment of clinically overt hyperthyroidism depends on the severity of the symptoms, the etiology, and the patient's age. Treatment options include medications, radioiodine treatment with iodine 131 (I-131), or thyroidectomy. In general, if the patient has overt hyperthyroidism, medications are initiated to decrease the production of thyroid hormones. The two most commonly used medications are in the class of thionamides: propylthiouracil (PTU) 100 to 300 mg/day divided three times daily, and methimazole (Tapazole) 10 to 40 mg/day divided twice or three times daily. A potentially fatal complication with the use of this class of drugs is agranulocytosis, the incidence of which fortunately is less than 0.5%. Other side effects of thionamides are generally minor and include rash, arthralgia, myalgia, neuritis, and hypothyroidism. If the patient has palpitations and tachycardia, a beta-blocker may be added. Propranolol is generally the preferred beta-blocker, because unlike other beta-blockers, it has some inhibitory effect on peripheral conversion of the inactive thyroid hormone T_4 to the active hormone T_3. Because propranolol is a nonselective beta-blocker, a contraindication to its use is the presence of restrictive pulmonary disease, such as asthma. Once the patient's thyrotoxicosis improves with medications, the long-term management can be determined. Because remission is achieved in approximately one third of Graves disease patients treated with thionamides, continuing the pharmacotherapy with close monitoring for side effects is one option. I-131 is a highly effective treatment for Graves disease.[92,93] However, some young patients, especially women of childbearing age, prefer thyroidectomy over I-131. In the elderly, thyroidectomy is generally performed for failed I-131 treatment or the presence of a malignant nodule. The relapse rate for treating toxic multinodular goiters with pharmacotherapy is high. Takats and colleagues[92] compared the efficacy of antithyroid medications to I-131 for treatment of toxic multinodular goiter, and reported a 46% relapse rate with methimazole treatment because of noncompliance or dose reduction by the physician.[13] They preferred I-131 or thyroidectomy as the definitive treatment for toxic multinodular goiter. Although I-131 can be effective for treatment of toxic goiters, a larger dose than what is conventionally used to treat Graves disease is generally necessary. In the same study by Takats and colleagues 79% of those treated with high doses of I-131 achieved euthyroidism, whereas 21% required re-treatment or continuation of methimazole. Furthermore, when low doses of I-131 were used, only 29% achieved euthyroidism and 64% required re-treatment. The authors also stressed that if I-131 is to be used for treatment of toxic nodular goiters, the goal should be to use high doses to achieve hypothyroidism, which can be controlled with thyroxine replacement, rather than trying to achieve euthyroidism because of the significant risk of relapse. In young patients with toxic nodular goiters who are low anesthesia risks, excellent results can also be achieved with surgery, and therefore is a good alterative to high-dose I-131 therapy. Surgery is best for the patient with toxic multinodular goiters if compressive symptoms or cold nodules are present. In elderly patients, I-131 has been the preferred treatment for toxic goiters, because they frequently have comorbidities that increase their risk of perioperative complications. The indications for thyroidectomy in elderly patients with toxic multinodular goiter include very large goiters with significant tracheal compression, the presence of a large or cold nodule that may be suspicious for malignancy, failed I-131 treatment, and patient preference. Whether the treatment of choice is I-131 or thyroidectomy, it is preferable to first treat the patient with thionamides so that the patient becomes euthyroid, or close to euthyroid, to reduce the risk of developing thyroid storm from the surgery or I-131. When operating on patients with Graves disease, an iodine preparation such as Lugol solution (5 to 10 drops t.i.d.) or saturated solution of potassium iodide (SSKI) (100–200 mg t.i.d.) can be started approximately 10 days preoperatively to decrease the vascularity of the gland and help achieve a euthyroid state.

Toxic adenomatous nodules are more common in younger patients. A young asymptomatic patient with a toxic nodule can be observed. In a young symptomatic patient, the preferred treatment is hemithyroidectomy. It is better to institute some form of treatment in an older patient with a toxic nodule because of the risk of potential complications, such as cardiac arrhythmias and osteoporosis. In the elderly patient, the treatment options are thionamides, I-131, or surgery, depending on the patient's preference and anesthesia risk.

Whether or not subclinical hyperthyroidism should be treated has been a topic of considerable controversy. The natural history of untreated subclinical hyperthyroidism is variable and appears to depend on the etiology. The suppressed TSH in Graves disease with subclinical thyroidism tends to return to normal levels with time; however, it often will remain elevated if the etiology is toxic multinodular goiter.[94] In elderly patients, persistent subnormal TSH levels can be associated with increased risk of cardiac complications and fractures. Therefore, it would seem prudent to treat subclinical hyperthyroidism in this age group; however, no controlled prospective studies have provided evidence to support this approach. In a recent survey of endocrinologists, 84% recommended observation rather than active treatment for a young patient with a low but detectable serum TSH level and 58% recommended observation alone for undetectable serum TSH level. For an older woman with a low but detectable serum TSH value, 63% recommended observation; however, 66% favored treatment if the serum TSH is undetectable.[95] These opinions are also consistent with the recommendations of the ATA Guidelines Task Force of 2005.[69]

Inflammatory Thyroid Conditions

Thyroiditis can be classified as (1) chronic thyroiditis, which encompasses Hashimoto thyroiditis and Riedel struma; (2) subacute, which includes granulomatous and lymphocytic painless thyroiditis: and (3) acute suppurative, which is exceedingly rare.

Hashimoto Thyroiditis

By far the most common of all inflammatory thyroid disorders, Hashimoto thyroiditis affects approximately 2% of the general population. It is an autoimmune disease, and a close association with the human leukocyte antigen (HLA) system, most frequently HLA-DR5, HLA-DR3, and HLA-DRB8, has been demonstrated.[96] Histologically, the gland is infiltrated with a polymorphous population of lymphocytes, and destruction of thyroid follicles and formation of lymphoid follicles is seen. Unlike painless lymphocytic thyroiditis (see below), oxyphilic (Hürthle cell) changes and areas of glandular fibrosis are also seen. The clinical presentation varies, depending on the stage at the time of presentation. The patient may be completely asymptomatic or may present with symptoms of hypothyroidism. The gland is generally enlarged, symmetrical, and finely nodular without any discrete palpable nodules. Rarely, the patient may present with pain and the gland may be tender to palpation, mimicking the clinical features of subacute thyroiditis.[97,98] Thyroid hormone levels also will vary at the time of presentation. They may be normal with a normal TSH (euthyroid), low with an elevated TSH (hypothyroid), or normal with an elevated TSH (subclinically hypothyroid). Thyroglobulin antibodies and antithyroid peroxidase antibodies are often elevated. Thyroid uptake scan shows an irregular pattern of uptake, and the 24-hour uptake may be normal or reveal increased uptake. On thyroid sonography, the gland appears enlarged with innumerable tiny hypoechoic solid nodules and coarse echogenic bands.[25] The clinical course of Hashimoto thyroiditis is variable. Up to 50% of patients can become subclinically hypothyroid, and 5 to 40% can become clinically hypothyroid, emphasizing the importance of following thyroid function tests in these patients.[99–101] Patients with Hashimoto thyroiditis have a higher frequency of other autoimmune disorders, such as adrenal insufficiency, diabetes mellitus, Sjögren syndrome, celiac disease, rheumatoid arthritis, and lupus erythematous. They also have an increased risk of developing B-cell lymphoma of the thyroid.[102–104] Rapid growth in the setting of Hashimoto thyroiditis should alert the clinician to the possibility of thyroid lymphoma.

Subacute Painless Lymphocytic Thyroiditis

There are two forms of painless thyroiditis, sporadic and postpartum, both sharing very similar features. It is characterized by destruction of the thyroid gland by lymphocytes, absence of pain, and temporary thyroid dysfunction. It is much more common in women. The etiology is uncertain, but it is clear that the immune system is involved because it has been found in patients with a wide variety of autoimmune diseases. HLA-DR3 is present in increased frequency in both sporadic and postpartum forms.[105] In addition to HLA-DR3, HLA-DR5 is also increased in frequency in postpartum thyroiditis.[105] Histologically, the gland is prominently infiltrated with lymphocytes, and areas of follicle destruction are prominent.[106] Clinically, the patient typically passes through four phases: thyrotoxic, euthyroid, hypothyroid, and euthyroid. The initial thyrotoxicosis is caused by a release of preformed hormone and not because of sustained overproduction of the hormone, and therefore is not true hyperthyroidism. It typically lasts 3–6 months but may persist for 1 year.[100] Symptoms are generally mild, although in some cases they may be quite severe and require hospitalization. The initial thyrotoxic phase of postpartum thyroiditis is usually milder than sporadic thyroiditis. The gland is usually symmetrical and may be slightly to moderately enlarged. It is completely painless to palpation. Thyroid function tests reflect the degree of hypo- or hyperthyroidism at the time of testing. The thyroglobulin levels are elevated, as are antimicrosomal antibodies. Unlike subacute granulomatous thyroiditis, the erythrocyte sedimentation rate is generally normal. I-131 uptake is low, usually below 5%. Because the hyperthyroid phase of the disease is usually transient and is mild in nature, most patients do not require treatment. If the cardiac symptoms are prominent, they can be controlled with beta-blockers.

Subacute Granulomatous Thyroiditis

Also known as painful thyroiditis and granulomatous thyroiditis, this disorder is characterized by the sudden onset of anterior neck pain, localized over the thyroid gland, which may radiate to one or both ears or jaws. It may be associated with antecedent viral illness. There is a female preponderance. The patients frequently report malaise, weakness, and fatigue as well as symptoms of thyrotoxicosis, such as palpitations, nervousness, tremor, heat intolerance, and weight loss. The most prominent physical finding is an enlarged thyroid gland that is exquisitely tender to palpation. Frequently, patients present with tachycardia and hyperpyrexia, with the temperature elevated up to 102°F. The erythrocyte sedimentation rate is consistently high and the white blood cell count may be elevated. Thyroid function tests may be normal, elevated, or low, depending on the stage of the disease at the time of presentation. Similar to painless thyroiditis, patients go through the initial phases of thyrotoxicosis for 1 to 3 months, which is a result of the release of stored thyroid hormones from acute destruction of the thyroid parenchyma. Subsequent to that they become euthyroid. In severe cases, after returning to the euthyroid state the patient can then develop hypothyroidism, which usually lasts 2 to 6 months. This phase of hypothyroidism is usually transient, with approximately 90% of the patients recovering and returning to an euthyroid state. Pathologically, the thyroid is infiltrated with neutrophils, lymphocytes, and large monocytes. Multinuclear giant cells with granuloma formation are also seen. Thyroid follicles become hyperplastic, and areas of follicular disruption are seen. In the late stage of the disease, follicular regeneration is evident with only minimal fibrosis.

Acute Suppurative Thyroiditis

This rare entity usually occurs from a bacterial infection, and rarely from nonbacterial infections of the thyroid. It tends to affect a younger age group, the 30- to 40-year age range, and not infrequently affects children. Infection may reach the gland via blood, lymphatics, or directly through a persistent thyroglossal duct or a nearby internal fistula such as a piriform sinus fistula. History of an antecedent infection, such as pharyngitis can frequently be elicited. Patients typically present with symptoms very similar to those of subacute thyroiditis, in that there is usually anterior neck pain and fever. The patient may experience dysphagia, and, if left untreated, may progress to dyspnea. Physical findings include tenderness over the thyroid with localized erythema and warmth. Pyriform sinus fistula is a common finding in children.[107] The white blood cell count is usually elevated. The bacterial pathogens are staphylococcus, streptococcus, and a variety of gram-negative organisms, particularly oral pathogens.[108–110] Nonbacterial infection of the thyroid gland is very rare, which can result from *Aspergillus, Coccidioides immitis,* and *Candida.*[108] Treatment consists of appropriate antimicrobial therapy and analgesics.

Riedel Struma

Also known as invasive fibrous thyroiditis, this exceedingly rare disorder is characterized by intense infiltration of the thyroid parenchyma by inflammatory cells and subsequent replacement by dense fibrosis and collagen.[111] It is not a primary disorder of the thyroid but involves the thyroid and represents part of a systemic disease. It may affect only the thyroid gland, or also involve other sites such as the mediastinum, retroperitoneum, orbit, and biliary tract. It generally affects women in the fourth to fifth decade of life. Patients typically present with a painless thyroid mass that feels hard and fixed. With time the fibrosis extends beyond the thyroid capsule and infiltrates into the surrounding structures, including the strap muscles. Vasculitis and phlebitis may also be seen. Thyroid function tests reflect euthyroidism in approximately two thirds of the patients; however, they may also reflect hypothyroidism when the gland is sufficiently replaced by the fibroid tissue. The clinical presentation may be confused with that of an aggressive thyroid malignancy such as anaplastic carcinoma. Imaging studies and FNA can help differentiate the two. Unlike the CT findings of most thyroid malignancies, the thyroid gland with Riedel appears as an infiltrative mass that is isodense with the neck muscles, hypodense with the normal thyroid tissue, and does not enhance with contrast.[112] This condition is benign and usually self-limiting. However, as it progresses and encases the trachea, the patient may develop dyspnea. If symptomatic, a wedge resection of the isthmus and insertion of tracheotomy can be performed. High-dose glucocorticoid and levothyroxine treatment has been reported to be effective for reducing the symptoms from Riedel.[113] Tamoxifen therapy has also been shown to be effective in reducing the mass effect on the airway.[114,115]

Conclusion

The suggestions made in this chapter are general recommendations based on information from the literature and should be interpreted as such. Management decisions should be individualized based on the patient's clinical situation and the clinician's experience.

References

1. Vanderpump MP, Tunbridge WM, French JM, et al. The incidence of thyroid disorders in the community: a twenty-year follow-up of the Whickham Survey. Clin Endocrinol (Oxf) 1995;43:55–68

2. Mortensen JD, Woolner LB, Bennett WA. Gross and microscopic findings in clinically normal thyroid glands. J Clin Endocrinol 1955;15:1270–1280

3. Mazzaferri EL. Management of the solitary thyroid nodule. N Engl J Med 1993;328:553–558

4. Lin J-D, Chao T-Z, Huang B-Y, Chen S-T, Chang H-Y, Hsueh C. Thyroid cancer in the thyroid nodules evaluated by ultrasonography and fine-needle aspiration cytology. Thyroid 2005;15:708–717

5. Cooper DS, Doherty GM, Haugen BR, et al. Management guidelines for patients with thyroid nodules and differentiated thyroid cancer. Thyroid 2006;16:109–142

6. Hegedus L. Clinical practice. The thyroid nodule. N Engl J Med 2004;351:1764–1771

7. Wong CKM. Thyroid nodules: rational management. World J Surg 2000;24:934–941

8. Roman SA. Endocrine tumors: evaluation of the thyroid nodule. Curr Opin Oncol 2003;15:66–70

9. Favus MJ, Schneider AB, Stachura ME, et al. Thyroid cancer occurring as a late consequence of head and neck irradiation: evaluation of 1,056 patients. N Engl J Med 1976;294:1019–1025

10. Sklar C, Whitton J, Mertens A, et al. Abnormalities of the thyroid in survivors of Hodgkin's disease; data from the childhood cancer survivor study. J Clin Endocrinol Metab 2000;85:3227–3232

11. Curtis RE, Rowlings PA, Deeg HJ, et al. Solid cancers after bone marrow transplantation. N Engl J Med 1997;336:897–904

12. Cohen A, Rovelli A, VanLint MT, et al. Secondary thyroid carcinoma after allogenic bone marrow transplantation during childhood. Bone Marrow Transplant 2001;28:1125–1128

13. Heidenreich WF, Bogdanova TI, Biryukov AG, Tronko ND. Time trends of thyroid cancer incidence in Ukraine after the Chernobyl accident. J Radiol Prot 2004;24:283–293

14. Pacini F, Volrontsova T, Demidchik E, et al. Post-Chernobyl thyroid carcinoma in Belarus children and adolescents: comparison with naturally occurring thyroid carcinoma in Italy and France. J Clin Endocrinol Metab 1997;82:3563–3569

15. Williams ED, Abrosimov A, Bogdanova T, et al. Thyroid carcinoma after Chernobyl latent period, morphology and aggressiveness. Br J Cancer 2004;90:2219–2224

16. Lee S, Hong SW, Shin SJ, et al. Papillary thyroid carcinoma associated with familial adenomatous polyposis: molecular analysis of pathogenesis in a family and review of the literature. Endocr J 2004;51:317–323

17. Alsanea O, Clark OH. Familial thyroid cancer. Curr Opin Oncol 2001;13:44–51

18. Harach HR, Soubeyran I, Brown A, Bonneau D, Longy M. Thyroid pathologic findings in patients with Cowden disease. Ann Diagn Pathol 1999;3:331–340

19. Stratakis CA, Kirschner LS, Carney JA. Clinical and molecular features of the Carney complex: diagnostic criteria and recommendations for patient evaluation. J Clin Endocrinol Metab 2001;86:4041–4046

20. Fugazzola L, Cerutti N, Mannavola D, et al. Differential diagnosis between Pendred and pseudo-Pendred syndromes: clinical, radiologic, and molecular studies. Pediatr Res 2002;51:479–484

21. Kuma K, Matsuzuka F, Yokozawa T. Fate of untreated benign thyroid nodules: results of long term follow up. World J Surg 1994;18:495–498

22. Marqusee E, Benson CB, Frates MC, et al. Usefulness of ultrasonography in the management of nodular thyroid disease. Ann Intern Med 2000;133:696–700

23. Weiss RE, Lado-Abeal J. Thyroid nodules: diagnosis and therapy. Curr Opin Oncol 2002;14:46–52

24. Ezzat S, Sarti DA, Cain DR, Braunstein GD. Thyroid incidentalomas. Prevalence by palpation and ultrasonography. Arch Intern Med 1994;154:1838–1840

25. Reading CC, Charboneau JW, Hay ID, Sebo TJ. Sonography of thyroid nodules: A "classic pattern" diagnostic approach. Ultrasound Q 2005;21:157–165

26. Seiberling KA, Dutra JC, Grant T, Bajramovic S. Role of intrathyroidal calcifications as a marker of malignancy. Laryngoscope 2004;114:1753–1757

27. Ravetto C, Columbo L, Dottorini ME. Usefulness of fine-needle aspiration in the diagnosis of thyroid carcinoma. A retrospective study of 37,895 patients. Cancer 2000;90:357–363

28. Raab SS, Silvereman JF, Elsheikh TM, Thomas PA, Wakely PE. Disease demographics and clinical management as determined by fine needle aspiration biopsy. Pediatrics 1995;95:46–49

29. Corrias A, Einaudi S, Chiorboli E, et al. Accuracy of fine needle aspiration biopsy of thyroid nodules in detecting malignancy in childhood: comparison with conventional clinical, laboratory and imaging approaches. J Clin Endocrinol Metab 2001;86:4644–4648

30. Halac I, Zimmerman D. Thyroid nodules and cancers in children. Endocrinol Metab Clin North Am 2005;34:725–744

31. Vini L, Hyer S, Marshall J, A' Hern R, Harmer C. Long-term results in elderly patients with differentiated thyroid carcinoma. Cancer 2003;97:2736–2742

32. Hundahl SA, Cady B, Cunningham MP, et al. Initial results from a prospective cohort study of 5583 cases of thyroid carcinoma treated in the United States during 1996. Cancer 2000;89:202–217

33. Silver RJ, Parangi S. Management of thyroid incidentalomas. Surg Clin North Am 2004;84:907–919

34. Newkirk KA, Ringel MD, Jelinek J, et al. Ultrasound-guided fine-needle aspiration and thyroid disease. Otolaryngol Head Neck Surg 2000;123:700–705

35. Danese D, Sciacchitano S, Farsetti A, Andreoli M, Pontecorvi A. Diagnostic accuracy of conventional versus sonography-guided fine-needle aspiration biopsy of thyroid nodules. Thyroid 1998;8:15–21

36. Baloch ZW, Tam D, Langer J, Mandel S, LiVolsi VA, Gupta PK. 2000 Ultrasound-guided fine-needle aspiration biopsy of the thyroid: role of on-site assessment and multiple cytologic preparations. Diagn Cytopathol 2000;23:425–429

37. Yang GC, Liebeskind D, Messina AV. Ultrasound-guided fine-needle aspiration of the thyroid assessed by ultrafast Papanicolaou stain: data from 1135 biopsies with a two-to six-year follow-up. Thyroid 2001;11:581–589

38. Baloch ZW, Fleisher S, LiVolsi VA, Gupta PK. Diagnosis of "follicular neoplasm": a gray zone in thyroid fine-needle aspiration cytology. Diagn Cytopathol 2002;26:41–44

39. Sclabas GM, Staerkel GA, Shapiro SE, et al. Fine-needle aspiration of the thyroid and correlation with histopathology in a contemporary series of 240 patients. Am J Surg 2003;186:702–709

40. Goldstein RE, Netterville JL, Burkey B, Johnson JE. Implications of follicular neoplasms, atypia and lesions suspicious for malignancy diagnosed by fine-needle aspiration of thyroid nodules. Ann Surg 2002;235:656–662

41. Shindo ML, Tanzella F. Thyroid diseases in the elderly. In: Calhoune KE, Eibling DE, eds. Geriatric Otolaryngology. New York: Marcel Dekker, 2006:491–500

42. De los Santos ET, Keyhani-Rofaga S, Cunningham JJ, Mazzaferi EL. Cystic thyroid nodules: the dilemma of malignant lesions. Arch Intern Med 1990;150:1422–1427

43. Monchik JM, De Petris G, De Crea C. Occult papillary carcinoma of the thyroid presenting as a cervical cyst. Surgery 2001;129:429–432

44. Abbas G, Heller KS, Khoynezhad A, et al. The incidence of carcinoma in cytologically benign thyroid cysts. Surgery 2001;130:1035–1038

45. Hatabu H, Kasagi K, Yamamoto K, et al. Cystic papillary carcinoma of the thyroid gland: a new sonographic sign. Clin Radiol 1991;43:121–124

46. Massoll N, Nizam MS, Mazzaferri EL. Cystic thyroid nodules: diagnostic and therapeutic dilemmas. Endocrinologist 2002;12:185–198

47. Braga M, Cavalcanti TC, Collaco LM, Graf H. Efficacy of ultrasound-guided fine-needle aspiration biopsy in the diagnosis of complex thyroid nodules. J Clin Endocrinol Metab 2001;86:4089–4091

48. Meko JB, Norton JA. Large cystic/solid thyroid nodules: a potential false-negative fine-needle aspiration. Surgery 1995;118:996–1003

49. Nakagawa T, Takashima T, Tomiyama K. Differential diagnosis of a lateral cervical cyst and solitary cystic lymph node metastasis of occult thyroid papillary carcinoma. J Laryngol Otol 2001;115:240–242

50. Hegedus L, Bonnema SJ, Bennedbaek FN. Management of simple nodular goiter: current status and future perspectives. Endocr Rev 2003;24:102–132

51. Brix TH, Hegedüs L. 2000 Genetic and environmental factors in the aetiology of simple goitre. Ann Med 2000;32:153–156

52. Medeiros-Neto G. Iodine deficiency disorders. In: deGroot LJ, Jameson JL, eds. Endocrinology. Philadelphia: WB Saunders, 2000:1529–1539

53. Gaitan E. Goitrogens in food and water. Annu Rev Nutr 1990;10:21–39

54. Bertelsen JB, Hegedus L. Cigarette smoking and the thyroid. Thyroid 1994;4:327–331

55. Brix TH, Hansen PS, Kyvic KO, Hegedus L. Cigarette smoking and the risk of overt thyroid disease. Arch Intern Med 2000;160:661–666

56. Surks MI, Sievert R. Drugs and thyroid function. N Engl J Med 1995;333:1688–1694

57. Orenstein H, Peskind A, Raskind MA. Thyroid disorders in female psychiatric patients with panic disorder or agoraphobia. Am J Psychiatry 1988;145:1428–1430

58. Neumann S, Willgerodt H, Ackermann F, et al. Linkage of familial euthyroid goiter to the multinodular goiter-1 locus and exclusion of the candidate genes thyroglobulin, thyroperoxidase and Na+/I-symporter. J Clin Endocrinol Metab 1999;84:3750–3756

59. Bignell GR, Canzian F, Shayeghi M, et al. Familial nontoxic multinodular thyroid goiter locus maps to chromosome 14q but does not account for familial nonmedullary thyroid cancer. Am J Hum Genet 1997;61:1123–1130

60. Tomer Y, Barbesino G, Keddache M, Greenberg DA, Davies TF. Mapping of a major susceptibility locus for Graves' disease (GD-1) to chromosome 14q31. J Clin Endocrinol Metab 1997;82:1645–1648

61. Capon F, Tacconelli A, Giardina E, et al. Mapping a dominant form of multinodular goiter to chromosome Xp22. Am J Hum Genet 2000;67:1004–1007

62. Gabriel EM, Bergert ER, Grant CS, van Hardeen JA, Thompson GB, Morris JC. Germline polymorphism of codon 727 of human thyroid stimulating hormone receptor is associated with toxic multinodular goiter. J Clin Endocrinol Metab 1999;84:3328–3335

63. Smyth PPA, McMullan NM, Grubeck-Loebenstein B, et al. Thyroid growth-stimulating immunoglobulins in goitrous disease: relationship to thyroid stimulating immunoglobulins. Acta Endocrinol (Copenh) 1986;111:321–330

64. Yaturu S, McDonald J. Levels of soluble human leukocyte antigen class 1 are increased in Graves' disease and toxic multinodular goiter and correlate with the levels of triiodothyronine. Thyroid 2002;12:679–682

65. Tamura M, Kimura H, Koji T, et al. Role of apoptosis of thyrocytes in a rat model of goiter. A possible involvement of Fas system. Endocrinology 1998;139:3646–3653

66. Elte JW, Bussemaker JK, Haak A. The natural history of euthyroid multinodular goitre. Postgrad Med J 1990;66:186–190

67. Berghout A, Wiersinga WM, Drexhage HA, Smits NJ, Touber LJ. Comparison of placebo with L-thyroxine alone or the carbimazole for treatment of non-toxic goiter. Lancet 1990;336:193–197

68. Chin SC, Rice H, Som PM. Spread of goiters outside the thyroid bed. Arch Otolaryngol Head Neck Surg 2003;129:1198–1202

69. Bonnema SJ, Bennedbaek FN, Ladenson PW, Hegedus L. Management of the non-toxic multinodular goiter: a North American survey. J Clin Endocrinol Metab 2002;87:112–117

70. Guglielmi R, Pacella C, Bianchini A, et al. Percutaneous ethanol injection treatment in benign thyroid lesions: role and efficacy. Thyroid 2004;14:125–131

71. Zingrillo M, Torlantano M, Chiarella R, et al. Percutaneous ethanol injection may be a definitive treatment for symptomatic thyroid cystic nodules not treatable by surgery: Five-year follow-up study. Thyroid 1999;9:763–767

72. Del Prete S, Caraglia D, Vitale G, et al. Percutaneous ethanol injection efficacy in the treatment of large symptomatic thyroid cystic nodules: ten-year follow-up of large series. Thyroid 2002;12:815–821

73. Lee SJ, Ahn IM. Effectiveness of percutaneous ethanol injection therapy in benign nodular and cystic thyroid diseases: long-term follow-up experience. Endocr J 2005;52:455–462

74. Valcavi R, Frasoldati A. Ultrasound-guided percutaneous ethanol injection therapy in thyroid cystic nodules. Endocr Pract 2004;10:269–275

75. Zielezник W, Kawczyk-Krupka A, Barlik MP, Cebula W, Sieron A. Modified percutaneous ethanol injection in the treatment of viscous cystic thyroid nodules. Thyroid 2005;15:683–684

76. Freitas JE. Therapeutic options in the management of toxic and nontoxic nodular goiter. Semin Nucl Med 2000;30:88–97

77. Kunori T, Shinya H, Satomi T, et al. Management of nodular goiters and their operative indications. Surg Today 2000;30:722–726

78. Lahey FH, Swinton MW. Intrathoracic goiter. Surg Gynecol Obstet 1934;59:627–637

79. Reeves TS, Rubinstein C, Rundle FF, et al. The investigation and arrangement of intrathoracic goiter. Surg Gynecol Obstet 1962;115:223–229

80. Reeves TS, Rubinstein C, Rundle FF. Intrathoracic goiter: its prevalence in Sydney metropolitan mass x-ray surveys. Med J Aust 1957;2:148–152

81. Higgins CC. Intrathoracic goiter. Arch Surg 1927;15:895–912

82. Cohen JP, Cho HT. Surgery for substernal goiter. In: Freidman M, ed. Operative Techniques in Otolaryngology and Head and Neck Surgery. Philadelphia: WB Saunders, 1994:118–125

83. Netterville JL, Coleman SC, Smith JC, Smith MM, Day TA, Burkey BB. Management of substernal goiter. Laryngoscope 1998;108:1611–1617

84. Newman E, Shaha AR. Substernal goiter. J Surg Oncol 1995;60:207–212

85. Pulli RS, Coniglio JU. Surgical management of the substernal thyroid gland. Laryngoscope 1998;108:358–361

86. Torre G, Borgonovo G, Amato A, et al. Surgical management of substernal goiter: analysis of 237 patients. Am Surg 1995;61:826–831

87. Sanders LE, Rossi RL, Shahian DM, Williamson WA. Mediastinal goiters: the need for an aggressive approach. Arch Surg 1992;127:609–613

88. Singh B, Lucente FE, Shaha AR. Substernal goiter: a clinical review. Am J Otolaryngol 1994;15:409–416

89. Wesche MF, Tiel V, Buul MM, Lips P, Smits MJ, Wiersinga WM. A randomized trial comparing levothyroxine and radioactive iodine in the treatment of sporadic nontoxic goiter. Clin Endocrinol Metab 2001;86:998–1005

90. Nygaard B, Faber J, Hegedus L, Hansen JM. 131I treatment of nontoxic nodular goitre. Eur J Endocrinol 1996;134:15–20

91. Le Moli R, Wesche MF, Tiel-Van Buul MM, Wiersinga WM. Determinants of longterm outcome of radioiodine therapy of sporadic non-toxic goitre. Clin Endocrinol (Oxf) 1999;50:783–789

92. Takats KI, Szabolcs I, Foldes J, et al. The efficacy of long term thyrostatic treatment in elderly patients with toxic nodular goiter compared to radioiodine therapy with different doses. Exp Clin Endocrinol Diabetes 1999;107:70–74

93. Kok SW, Smit JW, De Craen AJM, Goslings BM, Van Eck-Smit BLF, Romijn JA. Clinical outcome after standardized versus dosimetric radioiodine treatment of hyperthyroidism: an equivalence study. Nucl Med Commun 2000;21:1071–1078

94. Woeber KA. Observations concerning the natural history of subclinical hyperthyroidism. Thyroid 2005;15:687–691

95. McDermott MT, Woodmansee WW, Haugen BR, Smart A, Ridgway EC. The management of subclinical hyperthyroidism by thyroid specialists. Thyroid 2003;13:1133–1139

96. Weetman AP. Autoimmune thyroiditis; predisposition and pathogenesis. Clin Endocrinol (Oxf) 1992;36:307–323

97. Shigemasa C, Ueta Y, Mitani Y, et al. Chronic thyroiditis with painful tender thyroid enlargement and transient thyrotoxicosis. J Clin Endocrinol Metab 1990;70:385–390

98. Ishihara T, Mori T, Waseda N, Ikekubo K, Akamizu T, Imura H. Histological, clinical and laboratory findings of acute exacerbation of Hashimoto's thyroiditis-comparison with those of subacute granulomatous thyroiditis. Endocrinol Jpn 1987;34:831–841

99. Hayashi Y, Tamai H, Fukata S, et al. A long term clinical, immunological and histological follow-up study of patients with goitrous chronic lymphocytic thyroiditis. J Clin Endocrinol Metab 1985;61:1172–1178

100. Woolf PD. Thyroiditis. In: Falk SA, ed. Thyroid Disease. Philadelphia: Lippincott-Raven, 1997:393–410

101. Maenpaa J, Raatikka M, Rasanen J, Taskenen E, Wagner O. Natural course of juvenile autoimmune thyroiditis. J Pediatr 1985;107:898–904

102. Holm LE, Blomgreh H, Lowhagen T. Cancer risks in patients with chronic lymphocytic thyroiditis. N Engl J Med 1985;312:601–604

103. Matsuzuka F, Kuma K, Tomingaga S. Chronic thyroiditis as a risk factor of B-cell lymphoma in the thyroid gland. Jpn J Cancer Res 1985;76:1085–1090

104. Rizvi AA. Primary thyroid lymphoma: review of clinical features and diagnostic evaluation. Endocrinologist 2004;14:144–147

105. Farid NR, Hawe BS, Walfish PG. Increased frequency of HLA-DR3 and 5 in the syndromes of painless thyroiditis and transient thyrotoxicosis: evidence for an autoimmune aetiology. Clin Endocrinol (Oxf) 1983;19:699–704

106. Mizukami Y, Michigishi T, Nonomura A, et al. Postpartum thyroiditis. A clinical, histologic and immunologic study of 15 cases. Am J Clin Pathol 1993;100:200–205

107. Miyauchi A, Matsuzuka F, Kuma K, Takai S. Piriform sinus fistula: an underlying abnormality common in patients with acute suppurative thyroiditis. World J Surg 1990;14:400–405

108. Berger SA, Zonszein J, Villamena P, Mittman N. Infectious diseases of the thyroid gland. Rev Infect Dis 1983;5:108–122

109. Jeng LB, Lai JB, Chen MF. Acute suppurative thyroiditis: a 10-year review in a Taiwanese hospital. Scand J Infect Dis 1994;26:297–300

110. Musharrafieh UM, Nassar NT, Azar ST. Acute suppurative thyroiditis: a forgotten entity: case report and literature review. Endocrinologist 2002;12:173–177

111. Schwaegerle SM, Bauer TW, Esselstyn CB. Riedel's thyroiditis. Am J Clin Pathol 1988;90:715–722

112. Ozgen A, Cila A. Riedel's thyroiditis in multifocal fibrosclerosis: CT and MR imaging findings. AJNR Am J Neuroradiol 2000;21:320–321

113. Lo JC, Loh K, Rubin AL, et al. Riedel's thyroiditis presenting with hypothyroidism and hypoparathyroidism: dramatic response to glucocorticoid and thyroxine therapy. Clin Endocrinol (Oxf) 1998;48:815–818

114. Few J, Thompson NW, Angelos P, et al. Riedel's thyroiditis: treatment with tamoxifen. Surgery 1996;120:993–999

115. Pritchyk K, Newkirk K, Garlich P, Deeb Z. Tamoxifen therapy for Riedel's thyroiditis. Laryngoscope 2004;114:1758–1760

7 Medical Management of Benign Thyroid Diseases

Matthew I. Kim and Ralph P. Tufano

Goiter

A suspected goiter should be evaluated with a dedicated ultrasound to determine (1) if there is any definable enlargement of one or both lobes, and (2) if definable enlargement has been caused by diffuse expansion of tissue or the aggregate growth of multiple nodules.[1] A patient with significant redundant skin and soft tissue in the lower anterior region of the neck who appears to have a goiter may prove to have a normal sized thyroid on ultrasound. This presentation, which may be classified as a pseudogoiter, does not require any specific attention beyond reassurance. Laboratory tests that should be checked to characterize the status of a goiter include (1) thyroid-stimulating hormone (TSH), levothyroxine (T_4), and triiodothyronine (T_3) levels to distinguish between functional hypothyroid, thyrotoxic, and euthyroid states (**Table 7.1**); and (2) antithyroid peroxidase and antithyroglobulin antibody titers to determine whether autoimmune thyroiditis is present. Characterization of a goiter as diffuse or nodular in tandem with delineation of its functional and autoimmune status may help to guide the course of evaluation focused on the identification and treatment of specific disorders.

Diffuse Goiter

Hypothyroid

The most common underlying cause of a diffuse goiter presenting with hypothyroidism in the United States is chronic lymphocytic thyroiditis. This disorder, also known as Hashimoto thyroiditis, is an autoimmune condition characterized by lymphocytic infiltration and destruction of thyroid tissue that compromises the synthesis and secretion of normal amounts of T_4 and T_3. This in turn leads to increased secretion of TSH from the pituitary that may stimulate growth and expansion of residual functioning thyroid tissue. Ultrasound often reveals a diffuse heterogeneous echotexture extending throughout both lobes.[2] Care must be taken to ensure that foci of heterogeneity identified on ultrasound are distinguished from discrete nodules that may also be present. Confirmation of a suspected diagnosis of chronic lymphocytic thyroiditis relies on the detection of elevated antithyroid antibody titers. Antithyroid peroxidase antibody titers have proven to be the most sensitive and specific indicators in this setting.[3] Treatment is based on providing adequate thyroid hormone replacement in the form of levothyroxine administered orally in doses targeted to normalize TSH levels.[4] Levothyroxine is available in doses ranging from 25 to 300 μg. A healthy young adult can usually be started on a full replacement dose calculated to provide approximately 0.8 μg/lb of body weight daily. A TSH level should be checked 6 weeks after starting treatment to assess the adequacy of replacement. If a dose needs to be adjusted, a subsequent TSH level should be checked 4 weeks later to assess the impact of the change. A patient with known or suspected atherosclerotic heart disease should be started on a lower dose of 25 to 50 μg daily that can then be gradually increased in 12.5- to 25-μg increments every 2 weeks based on measurement of TSH levels and assessments of tolerance.

A diffuse goiter that develops in association with hypothyroidism detected in a young woman after a recent pregnancy may be a manifestation of postpartum or silent thyroiditis.[5] This represents a more acute form of autoimmune thyroiditis that may develop in 5 to 8% of all women after delivery. It typically progresses through thyrotoxic and hypothyroid phases before resolving over the course of several weeks. Detection of elevated antithyroid antibody titers may confirm a suspected diagnosis. Management should focus on periodic measurement of TSH levels to detect transitions between phases. In particularly severe cases, levothyroxine can be administered in supportive doses on a temporary basis to help alleviate symptoms of hypothyroidism. Up to of 25% of patients may develop permanent hypothyroidism necessitating ongoing treatment with full replacement doses.[6]

In rare instances, underlying iodine deficiency may lead to the development of hypothyroidism associated with a diffuse goiter.[7] Although iodine deficiency has been identified

Table 7.1 Functional States

State	TSH	T_4	T_3
Euthyroid	Normal	Normal*	Normal*
Hypothyroid	Elevated	Decreased**	Decreased**
Thyrotoxic	Decreased	Elevated***	Elevated***

Abbreviation: TSH, thyroid-stimulating hormone.
*Total levels may be elevated in euthyroid hyperthyroxinemic states or decreased in euthyroid hypothyroxinemic states.
**Total and free levels may be normal in subclinical hypothyroid states.
***Total and free levels may be normal in subclinical thyrotoxic states.

as the most common cause of hypothyroidism worldwide, it is relatively rare in the United States due to the addition of iodine to table salt and stabilizers incorporated in baked goods. Most cases are detected in recent immigrants from iodine-deficient regions of the world. A suspected diagnosis can be confirmed by detection of a low urine iodine level.[8] Dietary iodine supplementation provides effective treatment.[9]

Thyrotoxic

Thyrotoxicosis identified in association with a diffuse goiter may be caused by (1) increased synthesis and secretion of thyroid hormone due to underlying Graves disease, or (2) release of stored thyroid hormone precipitated by inflammation characteristic of the thyrotoxic phase of subacute or silent thyroiditis. When feasible, a radionuclide thyroid uptake and scan study should be checked to distinguish between these conditions.[10] Graves disease is characterized by higher than normal quantitative uptake of radionuclide over a defined interval with scan images that demonstrate intense bilateral tracer uptake with definition of a midline pyramidal lobe. Thyroiditis is characterized by low to undetectable quantitative uptake of radionuclide with scan images that show little or no tracer uptake in the region of the thyroid bed.[11] Subacute thyroiditis represents granulomatous inflammation of the thyroid associated with marked tenderness to palpation and localized pain that may progress in a migratory or radiating pattern. It can be distinguished from other forms of thyroiditis by detection of an elevated erythrocyte sedimentation rate (ESR). Treatment should focus on relief of discomfort through administration of acetaminophen at doses of up to 1000 mg four times daily or aspirin at doses of up to 650 mg four times daily. Refractory pain and tenderness may respond to limited courses of treatment with prednisone started at a dose of 40 mg daily and tapered gradually over 4 to 8 weeks. Pronounced hyperadrenergic symptoms associated with the thyrotoxic phase of either form of thyroiditis may respond to temporizing treatment with beta-blockers (**Table 7.2**).[12] In rare instances, a TSH-secreting pituitary adenoma may present with a diffuse goiter that demonstrates increased quantitative uptake of radionuclide in association with thyroid function tests that reveal a pattern of elevated T_4 and T_3 levels in tandem with an inappropriately elevated TSH level.[13]

Euthyroid

A diffuse goiter identified in a patient with normal thyroid function and no evidence of underlying autoimmune thyroiditis can be classified as a simple or nontoxic goiter. Medical treatment in this setting is currently limited to the administration of levothyroxine in supratherapeutic doses targeted to suppress TSH levels in an effort to limit growth and expansion of thyroid tissue.[14] Doses of levothyroxine that are slightly higher than predicted requirements should be adjusted based on tolerance to maintain TSH levels in

Table 7.2 Beta-Blockers

Agent	Name	Available Doses	Usual Starting Dose
Propranolol: regular	Inderal	10, 20, 40, 80 mg	10–20 mg po t.i.d.
Propranolol: sustained release	Inderal-LA	60, 80, 120, 160 mg	*
Atenolol	Tenormin	25, 50, 100 mg	25–50 mg po qd
Metoprolol: regular	Lopressor	50, 100 mg	25–50 mg po b.i.d
Metoprolol: sustained release	Toprol-XL	50, 100, 200 mg	*

*Usual dose approximates the total daily dose of the regular preparation.

the 0.1- to 0.5-mU/L range. Objective measurements of the dimensions of each lobe should be tracked over time with serial ultrasounds to determine whether suppression leads to any significant decrease in volume.

Nodular Goiter

Thyrotoxic

A nodular goiter presenting with thyrotoxicosis may represent (1) a toxic multinodular goiter composed of multiple autonomously functioning thyroid nodules, or (2) nonfunctioning thyroid nodules identified in the setting of concurrent Graves disease. A radionuclide scan may help to distinguish between these conditions. Most toxic multinodular goiters demonstrate patterns of heterogeneous tracer distribution characterized by hotter spots of intense uptake of tracer that correspond to foci of increased autonomy, interspersed with cold areas that correspond to suppressed or nonfunctioning thyroid tissue. In contrast, Graves disease is more likely to show intense bilateral uptake of tracer marked by cold spots that indicate the location of nonfunctioning thyroid nodules. Beta-blockers can be used to treat hyperadrenergic symptoms associated with either disorder (**Table 7.2**).[15] Antithyroid drugs can be used to control hyperthyroidism that develops with progressive growth of a toxic multinodular goiter (**Table 7.3**). An antithyroid drug may be used as definitive therapy, or as a temporizing measure aimed at reducing thyroid hormone levels in anticipation of more definitive treatment with radioactive iodine. When used for this purpose, methimazole may be less likely

Table 7.3 Antithyroid Drugs

Agent	Name	Available Doses	Usual Starting Dose
Methimazole	Tapazole	5, 10 mg	10–40 mg po qd
Propylthiouracil	PTU	50 mg	50–100 mg po b.i.d.–t.i.d.

to blunt the efficacy of treatment.[16] Administration of radioactive iodine in therapeutic doses has proven to be a safe and effective means of treating toxic multinodular goiters.[17] In most cases a single empiric dose of orally administered iodine 131 (I-131) effectively ablates autonomously functioning nodules while leaving a critical mass of normal tissue intact. Effective treatment with radioactive iodine may shrink the size of a toxic multinodular goiter by up to 50%. This secondary effect may be of particular benefit in cases where expansive substernal growth of autonomously functioning nodules may predispose to development of problems with tracheal or esophageal compression. Thyroid function tests should be measured after treatment to confirm resolution of hyperthyroidism and at regular intervals thereafter to monitor for possible transition to a hypothyroid state.[18] Up to 30% of patients may develop postablative hypothyroidism within 5 years of treatment.

Euthyroid

Radioactive iodine has been used to treat nontoxic nodular goiters causing compressive symptoms in a range of trials with varying degrees of success.[19,20] Most have reported appreciable decrements in the size of nontoxic nodular goiters with a low incidence of complicating radiation thyroiditis and transient hyperthyroidism following administration of therapeutic doses of I-131. Attempts to bolster the efficacy of treatment by administering preparatory doses of recombinant TSH to augment uptake of radioactive iodine have demonstrated more mixed results.[21,22] Although this strategy does appear to increase the efficacy of treatment based on objective measurements of thyroid volume, its adoption has been limited to date due to reports of complications related to exacerbations of neck pain, hyperthyroidism, and transient increases in the size of nontoxic nodular goiters following administration of recombinant TSH.[23,24]

Administration of levothyroxine in supratherapeutic doses targeted to suppress TSH levels has proven to be a relatively effective means of controlling the growth and expansion of nontoxic nodular goiters.[25] This approach is particularly effective in preventing the regrowth of nodules in patients with a history of childhood neck irradiation.[26] Extended use of suppressive doses of levothyroxine may be limited by concerns about the increased risk of developing atrial arrhythmias and osteopenia associated with iatrogenic thyrotoxicosis. Surgery continues to be the mainstay for treatment of compressive nontoxic nodular goiters.

Thyroid Nodule

Thyroid nodules palpated on physical examination or incidentally noted on radiographic studies should be evaluated with a dedicated thyroid ultrasound to determine (1) if a discrete nodule is indeed present, (2) if any additional undetected nodules may be present, and (3) if any suspicious

cervical lymph nodes may be present.[27] An adequate study should delineate the relative position, dimensions, and appearance of each structure identified with specific notation of whether nodules are solid or variably cystic. A profile of laboratory tests including TSH, T_4, and T_3 levels should be checked to characterize the functional status of the thyroid (**Table 7.1**). Distinction between functional hypothyroid, thyrotoxic, and euthyroid states may help to guide the course of evaluation (**Fig. 7.1**).

Hypothyroid

An ultrasound that reveals a diffuse heterogeneous echotexture extending throughout both lobes in the setting of hypothyroidism is most likely to reflect changes associated with chronic lymphocytic thyroiditis. This condition may be mistaken for a discrete thyroid nodule when it leads to predominant enlargement of one lobe that can be readily palpated on physical examination, or when lower-resolution imaging studies identify regions of heterogeneity that are interpreted as distinct entities. Antithyroid peroxidase and antithyroglobulin antibody titers can be checked to determine whether underlying autoimmune thyroiditis is present. Treatment is based on providing adequate thyroid hormone replacement in the form of levothyroxine. Discrete thyroid nodules identified on ultrasound should be evaluated to determine whether they warrant investigation with fine needle aspiration.

Thyrotoxic

A single thyroid nodule confirmed on ultrasound in the setting of thyrotoxicosis may represent (1) an autonomously functioning toxic adenoma that is synthesizing and secreting excessive amounts of thyroid hormone, or (2) a nonfunctioning thyroid nodule identified in a patient presenting with concurrent Graves disease. A radionuclide thyroid scan can help to determine which condition is present. Scan images of a toxic adenoma typically reveal an intense focus of tracer uptake co-localized to the nodule with suppression of uptake in any surrounding tissue. Medical management of a toxic adenoma may involve the use of antithyroid drugs administered at doses targeted to attenuate the hyperthyroidism associated with this condition (**Table 7.3**).[28] This approach may be a temporizing measure at best, as discontinuation of treatment inevitably leads to recurrence of hyperthyroidism. A calculated dose of I-131 can be administered as more definitive treatment.[29] Treatment with radioactive iodine may ablate a toxic adenoma without damaging normal functioning thyroid tissue. Scan images that show intense uptake of tracer surrounding a cold spot that corresponds to a nonfunctioning thyroid nodule are more likely to represent concurrent Graves disease. In this setting, fine-needle aspiration of the nonfunctioning nodule should be considered to help determine whether definitive treatment should focus on medical or surgical management.

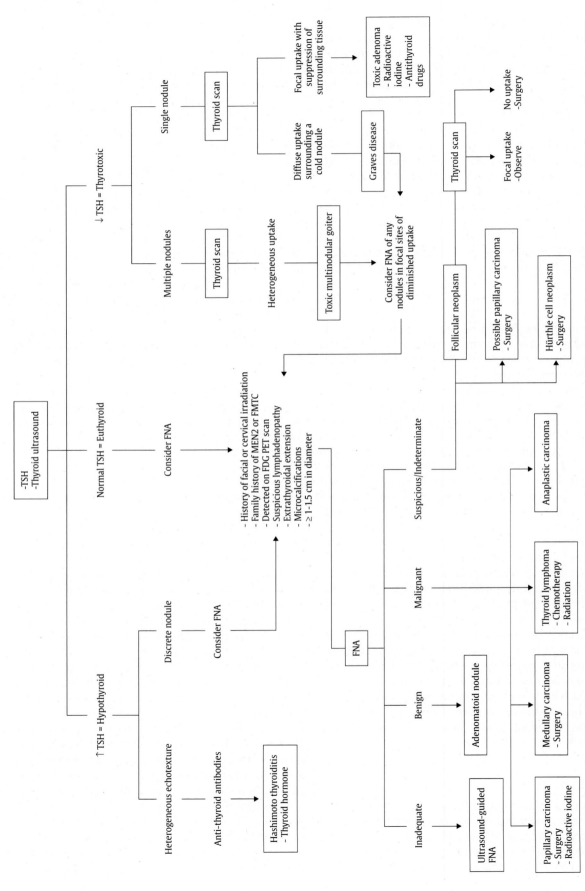

Fig. 7.1 Evaluation of a thyroid nodule. *Abbreviations:* FDG-PET, fluorodeoxyglucose positron emission tomography; FMTC, familial medullary thyroid cancer; FNA, fine-needle aspiration; MEN, multiple endocrine neoplasia; TSH, thyroid-stimulating hormone.

Multiple thyroid nodules noted on ultrasound in the setting of thyrotoxicosis are likely to indicate the presence of a toxic multinodular goiter. A radionuclide thyroid scan can help to confirm a suspected diagnosis and identify nodules corresponding to cold spots that may need to be evaluated with fine-needle aspiration.

Euthyroid

Fine-needle aspiration biopsy has emerged as the most reliable means of evaluating the malignant potential of thyroid nodules. The marked increase in the rate of detection of incidental thyroid nodules associated with widespread use of different imaging modalities has prompted professional organizations to define specific criteria to guide sampling.[30,31] A range of different radiographic features has been investigated as possible indicators of the likelihood that a given thyroid nodule may represent a malignancy. Those that have proven to be most informative include (1) the presence of microcalcifications, (2) evidence of extrathyroidal extension, (3) evidence of suspicious lymphadenopathy, and (4) initial detection of the thyroid nodule on a fluorodeoxyglucose positron emission tomography (FDG-PET) scan.[32-34] Ultrasound guidance should be used to direct fine-needle aspiration of nonpalpable, deeply situated, or partially cystic thyroid nodules. This technique has been proven to increase the diagnostic yield of samples returned from initial and repeat biopsies.[35] Although the terminology used to report results often varies among institutions, cytopathology readings are generally divided into four distinct categories: benign, malignant, suspicious/indeterminate, and unsatisfactory. An unsatisfactory designation usually indicates that an inadequate amount of cellular material was submitted for analysis. In most cases a repeat biopsy should be attempted using ultrasound guidance.[36]

A malignant designation indicates confirmation of cytologic features consistent with papillary thyroid carcinoma, anaplastic thyroid carcinoma, medullary thyroid carcinoma, or a diffuse large B-cell thyroid lymphoma. Flow cytometric analysis of aspirated lymphocytes may be required to distinguish other types of thyroid lymphoma from the infiltrates characteristic of chronic lymphocytic thyroiditis. Thyroid lymphoma is the only malignancy principally treated with medical management. Cases that present without evidence of tracheal compression may be effectively treated with combination chemotherapy and external beam radiation.[37]

A benign designation indicates that (1) an adequate amount of cellular material was submitted for review, (2) inspection revealed findings consistent with an adenomatoid nodule or thyroid cyst, and (3) inspection did not reveal any cytologic findings concerning for specific malignancies. A sample composed of proteinaceous colloid intermingled with sheets and clusters of follicular epithelial cells with normal nuclear features may be interpreted as representative of an adenomatoid nodule. The presence of hemosiderin-laden macrophages may reflect the onset of cystic degenerative changes. Although benign adenomatoid nodules are unlikely to transform into malignancies, they may continue to grow in a progressive fashion.[38] Administration of levothyroxine in supratherapeutic doses targeted to suppress TSH levels has long been employed as a mainstay of therapy directed toward shrinking enlarged or expanding adenomatoid nodules. The viability of this strategy has been called into question as randomized controlled trials and meta-analyses of levothyroxine suppression therapy have shown that it has a limited impact on the growth of solitary thyroid nodules.[39] In cases where it can be safely considered on a trial basis, doses of levothyroxine that are slightly higher than predicted requirements should be adjusted based on tolerance to maintain TSH levels in the 0.1- to 0.5-mU/L range. Objective measurements should be tracked over time to determine whether suppression leads to any significant decrease in nodule volume. Experimental treatments that may eventually be used to control the growth of thyroid nodules include protocols that employ laser thermal probes and high-intensity focused ultrasound to ablate demarcated volumes of tissue.[40,41] Although thyroid cysts can be drained by aspiration, a significant number will eventually reaccumulate fluid over time. Sclerotherapy involving injection of ethanol has been used to collapse drained thyroid cysts.[42]

A suspicious/indeterminate designation indicates that (1) an adequate amount of cellular material was submitted for review, and (2) inspection revealed cytologic findings that could be consistent with either a benign or malignant process. A sample composed of spherical clusters of follicular epithelium that form microfollicles with little or no background colloid present may be identified as a follicular neoplasm that could represent a benign follicular adenoma or a malignant follicular thyroid carcinoma.[43] Definitive diagnosis requires surgical removal to allow for complete pathologic examination of its perimeter. Detection of a focus of invasion into surrounding tissue will distinguish a follicular thyroid carcinoma from a follicular adenoma. A follicular neoplasm that demonstrates focal tracer uptake on a thyroid scan is more likely to represent a follicular adenoma. A suspicious/indeterminate thyroid nodule that has been classified as a Hürthle cell neoplasm or a possible focus of papillary thyroid carcinoma should be removed.[44]

Graves Disease

A suspected diagnosis of Graves disease may be confirmed when clinical evaluation and physical examination reveal a constellation of (1) thyroid function test profiles consistent with a thyrotoxic state; (2) diffuse goitrous enlargement of the thyroid; and (3) specific findings consistent with complicating thyroid eye disease, dermopathy, or acropachy. In situations where physical examination findings are equivocal, a radionuclide thyroid uptake and scan study should be performed to determine whether there is evidence of increased uptake in a diffuse distribution consistent with hyperthyroidism ascribed to Graves disease.[45]

Beta-Blockers

Beta-blockers can be used as temporizing agents to help control the hyperadrenergic manifestations of hyperthyroidism in patients with active Graves disease (**Table 7.2**). With effective treatment, there is usually a substantial decrease in the intensity of reported palpitations, anxiety, and tremors. Propranolol offers the theoretic advantage of acting to partially inhibit the peripheral conversion of T_4 to T_3. This may only be of issue in cases of severe hyperthyroidism. In practice, propranolol is short-acting enough to allow for rapid titration of doses administered three times daily to determine the total daily dose needed to ameliorate symptoms. When an effective dose has been determined, patients can be switched to an equivalent daily dose of the sustained release preparation. Longer-acting cardioselective agents that are also commonly used to treat thyrotoxicosis include atenolol and metoprolol. After a starting dose of an agent has been selected, the daily dose should be adjusted over the course of several days to a level that maintains a resting heart rate <90 beats per minute while reducing symptoms to a tolerable level.

Antithyroid Drugs

Thionamide antithyroid drugs work to decrease thyroid hormone synthesis by inhibiting the organification of iodine and the coupling of iodotyrosines necessary to produce T_4 and T_3. The two agents available for use in the United States are methimazole and propylthiouracil (**Table 7.3**). For mild to moderate hyperthyroidism, methimazole is usually started at a dose of 10 to 40 mg daily. For the same indication, propylthiouracil is usually started at a dose of 50 to 100 mg two to three times daily. It may take up to 4 weeks to see the full effect of treatment as previously synthesized T_4 and T_3 continue to be released. In the early stages of treatment, it is best to follow T_4 and T_3 levels to determine the adequacy of dosing and need for adjustment, as TSH levels may remain suppressed for several weeks after T_4 and T_3 levels have normalized.

Side effects that may be encountered with use of the thionamides include fever, rash, and pruritus. If any of these occur with either agent, it is best to switch to a trial of the alternate agent before discontinuing therapy. Hepatotoxicity may occur with use of higher doses. A rare but potentially life-threatening toxicity is agranulocytosis, which may develop in 0.2 to 0.5% of cases of treatment. Any patient taking methimazole or propylthiouracil should be cautioned to stop taking the drug and to seek medical attention if they develop a high fever, severe pharyngitis, or abdominal pain and jaundice during a course of treatment.

Radioactive Iodine

The uptake and concentration of iodine in the thyroid gland allows for the use of a radioactive isotope of iodine to definitively treat hyperthyroidism ascribed to Graves disease. When administered orally in therapeutic doses, I-131 is taken up and concentrated in hyperfunctioning thyroid tissue where it delivers β-radiation that causes localized tissue destruction over the course of several weeks. In the setting of Graves disease, a high level of uptake in a diffuse distribution allows for precise calculation of a dose based on estimated gland weight and measured uptake of I-123.

Management

Approaches to the management of Graves disease should be based on evaluation that takes into account a range of factors including the severity and duration of hyperthyroidism, likelihood of spontaneous remission, significant complications, comorbidities, and patient preferences regarding modes of therapy. Different strategies may be employed that incorporate the use of beta-blockers, antithyroid drugs, and radioactive iodine.

Mild Graves disease that presents with a minimal degree of hyperthyroidism has a greater probability of progressing to a state of spontaneous remission. As such, it can usually be treated with an antithyroid drug alone.[46] Factors identified on presentation that may predict a greater likelihood of remission include minimal goitrous enlargement of the thyroid gland, age >40, and low titers of anti-TSH receptor antibodies.[47] Treatment is usually started with methimazole (though propylthiouracil can be used if cost is a significant consideration). Over the course of several months the dose should be adjusted in increments of 5 to 10 mg per dose (25 to 50 mg per dose for propylthiouracil) until a daily dose is identified that normalizes the TSH level. After treatment has been continued for 9 months to a year, it can be held to see if hyperthyroidism recurs. If hyperthyroidism does recur, a second course of treatment with an antithyroid drug may be tried, though it is often recommended that patients proceed to more definitive treatment with radioactive iodine.

Graves disease that presents with an appreciable degree of thyrotoxicosis without evidence of significant complications or comorbid conditions can usually be treated directly with radioactive iodine.[48] A beta-blocker can be started to help control symptoms prior to administration of radioactive iodine. To calculate an effective dose, iodine uptake in the thyroid gland should measured with I-123. Treatment with saturated solution of potassium iodide can be started after radioactive iodine has been given to help reduce the interim level of hyperthyroidism. After a dose of I-131 has been administered, it may take up to 3 months to see the full effects of treatment. Patients should followed with frequent thyroid function tests during this time with the expectation that the majority will eventually progress to become hypothyroid, requiring treatment with replacement doses of levothyroxine. A percentage of patients who show an initial response to treatment may subsequently relapse with recurrence of hyperthyroidism. These cases are usually adequately treated with a second course of radioactive iodine.

Patients who present with severe hyperthyroidism or significant cardiovascular or ophthalmologic complications may require a period of cooling off with antithyroid drugs before proceeding to more definitive treatment with radioactive iodine.[49] This is indicated due to the slight risk of a transient increase in thyrotoxicosis associated with the use of radioactive iodine that may precipitate a crisis. A beta-blocker can be started with doses escalated as needed to help attenuate symptoms and control any arrhythmias that may develop. Treatment with methimazole or propylthiouracil can be initiated at higher starting doses and continued until there is an appreciable decline in symptoms and signs of thyrotoxicosis with a concomitant decline in T_4 and T_3 levels.[50] When it is deemed safe to proceed with radioactive

iodine therapy, antithyroid drugs should be stopped prior to planned treatment. After a dose of I-131 has been administered, an antithyroid drug can be restarted after an interval at a lower dose and continued while the patient is being followed and monitored. With successful treatment, there is usually a substantial decrease in the size and prominence of the thyroid. In patients with evidence of thyroid eye disease, there is some concern that treatment with radioactive iodine may exacerbate this condition. Glucocorticoids can be administered in tapering doses over 4 to 6 weeks following treatment in an attempt to minimize complications.

References

1. Knudsen N, Bols B, Bulow I, et al. Validation of ultrasonography of the thyroid gland for epidemiological purposes. Thyroid 1999;9:1069–1074

2. Raber W, Gessl A, Nowotny P, Vierhapper H. Thyroid ultrasound versus antithyroid peroxidase antibody determination: a cohort study of four hundred fifty-one subjects. Thyroid 2002;12:725–731

3. Mariotti S, Caturegli P, Piccolo P, Barbesino G, Pinchera A. Antithyroid peroxidase autoantibodies in thyroid diseases. J Clin Endocrinol Metab 1990;71:661–669

4. Hegedus L, Hansen JM, Feldt-Rasmussen U, Hansen BM, Hoier-Madsen M. Influence of thyroxine treatment on thyroid size and anti-thyroid peroxidase antibodies in Hashimoto's thyroiditis. Clin Endocrinol (Oxf) 1991;35:235–238

5. Lucas A, Pizarro E, Granada ML, Salinas I, Foz M, Sanmarti A. Postpartum thyroiditis: epidemiology and clinical evolution in a nonselected population. Thyroid 2000;10:71–77

6. Othman S, Phillips DI, Parkes AB, et al. A long-term follow-up of postpartum thyroiditis. Clin Endocrinol (Oxf) 1990;32:559–564

7. Andersson M, Takkouche B, Egli I, Allen HE, de Benoist B. Current global iodine status and progress over the last decade towards the elimination of iodine deficiency. Bull World Health Organ 2005;83:518–525

8. PAHO/WHO Technical Group on Endemic Goiter Cretinism and Iodine Deficiency. Fifth meeting, 1983, Lima Peru). In: Dunn JT, ed. Towards the Eradication of Endemic Goiter, Cretinism, and Iodine Deficiency: Proceedings of the Vth Meeting of the PAHO/WHO Technical Group on Endemic Goiter, Cretinism, and Iodine Deficiency. Washington, DC: Pan American Health Organization Regional Office of the World Health Organization, 1986

9. Dunn JT, Haar Fvd. A practical guide to the correction of iodine deficiency. Netherlands: International Council for Control of Iodine Deficiency, 1990

10. Tollin SR, Fallon EF, Mikhail M, Goldstein H, Yung E. The utility of thyroid nuclear imaging and other studies in the detection and treatment of underlying thyroid abnormalities in patients with endogenous subclinical thyrotoxicosis. Clin Nucl Med 2000;25:341–347

11. Intenzo CM, Park CH, Kim SM, Capuzzi DM, Cohen SN, Green P. Clinical, laboratory, and scintigraphic manifestations of subacute and chronic thyroiditis. Clin Nucl Med 1993;18:302–306

12. Bryer-Ash M. Evaluation of the patient with a suspected thyroid disorder. Obstet Gynecol Clin North Am 2001;28:421–438

13. Beck-Peccoz P, Persani L. Medical management of thyrotropin-secreting pituitary adenomas. Pituitary 2002;5:83–88

14. Berghout A, Wiersinga WM, Drexhage HA, Smits NJ, Touber JL. Comparison of placebo with L-thyroxine alone or with carbimazole for treatment of sporadic non-toxic goitre. Lancet 1990;336:193–197

15. Geffner DL, Hershman JM. Beta-adrenergic blockade for the treatment of hyperthyroidism. Am J Med 1992;93:61–68

16. Imseis RE, Vanmiddlesworth L, Massie JD, Bush AJ, Vanmiddlesworth NR. Pretreatment with propylthiouracil but not methimazole reduces the therapeutic efficacy of iodine-131 in hyperthyroidism. J Clin Endocrinol Metab 1998;83:685–687

17. Nygaard B, Hegedus L, Ulriksen P, Nielsen KG, Hansen JM. Radioiodine therapy for multinodular toxic goiter. Arch Intern Med 1999;159:1364–1368

18. Ceccarelli C, Bencivelli W, Vitti P, Grasso L, Pinchera A. Outcome of radioiodine-131 therapy in hyperfunctioning thyroid nodules: a 20 years' retrospective study. Clin Endocrinol (Oxf) 2005;62:331–335

19. Le Moli R, Wesche MF, Tiel-Van Buul MM, Wiersinga WM. Determinants of longterm outcome of radioiodine therapy of sporadic non-toxic goitre. Clin Endocrinol (Oxf) 1999;50:783–789

20. Bonnema SJ, Bertelsen H, Mortensen J, et al. The feasibility of high dose iodine 131 treatment as an alternative to surgery in patients with a very large goiter: effect on thyroid function and size and pulmonary function. J Clin Endocrinol Metab 1999;84:3636–3641

21. Huysmans DA, Nieuwlaat WA, Hermus AR. Towards larger volume reduction of nodular goitres by radioiodine therapy: a role for pretreatment with recombinant human thyrotropin? Clin Endocrinol (Oxf) 2004;60:297–299

22. Albino CC, Mesa CO, Olandoski M, et al. Recombinant human thyrotropin as adjuvant in the treatment of multinodular goiters with radioiodine. J Clin Endocrinol Metab 2005;90:2775–2780

23. Nielsen VE, Bonnema SJ, Boel-Jorgensen H, Grupe P, Hegedus L. Stimulation with 0.3-mg recombinant human thyrotropin prior to iodine 131 therapy to improve the size reduction of benign nontoxic nodular goiter: a prospective randomized double-blind trial. Arch Intern Med 2006;166:1476–1482

24. Silva MN, Rubio IG, Romao R, et al. Administration of a single dose of recombinant human thyrotrophin enhances the efficacy of radioiodine treatment of large compressive multinodular goitres. Clin Endocrinol (Oxf) 2004;60:300–308

25. Ross DS. Thyroid hormone suppressive therapy of sporadic nontoxic goiter. Thyroid 1992;2:263–269

26. Fogelfeld L, Wiviott MB, Shore-Freedman E, et al. Recurrence of thyroid nodules after surgical removal in patients irradiated in childhood for benign conditions. N Engl J Med 1989;320:835–840

27. Wiest PW, Hartshorne MF, Inskip PD, et al. Thyroid palpation versus high-resolution thyroid ultrasonography in the detection of nodules. J Ultrasound Med 1998;17:487–496

28. Vidal-Trecan GM, Stahl JE, Eckman MH. Radioiodine or surgery for toxic thyroid adenoma: dissecting an important decision. A cost-effectiveness analysis. Thyroid 2004;14:933–945

29. Nygaard B, Hegedus L, Nielsen KG, Ulriksen P, Hansen JM. Long-term effect of radioactive iodine on thyroid function and size in patients with solitary autonomously functioning toxic thyroid nodules. Clin Endocrinol (Oxf) 1999;50:197–202

30. American Association of Clinical Endocrinologists and Associazione Medici Endocrinologi. Medical guidelines for clinical practice for the diagnosis and management of thyroid nodules. Endocr Pract 2006;12:63–102

31. Frates MC, Benson CB, Charboneau JW, et al. Management of thyroid nodules detected at US: Society of Radiologists in Ultrasound consensus conference statement. Radiology 2005;237:794–800

32. Iannuccilli JD, Cronan JJ, Monchik JM. Risk for malignancy of thyroid nodules as assessed by sonographic criteria: the need for biopsy. J Ultrasound Med 2004;23:1455–1464

33. Ishigaki S, Shimamoto K, Satake H, et al. Multi-slice CT of thyroid nodules: comparison with ultrasonography. Radiat Med 2004;22:346–353

34. Kim TY, Kim WB, Ryu JS, Gong G, Hong SJ, Shong YK. 18F-fluorodeoxyglucose uptake in thyroid from positron emission tomogram (PET) for evaluation in cancer patients: high prevalence of malignancy in thyroid PET incidentaloma. Laryngoscope 2005;115:1074–1078

35. Deandrea M, Mormile A, Veglio M, et al. Fine-needle aspiration biopsy of the thyroid: comparison between thyroid palpation and ultrasonography. Endocr Pract 2002;8:282–286

36. Alexander EK, Heering JP, Benson CB, et al. Assessment of nondiagnostic ultrasound-guided fine needle aspirations of thyroid nodules. J Clin Endocrinol Metab 2002;87:4924–4927

37. McDougall IR, Berry GJ. Management of Thyroid Cancer and Related Nodular Disease. London: Springer, 2006

38. Alexander EK, Hurwitz S, Heering JP, et al. Natural history of benign solid and cystic thyroid nodules. Ann Intern Med 2003;138:315–318

39. Castro MR, Caraballo PJ, Morris JC. Effectiveness of thyroid hormone suppressive therapy in benign solitary thyroid nodules: a meta-analysis. J Clin Endocrinol Metab 2002;87:4154–4159

40. Papini E, Guglielmi R, Bizzarri G, Pacella CM. Ultrasound-guided laser thermal ablation for treatment of benign thyroid nodules. Endocr Pract 2004;10:276–283

41. Esnault O, Franc B, Monteil JP, Chapelon JY. High-intensity focused ultrasound for localized thyroid-tissue ablation: preliminary experimental animal study. Thyroid 2004;14:1072–1076

42. Valcavi R, Frasoldati A. Ultrasound-guided percutaneous ethanol injection therapy in thyroid cystic nodules. Endocr Pract 2004;10:269–275

43. Castro MR, Gharib H. Continuing controversies in the management of thyroid nodules. Ann Intern Med 2005;142:926–931

44. Chen H, Nicol TL, Zeiger MA, et al. Hürthle cell neoplasms of the thyroid: are there factors predictive of malignancy? Ann Surg 1998;227:542–546

45. Werner SC, Ingbar SH, Braverman LE, Utiger RD. Werner & Ingbar's The Thyroid: A Fundamental and Clinical Text, 9th ed. Philadelphia: Lippincott Williams & Wilkins, 2005

46. Cooper DS. Antithyroid drugs. N Engl J Med 2005;352:905–917

47. Vitti P, Rago T, Chiovato L, et al. Clinical features of patients with Graves' disease undergoing remission after antithyroid drug treatment. Thyroid 1997;7:369–375

48. Solomon B, Glinoer D, Lagasse R, Wartofsky L. Current trends in the management of Graves' disease. J Clin Endocrinol Metab 1990;70:1518–1524

49. Cooper DS. Medical Management of Thyroid Disease. New York: M. Dekker, 2001

50. Braga M, Walpert N, Burch HB, Solomon BL, Cooper DS. The effect of methimazole on cure rates after radioiodine treatment for Graves' hyperthyroidism: a randomized clinical trial. Thyroid 2002;12:135–139

8 Surgical Management of Benign Thyroid Diseases

William H. Moretz III, Christine G. Gourin, and David J. Terris

Thyroid surgery offers definitive treatment for benign thyroid disease with relatively low complication rates. Currently, most thyroid surgery is performed for glands suspicious for carcinoma; however, surgery for benign disease has become a more appealing option for patients as a result of minimally invasive techniques. These techniques can be safely applied for the treatment of benign thyroid disease, resulting in smaller postoperative scars and reduced postoperative pain compared with standard open methods. This chapter includes a detailed discussion of two different minimally invasive approaches for benign thyroid disease.

The thyroid surgeon should have a close working relationship with the endocrinologist or primary care physician, as perioperative medical management is crucial to prevent complications. The management strategy for benign diseases, such as toxic solitary nodules, multinodular goiters, and Graves disease, should be decided by the patient in conjunction with all members of the treating medical team. Although nonsurgical treatment options are discussed briefly in this chapter, a detailed discussion of the medical management of benign thyroid disease can be found in Chapter 7.

Toxic Solitary Nodule

Solitary autonomously functioning toxic nodules are independent of thyroid-stimulating hormone (TSH) control and produce clinical or subclinical hyperthyroidism. Radionuclide imaging displays an increased uptake of radioactive iodine by the toxic nodule. Definitive treatment for the toxic solitary nodule includes sclerosing therapy, iodine-131 (I-131) ablation, and surgical resection. Thionamides offer only temporary control of toxic solitary nodules.

Sclerosing therapy, popular as a treatment modality in Europe, involves the percutaneous injection of ethanol directly into the toxic nodule, typically under ultrasound guidance. Monzani and colleagues[1] reported a permanent cure rate of 70.6% when sclerosing therapy is used for toxic adenomas. Sclerosing therapy, however, may require multiple treatment sessions.

Treatment with radioactive iodine is the most common treatment for toxic solitary nodules in the United States. Doses of I-131 can vary, depending on the size of the toxic nodule. Smaller doses of I-131 are associated with a lower incidence of posttreatment hypothyroidism, but relapse rates are correspondingly higher. The reverse trend is seen with larger treatment doses. Up to 75 to 90% of patients are cured within 3 months of I-131 ablation.[2,3] Rates of posttreatment hypothyroidism range from 8 to 60%, depending on the dose of I-131.[2-6] With a typical dose of 20 mCi, approximately 15% of patients require more than one treatment for cure.

Surgical treatment of toxic solitary nodules offers a definitive cure with a very low postoperative risk of hypothyroidism.[4,7] Complete surgical resection typically involves a unilateral thyroid lobectomy, resulting in resolution of hyperthyroidism. Surgery is preferred for children, adolescents, and pregnant patients with toxic thyroid nodules to avoid the potential long-term risks of radioactive iodine. Large toxic nodules are typically treated with surgery, to obviate the need for the large doses of radioactive iodine that would be required for ablation. Complications are rare after unilateral thyroid lobectomy for benign toxic disease, with essentially no risk of hypoparathyroidism and a 0.2 to 0.6% risk of permanent vocal cord paralysis.[7-9]

Multinodular Goiter

Multinodular goiter occurs in 4% of the United States population. Surgery provides definitive treatment with low complication rates and immediate resolution of symptoms associated with upper aerodigestive tract compression. Histologic examination of removed tissue allows the detection of potential malignancy, which is present in approximately 8.3% of cervical and substernal goiters.[10] Large multinodular goiters generally are not amenable to minimally invasive surgical techniques. Substernal goiters are discussed in greater detail in Chapter 9.

Surgery for toxic multinodular goiter may be preferable to I-131 in healthy patients, resulting in the immediate resolution of hyperthyroidism and compressive symptoms when present. Large and often multiple doses of radioactive iodine are required to control hyperthyroidism in toxic multinodular goiter.

Graves Disease

Radioiodine is the most common method used to treat Graves disease in the United States because of the high efficacy, ease of use, and low cost. Radioiodine is contraindicated in patients who are pregnant or nursing. Caution must be exercised when considering treatment with radioiodine in children because of the concern for a subsequent increased risk of malignancy.[11]

Thyroidectomy is usually indicated in patients with Graves disease who have a large goiter or coexistent suspicious thyroid nodules. Mazzaferri[12] reported that well-differentiated thyroid cancer is approximately twice as prevalent in patients with Graves disease as in the general population. Cancer in this setting is associated with higher rates of regional lymph node metastases and local invasion.[13] Surgery is also preferred in pregnant women whose hyperthyroidism is not controlled with antithyroid drugs. The optimal timing for surgery is in the second trimester to minimize the risk to the fetus.[14] When surgery is indicated for Graves disease, total thyroidectomy is promptly curative, with relatively low complication rates.[15] Total thyroidectomy is preferred over subtotal thyroidectomy to avoid the risk of recurrent hyperthyroidism.[16] Total thyroidectomy is associated with a 2 to 3% incidence of transient vocal cord paralysis, which is permanent in 1% of patients, and temporary hypoparathyroidism in 10 to 15% of cases, which is permanent in 2 to 3%.[9,17,18]

Preoperative Preparation

In addition to achieving a stable medical state prior to surgery, it is important to ensure that the patient is euthyroid to minimize the risk of thyroid storm, a potential complication of surgery for hyperthyroidism. The pathogenesis of thyroid storm is unclear but is precipitated by stress or trauma such as surgery in hyperthyroid patients and manifests as extreme thyrotoxicosis associated with a hypermetabolic state, resulting in cardiac arrhythmias, hyperpyrexia, congestive heart failure, and cardiovascular collapse. Treatment for hyperthyroidism usually starts 4 to 6 weeks prior to surgery with an antithyroid drug, such as methimazole (10–30 mg/day) or propylthiouracil (100–300 mg, three times daily). Potassium iodide (Lugol solution) may be administered 7 to 10 days prior to surgery in doses of 5 to 10 drops two to three times a day to decrease the vascularity of the thyroid gland. Inorganic iodine treatment inhibits thyroid hormone secretion and decreases thyroid blood flow, possibly reducing bleeding during surgery.[19] Beta-blockers are often added to the preparation regimen to control symptoms of hyperthyroidism such as tachycardia, anxiety, tremor, and heat intolerance. Propranolol, an adrenergic blocking agent, inhibits peripheral conversion of T_4 to T_3, and is prescribed in doses of 40 to 120 mg, up to four times a day. Propranolol is continued for up to a week after surgery because the half-life of thyroxine is 7 days. Beta-blockers have been used alone for preoperative preparation, although higher rates of perioperative thyrotoxicosis are associated with this single-drug regimen.[19]

Conventional Thyroidectomy

Thyroid lobectomy is the standard surgical procedure for a unilateral solitary nodule. The surgical technique begins with an incision in a relaxed skin tension line, just above the sternal notch. It is preferable to mark the patient preoperatively while he or she is in a sitting position in the hold-ing area, to optimize the location of the incision while the patient is positioned naturally.[20] Dissection is carried down to the subplatysmal fascial plane. The midline of the strap muscles is identified and separated to expose the underlying thyroid gland. The gland is dissected bluntly from the overlying sternothyroid muscle. Medial retraction of the thyroid lobe allows identification of the middle thyroid vein, which is isolated and ligated. The superior pole is isolated and the superior thyroid artery and vein are either ligated individually or as a bundle on the surface of the gland capsule. Care is exercised to avoid injury to the external branch of the superior laryngeal nerve. This nerve is not routinely identified.

Dissection of the recurrent laryngeal nerve (RLN) begins near the inferior pole of the gland, in the tracheoesophageal groove. Identification of the RLN during thyroidectomy reduces the incidence of nerve injury.[21,22] The right RLN enters the tracheoesophageal groove more obliquely than the left.[23] Identification is facilitated by medial retraction of the thyroid lobe and dissection with blunt elevators in a direction perpendicular to the direction of the nerve (**Fig. 8.1**). Once

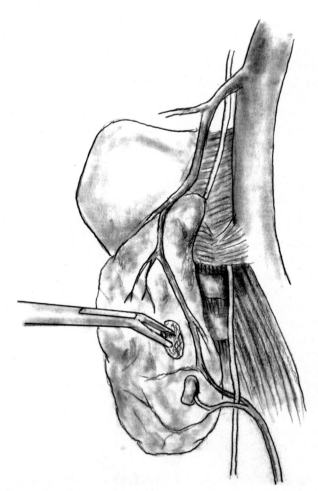

Fig. 8.1 Identification of the left recurrent laryngeal nerve in the tracheoesophageal groove. Medial retraction of the thyroid lobe allows for visualization of the nerve using this approach.

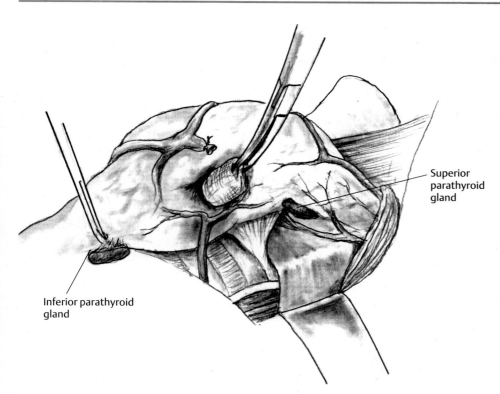

Inferior parathyroid gland

Superior parathyroid gland

Fig. 8.2 Meticulous dissection of the parathyroid glands from the thyroid capsule to preserve the vascular supply, avoiding postoperative hypoparathyroidism.

the nerve is identified by careful dissection, it is followed superiorly. The RLN crosses the inferior thyroid artery in a variable fashion, making the inferior thyroid artery an unreliable landmark for RLN identification.[24] The possibility of a nonrecurrent laryngeal nerve should be considered if the nerve is not located in the tracheoesophageal groove.

The inferior thyroid pole is mobilized and retracted superomedially to identify the inferior parathyroid gland. The gland is preserved along with its blood supply (a branch of the inferior thyroid artery) by meticulous dissection laterally away from the thyroid capsule (**Fig. 8.2**). The superior parathyroid gland is similarly identified and gently dissected from the thyroid gland. The superior parathyroid glands receive their blood supply from branches of the inferior thyroid artery but may infrequently be supplied by branches of the superior thyroid artery or from an anastomosis between the inferior and superior thyroid arteries. Terminal branches of both the inferior and superior thyroid vessels are ligated as close to the thyroid capsule as possible to ensure preservation of the parathyroid blood supply.

The thyroid gland is dissected free from the posterior suspensory ligament of Berry, the most vulnerable area for RLN injury. The RLN typically passes deep to this ligament; however, it may pass through or in front of the ligament.[25] Division of the Berry ligament should be performed while carefully visualizing the nerve to avoid inadvertent nerve injury. The RLN frequently branches prior to entering the larynx (**Fig. 8.3**). Up to 65% of RLNs demonstrate extralaryngeal branching, with two to three terminal branches noted in the majority of cases.[26] The thyroid lobe is divided at the isthmus and removed.

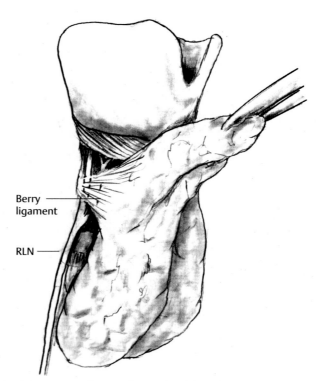

Berry ligament

RLN

Fig. 8.3 Recurrent laryngeal nerve (RLN) branching at the level of the Berry ligament requires special attention during dissection to avoid inadvertent injury.

If a total thyroidectomy is indicated, the contralateral gland is removed in the same fashion as the ipsilateral lobe. Special attention should be directed to identification and preservation of all parathyroid glands because the patient is at risk for postoperative hypoparathyroidism. Rates of permanent hypoparathyroidism after total thyroidectomy have been reported to occur in approximately 2 to 3% of cases performed by experienced surgeons.[17,18] Reimplantation of parathyroid tissue of questionable viability is recommended, and has been shown to result in a lower incidence of permanent postoperative hypoparathyroidism.[27,28]

Minimally Invasive Techniques

Minimally invasive techniques can be safely applied for the treatment of benign thyroid disease. Several distinct versions of minimally invasive surgery have been described.[29–39] The advantages common to these methods include an improved postoperative cosmetic result and reduced postoperative pain compared with conventional open surgery.[40,41] Two approaches are discussed in this chapter, along with their indications, technical descriptions, and complications.

Minimally Invasive Nonendoscopic Thyroidectomy

This technique has been previously described in detail[30] and is particularly valuable for the inexperienced minimal access thyroid surgeon. Transection of the strap muscles can occasionally be done to facilitate exposure within the limited surgical field. Patient selection is important. Obese patients pose a challenge because of a greater depth of the operative field, which may hinder exposure through a smaller incision. The presence of thyroiditis may result in troublesome bleeding and difficult dissection of tissue planes secondary to adhesions. Large multinodular goiters pose a relative contraindication to the use of minimally invasive techniques.

Surgical Technique

The patient is positioned with no or only minimal neck extension, and a 3- to 6-cm incision is created in a relaxed skin tension line (the precise length dictated by the clinical circumstances). Again, the location is determined presurgically with the patient sitting upright. The sternohyoid and sternothyroid musculature is exposed and either retracted laterally or in some cases transected horizontally to expose the thyroid gland.

The superior pole of the thyroid is first isolated and the vessels are ligated with the ultrasonic shears (Harmonic Shears, model #CS-14C or ACE 23P; Ethicon Endo-Surgery). The superior lobe is mobilized, and the superior parathyroid gland identified. The middle thyroid vein is identified and ligated, and the inferior lobe is mobilized sufficiently to identify the inferior parathyroid gland and the recurrent laryngeal nerve. The inferior pole vessels are ligated at the capsule of the thyroid gland, and the gland is dissected off

the trachea. During this dissection, the recurrent laryngeal nerve is visualized to avoid injury. The isthmus is divided adjacent to the contralateral lobe for unilateral lobectomy. For total thyroidectomy, the dissection is performed in the same manner on the contralateral thyroid lobe.

Following thyroidectomy, the sternohyoid and sternothyroid muscles are reapproximated (if they were transected) using interrupted figure-of-eight 3–0 Vicryl sutures (Ethicon, Inc., Somerville, NJ). The subcutaneous tissues are approximated with interrupted 4–0 Vicryl sutures, and the skin is closed with liquid skin adhesive (Dermabond, Ethicon, Inc.). A drain is rarely required.[29,30]

This minimally invasive approach is safe,[29,30] with no increased risk of permanent hypocalcemia or recurrent laryngeal nerve paralysis compared with conventional open surgery. Cosmetic results are superior, with an incision as small as 3.0 cm.

Endoscopic Thyroidectomy

Indications

The endoscopic or minimally invasive video-assisted thyroidectomy (MIVAT) was pioneered in Italy[31,32] and subsequently introduced in North America.[29,42,43] The indications for endoscopic thyroidectomy are relatively narrow, and include thyroid nodules no larger than 25 to 30 mm in glands with volume less than 20 cc. Some authors have expanded these indications to include patients with Graves disease whose thyroid glands are smaller than 20 to 30 cc, and those with low-risk papillary thyroid carcinomas as large as 35 mm.[31,32] A prospective, randomized study by Miccoli et al[44] found that a MIVAT is at least as thorough and complete as open thyroidectomy for patients with small, isolated papillary thyroid carcinoma (less than 3.5 cm) based on thyroid uptake studies and thyroglobulin levels. Patients who require lymph node dissection or have invasive thyroid carcinoma are generally not considered candidates for endoscopic approaches, although central compartment neck dissection has been described using the minimally invasive technique.[45] A history of thyroiditis, previous neck surgery or irradiation, and substernal extension are relative contraindications to the endoscopic technique. In high-volume institutions, between 12 and 29% of patients undergoing thyroidectomies are candidates for an endoscopic approach.[42,46,47]

Technical Considerations

The pursuit of an endoscopic approach has been greatly facilitated by ultrasonic technology.[48] The Harmonic scalpel cuts and coagulates with ultrasonic vibrations of the blade at a speed of 55,500 Hz. Mechanical vibration from the device creates frictional energy, denaturing proteins by breaking the hydrogen bonds at temperatures between 50° and 100°C. A coagulum, formed from denatured proteins, seals vessels of up to 5 mm in diameter. No electrical energy is transferred to the patient, reducing the risk of thermal injury to

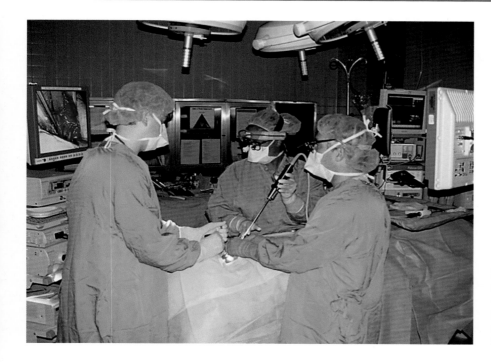

Fig. 8.4 The operating room setup for endoscopic thyroidectomy. Table is rotated 180 degrees to allow room for the surgeon and two assistants (one holding the endoscope and one holding the retractors), as well as the endoscopic and ultrasonic equipment.

important structures such as the RLN and parathyroid glands.[49–52] Other essential instruments utilized during endoscopic thyroidectomy include deep retractors, blunt elevators, and a 5-mm 30-degree laparoscope.

The operating room table should be rotated 180 degrees to allow ample space for the surgeon and two assistants (one holding the endoscope, and one holding retractors), as well as the endoscopic and ultrasonic equipment (**Fig. 8.4**).

Surgical Technique

The patient is marked while in the upright position for a 15- to 30-mm horizontal cervical incision in a relaxed skin tension line at the midline. In the operating room, the patient is placed in the supine position with no or only slight cervical extension without a shoulder roll. The incision is made through the skin and subcutaneous tissues (**Fig. 8.5**), and the midline raphe between the strap muscles is identified. A protected and extended electrocautery tip facilitates dissection at midline down to the thyroid isthmus.

A plane between the sternothyroid muscle and the thyroid gland is developed bluntly with an elevator (**Fig. 8.6**). The gland is carefully mobilized away from the sternothyroid muscle. The middle thyroid vein branches are isolated and ligated with the ultrasonic shears. Retractors are placed against the sternothyroid muscle and the thyroid gland to facilitate visualization of the superior thyroid vessels.

The endoscopic component of the technique begins as the laparoscope is angled upward just within the wound for visualization of the superior pole. No carbon dioxide insufflation is necessary. The operating room setup ensures appropriate placement of monitors for the surgeon and assistant (**Fig. 8.4**).

A small portion of the sternothyroid muscle is divided with the ultrasonic shears superficial to the superior pole vessels to improve visualization. This is the only muscle that is cut during the operation. Dissection and isolation of the superior thyroid artery and vein is performed using blunt elevators.

The ultrasonic shears are used to seal and divide the vessels (**Fig. 8.7**), while a suction elevator evacuates the steam created. Alternatively, the terminal branches of the superior pole vessels may be ligated in a bundle as they enter the capsule of the gland. The superior laryngeal nerve may be visualized as it crosses lateral to medial in relation to the vessels. The superior parathyroid gland is identified and dissected away from the thyroid gland as the gland is mobilized inferiorly.

The laparoscope is then angled downward, and the inferior pole of the thyroid is mobilized and retracted medially to facilitate endoscopic identification of the RLN. The nerve is identified in the tracheoesophageal groove and traced out for a length of 15 to 20 mm. The inferior parathyroid gland is identified and gently mobilized away from the thyroid gland. Once the recurrent laryngeal nerve is identified, the inferior thyroid artery and vein may be isolated, sealed, and divided.

The remaining steps are performed in an open fashion. The isthmus is dissected from the trachea and divided using either electrocautery or the ultrasonic shears. Sequential placement of a series of clamps on the superior pole of the gland is accomplished to allow delivery of the thyroid (**Fig. 8.8**). Any remaining attachments at the superior pole are divided,

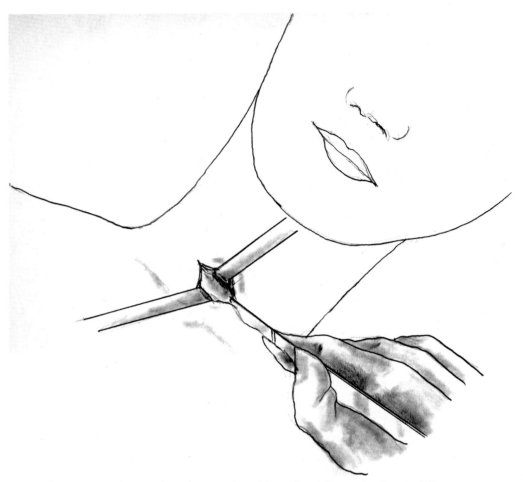

Fig. 8.5 An incision is made approximately 2 cm above the sternal notch in a relaxed skin tension line at midline.

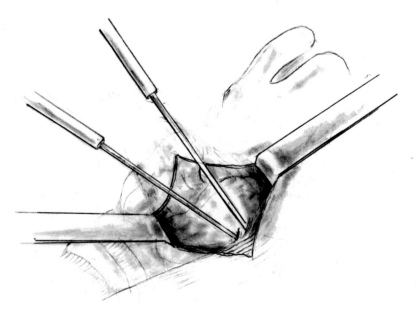

Fig. 8.6 A plane between the sternothyroid muscle and the thyroid gland is developed bluntly with an elevator.

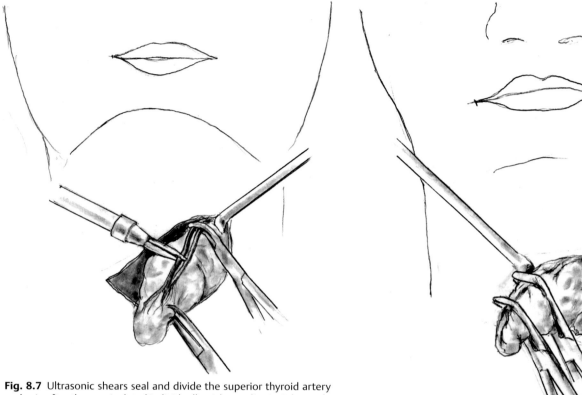

Fig. 8.7 Ultrasonic shears seal and divide the superior thyroid artery and vein after they are isolated individually with a pediatric right-angle clamp. An alternate method is to ligate the terminal branches in a bundle as they enter the capsule of the gland.

Fig. 8.8 Sequential placement of clamps, on the superior pole, facilitates the delivery of the thyroid gland.

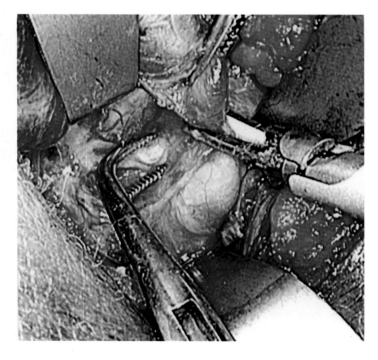

Fig. 8.9 The recurrent laryngeal nerve is traced to its entrance at the larynx using a pediatric right-angle clamp, and the connective tissue attachments between the gland and trachea (the ligament of Berry) are divided using the ultrasonic shears.

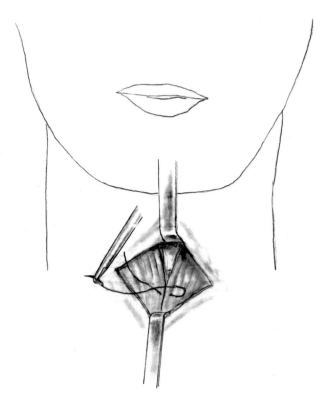

Fig. 8.10 Two interrupted sutures of 4–0 Vicryl are used to approximate the subcutaneous tissues. Liquid tissue sealant (Dermabond) is used to close the wound without a drain.

and the gland is mobilized inferiorly and exteriorized. The recurrent laryngeal nerve is traced to its entrance at the larynx, and the ligament of Berry is divided using the ultrasonic shears (**Fig. 8.9**).

Surgicel is placed into the thyroid bed, and the strap muscles are reapproximated with a figure-of-eight suture of 3–0 Vicryl (**Fig. 8.10**). A single 4–0 Vicryl suture is used to approximate the subcutaneous tissues, and Dermabond is used to close the skin. No drain or skin sutures are required.[29,30] Patients are usually discharged after recovering in the postanesthesia unit (see Chapter 22).

Complications

The complication rates associated with endoscopic thyroid surgery are similar to those described for conven-

tional surgery, including the rates of transient and permanent recurrent laryngeal nerve palsy, transient and permanent hypocalcemia, postoperative hematoma, and wound infection.[29,31,32,42–44]

Conclusion

Improvements in the technique of thyroidectomy have made thyroid surgery a more appealing option in the treatment of benign thyroid disease. Minimally invasive thyroidectomy has been demonstrated to be safe and is cosmetically superior to conventional open techniques. Technological advances will undoubtedly fuel continued refinements in minimal access surgery.

References

1. Monzani F, Caraccio N, Goletti O, et al. Treatment of hyperfunctioning thyroid nodules with percutaneous ethanol injection: eight years' experience. Exp Clin Endocrinol Diabetes 1998;106:S54–S58
2. Nygaard B, Hegedus L, Nielsen KG, et al. Long-term effect of radioactive iodine on thyroid function and size in patients with solitary autonomously functioning toxic thyroid nodules. Clin Endocrinol (Oxf) 1999;50:197–202
3. Ross DS, Ridgway EC, Daniels GH. Successful treatment of solitary toxic thyroid nodules with relatively low-dose iodine-131, with low prevalence of hypothyroidism. Ann Intern Med 1984;101:488–490

4. O'Brien T, Gharib H, Suman VJ, et al. Treatment of toxic solitary thyroid nodules: surgery versus radioactive iodine. Surgery 1992;112:1166–1170
5. Goldstein R, Hart IR. Follow-up of solitary autonomous thyroid nodules treated with [131]I. N Engl J Med 1983;309:1473–1476
6. Ceccarelli C, Bencivelli W, Vitti P, et al. Outcome of radioiodine-131 therapy in hyperfunctioning thyroid nodules: a 20 years' retrospective study. Clin Endocrinol (Oxf) 2005;62:331–335
7. Eyre-Brook IA, Talbot CH. The treatment of autonomous functioning thyroid nodules. Br J Surg 1982;69:577–579

8. Chiang FY, Wang LF, Huang YF, et al. Recurrent laryngeal nerve palsy after thyroidectomy with routine identification of the recurrent laryngeal nerve. Surgery 2005;137:342–347

9. Rosato L, Avenia N, Bernante P, et al. Complications of thyroid surgery: analysis of a multicentric study on 14,934 patients operated on in Italy over 5 years. World J Surg 2004;28:271–276

10. Singh B, Lucente F, Shaha AR. Substernal goiter: a clinical review. Am J Otolaryngol 1994;15:409–416

11. Kaplan MM, Meier DA, Dworkin HJ. Treatment of hyperthyroidism with radioactive iodine. Endocrinol Metab Clin North Am 1998;27:205–223

12. Mazzaferri EL. Thyroid cancer and Graves' disease. J Clin Endocrinol Metab 1990;70:826–829

13. Belfiore A, Garofalo MR, Giuffrida D, et al. Increased aggressiveness of thyroid cancer in patients with Graves' disease. J Clin Endocrinol Metab 1990;70:830–835

14. Masiukiewicz US, Burrow GN. Hyperthyroidism in pregnancy: diagnosis and treatment. Thyroid 1999;9:647–652

15. Palit TK, Miller CC, Miltenburg DM. The efficacy of thyroidectomy for Graves' disease: a meta-analysis. J Surg Res 2000;90:161–165

16. Schussler-Fiorenza CM, Bruns CM, Chen H. The surgical management of Graves' disease. J Surg Res 2006;133:207–214

17. Bron LP, O'Brien CJ. Total thyroidectomy for clinically benign disease of the thyroid gland. Br J Surg 2004;91:569–574

18. Bellantone R. Total thyroidectomy for management of benign thyroid disease: Review of 526 cases. World J Surg 2002;26:1468–1471

19. Lennquist S, Jortso E, Anderberg B, et al. Beta-blockers compared with antithyroid drugs as preoperative treatment in hyperthyroidism: drug tolerance, complication, and postoperative thyroid function. Surgery 1985;98:1141–1147

20. Terris DJ, Seybt MW, Chin E. Cosmetic thyroid surgery: defining the essential principles. Laryngoscope 2007;117:1168–1172

21. Herranz-Gonzalez J, Gavilan J, Matinez-Vidal J, et al. Complications following thyroid surgery. Arch Otolaryngol Head Neck Surg 1991;117:516–518

22. Riddell V. Thyroidectomy: Prevention of bilateral recurrent nerve palsy. Results of identification of the nerve over 23 consecutive years (1946–69) with description of an additional safety measure. Br J Surg 1970;57:1–11

23. Wheeler MH. Thyroid surgery and the recurrent laryngeal nerve. Br J Surg 1999;86:291–292

24. Hisham AN, Lukman MR. Recurrent laryngeal nerve in thyroid surgery: a critical appraisal. ANZ J Surg 2002;72:887–889

25. Loré JM. Practical anatomical considerations in thyroid tumor surgery. Arch Otolaryngol 1983;109:568–574

26. Karlan MS, Catz B, Dunkelman D, et al. A safe technique for thyroidectomy with complete nerve dissection and parathyroid preservation. Head Neck Surg 1984;6:1014–1019

27. Lo CY, Lam KY. Postoperative hypocalcemia in patients who did or did not undergo parathyroid autotransplantation during thyroidectomy: a comparative study. Surgery 1998;124:1081–1087

28. Shaha AR, Jaffe BM. Parathyroid preservation during thyroid surgery. Am J Otolaryngol 1998;19:113–117

29. Terris DJ, Gourin CG, Chin E. Minimally invasive thyroidectomy: basic and advanced techniques. Laryngoscope 2006;116:350–356

30. Terris DJ, Bonnett A, Gourin CG, et al. Minimally invasive thyroidectomy using the Sofferman technique. Laryngoscope 2005;115:1104–1108

31. Miccoli P, Berti P, Raffaelli M, et al. Minimally invasive video-assisted thyroidectomy. Am J Surg 2001;181:567–570

32. Miccoli P, Berti P, Frustaci GL, et al. Video-assisted thyroidectomy: indications and results. Langenbecks Arch Surg 2006;391:68–71

33. Ishii S, Ohgami M, Arisaka Y, et al. Endoscopic thyroidectomy with precordial approach. JSES 1998;3:159–163

34. Kitano H, Fujimura M, Kinoshita T, et al. Endoscopic thyroid resection using cutaneous elevation in lieu of insufflation. Surg Endosc 2002;16:88–91

35. Maeda S, Uga T, Hayashida N, et al. Video-assisted subtotal or near-total thyroidectomy for Graves' disease. Br J Surg 2006;93:61–66

36. Yeung HC, Ng WT, Kong CK. Endoscopic thyroid and parathyroid surgery. Surg Endosc 1997;11:1135

37. Ohgami M, Ishii S, Arisawa Y, et al. Scarless endoscopic thyroidectomy: breast approach for better cosmesis. Surg Laparosc Endosc Percutan Tech 2000;10:1–4

38. Ikeda Y, Takami H, Sasaki Y, et al. Endoscopic resection of thyroid tumors by the axillary approach. J Cardiovasc Surg (Torino) 2000;41:791–792

39. Shimizu K, Akira S, Jasmi AY, et al. Video-assisted neck surgery: endoscopic resection of thyroid tumors with a very minimal neck wound. J Am Coll Surg 1999;188:697–703

40. Miccoli P, Berti P, Raffaelli M, et al. Comparison between minimally invasive video-assisted thyroidectomy and conventional thyroidectomy: a prospective randomized study. Surgery 2001;130:1039–1043

41. Lombardi CP, Raffaelli M, Princi P, et al. Safety of video-assisted thyroidectomy versus conventional surgery. Head Neck 2005;27:58–64

42. Terris DJ, Chin E. Clinical implementation of endoscopic thyroidectomy in selected patients. Laryngoscope 2006;116:1745–1748

43. Terris DJ, Angelos P, Steward D, Simental A. Minimally invasive video-assisted thyroidectomy: a multi-institutional North American experience. Arch Otolaryngol Head Neck Surg 2008;134:81–84

44. Miccoli P, Elisei R, Materazzi G, et al. Minimally invasive video-assisted thyroidectomy for papillary carcinoma: a prospective study of its completeness. Surgery 2002;132:1070–1073

45. Bellantone R, Lombardi CP, Raffaelli M, et al. Central neck lymph node removal during minimally invasive video-assisted thyroidectomy for thyroid carcinoma: a feasible and safe procedure. J Laparoendosc Adv Surg Tech A 2002;12:181–185

46. Lombardi CP, Raffaelli M, Princi P, et al. Video-assisted thyroidectomy: report of a 7-year experience in Rome. Langenbecks Arch Surg 2006;391:174–177

47. Miccoli P, Berti P, Materazzi G, Minuto M, Barellini L. Minimally invasive video-assisted thyroidectomy: five years of experience. J Am Coll Surg 2004;199:243–248

48. Terris DJ, Seybt MW, Gourin CG, et al. Ultrasonic technology facilitates minimal access thyroid surgery. Laryngoscope 2006;116:851–854

49. Miccoli P, Berti P, Raffaelli M, et al. Impact of harmonic scalpel on operative time during video-assisted thyroidectomy. Surg Endosc 2002;16:663–666

50. Siperstein AE, Berber E, Morkoyun E. The use of the harmonic scalpel vs conventional knot tying for vessel ligation in thyroid surgery. Arch Surg 2002;137:137–142

51. Voutilainen PE, Haglund CH. Ultrasonically activated shears in thyroidectomies: a randomized trial. Ann Surg 2000;231:322–328

52. Shemen L. Thyroidectomy using the harmonic scalpel: analysis of 105 consecutive cases. Otolaryngol Head Neck Surg 2002;127:284–288

9 Surgical Management of Substernal Goiter

Brian Hung-Hin Lang, Chung-Yau Lo, and Gregory W. Randolph

With an improved understanding of the neck base anatomy and refinement of surgical technique, goiter surgery has been transformed from "horrid butchery," to the elegant operation with negligible morbidity of today.[1] In fact, at the turn of the 20th century thyroid surgery was described by William Stewart Halsted as the "supreme triumph of the surgeon's art." On the other hand, thyroid surgery for certain pathologies remains a great challenge to the operating surgeon. The extension of a goiter from its original cervical position into the mediastinum, known as substernal goiter, represents one of these challenges. Although this condition was first described in 1749, it was not until 1820 that the first successful surgical removal of a substernal goiter was documented.[2,3] Distorted neck base anatomy, restricted surgical access of the thoracic inlet, mediastinal extension, increased size of the thyroid gland, and the increased glandular vascularity all contribute to the increased technical demand and serve to make the operation more hazardous and unpredictable than that of a cervical goiter.

Definition and Classification of a Substernal Goiter

The word *goiter* is derived from the Latin word *guttur*, meaning throat, and is generally referred to as an enlargement of the thyroid gland. On the other hand, the definition of a substernal goiter is less clear. Various definitions have been proposed. A substernal goiter has been variously defined as an enlarged gland "with the greatest diameter of the intrathoracic component by x-ray well below the upper aperture of the thoracic inlet,"[4] with extension down to the aortic arch,[5] with its lower border reaching the transverse process of the fourth thoracic vertebra or below,[6] or with greater than 50% of the goiter volume presenting behind the sternum.[7,8] Recently, goiter has been defined more loosely as substernal when it requires mediastinal exploration and dissection for removal,[9] when an intrathoracic goiter is clearly found while the neck is extended at operation,[10] or when the intrathoracic component appears to extend more than 3 cm from the thoracic inlet.[11]

In addition, several authors have attempted to offer various classification schemes for substernal goiter to objectively describe the degree of substernal extension. Substernal goiters were classified into two grades by Lahey according to the relationship to the aortic arch: grade I includes those extending nearly to the arch of the aorta, and grade II includes those extending to the arch of the aorta or beyond.[4] Higgins[12] described a classification scheme based on the percentage of goiter in the chest; goiters with greater than 50% in the neck are substernal, those with greater than 50% in the chest are partially intrathoracic, and those with greater than 80% in the chest are completely intrathoracic.[12] Similarly, Cohen and Cho[13] graded substernal goiters according to the percentage of the mediastinal or intrathoracic component of the goiter (grade 1, 0–25%; grade 2, 26–50%; grade 3, 51–75%; grade 4: >75%).[13] **Table 9.1** shows a practical classification scheme with associated anatomic correlates proposed by Randolph.[14]

Pathogenesis of Substernal Goiter

It is generally recognized that the vast majority of substernal goiters (over 98%) derive from a caudal migration of cervical goiters. The substernal components tend to migrate anterior to the trachea, esophagus, recurrent laryngeal nerve, and subclavian vessels in 85 to 90% of cases.[11,15] They may extend evenly on both sides but more commonly, asymmetrically. Some series reported a higher incidence of substernal extension on the left side,[9,10] whereas others reported the exact opposite phenomenon.[16,17] This downward migration of cervical goiters into the thorax has been attributed to a combination of factors such as the negative intrathoracic pressure generated during inspiration, repetitive forces of deglutition, the effect of gravity, and the large potential space of the mediastinum acting in concert.

An uncommon type of substernal goiter accounting for approximately 1% of substernal goiters is the so-called primary or "true intrathoracic" goiter (i.e., substernal goiter type III, see **Table 9.1**). This substernal goiter maintains no cervical connection with the orthotopic thyroid gland. Several interesting theories have been put forward to explain the pathogenesis of such goiters. The first proposes that at least some of these goiters develop from thyrothymic congenital rests in the thyrothymic ligament and grow after the removal of the cervical goiter.[18] Sackett et al[19] reported an incidence of these rests of up to 53% in 100 consecutive patients who underwent thyroid or parathyroid surgery. Other theories of substernal goiter formation include embryologic fragmentation of thyroid anlagen with hyperdescent. Another theory proposes that such goiters start as exophytic nodules from

Table 9.1 A Substernal Goiter Classification Based on Anatomical Relationships[14]

Type	Location	Anatomy	Prevalence	Approach
I	Anterior mediastinum	Anterior to great vessels, trachea, recurrent laryngeal nerve	85%	Transcervical (sternotomy, only if intrathoracic goiter diameter is greater than thoracic inlet diameter)
II	Posterior mediastinum	Posterior to great vessels, trachea, recurrent nerve	15%	As above; also consider sternotomy or right posterolateral thoracotomy if type IIB
IIA	Ipsilateral extension			
IIB	Contralateral extension			
IIB1	Extension posterior to both trachea and esophagus			
IIB2	Extension between trachea and esophagus			
III	Isolated mediastinal goiter	No connection to orthotopic gland; may have mediastinal blood supply	<1%	Transcervical or sternotomy

the thyroid inferior pole, and over time there is attenuation of the nodule-thyroid stalk.[14] Early recognition of this type of goiter is useful in preoperative planning as these goiters tend to derive their blood supply from the internal mammary and innominate arteries, or directly from the intrathoracic aorta rather than from the cervical sources, unlike most other substernal goiters, which typically maintain their cervical blood supply. This thoracic blood supply may necessitate a thoracotomy or a median sternotomy in contrast to those substernal goiters deriving from caudal migration of cervical goiters.[20,21] **Fig. 9.1** shows the imaging findings and the management of a patient suffering from a mediastinal goiter recognized after a hemithyroidectomy over 20 years earlier.

Incidence and Prevalence

Benign enlargement of the thyroid gland is a very common clinical problem. The worldwide incidence is approximately 5 to 10% but appears to be steadily decreasing primarily due to multiple factors including the routine use of iodized salt and earlier surgical intervention.[22] The actual incidence of substernal goiters in the general population is difficult to document because the number of substernal goiters treated nonsurgically remains largely unknown, with reported incidence derived from surgical series. However, based on chest radiograph screening of the general population in Australia, Reeve et al[23] detected substernal goiters in 0.02% of the population and in 0.05% of women older than age 40. In the United States, Rundle et al[24] reported a similar incidence of 0.02% during a tuberculosis radiography screening in 1959. Pemberton[25] in 1921 reported a surgical series of 4006 patients with thyroid goiters, and 13.5% were noted to be substernal. In 1934, Lahey and Swinton[4] reviewed 5131 thyroidectomies and found that 21% had substernal goiters. In 1992, Wax and Briant[26] reported the incidence in their surgical series of 939 patients to be 2.6%. More recently, Chow et al[24] reported a series of 287 patients from 2000 to 2003, in which 24 patients (9.4%) had substernal goiters. Similarly, Ahmed et al[17] reported that in 40 of 267 patients (5%) in

their series, the goiters were substernal. In our experience, the incidence of substernal goiters in our patients undergoing thyroidectomies ranged from 8 to 16%.[28–30]

Clinical Presentation

The majority of substernal goiters grow slowly and are infrequently malignant. Depending on the series, only 3 to 16% of cases are associated with malignancy.[31] Most patients present typically in their fifth decade, though some may present as early as 15 years old or as late as 90 years old.[32] There is a female preponderance, with a female to male ratio of 3 to 1. A positive family history can be present in up to 30% of patients.[33] The majority of patients are asymptomatic, with their goiters detected incidentally during radiologic examinations. Others present with a palpable neck mass (60–70%) or with respiratory symptoms (40–90%) varying from a simple irritative cough, to hoarseness, inspiratory stridor, or frank shortness of breath.[7,15,34] Acute airway obstruction is an uncommon but life-threatening emergency for benign goiters and occurs almost exclusively in patients with substernal extension.[35] The exact reason for the sudden onset of airway obstruction is unclear, but it has been thought to be related to sudden enlargement of the goiter due to hemorrhage, cystic degeneration, or malignant change within the substernal component.[36] In addition to respiratory distress, dysphagia and globus sensation are symptoms suggestive of local compression. When neck vasculature is compressed, superior vena cava (SVC) syndrome or even cerebral edema may occur.[31] True SVC syndrome, we have found, is almost exclusively associated with substernal malignancy, and preoperatively it should be carefully assessed radiographically. Hematemesis (secondary to downstream esophageal varices),[37] abscess formation,[38] chylothorax secondary to thoracic obstruction,[35] transient ischemic attack through "thyroid steal syndrome," venous thrombosis, and Horner syndrome[34] have all been reported as initial presentations or complications of substernal goiters. In addition, symptoms of hypothyroidism and hyperthyroidism should be actively sought during the history taking.

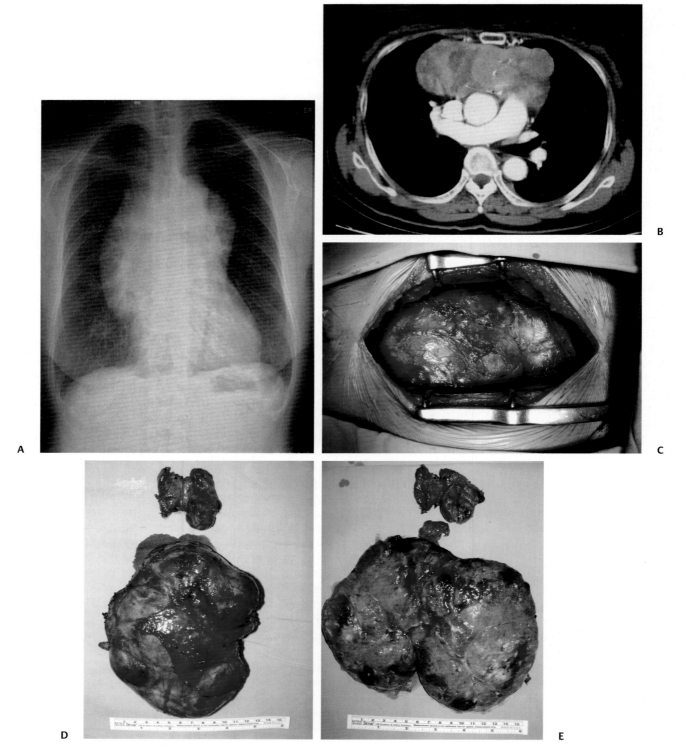

Fig. 9.1 A posteroanterior (PA) chest radiograph (**A**) and a computed tomography (CT) film (**B**) of a large mediastinal goiter developed after a hemithyroidectomy over 20 years ago. An additional median ster- notomy (**C**) was required for the complete removal of the mediastinal component (**D,E**).

Physical Examination

Physical examination of a patient with a substernal goiter should be similar to that for any thyroid lesion. Patients may have a neck scar due to previous surgery. The consistency, fixation, and size of the thyroid swelling in the neck should be documented. The larynx and trachea should be examined for any deviation from midline. A large asymmetrically enlarged cervical goiter with substernal extension would typically push the larynx and trachea to the contralateral side. However, substernal goiters might not be apparent in the neck or manifest with deviation of the airway because of the mass effect on the mediastinal trachea. Interestingly, up to 30% of patients with substernal goiters may have no palpable cervical component.[9,15] In patients with short necks, palpation of cervical goiter is difficult. For that reason, if one clinically suspects a substernal goiter because of the inability to define the lower border of a thyroid mass, axial imaging of the neck and upper chest should be performed. It is of note that with recurrent goiter the physical exam typically underestimates goiter extent, given a prior perithyroid restrictive blanketing scar. The neck should also be examined for any cervical lymphadenopathy. It is imperative to examine the vocal cords endoscopically for all patients with a substernal goiter. Vocal cord palsy without previous surgery is suggestive of the presence of invasive thyroid malignancy until proven otherwise. Occasionally, vocal cord paralysis may occur as a result of the mass effect of the large goiters, and bilateral vocal cord paralysis in a nonmalignant substernal goiter has been reported.[39] Patients should be asked to raise both arms above the neck to elicit the Pemberton sign (flushing of the face, dilation of the external jugular veins, and/or symptomatic airway compression).[21,31] Other clinical features such as Horner syndrome can occur occasionally.[34]

Preoperative Assessment

After a complete history and physical examination, patients with substernal goiters should have their thyroid function checked biochemically. Hyperthyroidism is slowly evolving in patients with long-standing multinodular goiters and may develop acutely in response to significant iodine load (such as with computed tomography [CT] contrast) or introduction of iodized salt in endemic goiter regions. Subclinical hyperthyroidism is not uncommon in substernal goiters. Hyperthyroidism can occur in up to 50% of patients undergoing surgical treatments for substernal goiters.[15,21,38,40,41] Hypothyroidism has also been reported in up to 16% of cases.[15] A fibrotic variant of Hashimoto disease can result in a massive firm goiter that can descend inferiorly.

The routine use of fine-needle aspiration (FNA) is controversial in substernal goiters. Because there is already an indication for surgery on the basis of a substernal goiter, an FNA can be omitted if it would not alter the plan of management.[9,10,42,43] Furthermore, there is a small potential risk of bleeding into a substernal nodule, which may convert a compromised airway to an acute obstruction. However, if there is any suspicion of malignancy during history taking, physical examination, or radiographic evaluation, FNA evaluation may enhance an accurate preoperative diagnosis and facilitate perioperative planning.

Plain chest radiography is commonly employed as the first investigation for a patient with suspected substernal goiter. It is useful in showing the degree of tracheal compression or deviation, but provides limited information on the size or extent of the substernal goiter. Up to 41% of patients with substernal goiters have a normal chest radiograph preoperatively.[15,41,44–46] Interestingly, tracheal diameter estimated on plain chest radiography films is significantly larger than that measured on axial CT scan and in cadaveric studies.[47,48] CT scans are very helpful in the assessments of patients with large cervical or substernal goiters.[49] It provides important information such as tracheal deviation, tracheal compression, retrotracheal extension right down to the level of the aortic arch, as well as esophageal and major vessel displacement or compression.[50] **Fig. 9.2** shows a massive substernal goiter causing significant tracheal compression and lateral displacement of the carotid artery and internal jugular vein. The demonstration of these relationships by preoperative CT assists not only in surgical planning but also in anesthesia's intubation approach. In addition, CT findings may also be useful in predicting the need for sternotomy,[50] providing information for diagnosing invasive malignancy, and determining the relationships of mediastinal structures to allow safe operative management for large posterior mediastinal goiters. Surgical candidacy may in fact derive from CT scan information. Preoperative TSH is recommended before CT scan with contrast. Nonetheless, the cost-effectiveness of a preoperative CT scan has recently been challenged.[15]

Functional tests such as pulmonary studies and flow volume loops have not been considered a routine part of a preoperative workup. Although the presence of airway obstruction can be accurately determined, it does not significantly affect the management of patients.

Surgical Technique in Substernal Goiter

Most authors have convincingly demonstrated the feasibility and safety of operating and delivering a substernal goiter through a standard cervical approach in the vast majority of cases.[7–9,17,31,42,49,50] Sand et al[51] advocated a more liberal use of sternotomy because it did not increase surgical morbidity and seemed to prevent postoperative complications, such as injury to the recurrent laryngeal nerve, parathyroid glands, and adjacent organs as well as hemorrhage from excessive traction through a cervical incision. However, with experience, equally low morbidity and mortality can be achieved through a cervical incision alone.[7–9,17,31,49,50] In fact, the routine or liberal use of a sternotomy or thoracotomy should be avoided unless it is absolutely necessary.

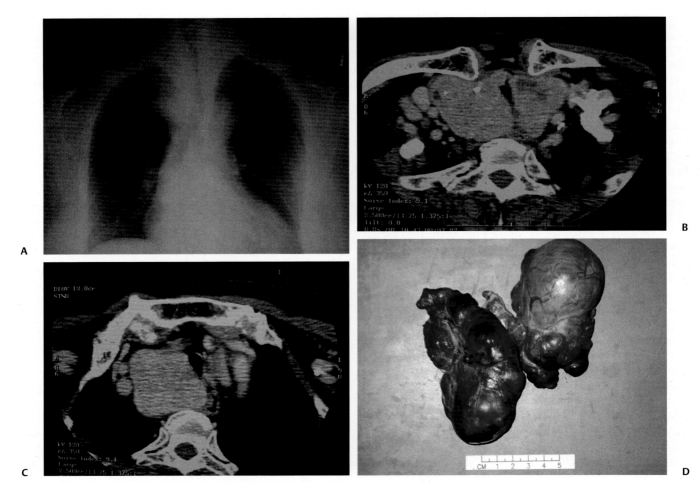

Fig. 9.2 A PA chest radiograph (**A**), CT scans (**B,C**), and a specimen photograph (**D**) of a typical substernal goiter descending from the neck.

Most of the surgical principles in thyroid surgery originally defined by Theodor Kocher remain extremely relevant to goiter surgery and should be similarly applied in substernal goiter procedures.[52] Despite some controversies, total thyroidectomy is now preferred over less extensive thyroid resections based on several reasons. First, a preoperative diagnosis of malignancy is often not possible. Second, there is a relatively higher incidence of underlying occult malignancy of up to 20% in substernal goiters. Third, there is a higher risk of future thyroid remnant recurrence after incomplete thyroidectomy.[11,15,31,49,53] On the other hand, in experienced centers, the rates of permanent recurrent laryngeal nerve paralysis and hypoparathyroidism for total thyroidectomy did not appear to be significantly greater than those undergoing less extensive thyroid resections.[54] Therefore, a total thyroidectomy is recommended as the procedure of choice in experienced centers for a majority of patients with substernal goiters with bilateral disease.

Positioning of the Patient

Upon induction of general anesthesia and endotracheal intubation, an inflatable bag is placed under the patient's shoul-

ders to hyperextend the neck slightly. The patient is then placed in a semisitting position to reduce the neck venous congestion or engorgement because substernal goiters may extend into the thorax, compress, and cause venous engorgement.

Skin Incision

A generous collar skin incision should be made extending from the lateral edge of both sternocleidomastoid muscles. Although it might sound paradoxical at first, a slightly higher skin incision is useful in a low-lying goiter because it allows a better access of the lobe inferiorly by facilitating upward traction of the gland after ligation and division of the upper pole vessels.[55] The upper and lower subplatysmal flaps are developed and sutured in place.

Strap Muscles

The strap muscles can be mobilized from the sternocleidomastoid muscles to facilitate subsequent mobilization of the thyroid lobes. Strap muscles are separated in the midline. Some surgeons routinely transect the strap muscle to improve access to the gland.[10,17] Routine transection of the

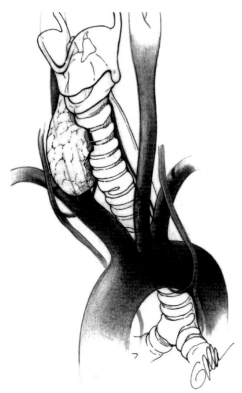

Fig. 9.3 View of the cervical–mediastinal continuity of great vessels that are important in substernal goiter surgery.

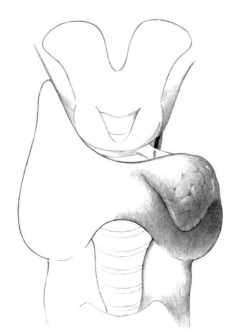

Fig. 9.4 The superior approach to the recurrent laryngeal nerve (RLN).

strap muscle is frequently not necessary in the substernal goiter. In case of strap transection, the muscles should be divided as cranially as possible so as to lessen the effect of nerve denervation. The transected ends are retracted cranially and caudally to optimize exposure.

Thyroid Mobilization

To ensure full mobilization of the anterolateral aspect of the thyroid lobe, as an important first step in goiter surgery, it is essential to identify the carotid sheath contents because this is usually the landmark for the outer lateral boundary. Knowledge of the carotid sheath contents also allows a surgery to "follow the neck into the chest" and become oriented as to the best approach for the specific goiter one is treating (**Fig. 9.3**). It is not necessary to deliberately look for and ligate the middle thyroid vein as the first step unless it helps to facilitate the upper pole mobilization because the vein(s) is often pushed and compressed by the enlarged thyroid lobe. Dissection should be kept close to the thyroid capsule and moved cranially toward the upper pole. Once the lateral aspect of the upper pole has been mobilized, the medial space between the cricothyroid muscle and thyroid lobe is opened and this step is best facilitated by gentle lateral retraction of the upper pole. The usual precaution of identifying and preserving the external branch of the superior laryngeal nerve (ESLN) should be taken. The greater the superior pole's

cranial development, the more likely the ESLN will be brought into a type IIB configuration. Once the upper pole has been mobilized and delineated, the upper pole vessels are doubly ligated close to the thyroid capsule. The superior parathyroid gland should be identified next and should be considered for reimplantation if its viability is doubtful. Sometimes it is possible to identify the recurrent laryngeal nerve (RLN) entering the larynx once the upper pole has been fully reflected (**Fig. 9.4**). The RLN can then be dissected retrograde off the posterior surface of the gland.

The substernal component can then be retracted into the neck base. A Kocher clamp is then applied to the upper pole, or the operator's fingers can be applied for upward traction of the thyroid lobe. This upward traction allows rotation of the cervical portion of the gland from lateral to medial and also facilitates gentle, blunt finger dissection on the surface of the capsule through areolar planes around all borders of the goiter. The surgeon's finger should be used to confirm that all palpable adhesions have been divided and the substernal component could now be delivered into the neck. Apart from using the surgeon's finger, instruments such as a sterile tablespoon, a delivery forceps, and a Foley catheter have been employed to facilitate the delivery of the substernal portion out to the cervical wound.[56,57] A sterile tablespoon is particularly useful because it can reach more inferiorly than the longest surgeon's finger, as it occupies less space. Once the intrathoracic component has been delivered into the wound, the gland is retracted medially, and the rest of the operation, including "subcapsular dissection," is performed as with any thyroid operation.[58]

Other Useful Maneuvers

In situations when the substernal component cannot be brought into the neck despite all these maneuvers, the smaller contralateral lobe may be excised first to provide more room for mobilization in the neck. Morcellation of the substernal component has been advocated because of the frequent benign nature of the goiters and the ability to control its feeding vessels frequently derived from the neck. However, most surgeons would avoid a blind morcellation because of excess bleeding and would proceed to a partial or a complete sternotomy, failing all these maneuvers to facilitate a safe mediastinal approach to the removal of the substernal goiter. The use of sternotomy was described originally by Dunhill[59] and later popularized by Taylor.[60] In fact, this approach is rarely required, and has been reported in 0 to 37.1% of patients undergoing surgical treatment for substernal goiters. **Table 9.2** shows a comparison of the rate of substernal goiters, sternotomies/thoracotomies, tracheostomies, and the number of in-hospital deaths in most substernal goiter surgeries reported in the past two decades. The adoption of more routine sternotomy appears to be associated with an increase in operative morbidity and length of hospital stay.[42] It is, nevertheless, indicated for extraordinarily large or low-lying intrathoracic goiters and in

Table 9.2 A Comparison of the Proportion of Substernal Goiters, Need of Sternotomies/Thoracotomies/Tracheostomies and the Number of In-Hospital Deaths in Substernal Goiters Surgical Series Reported in the Past Two Decades

First Author (Year)	No. of Thyroid Resections	No. (%) of Substernal Goiters	No. (%) of Sternotomies/ Thoracotomies	No. of Postoperative Tracheostomies	No. of Hospital Deaths
Sand (1983)[51]	n/a	31	6 (19.4)	0	0
Allo (1983)[31]	872	50 (5.7)	1 (2.0)	0	0
Katlic (1985)[7]	n/a	80	2 (2.5)	0	0
Melliere (1988)[68]	2908	58 (2.0)	5 (8)	0	0
Michel (1988)[41]	170	34 (20.0)	4 (11.8)	1	0
Shaha (1989)[69]	370	72 (19.5)	1 (13.9)	2	0
Madjar (1995)[21]	222	44 (19.8)	6 (13.6)	0	0
Torre (1995)[67]	3338	237 (7.1)	8 (3.4)	5	2
Hsu (1996)[54]	1585	234 (14.8)*	4 (1.7)	3	0
Moron (1998)[70]	234	16 (6.8)	3 (1.9)	0	0
Nervi (1998)[71]	5263	621 (11.8)	44 (7.1)	1	0
Netterville (1998)[49]	150	23 (15.3)	0 (0.0)	0	0
Pulli (1998)[42]	n/a	21	3 (14.3)	0	0
Vadasz (1998)[62]	1458	175 (12.0)	42 (24.0)	2	2
Rodriguez (1999)[34]	780	72 (9.2)	7 (9.7)	0	0
Abdel Rahim (1999)[64]	n/a	103	0 (0.0)	13	0
Dedivitis (1999)[72]	204	32 (15.7)	2 (6.3)	0	1
Ozdemir (2000)[73]	1320	30 (2.3)	2 (6.7)	0	0
Mussi (2000)[16]	7480	374 (5.0)	43 (11.5)	0	0
Hedayati (2002)[11]	381	116 (30.4)	2 (1.7)	2	1
Erbil (2004)[15]	2650	170 (6.4)	12 (7.1)	0	0
Shen (2004)[8]	n/a	60	1 (1.7)	0	1
Chow (2005)[27]	287	24 (8.4)	2 (8.3)	1	0
Sancho (2006)[74]	n/a	35	13 (37.1)	3	2
Chauhan (2006)[10]	755	199 (26.4)	0 (0.0)	0	0
Ahmed (2006)[17]	267	40 (15.0)	9 (22.5)	5	0

n/a = not available.
*Recurrent substernal goiters.

situations where excessive uncontrollable bleeding is encountered during traction of the gland. In addition, the rare truly ectopic intrathoracic goiter (with its major blood supply derived often from intrathoracic vessels) and recurrent substernal goiters requiring reoperations may more frequently necessitate this surgical approach. In fact, certain preoperative predictors for sternotomy or thoracotomy including atypical neck anatomy, dense adhesions, primary intrathoracic goiter, recurrent intrathoracic goiter, or carcinoma have been identified.[17,38,42,45,61] Another potential but rare situation requiring a sternotomy or a thoracotomy is the so-called crossed substernal or posterior mediastinal goiter (type IIB). This is a rare variant of substernal goiter in which there is extension from one side to the opposite side of the posterior mediastinum. A right anterolateral thoracotomy through the fourth interspace is recommended for this type of substernal goiter.[62]

Tracheomalacia and Tracheostomy

At the end of the thyroidectomy prior to wound closure, the surgeon should check the integrity of the trachea by observation during the respiratory cycle and by gentle pressure between the thumb and index finger. This can be done more effectively by asking the anesthesiologist to pull out the endotracheal tube slightly while the surgeon applies gentle pressure to the trachea. An obvious collapse or softening of the tracheal rings indicates tracheomalacia, a condition that is poorly understood, extremely rare, and apparently reversible.[8,63–65] Tracheomalacia manifests as postoperative airway obstruction with paradoxical collapse of the airway during inspiration because the tracheal ring softens and loses strength secondary to chronic extrinsic compression. The reported incidence of tracheomalacia secondary to large goiters ranged from 0.001 to 1.5% in surgical series.[38,44,65] With the advance in anesthesia technique and the early treatment of large substernal goiters, the true incidence of tracheomalacia from goiter compression should be even much lower. In situations when the presence of tracheomalacia is certain, some authors would recommend keeping the endotracheal tube for 24 to 48 hours before controlled extubation afterward.[66] Other options, including continuous positive pressure ventilation, Marlex mesh tracheopexy, and postoperative tracheostomy, have been adopted and described.[67] One must keep in mind that some cases of "tracheomalacia" are likely misdiagnosed bilateral vocal cord paralysis.

Although tracheostomy is rarely indicated in the postoperative period after thyroidectomy, the incidence ranged from 0 to 12.6% in reported thyroidectomy series for substernal goiters (**Table 9.2**). **Fig. 9.5** shows a patient needing a preoperative tracheostomy due to airway obstruction from a substernal goiter. **Fig. 9.6** shows the chest radiograph and CT scan of the same patient with the tracheostomy in situ. Apart from tracheomalacia, other indications for tracheostomy would include bilateral vocal cord palsies, laryngeal edema, postoperative bleeding, and traumatic endotracheal intubation.[54,64]

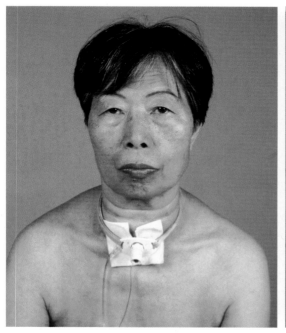 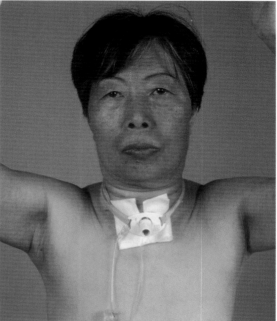

A **B**

Fig. 9.5 Clinical photographs of a patient presenting with acute airway obstruction caused by a large substernal goiter. An emergency tracheostomy (**A**) before referral was required and a positive Pemberton sign with facial flushing on raising both arms (**B**) was elicited.

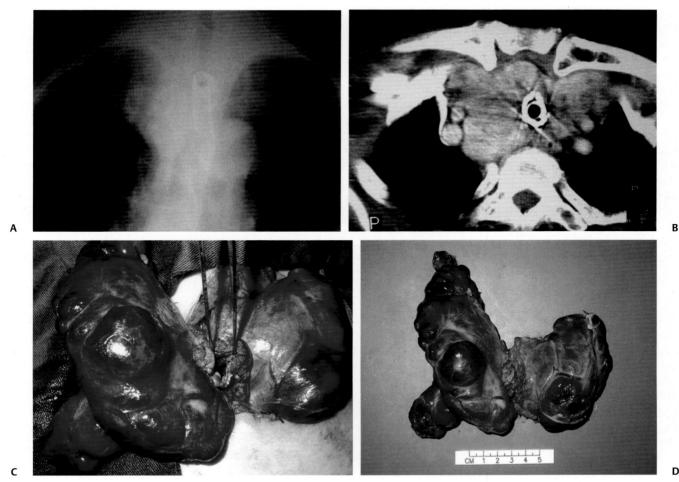

Fig. 9.6 A PA chest radiograph (**A**) and a CT scan (**B**) of a substernal goiter with a tracheostomy tube in situ. Operative photos show the tracheostomy track through the thyroid isthmus (**C**) and the resected specimen (**D**).

Conclusion

Surgical management of substernal goiters poses a challenge to the thyroid surgeons but reflects an ultimate triumph of the surgeon's art in thyroid surgery. Despite the condition being described more than a century ago, the need for a precise preoperative diagnosis and workup, understanding of the important anatomic landmarks, the adoption of different surgical strategies, the application of good anesthesia and surgical skills, as well as perioperative care would remain important components in ensuring a safe and excellent outcome in patients undergoing thyroidectomies for substernal goiters. Although the incidence of substernal goiters ranges in various surgical series because of differences in case selection and variations in definition, the outcome of thyroidectomy for substernal goiter is excellent in experienced hands. The majority of the procedures can be accomplished through a cervical incision, and an additional sternotomy, thoracotomy, or tracheostomy is reserved for a small subset of patients only.

References

1. Singh B, Lucente FE, Shaha AR. Substernal goiter: a clinical review. Am J Otolaryngol 1994;15:409–416
2. Haller A. Disputationes Anatomica Selectae. Gottingen, Germany: Vendenhoeck, 1749:96
3. Klein F. Veber die Austrotting verschiedener geschwulste, besonders jener der Ohrspercheldruse und der Schiddruse; Aussachalung der Schilddruse. J Chir Augenlleillk 1820;12:106–113
4. Lahey FH, Swinton NW. Intrathoracic goiter. Surg Gynecol Obstet 1934;59:627–637
5. Crile G. Intrathoracic goiter. Cleve Clin Q 1939;6:313–322
6. Lindskog GE, Goldenberg IS. Definitive diagnosis, pathology and treatment of substernal goiter. JAMA 1957;163:327–329
7. Katlic MR, Grillo HC, Wang CA. Substernal goiter. Analysis of 80 patients from Massachusetts General Hospital. Am J Surg 1985;149:283–287
8. Shen WT, Kebebew E, Duh QY, Clark OH. Predictors of airway complications after thyroidectomy for substernal goiter. Arch Surg 2004;139:656–659

9. Sanders LE, Possi RL, Shahian DM, Williamson WA. Mediastinal goiters: the need for an aggressive approach. Arch Surg 1992;127:609–613

10. Chauhan A, Serpell JW. Thyroidectomy is safe and effective for retrosternal goitre. ANZ J Surg 2006;76:238–242

11. Hedayati N, McHenry CR, Prinz RA, DeJong SA. The clinical presentation and operative management of nodular and diffuse substernal thyroid disease. Am Surg 2002;68:245–252

12. Higgins CC. Intrathoracic goitre. Arch Surg 1927;15:895–901

13. Cohen JP, Cho HT. Surgery for substernal goiter. In: Friedman M, ed. Operative Techniques in Otolaryngology and Head and Neck Surgery. Philadelphia: WB Saunders, 1994:118–125

14. Randolph G. Surgery of Cervical and Substernal Goiter. In: Randolph G, ed. Surgery of the Thyroid and Parathyroid. Philadelphia: WB Saunders, 2003:70–99

15. Erbil Y, Bozbora A, Barbaros U, Ozarmagan S, Azezli A, Molvalilar S. Surgical management of substernal goiters: clinical experience of 170 patients. Surg Today 2004;34:732–736

16. Mussi A, Ambrogi MC, Iacconi P, Spinelli C, Miccoli P, Angeletti CA. Mediastinal goiters: when the transthoracic approach? Acta Chir Belg 2000;100:259–263

17. Ahmed ME, Ahmed EO, Mahadi SI. Substernal goiter: the need for median sternotomy. World J Surg 2006;30:1945–1948

18. Snook KL, Stalberg PL, Dishu SB, Sywak MS, Edhouse P, Delbridge L. Recurrance after total thyroidectomy for benign modular goiter. World J Surg 2007;31:593–600

19. Sackett WR, Reeve TS, Barraclough B, Delbridge L. Thyrothymic thyroid rests: incidence and relationship to the thyroid gland. J Am Coll Surg 2002;195:635–640

20. Newman E, Shaha AR. Substernal goiter. J Surg Oncol 1995;60:207–212

21. Madjar S, Weissberg D. Retrosternal goiter. Chest 1995;108:78–82

22. Hegedüs L, Bonnema SJ, Bennedbaek FN. Management of simple nodular goiter: current status and future perspectives. Endocr Rev 2003;24:102–132

23. Reeve TS, Rubinstein C, Rundle FF. Intrathoracic goiter: its prevalence in Sydney metropolitan mass radiography surveys. Med J Aust 1957;44:149–156

24. Rundle FF, De Lambert RN, Epps RG. Cervicothoracic tumors: the technical aid to their roentgenologic localization. Am J Roentgenol Radium Ther Nucl Med 1959;81:316–321

25. Pemberton J. Surgery of substernal and intrathoracic goiter. Arch Surg 1921;2:1

26. Wax MK, Briant TD. Management of substernal goiter. J Otolaryngol 1992;21:165–170

27. Chow TL, Chan TTF, Suen DTK, Chu DW, Lam SH. Surgical management of substernal goiter: local experience. Hong Kong Med J 2005;11:360–365

28. Lo CY, Lam KY. Postoperative hypocalcemia in patients who did or did not undergo parathyroid autotransplantation during thyroidectomy: a comparative study. Surgery 1998;124:1081–1087

29. Lang BH, Lo CY. Total thyroidectomy for multinodular goiter in the elderly. Am J Surg 2005;190:418–423

30. Chan WF, Lang BH, Lo CY. The role of intraoperative neuromonitoring of recurrent laryngeal nerve during thyroidectomy: a comparative study on 1000 nerves at risk. Surgery 2006;140:866–872

31. Allo MD, Thompson NW. Rationale for the operative management of substernal goiters. Surgery 1983;94:969–977

32. Johnston JH, Twente GE. Surgical approach to intrathoracic (mediastinal) goiter. Ann Surg 1956;143:572–579

33. Wychulis AR, Payne WS, Cagall OT, Woolner LB. Surgical treatment of mediastinal tumours: a 40 year experience. J Thorac Cardiovasc Surg 1971;62:379–385

34. Rodriguez JM, Hernandez Q, Pinero A, et al. Substernal goiter: clinical experience of 72 cases. Ann Otol Rhinol Laryngol 1999;108:501–504

35. Abraham D, Singh N, Lang B, Chan WF, Lo CY. Benign nodular goitre presenting as acute airway obstruction. ANZ J Surg 2007;77:364–367

36. Torres A, Arroyo J, Kastanos N, Estopa R, Rabaseda J, Agusti-Vidal A. Acute respiratory failure and tracheal obstruction in patients with intrathoracic goiter. Crit Care Med 1983;11:265–266

37. Bedard ELR, Deslauriers J. Bleeding "downhill" varices: a rare complication of intrathoracic goiter. Ann Thorac Surg 2006;81:358–360

38. Mack E. Management of patients with substernal goiters. Surg Clin North Am 1995;75:377–379

39. Souza JW, Williams JT, Ayoub MM, Jerles ML, Dalton ML. Bilateral recurrent nerve paralysis associated with multinodular substernal goiter: a case report. Am Surg 1999;65:456–459

40. De Andrade MA. A review of 128 cases of posterior mediastinal goiter. World J Surg 1977;1:789–794

41. Michel LA, Bradpiece HA. Surgical management of substernal goiter. Br J Surg 1988;75:565–569

42. Pulli RS, Coniglio JU. Surgical management of the substernal thyroid gland. Laryngoscope 1998;108:358–361

43. Hashmi SM, Premachandra DJ, Bennett AMD, Parry W. Management of retrosternal goiters: results of early surgical intervention to prevent airway morbidity and a review of the English literature. J Laryngol Otol 2006;120:644–649

44. Makeieff M, Marlier F, Khudjadze M, Garrel R, Crampetter L, Guerrier B. Substernal goiter: report of 212 cases. Ann Chir 2000;125:18–25

45. Armour RH. Retrosternal goitre. Br J Surg 2000;87:519

46. Wright CD, Mathisen DJ. Mediastinal tumors: diagnosis and treatment. World J Surg 2001;25:204–209

47. Dekker E, Ledeboer RC. Compression of the tracheobronchial tree by the action of voluntary respiratory musculature in normal individuals and in patients with asthma and emphysema. Am J Roentgenol Radium Ther Nucl Med 1961;85:217–228

48. Barker P, Mason RA, Thorpe MH. Computed axial tomography of the trachea. A useful investigation when a retrosternal goiter causes symptomatic tracheal compression. Anaesthesia 1991;46:195–198

49. Netterville JL, Coleman SC, Smith JC, Smith MM, Day T, Burkey BB. Management of substernal goiter. Laryngoscope 1998;108:1611–1617

50. Grainger J, Saravanappa N, D'Souza A, Wilcock D, Wilson PS. The surgical approach to retrosternal goiters: the role of computed tomography. Otolaryngol Head Neck Surg 2005;132:849–851

51. Sand ME, Laws HL, McElvein RB. Substernal and intrathoracic goiter. Reconsideration of surgical approach. Am Surg 1983;49:196–202

52. Kocher T. In: Textbook of Operative Surgery, 4th ed. Translated by H.J. Styles. London: A&C Vlack, 1903:133–151

53. Reeve TS, Delbridge L, Cohen A, et al. Total thyroidectomy—the preferred option for multinodular goiter. Ann Surg 1987;206:782–786

54. Hsu B, Reeve TS, Guinea AI, Robinson B, Delbridge L. Recurrent substernal nodular goiter: incidence and management. Surgery 1996;120:1072–1075

55. Wheeler MH. Retrosternal goiter. Br J Surg 1999;86:1235–1236

56. Landreneau RJ, Nawarawong W, Boley TM, Johnson JA, Curtis JJ. Intrathoracic goiter: approaching the posterior mediastinal mass. Ann Thorac Surg 1991;52:134–135

57. Pandya S, Sanders LE. Use of a Foley catheter in the removal of a substernal goiter. Am J Surg 1998;175:155–157

58. Delbridge L. Total thyroidectomy: the evolution of surgical technique. ANZ J Surg 2003;73:761–768

59. Dunhill TP. Removal of intrathoracic tumours by the transsternal route. Br J Surg 1922;10:4–14

60. Taylor S. Thyroid. In: Taylor S, Chisholm GD, O'Higgins N, Shields R, eds. Surgical Management. London: Heinemann, 1984:513–524

61. Monchik JM, Materazzi G. The necessity for a thoracic approach in thyroid surgery. Arch Surg 2000;135:467–472

62. Vadasz P, Kotsis L. Surgical aspects of 175 mediastinal goiters. Eur J Cardiothorac Surg 1998;14:393–397

63. Geelhoed GW. Tracheomalacia from compressing goiter: management after thyroidectomy. Surgery 1988;104:1100–1108

64. Abdel Rahim AA, Ahmed ME, Hassan MA. Respiratory complications after thyroidectomy and the need for tracheostomy in patients with a large goiter. Br J Surg 1999;86:88–90

65. Bennett AMD, Hashmi SM, Premachandra DJ, Wright MM. The myth of tracheomalacia and difficult intubation in cases of retrosternal goiter. J Laryngol Otol 2004;118:778–780

66. Shaha AR. Surgery for benign thyroid disease causing tracheoesophageal compression. Otolaryngol Clin North Am 1990;23:391–401

67. Torre G, Borgonovo G, Amato A, et al. Surgical management of substernal goiter: analysis of 237 patients. Am Surg 1995;61:826–831

68. Melliere D, Saada F, Etienne G, Becquemin JP, Bonnet F. Goiter with severe respiratory compromise: evaluation and treatment. Surgery 1988;103:367–373

69. Shaha AR, Alfonso AE, Jaffe BM. Operative treatment of substernal goiters. Head Neck 1989;11:325–330

70. Moron JC, Singer JA, Sardi A. Retrosternal goiter: a six-year institutional review. Am Surg 1998;64:889–893

71. Nervi M, Iacconi P, Spinelli C, Janni A, Miccoli P. Thyroid carcinoma in intrathoracic goiter. Langenbecks Arch Surg 1998;383:337–339

72. Dedivitis RA, Guimaraes AV, Machado PC, Suehara AN, Noda E. Surgical treatment of the substernal goiter. Int Surg 1999;84:190–192

73. Ozdemir A, Hasbahceci M, Hamaloglu E, Ozenc A. Surgical treatment of substernal goiter. Int Surg 2000;85:194–197

74. Sancho JJ, Kraimps JL, Sanchex-Blanco JM, et al. Increased mortality and morbidity associated with thyroidectomy for intrathoracic goiters reaching the carina tracheae. Arch Surg 2006;141:82–85

Thyroid Malignancy

10 Medical Management of Aggressive Forms of Differentiated Thyroid Cancer

Jennifer Sipos and Ernest L. Mazzaferri

Epidemiology

Thyroid cancer comprises a group of tumors with remarkably different features. Tumors of the thyroid follicular cell, which include papillary thyroid cancer (PTC), follicular thyroid cancer (FTC), and Hürthle cell thyroid cancer (HTC), retain many of the characteristics of their normal progenitor cells, including the capacity to synthesize thyroglobulin (Tg) and sometimes thyroid hormone. These tumors ordinarily retain functioning thyrotropin (thyroid-stimulating hormone, TSH) receptors and iodide symporters that facilitate the transport of radioactive iodine into the malignant follicular cells, thus playing key roles in both diagnosis and treatment. This group of follicular cell tumors, although often collectively referred to as differentiated thyroid cancer (DTC), has many important diagnostic, therapeutic, and prognostic differences. This chapter provides an overview of the management of the more aggressive forms of DTC.

Incidence and Mortality Rates

Incidence Rates

Historical Changes in Incidence Rates

Over the past three decades the incidence rates of thyroid cancer have increased around the world.[1] Between 1973 and 2001, the incidence rates more than doubled in the United States, going from approximately 3.6 per 100,000 in 1973 to 8.7 per 100,000 in 2002—a 2.4-fold increase due almost entirely to a rise in the incidence of PTCs, many of which are tumors smaller than 1 cm, without a concurrent increase in FTCs.[2] A study from France found a similar increase between 1978 and 1997 that was also mainly due to PTC.[3] Similar observations made elsewhere around the world have been attributed to ionizing radiation,[4] iodine prophylaxis,[5] and alterations in histologic diagnostic criteria,[6] but the main reason for the increasing incidence is most likely the increasing use of neck ultrasonography for a variety of purposes, leading to the discovery of asymptomatic thyroid cancers, termed "incidentalomas," which are usually early-stage cancers.[2,7]

Contemporary Incidence Rates

Thyroid cancer occurs in persons of all ages, but only accounts for approximately 1% of all new cancer cases in the United States.[8] Still, it is the most rapidly rising form of cancer in women.[9] Its incidence is the same in both genders in the first decade of life, but thereafter is threefold higher in women, its onset peaking in midlife (approximately 40 years of age), about two decades earlier than it does in men.

Mortality Rates

Historical Changes in Mortality Rates

Despite the significant rise in the incidence of thyroid cancer, its mortality rates have declined significantly in the past three decades, more than almost any other cancer.[10] This improved outcome is most apparent in women aged 40 years or older at the time of diagnosis.[9] Why this occurred is unknown, but is likely due to earlier diagnosis and treatment of less advanced tumors.[2,9] In sharp contrast, thyroid cancer mortality rates in men have increased in the past three decades and are now twice those in women, largely because men present at an older age with more advanced tumors than those in women, making it the most rapidly rising cause of cancer death in men in the United States.[10] This is due to late detection and delayed therapy, which reflects how men underutilize the health care system. A study from France[7] found that the proportion of women referred for evaluation of a thyroid nodule has increased over the past two decades, which did not happen in men, a finding attributed to two facts: thyroid disorders are more common in women, and women are the main consumers of health care.[11]

Contemporary Mortality Rates

Ten-year thyroid cancer mortality rates among 53,856 patients treated between 1985 and 1995 in the United States were lowest for PTC and highest for anaplastic thyroid cancer (ATC) (**Table 10.1**).[12] Still, the majority of deaths (53%) are from PTC, simply because it comprises the majority of thyroid cancers.[12]

Causes of Death from Thyroid Cancer

There are few explicit clinical descriptions of how patients die from their thyroid tumor. A study of 161 fatal cases found that respiratory insufficiency accounted for most deaths (43%), followed by circulatory failure (15%), hemorrhage (15%), and airway obstruction (13%).[13] Respiratory insufficiency is due to bulky pulmonary metastases that replace

Table 10.1 Distribution of Histologic Tumor Types and Deaths Due to Thyroid Cancer among 53,856 Patients Treated Between 1985 and 1995 in the United States*

Type of Tumor	Patients(n)	Percent of All Thyroid Cancers	10-year Relative Survival	Cancer Deaths(n)	Deaths Due to Tumor Type†(%)
Papillary	42,686	79%	93%	2988	53%
Follicular	6764	13%	85%	1015	18%
Hürthle	1585	2%	76%	380	7%
Medullary	1928	4%	75%	482	9%
Anaplastic	893	2%	14%	768	14%
Total	53,856			5633	

†The total number of deaths attributable to each type of thyroid cancer between 1985 and 1995.
*Data from Hundahl SA, Fleming ID, Fremgen AM, Menck HR. A National Cancer Data Base report on 53,856 cases of thyroid carcinoma treated in the US, 1985–1995. Cancer 1998;83:2638–2648. Percentages rounded to nearest integer.

normal lung tissue, whereas massive hemorrhage and airway obstruction are due to uncontrolled tumor growth in the neck and mediastinum.[13] Circulatory failure is caused by compression of the vena cava by mediastinal or sternal metastases.[13] These observations provide guidance for improving survival and the quality of life for patients with advanced cancer.

Pathogenetic Factors

Gene Mutations and Familial Syndromes

Familial Nonmedullary Thyroid Cancer

Although the causative gene(s) has yet to be identified, familial nonmedullary thyroid cancer (FNMTC) is recognized as a distinct clinical entity in which almost all of the tumors are PTC.[14] Yet sporadic PTC is so prevalent that up to 69% of two-hit families actually have sporadic not familial tumor.[15] An estimated 1 of 338 persons with thyroid cancer (approximately 3%) carries the genetic trait for FNMTC, and its presence is most certain in families with three to five affected members, in which case there is a 96% likelihood it is an affected kindred.[15] Hemminki et al[16] studied the Swedish Cancer Registry by defining familial risk for offspring by means of standardized incidence ratios.[1] When either parent had thyroid cancer, the risk was 4.98 for sons and 3.44 for daughters. The risk for thyroid cancer was 6.24 when a sibling had the disease, which climbed to 11.19 when it was a sister.

Familial nonmedullary thyroid cancer is characterized by an earlier age of onset and more aggressive phenotype[17] than sporadic DTC. One study of 258 cases[18] found that although patient gender, age, and tumor histology were similar to that of sporadic DTC, FNMTC tumors were more likely to have intrathyroidal dissemination (41% versus 29%) and higher recurrence rates (16% versus 10%) than sporadic tumors, without displaying significant differences in size, local invasion, or macroscopic metastasis. Locoregional recurrence was more frequent in FNMTC than sporadic tumors, but there

was no difference in the rate of distant metastases. Still, FNMTC was an independent predictor of shorter disease-free survival (risk ratio 1.9).

Familial nonmedullary thyroid cancer can be a component in some well-described heritable cancer syndromes that usually are transmitted as autosomal dominant disorders such as familial adenomatous polyposis, Cowden syndrome, Werner syndrome, and Carney complex, and probably also in Peutz-Jeghers syndrome and tuberous sclerosis.[19,20]

Familial Adenomatous Polyposis

Thyroid cancer occurs in approximately 2% of patients with familial adenomatous polyposis (FAP), most often in female carriers, who manifest the disease at about age of 28 years.[21] The PTC is frequently multicentric and regionally metastatic.[21] Unlike FNMTC, this hereditary tumor seems to have an excellent prognosis, particularly with rearranged during transfection (RET)/PTC activation.[22,23]

Cowden Syndrome

This autosomal dominant disorder, which is part of the *PTEN* hamartoma tumor syndrome,[20] is manifest by mucocutaneous polyps, hamartomas, and breast cancer, and is associated with a 3 to 10% risk of follicular-derived thyroid cancer,[19,20] which typically is PTC with a good prognosis.[24] The *PTEN* gene[25] codes for a dual-specificity phosphatase that is likely a tumor suppressor gene.[24]

Carney Complex

This syndrome, which comprises spotty skin pigmentation, myxomas, schwannomas, and multiple neoplasias affecting multiple glands, includes familial papillary thyroid cancer, which has a good prognosis.[26]

Surveillance recommendations for thyroid cancer in these syndromes vary, but we prefer annual neck ultrasonography to identify thyroid tumors early in their course.

Oncogenes

Tyrosine Kinase Oncogenes

The human genome contains approximately 90 protein tyrosine kinases (TKs), which are enzymes that catalyze the transfer of phosphate from adenosine triphosphate (ATP) to tyrosine residues in polypeptides that regulate cell proliferation, survival, differentiation, function, and motility.[27] The enormous clinical importance of TKs, which are now regarded as oncogenes, became suddenly quite clear with the success of imatinib mesylate (Gleevec), an inhibitor of the bcr-abl TK in chronic myeloid leukemia that provided the first major triumph of targeted cancer chemotherapy. TK inhibitors have become a common avenue of research for antithyroid cancer drugs.[28,29]

ret/ptc Oncogene

There is a high prevalence of chromosomal inversions in PTC. A single gene located on chromosome 10, the rearranged during transfection (*ret*) proto-oncogene that codes for a RET cell membrane TK receptor, is normally not expressed or is present in very low levels in follicular cells. In PTC, however, TK is activated by a chromosomal rearrangement resulting in the fusion of the 3′ portion of the *ret* gene coding for the TK domain to the 5′ portion of various genes, creating a group of chimeric oncogenes named *ret/ptc* (**Fig. 10.1**). Although there are several forms of this oncogene that differ according to the 5′ partner gene, the two most important are *ret/ptc1* [30] and *ret/ptc3*.[31,32]

ret/ptc is a key first step in thyroid cancer pathogenesis.[33–37] Transgenic mice with thyroid-targeted expression of *ret/ptc1* [38] and *ret/ptc3* [39] develop PTC. These intrachromosomal recombinations, particularly paracentric inversions, appear to be a fundamental mechanism of radiation-induced thyroid carcinogenesis. *ret/ptc3* rearrangements have been found in 66 to 87% of the post-Chernobyl tumors in children.[40–43] Nikiforova et al[37] proposed that spatial contiguity of RET and H4 may provide a structural basis for the generation of *ret/ptc1* rearrangement by allowing a single radiation track to produce a double-stranded break in each gene at the same site in the nucleus. *ret/ptc* oncogenes do not, however, seem to be specific to radiation-induced cancers, because they are also found in approximately 40% of sporadic pediatric PTCs and in 15 to 20% of adult cases, with considerable regional variability ranging from 5 to 40%. The prevalence of *ret/ptc* rearrangements in PTC, however, varies, and is influenced by the detection methods and genetic heterogeneity.[44]

BRAF Oncogene

RAF kinase is a component of the RAS→RAF→MEK→ERK/mitogen-activated protein kinase (MAPK) signaling pathway (**Fig. 10.2**), which plays a key role in the regulation of cell growth, division, and proliferation. Of the three RAF isoforms in the TK that map to chromosome 7q, BRAF is the strongest MAP kinase activator.

First found in malignant melanoma, the activating BRAF point mutation V600E (formerly designated V599E) occurs in 50 to 80% of adult PTCs including its tall cell variant[45–50] and in ATC, but not in other forms of thyroid cancer.[48,51] It is not a germline mutation in FNMTC[52] and is rarely found in children, including those exposed to radiation[53]

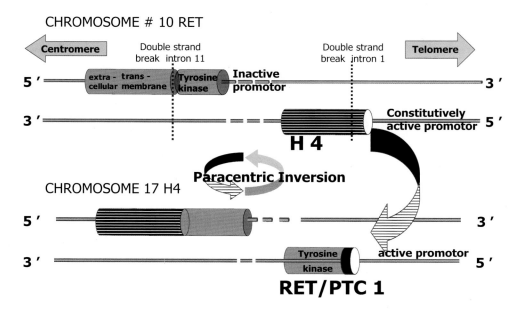

Fig. 10.1 *ret/ptc1* oncogene formed by paracentric inversion of *ret* and its fusion partner (either H4 or ELE1), leading to activation of the RET TK receptor that is critical to RET-mediated cellular transformation and dedifferentiation primarily through the RAS-RAF–mitogen-activated protein kinase (MAPK) pathway.

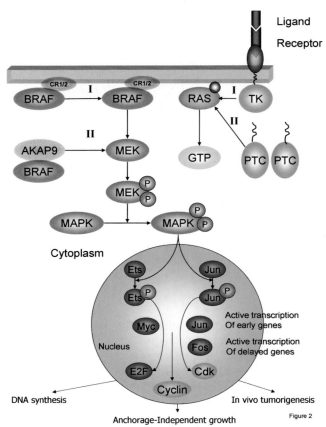

Fig. 10.2 The MAPK pathway. RAS→RAF→MEK→ERK/MAPK signaling pathway involved in the pathogenesis of papillary and anaplastic thyroid cancer. Once activated, tyrosine kinase (TK) receptors activate the monomeric G protein RAS (pathway I), which in turn binds the serine-threonine kinase BRAF by inducing a conformational change that allows its activation (pathway I) and hence activation of the MAPK pathway. The activation of the MAPK pathway results in DNA synthesis in response to the external mitogenic stimulus (pathway I). When the *ret/ptc* (pathway II) or the BRAF pathway (II) oncogenes are generated through chromosomal rearrangements, activation of the MAPK pathway becomes constitutive, and cells become able to proliferate indefinitely, to grow in an anchorage-independent manner, and to induce tumors after injection into athymic mice (pathway II). *Abbreviations:* GTP, guanosine triphosphate; L, ligand; MEK, MAPK/ERK kinase. (From Fusco A, Viglietto G, Santoro M. A new mechanism of BRAF activation in human thyroid papillary cancers. J Clin Invest 2005;115:20–23, with permission.)

even after they reach maturity.[54] Ciampi et al[55] identified a novel *akap9-braf* fusion oncogene in patients with radiation-induced PTCs, suggesting that chromosomal inversions represent a common genetic theme of radiation-associated thyroid cancer, which may account for the small number of BRAF mutations detected in radiation-induced thyroid cancers in children.[56]

A high prevalence of BRAF mutation is found in lymph node metastases from BRAF-positive primary tumors.[51] In some cases de novo formation of the mutation appears to occur in lymph node metastases, consistent with the notion that BRAF mutations facilitate metastasis to and progression

of PTC in lymph nodes.[57] Indeed most find a high prevalence of extrathyroidal tumor invasion,[48,58] distant metastases,[59] and lymph node metastases with this mutation.[60]

A large multicenter study[51] reported that the BRAF mutation is associated with a poor prognosis, including a significant association between the mutation and extrathyroidal tumor invasion, neck lymph node metastases, and more advanced initial tumor stage. In this study, BRAF-positive tumors had higher recurrence rates than tumors without the mutation (25% versus 9%, $p = .004$),[51] and tumor recurrences were more extensive and required more aggressive treatment than those without the mutation. Almost 70% of BRAF-positive tumors required at least one additional surgery or external beam radiotherapy (EBRT), whereas only 14% of the BRAF-negative recurrent tumors required additional surgery and none required EBRT.[51] More than half (54%) of BRAF-positive tumors lacked iodine-131 (I-131) avidity, whereas none of the BRAF-negative tumors failed to concentrate I-131. Patients continued to have active disease with BRAF-positive recurrent tumors that had lost I-131 avidity, even after repeated surgeries or EBRT, whereas all seven patients with BRAF-negative recurrent tumor were cured by repeated I-131 treatments.

One prospective analysis found that half the PTC nodules were correctly diagnosed by BRAF mutation analysis of FNAB cytology specimens; there were no false-positive findings.[50] These observations thus underscore the importance of BRAF mutations in the development of PTC and its variants and its diagnostic and prognostic utility. Still, about half of tumors, even those associated with distant metastases, do not have this mutation.

A study of 97 PTCs found that 42% were positive for BRAF, 18% were positive for RET/PTC, and 15% were positive for RAS mutations.[61] BRAF mutations were associated with older patient age, typical PTC appearance or the tall cell variant, a higher rate of extrathyroidal extension, and more advanced tumor stage at presentation than the tumors with the other mutations. RET/PTC-positive tumors presented at younger age and had predominantly typical PTC histology, frequent psammoma bodies, and a high rate of lymph node metastases. Tumors with RAS mutations were all follicular variant PTCs that had a significantly low rate of lymph node metastases.

Radiation Exposure

Ionizing radiation and familial factors are the most clearly delineated pathogenetic factors in the development of PTC. Still, the majority of thyroid cancer is sporadic and has no readily identifiable cause. Examining the risk of developing thyroid cancer after exposure to external beam radiation for acne and other benign disorders is complex because of the relatively small number of cases, and the time to develop thyroid cancer varies so widely among studies, ranging from 10 to over 40 years.[64–69] Likewise, the smallest amount of radiation necessary to develop thyroid cancer continues to be debated, although most authorities agree that doses as small as 10 cGy can induce thyroid cancer in children, and that the rate increases with the radiation dose, leveling off after 200 cGy when thyroid tissue is destroyed.[65,66,72]

Exposure to some radioactive isotopes such as I-131 also increases the risk of thyroid cancer. In the 5 years preceding the Chernobyl nuclear accident, there were 59 cases of thyroid cancer in the Ukraine among patients between the ages of birth to 18 years. In the years between 1986 and 1997, there were 577 cases, almost a 10-fold increase.[69] After the accident, the latent period for the development of thyroid cancer was 4 to 6 years.[70] Children younger than 1 year of age at the time of exposure were at highest risk of developing thyroid cancer, with the risk gradually declining through age 12 years.[71] The vast majority were PTCs with a follicular or solid growth pattern with extrathyroidal spread and lymph node metastases.[69,70,72] Many reports have shown that the post-Chernobyl PTCs were characterized by about a 60% frequency of RET rearrangements predominantly involving ELE1 producing the *ret/ptc3* oncogene.

Factors Influencing Prognosis

Patient Factors

Patient Age

Thyroid cancer death rates increase after about age 40 years and increase with each subsequent decade of life, dramatically rising after age 60 years. The pattern of tumor recurrence is quite different: recurrence rates are highest (40%) at the extremes of life, before age 20 and after age 60 years.[73-75] As a result, there is disagreement about how age should be factored into the treatment plan, especially in children and young adults. Children commonly present with more advanced disease than adults and have more tumor recurrences after therapy, but their prognosis for survival is good,[77] even with lung metastases.[76] Some believe that young age has such a favorable influence upon survival that it overshadows the prognosis predicted by the tumor characteristics.[79] Most, however, believe that the tumor stage and histologic differentiation are as important as the patient's age in determining prognosis and management.[74,75,78]

Gender

Thyroid cancer death rates in men are twice those in women,[74,77] and men should be regarded with high concern, especially those over age 50 years.

Graves Disease

Thyrotropin receptor antibodies may promote tumor growth in patients with Graves disease. Some find thyroid cancer in almost half of the palpable nodules in patients with Graves disease and report that the tumors are larger and display more invasiveness and metastases to regional lymph nodes than usual, even when the primary tumor is small.[79,80]

Tumor Factors

Papillary Thyroid Cancer

Tumor histology has a major impact upon survival. PTC, which comprises almost 80% of all thyroid cancers, has a 10-year cancer mortality rate of 7% (**Table 10.2**).[12] PTC is classically characterized by complex papillae with a central fibrovascular stalk interspersed with neoplastic follicles and psammoma bodies, calcific concentric spherical objects within the tumor that represent ghosts of follicular cells

Table 10.2 Correlation Between Clinicopathological Characteristics and BRAF Mutation Status in Patients with Papillary Thyroid Cancer (PTC)

	BRAF Positive	BRAF Negative	*p*-Value
N (total)	107	112	
Age at diagnosis (year)	43	45	.41
Male gender	43	29	.009
Tumor size (cm)	2.0	2.4	.49
Multifocality	45	42	<.001
Extrathyroidal extension	44	18	<.001
Lymph node metastases	58	24	<.002
Tumor stage			
I	44	39	
II	30	57	
III	29	15	
IV	2	1	
Tumor stage III/IV	31	16	.007
Tumor recurrence	23	9	.004
No. of I-131 treatments			
0	19	26	
1	68	67	
2	1	1	
Total I-131 given (mCi)	100 (32–100)	100 (0–101)	.96
Total follow-up (months)	16.5 (5–30)	14.0 (2–28)	.40

The standardized incidence ratio (SIR) is a single, summary ratio that allows a comparison of incidence rates among two different populations. An SIR of 1.0 implies that the rates are the same for the population of interest and the standard population. A SIR > 1.0 implies that the rate is greater for the population of interest compared with the standard population. A SIR < 1.0 implies that the incidence rate is lower for the population of interest compared with the standard population.
Source: Modified from Xing M, Westra WH, Tufano RP, et al. BRAF mutation predicts a poorer clinical prognosis for papillary thyroid cancer. J Clin Endocrinol Metab 2005;90:6373–6379.

that are pathognomonic of PTC.[81] The diagnosis is based on distinctive cellular features with overlapping and round or oval nuclei with indentations, folds, pseudo-inclusions, and grooves. The nucleus may appear empty, a feature known as "Orphan Annie eyes." Mitotic figures, although very uncommon, suggest a poor prognosis.[82]

Tumor Size

This factor has such a powerful prognostic effect that it is independent of age and other important variables in most studies.[83–85] A 4-cm tumor diameter is often used as the cutoff above which PTC and FTC display more aggressive behavior and develop distant metastases.[86–88] This tumor size is used in many thyroid cancer prognostic classification systems[89] and in diagnostic recommendations for evaluating thyroid nodules.[90] Still, this caveat does not provide a clear picture about the smallest primary tumors that produce metastases, the most important issue to the patient and physician.

A study by Machens et al[91] shows that the threshold for developing extrathyroidal tumor extension and lymph node metastases is 5 mm for PTC and 20 mm for FTC. The threshold for developing lung metastases from PTC and FTC is 20 mm and for bone metastases is 30 to 40 mm. The curve describing the risk of metastases was steeper for PTC than FTC, showing the important key effect of PTC tumor size on the development of metastases. The curve for lung metastases was steeper than that for bone metastases, implying that lung metastases occur with smaller primary tumors.

Local Tumor Invasion

About 5 to 10% of tumors extend directly through the thyroid capsule into surrounding tissues, increasing morbidity and mortality. Microscopic or gross tumor invasion, which can occur with both PTC and FTC,[74] may involve neck muscles, blood vessels, recurrent laryngeal nerves, larynx, pharynx, and esophagus, or tumor can extend into the spinal cord and brachial plexus. The symptoms are usually obvious and include hoarseness, cough, dysphagia, hemoptysis, and airway insufficiency or neurologic dysfunction. Extrathyroidal tumor extension usually leads to regional and distant metastasis.[92] In a study from our institution, the tumor was locally invasive in 115 patients, 8% with PTC and 12% with FTC. When this occurred, 10-year rates of persistent tumor were 1.5-times and cancer death rates were five times those of patients without local invasion. Nearly all those with tumor invasion died within a decade.[74]

Regional Metastases

Lymph node metastases occur in 50 to 80% of PTC cases, with the highest rates (up to 90%) occurring in children,[83,93,94] whereas FTC lymph node metastases occur in only 10 to 25% of patients.[74,95] Neck lymph node metastases are palpable in

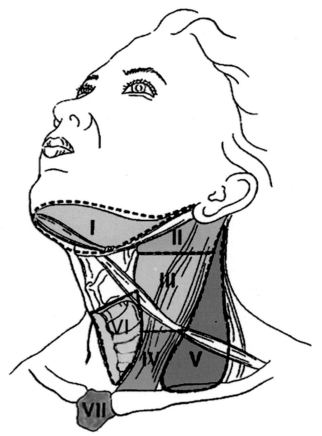

Fig. 10.3 Neck lymph node compartments.

only 15 to 40% of patients, whereas impalpable micrometastases are found in about twice as many patients.[96] About 25% of the neck metastases are bilateral.[97] The most common site (approximately 85%) is the central neck compartment (level VI), followed in descending order by midjugular (level III), supraclavicular, and subdigastric (level II) lymph nodes[97] (**Fig. 10.3**). Nevertheless, microscopic nodal metastases are often found at sites that have little relationship to the primary tumor location,[98] especially with multifocal primary microcancers.[99]

Neck physical examination is relatively unreliable in identifying metastatic lymph nodes, resulting in high false-positive and false-negative rates (20 to 30%).[96] At surgery sentinel lymph node metastases can be identified with isosulfan blue dye or preoperative injection of radiopharmaceuticals, which has an overall accuracy of approximately 90% but is not widely performed.[96,100] Neck ultrasonography in the hands of highly skilled operators is more accurate in detecting lymph node metastases than any other imaging studies[96,101] and should be routinely performed in patients undergoing surgery for thyroid cancer, including examination of the thyroid and major lymph node neck compartments. Not only should the sites most likely to contain metastatic lymph nodes (levels VI and III) be examined by ultrasonography, but also levels II, IV, and V should be studied.

Lymph node metastases as small as 2 or 3 mm can be identified by ultrasonography, the majority of which are round and have homogeneous internal echogenicity and punctate calcifications, internal Doppler flow, and absence of a normal hilum. Malignant lymph nodes often appear cystic with a thick outer wall, a finding that is characteristic of PTC, even in children,[102,103] and can be confused with a simple cyst. These lymph nodes may be identified as malignant, however, by measuring Tg levels in the washout from a fine-needle aspiration (FNA),[104] which is highly useful even in patients with serum antithyroglobulin antibodies.[105]

Although ultrasonography has several limitations, including diagnostic accuracy in evaluating deep level III and mediastinal lymph nodes and extracapsular tumor extension, and is very operator dependent,[96] it is the most cost-effective and accurate means of detecting neck lymph node metastases.[96,106,107] One study found that preoperative ultrasonography detected lymph node or soft tissue metastases in nearly 40% of patients thought to have uninvolved neck compartments by physical examination, thus altering the surgical procedure.[108] The 2006 guidelines from the National Cancer Center Network (NCCN)[109] and American Thyroid Association (ATA)[110] and the European Consensus Statement[111] on the management of thyroid cancer all advise neck ultrasonography as the primary test to identify neck metastases prior to surgery or with tumor recurrence.

After total thyroidectomy and I-131 ablation, approximately 15 to 20% of patients experience tumor recurrence, 60% of which are in cervical lymph nodes.[96,112,113] Although most studies demonstrate that lymph node metastases are a significant prognostic factor for recurrence and survival of patients with FTC,[95] debate continues about the clinical importance of PTC lymph node metastases. In a long-term study with a median follow-up of 16.6 years (range, 1–45 years), we found that lymph node metastases, especially bilateral cervical and mediastinal, were an independent variable that significantly affected recurrence and survival,[83] although not all studies find this to be true.[114] Podnos et al,[115] using a large multiinstitutional Surveillance Epidemiology and End Results (SEER) database to identify the prognostic implications of lymph node metastasis, identified 9904 PTC and FTC patients in whom lymph node status was known. Multivariate analysis found that age above 45 years, presence of distant metastasis, large tumor size, and lymph node metastases significantly predicted poor outcome. Overall survival at 14 years was 82% for node negative and 79% for node positive patients ($p < 0.05$), thus showing that survival of patients with DTC is adversely affected by lymph node metastases. A French study[116] found that after a mean follow-up of 8 years, eight patients (7%) with normal postablation whole body scans (RxWBSs) experienced tumor recurrence, and their 10-year disease-specific survival rate was 95% (confidence interval [CI], 97–100%). Significant risk factors for persistent disease included the number (>10), location (central neck), and extracapsular extension (>3 lymph nodes)

of lymph node metastases, and tumor size >4 cm. Significant risk factors for recurrent disease were the number (>10) and extracapsular extension of lymph node metastases (>3), and the Tg level measured 6 to 12 months after initial treatment after levothyroxine (T_4) withdrawal. Other studies have shown that extracapsular invasion of tumor from lymph node metastases is an especially important indicator of distant metastases and poor prognosis in patients with PTC.[117,118]

Distant Metastases

About 10% of patients with PTC, 25% with FTC, and 35% with HTC develop distant metastases.[75] Half are present at the time of initial surgery.[75] They occur more often in children and young adults,[78,121] and in patients over age 45 years at the time of initial diagnosis.[122] Among 1231 patients in 13 studies with DTC metastases, 49% were to lung alone, 25% to bone, and 15% in both sites and 10% in the central nervous system or other sites.[75] Much the same distribution was observed in a French study of 444 patients with distant metastases from PTC or FTC; the sites were lung alone (50%), bone only (26%), both lung and bone (18%), and other sites (5%).

Some patients survive for decades with distant metastases, especially younger patients, but about half die within 5 years regardless of tumor histology.[75] Outcome is influenced mainly by the patient's age at the time of initial diagnosis, tumor site(s), bulk and ability to concentrate I-131.[123,124] In a study from France, survival rates with distant metastases were 53% at 5 years, 38% at 10 years, and 30% at 15 years.[125] A later study from the same group found that, in response to I-131 therapy, negative I-131 RxWBS and conventional radiographs were achieved in 43% of 295 patients with I-131 uptake by tumor, most frequently in younger patients who had well-differentiated tumors and a limited extent of disease.[78] Negative imaging studies (96%) occurred after the administration 100 to 600 mCi of I-131, almost half of which occurred more than 5 years after commencing treatment of the metastases. Tumor recurrence was only 7% among patients with negative imaging studies after treatment. Overall survival at 10 years was 92% and 19% in patients who, respectively, had or had not achieved negative imaging studies. The authors of this study advised that patients should be treated until there is disappearance of any I-131 uptake by metastases or until a cumulative activity of 600 mCi has been administered, and that other treatment modalities should be employed when tumor progression has been documented.

Survival is longest in children and young adults with diffuse microscopic lung metastases seen only on post-treatment I-131 imaging and not by any other imaging study.[78,125–127] The prognosis is much worse when the metastases do not concentrate I-131 or appear as large lung nodules and is intermediate when the tumors are small nodules on x-ray that concentrate I-131.[123,127]

Papillary Thyroid Microcarcinoma

Papillary thyroid cancer <1 cm, termed microcarcinomas (PTMCs), are found in up to 36% of thyroid glands studied at autopsy.[126-131] They are often found unexpectedly by neck ultrasonography or during surgery for benign thyroid disorders. In one surgical series,[132] 4% of patients undergoing thyroidectomy for benign thyroid disorders had incidentally discovered PTMCs.[132] They also may be detected in multinodular goiter when sampling a small nodule adjacent to a larger one of interest.[133] These small tumors may rarely present with clinical signs, the commonest of which are cervical lymph node metastases; however, in others the first manifestation is a distant metastasis.[134] Although most PTMCs incidentally discovered at surgery pose no threat to survival and require no further surgery,[135] approximately 20% are multifocal and as many as 60% have cervical lymph node metastases[136] and some produce distant metastases.[118] In our series, 30-year recurrence rates with DTC smaller than 1.5 cm were less than one-third those associated with larger tumors,[74] but recurrences were still in the range of 10%. Lung metastases are most apt to occur with multifocal tumors that have cervical metastases, which are the only PTMCs with significant morbidity and mortality.[118,136] With these exceptions, the recurrence and cancer mortality rates are near zero.[135,136]

Multiple Intrathyroidal Papillary Thyroid Cancer Tumors

Found in approximately 20% of PTCs when the thyroid is examined routinely and in up to 80% when it is examined with great care,[83] multicentric PTC cannot be predicted on the basis of clinical risk stratification[138] and thus is not apparent until the final histologic sections of the entire thyroid have been studied. This argues for total thyroidectomy and thyroid I-131 remnant ablation. Half of those undergoing routine completion thyroidectomy have bilateral tumor,[83,137,138] and when multifocal tumors are found in the first lobe excised, the tumor is almost always bilateral.[139] Accordingly, residual DTC is found in 25% to almost half the contralateral lobes undergoing completion thyroidectomy.[118,137]

Still, some argue that multiple microscopic tumors are of little clinical consequence and thus do not require total thyroidectomy.[140] Yet recurrence rates of 5 to 20% in large thyroid remnants are reported, and lung metastases occur more often after subtotal than after total thyroidectomy.[141-143] Multicentric microcarcinomas have a higher incidence of recurrence in lymph node metastases than do single tumors.[118,144,145] Several studies show that PTC multicentricity and invasiveness are important tumor features that must be considered when planning therapy, despite small tumor size. Chow et al[118] found that despite their overall excellent prognosis, PTMCs were associated with a 1% disease-related mortality rate, a 5% lymph node recurrence

rate, and a 2.5% rate of distant metastasis. The risk of cervical lymph node recurrence increased about sixfold when either lymph node metastases or multifocal disease were present at the time of diagnosis, whereas age was not a significant factor in predicting recurrence or survival, suggesting that treatment of multifocal PTMC should be no different from that of patients with larger PTCs.

Regarded largely as intrathyroidal metastases in the past, multiple intrathyroidal tumors in the same thyroid gland were found often to contain different *ret/ptc* gene rearrangements, suggesting that they are individual tumors arising independently in a background of genetic or environmental susceptibility.[146] More recent studies using X-chromosome inactivation patterns in multifocal PTCs show discordant patterns in some tumors indicative of their independent origins[147] and monoclonal patterns in others confirming that intrathyroidal metastases can occur. These observations provide strong support for routinely performing bilateral thyroidectomy unless one can be absolutely certain that the tumor is a single isolated tumor confined to the thyroid, which as a practical matter is almost never apparent until the total thyroid has been removed.

Follicular Variant Papillary Thyroid Cancer

Among the several types of PTC, the two most common are classic PTC and FVPTC, comprising, respectively, from 55 to 66% and 23 to 41% of DTC.[148] FVPTC has typical nuclear features of PTC with a microfollicular architecture that on FNA biopsy (FNAB) may suggest a follicular neoplasm, or in the case of the macrofollicular encapsulated variant FVPTC, can mimic benign goiter.[149] With classic PTC there usually is an admixture of papillary architecture with some follicular features, which changes the diagnosis to classic PTC even if the papillary component is very small.[150] Given the difference in surgical management between follicular neoplasms and PTC, FVPTC often presents a major surgical dilemma. Still, the cellular features identify it as FVPTC.[151] Although FVPTC is more commonly encapsulated, it may be unencapsulated but its clinical behavior resembles that of classic PTC more than FTC.[148,152,153] One recent study of 160 patients, 29% of which had FVPTC, found that it presented with larger tumors (median 1.5 cm versus 1.0 cm) and thus higher tumor stage than PTC.[148] However, compared with FVPTC, PTC patients were more likely to have local invasion and local recurrence (0% versus 10% for both variables). There were no significant differences between the two in patient age, gender, vascular invasion, lymph node or distant metastases, surgical treatment, radioactive iodine therapy, remission rate, or mortality.

Diffuse Sclerosing Variant Papillary Thyroid Cancer

Comprising approximately 6% of PTC, diffuse sclerosing variant papillary (DSVP) thyroid cancer primarily affects young women and usually is clinically manifest as diffuse involvement of one or both thyroid lobes.[154] Serum antithyroid antibodies may be detected, confusing the diagnosis with Hashimoto disease. In addition, DSVP can be mistaken for nontoxic goiter, nonthyroidal malignant tumors, or undifferentiated thyroid cancer.[155] DSVP usually presents as diffuse thyroidal enlargement without an identifiable tumor mass, but most have lymph node metastases that are often bulky and bilateral, and up to 25% have lung metastases.[156] Many (approximately 10%) of the tumors found in the Chernobyl children were of this type.[70] Its histologic findings include intense fibrosis, a large number of psammoma bodies, primarily a solid growth pattern, lymphocytic infiltration, and extensive invasion of lymphatic spaces. Its nuclear features are typical of PTC. They are aggressive tumors that may have a poor prognosis; however, with total thyroidectomy and I-131 treatment, the prognosis is the same as with classical PTC.[157]

Encapsulated Papillary Thyroid Cancer

This variant accounts for 10 to 15% of PTCs[158,159] and is characterized by a well-defined fibrous capsule that completely surrounds the tumor, separating its cells from adjacent tissues. Patients with this variant present with a small tumor that is significantly less likely to cause compression symptoms or nodal metastases, and patients have a lower incidence of recurrence than do patients with unencapsulated PTC. The long-term prognosis is excellent.[158]

Tall Cell Variant

This tumor is marked by a papillary structure and PTC cells that are twice as tall as they are wide with intensely eosinophilic cytoplasm. According to LiVolsi,[156] at least 70% of the tumor should contain tall cells to fulfill this diagnosis. It tends to occur in older individuals,[160] typically presents at a late stage with extensive local and distant metastases, and subsequently carries a worse prognosis than classic PTC. One study of 332 consecutive PTC patients found that approximately 5% had the tall cell variant (TCV). At surgery, nodal metastases were found in half the patients and distant metastases were identified in 31%, fourfold that with classic PTC. TCV tends not to concentrate I-131,[161,162] and often contains the BRAF mutation, which may be the underlying reason for its poor prognosis.[163] The increased risk of distant metastasis associated with TCV warrants an extensive postoperative search for distant metastasis to facilitate early diagnosis and treatment of tumor deposits in distant organs.

Columnar Cell Variant

This rare and aggressive form of PTC is composed of columnar cells lacking typical nuclear features of PTC but they have papillae. It is distinguished from TCV by the lack of cellular eosinophilia and stratification of nuclei. Occasionally columnar cells are a component of TCV.[164] Similar to TCV, the tumor does not concentrate I-131 and it has a poor prognosis,[165] although an encapsulated form of the columnar cell variant may have a prognosis similar to that of classic PTC.[166]

Solid Variant

This rare PTC variant has a predominantly (>70%) solid growth pattern, cytologic features typical of classic PTC, and no tumor necrosis. It is associated with a slightly higher frequency of distant metastases and less favorable prognosis than classic PTC; however, it should be distinguished from poorly differentiated thyroid cancer, which has a lower survival rate than solid variant PTC.[167] It has been found in children affected by the Chernobyl accident, especially in Ukraine.[126]

Follicular Thyroid Cancer

In areas of sufficient iodine intake such as the United States, FTC represents approximately 13% of all thyroid cancers (**Table 10.1**),[12] whereas its prevalence is as high as 40% in regions of endemic iodine deficiency.[168] It is typically a solitary encapsulated tumor with a microfollicular histologic pattern that is slightly more aggressive than PTC and only occasionally metastasizes to regional lymph nodes. FTC metastasizes via hematogenous spread to the lungs, bone, brain, and liver more commonly than does PTC.[169] Widely invasive FTC, which is considerably less common than the encapsulated form, may completely lack a capsule and is characterized by gross invasion of extrathyroidal tissue. Its cytologic features are typically malignant, including high mitotic activity, solid areas, trabecular pattern, nuclear anaplasia, and necrosis.[170] Widely invasive tumors have a highly unfavorable prognosis and are easily recognized by their extensive growth into surrounding tissues. Up to 80% of patients with such tumors develop distant metastases and more than 15% die of their disease within 10 years.[12,83]

Most FTCs diagnosed in recent years are minimally invasive thickly encapsulated tumors that closely resemble follicular adenomas. The diagnosis can be made only by review of the permanent histologic sections and not by FNAB or frozen section study, which poses a serious management predicament at the time of surgery. Recently, Weber et al[171] found that the presence of three genes together, *CCND2*, *PLAB*, and *PCSK2*, facilitated differentiating FTC from follicular adenoma with 100% sensitivity and almost 95% specificity, but this test is not yet widely available. The principal diagnostic criteria for minimally invasive FTC are cells penetrating the tumor capsule or microscopically invading blood vessels within or beyond its capsule. The former has a worse prognosis than capsular penetration alone.[172] Still, a few patients with minimally invasive FTC have distant metastases or die of their disease.[173]

The poorer prognosis of FTC than PTC (**Table 10.1**) is more closely related to the older age of patients at the time of diagnosis and advanced tumor stage than its histology alone.[76] The survival rates with PTC and FTC are similar in patients of comparable age and disease stage.[74,83] Both have an excellent prognosis if they are confined to the thyroid, and are small (<20 mm)[91] or are minimally invasive.[74] Conversely, both have poor outcomes if they are large (≥20 mm) and widely invasive—PTC invading the thyroid capsule and adjacent structures and FTC invading blood vessels and the tumor capsule—or metastatic to distant sites.[74,83] Thirty-year cancer mortality rate in our study among patients with FTC was over twofold that of patients with PTC; however, FTC patients were older and had larger tumors and more advanced tumor at presentation than those with PTC. Patients with tumors of similar stage had 30-year recurrence and cancer-specific mortality rates that were the same, regardless of the tumor's papillary or follicular histology.[74]

Insular Variant

This uncommon tumor generally occurs in patients 45 years of age and older[174,175] but has been reported in adolescents.[176] The tumor is characterized by solid nests of tumor cells (acini) separated by vessels[177] that stain immunohistochemically for keratin and Tg and negatively for calcitonin.[178] Its clinical behavior ranges between that of well-differentiated PTC and FTC and undifferentiated (anaplastic) cancer, with rates of distant metastases ranging from approximately 50 to 85% and 10-year cancer-specific mortality rates ranging from approximately 33 to 68%, both well above those for PTC and FTC and below the 97% mortality rate for ATC.[175,179–180] Metastases may concentrate,[126,181] but its effect is questionable.[182]

Hürthle Cell Thyroid Cancer

Composed predominantly (>75%) or completely of follicular cells exhibiting oncocytic features including a large number of mitochondria and abundant acidophilic granular cytoplasm, Hürthle cell tumors have a broad clinical spectrum varying from encapsulated solitary adenomas to widely or minimally invasive cancers. The World Health Organization classifies HTC as a variant of FTC,[183] but more recent studies show that in some cases HTC may represent a variant of PTC, as many express *ret/ptc*.[184] Although some controversy has surrounded the diagnosis, management, and outcome of HTC, more recent large series clarify most of these issues. Some find these tumors to be aggressive, with mortality rates as high as 25% at 30 years;[185] however, others find it to behave similarly to FTC of the same stage. In one study, patients at low risk of cancer death by virtue of their age and sex, extent of metastases, and tumor size had a 20-year survival rate of 89% compared with 94% for FTC.[186]

Still, a large national study of 1585 cases of HTC found a 10-year cancer mortality rate of 25%, compared with a 15% rate in 5271 patients with FTC (**Table 10.1**).[12] Pulmonary metastases occur in 20 to 35% of patients with HTC, about twice the rate in FTC.[120] Hürthle-cell variant PTC is less common but may have higher than usual recurrence and mortality rates.[83]

Current Diagnostic Approach

Symptoms and Signs

Clinical Features of Advanced Disease

About 20% of patients with a thyroid nodule have symptoms that strongly suggest malignancy, such as a rapidly growing tumor, large cervical lymph nodes, compressive symptoms, vocal cord paralysis, and tumor fixed to surrounding tissues. These signs point to a diagnosis of thyroid cancer with an accuracy of 70 to 100% depending, respectively, on whether one or two suspicious findings are present.[187] Such high-risk patients should undergo surgery even if FNAB fails to document the diagnosis of thyroid cancer.[188] Nodules at intermediate risk for thyroid cancer are those in patients with a history of head and neck irradiation, new nodules in patients under age 14 or over age 65 years and in older men, and nodules larger than 4 cm that are partly cystic.[187] Patients with pulmonary metastases may develop hemoptysis, dyspnea, or stridor, and those with bone metastases may have localized pain, pathologic fracture, or damage to contiguous tissues such as the spinal cord or brain. Most patients with DTC, however, present with an asymptomatic solitary thyroid nodule; half are noticed by the physician and the other half by the patient. Nonetheless, approximately 5 to 10% of such low-risk patients have thyroid cancer.[74,188] In addition, a relatively large number of tumors are found by coincidence.

Clinical Significance of Thyroid Incidentalomas

Thyroid incidentalomas are impalpable asymptomatic nodules of any size that are discovered by neck imaging studies or at surgery. This is a pervasive problem stemming from the widespread use of neck imaging for nonthyroidal conditions. One facet of the problem is the high rate of small thyroid cancers (approximately 4%) in the population that pose little or no risk to survival, which when identified may prompt a cascade of studies and unnecessary surgery.[2] Still, a few others are thyroid cancers destined to create major problems for the patient.[189]

The prevalence of thyroid incidentalomas varies among studies as do the rates of thyroid cancer in these silent tumors. In two prospective studies, for example, the prevalence rates of incidentalomas were 13%[190] and 67%.[191] The malignancy rates in incidentalomas vary from 12 to 50%,[191–195] depending on how the nodules were discovered and how they were evaluated. For instance, positron emission tomographic (PET) scanning for nonthyroidal malignancy reveals a large number of incidental thyroid nodules that require close evaluation because 50% or more are thyroid cancers.[194,195]

The criteria used to perform FNAB weighs heavily on the malignancy rate of incidentalomas. A study of nodules discovered by computed tomography (CT) or magnetic resonance imaging (MRI) that managed all incidentalomas and palpable nodules larger than 1 cm with ultrasonographically-guided FNAB (US-FNAB) found a significantly higher rate of malignancy in the incidentaloma group than in the nonincidental group (17% and 3%, $p = .020$).[195] Studies that performed US-FNAB on sonographically suspicious incidentalomas, regardless of size, report even higher rates of malignancy ranging from approximately 30 to 40%.[196,198]

It is not surprising that the clinical importance of incidentalomas continues to be debated. In a study of 1475 patients, Kang et al[197] found that most of the malignant incidentalomas had favorable postoperative tumor, node, metastasis (TNM) stages, yet 20% were invading the thyroid capsule and 12% involved lymph nodes. In another study, Nam-Goong et al[198] found that 69% of incidentalomas had either extrathyroidal extension or regional node involvement and 39% were multifocal, suggesting that small size alone does not guarantee low risk in incidentally discovered thyroid cancers. These findings are consistent with the report by Chow et al,[118] in which 21% of 203 patients with PTC microcancers had local tumor extension, 25% had lymph node metastases, 2.5% had distant metastases, and 1.0% died of cancer, confirming that small tumor size, regardless of how it is found, does not always follow an indolent course.

Tests to Identify Malignant Nodules

Current Practice

Although FNAB has been advised for the past three decades as an essential preoperative test in the diagnosis of thyroid nodules,[188,199] one large study of 5583 cases of thyroid cancer treated in the United States in 1996 found that 40% of the patients underwent thyroidectomy without having had an FNAB.[200]

Fine Needle Aspiration Biopsy

According to 2006 ATA and NCCN thyroid cancer guidelines,[109,201] FNAB is the first step in the management of a patient with a normal or high TSH and a newly discovered thyroid nodule, whether it presents as an isolated tumor or a multinodular goiter, because the incidence of thyroid cancer in both is approximately 4%.[188,201,202] FNAB is a highly sensitive and specific test, but its effectiveness is dependent on the choice of nodules to biopsy, the expertise of the operator and the technique used to obtain an adequate specimen. The rate of inadequate cytology specimens, which ranges around 20% when palpation alone is used to guide FNAB, decreases significantly when it is done under ultrasound guidance and with on-site evaluation of the specimen for adequacy.[203,204] One study found that the inadequate cytology rate was reduced to 0.6% with the use of on-site cytologic evaluation of the cytology specimen.[205]

Thyroid Ultrasonography

Now a mainstay in the management of thyroid cancer, cervical ultrasonography assists in perhaps the most difficult diagnostic decision: choosing which nodules to biopsy. In the past, nodules larger than 1 cm underwent biopsy based on the notion that smaller nodules, even if malignant, pose little or no threat to the patients' survival. More recent studies suggest that this is a flawed concept (see the sections Papillary Thyroid Cancer Microcancer and Multiple Intrathyroidal Papillary Thyroid Cancer, earlier in chapter).[206,207] Several ultrasonographic nodule features provide a much better pretest probability of disease than size alone. Indeed, using size alone may well miss clinically relevant subcentimeter nodules. Machens et al[91] found that the threshold for developing extrathyroidal tumor extension and lymph node metastases is 5 mm for PTC.

Ultrasonography provides a high pre-FNAB test probability of cancer when the thyroid nodule has an irregular and blurred margin, or shows mixed hypoechoic-isoechoic areas and microcalcifications and an intranodular Doppler vascular pattern.[207] In lymph nodes, the best indicator of malignancy is its characteristic round appearance gauged by the Solbiati index (SI), the ratio of a nodule's largest to smallest diameter, which when near 1 is highly likely to represent malignancy. Other major indicators of malignancy are a complex echoic pattern or irregular hypoechoic small intranodular structures and irregular diffuse intranodular blood flow.[208] Using these features, ultrasonography can provide information that may alter the surgical approach.[108]

Cytology Categories

Cytology results are generally categorized into four broad types: (1) insufficient for diagnosis; (2) indeterminate, also reported as follicular tumor or neoplasm; (3) benign; and (4) malignant.[189,203]

Insufficient Cytology

According to the ATA and NCCN thyroid nodule and cancer guidelines,[109,110] FNAB should be repeated under ultrasound guidance with on-site evaluation for specimen adequacy, which will yield adequate cytology in at least 50% of the cases.[189,203] If repeated FNAB yields persistently nondiagnostic specimens, surgical removal of the nodule is advised.[109,110,189,203] Patients who cannot undergo surgery can be followed with serial ultrasonography.[209]

Benign Cytology

According to ATA and NCCN guidelines, benign cytology requires repeat ultrasonographic imaging at 6 to 18 months to monitor nodule growth.[109,110] Although benign nodules grow over time, only a small minority are found to be malignant on repeat FNAB.[210] According to the ATA guidelines, nodules showing more than a 20% increase in nodule volume or growing more than 2 mm in two diameters should be reaspirated to rule out malignancy.[211]

Indeterminate Cytology

About 80% of specimens in this category are from benign tumors,[189] but there is no widely accepted indicator that will preoperatively predict with certainty which are malignant, although finding a BRAF mutation[212] or other genes[176] in the specimen may soon fill this diagnostic gap. The current ATA and NCCN recommendations are that patients undergo hemithyroidectomy to remove the nodule[213] followed by completion thyroidectomy if the nodule is malignant.[213] In some European centers, serum calcitonin measurements are routinely done in the course of evaluating patients with multinodular goiter,[214] but this practice has not been fully embraced by American endocrinologists.[215]

Malignant Cytology

The ATA and NCCN guidelines indicate that malignant cytology and cytology that is suspicious for thyroid cancer require total or near-total thyroidectomy unless there is a contraindication to surgery.[109,110] A preoperative ultrasound should be done to search the lateral and central neck compartments for malignant lymph nodes.[109,110]

Initial Therapy

Delay in Treatment

A delay in the management of DTC accounts for many treatment failures. In our studies the median time from the detection of the tumor to initial therapy was 4 months, but ranged from less than 1 month to 20 years in some cases.[74] Cancer mortality increased in direct relation to time of delay until the patient underwent surgery. In patients who died of thyroid cancer the median delay was 18 months from the time a nodule was first discovered until the time of surgery, compared with 4 months in those still living at the time of last follow-up ($p < .001$). Cancer mortality was 4% in patients who underwent initial therapy within a year of the recognition of a nodule and 10% in the others; 30-year cancer mortality rates in these two groups, respectively, were 6% and 13% ($p < .001$). A retrospective study of 100 consecutive patients with thyroid cancer who had undergone preoperative FNAB found that 14 had cancers that were not detected by FNAB, three of whom developed widespread disease.[216] A single false-negative FNAB delayed surgical treatment by 28 months, sometimes despite clinical evidence suggesting malignancy. This group of patients had higher rates of tumor vascular and capsular invasion and was more likely to have persistent disease at follow-up (hazard ratio 2.28). In another study, 131 surgical patients who underwent completion thyroidectomy within 6 months of the primary operation had significantly fewer recurrences, fewer lymph node

metastases, and fewer hematogenous metastases, and they survived significantly longer than those in whom the second operation was delayed for longer than 6 months.[138] The authors of this study concluded that completion thyroidectomy should be performed as soon as possible after incomplete resection of the tumor and may improve prognosis, especially those with DTC tumor larger than 1 cm.

Thyroid Surgery

Optimal initial thyroid surgery for most patients is total or near-total thyroidectomy when DTC is identified preoperatively,[83,217] which is performed by the majority of surgeons in the United States.[200] Although the NCCN guidelines suggest lobectomy and isthmusectomy for patients aged 15 to 45 years, without prior radiation, cervical or distant metastases, extrathyroidal extension, or family history of thyroid cancer, and tumor <4 cm in diameter, this approach is associated with high recurrence rates,[83,218] including lung metastases in some patients, and there is no reliable way to promptly detect tumor outside the neck during follow-up. The ATA guidelines recommend total or near-total thyroidectomy if any of the following are present: primary thyroid cancer larger than 1 to 1.5 cm in diameter, contralateral thyroid nodules, regional or distant metastases, a history of radiation therapy to the head and neck, or a first-degree family member with a history of DTC. Also, older age (>45 years) may be a criterion for total or near-total thyroidectomy because of higher recurrence rates in this age group.

When thyroid lobectomy has been performed, completion thyroidectomy (removal of the contralateral lobe) is advised by the ATA and NCCN[109,110] if the ipsilateral tumor is larger than 1 cm, or when it is metastatic or invades surrounding tissues, or the patient has been exposed to radiation, or has familial thyroid cancer or multicentric tumor or an aggressive histologic variant.[83] Cancer is found in the contralateral lobe[83] about half the time unless the initially resected tumor is multifocal, in which case tumor is almost always found in the contralateral lobe.[139] Patients who undergo completion thyroidectomy within 6 months of the primary operation have significantly fewer recurrences, and fewer lymph node and hematogenous metastases, and they survive significantly longer than those in whom the second operation is delayed.[138] We thus advise completion thyroidectomy as soon as possible after hemithyroidectomy. At 30 years, the recurrence rate among 436 patients who had undergone subtotal thyroidectomy was significantly higher than that among 698 patients who had undergone total or near-total thyroidectomy (40% versus 26%, $p < .002$); cancer-specific mortality rates were also higher in the subtotal thyroidectomy group (9% and 6%, $p = .02$).[74]

Lymph Node Surgery

Systematic compartment-oriented dissection of lymph node metastases significantly improves recurrence ($p < .0001$) and survival (p <.005) rates in patients with T1 to T3 tumors.[219] Lymph node metastases increase the rate of distant metastases more than 11-fold.[118] We found that lymph node metastases, especially bilateral cervical or mediastinal, were an independent risk factor for persistent disease, distant metastases, and survival.[83] The ATA guidelines[110] recommend routine central compartment (level VI) lymph node dissection for patients with PTC and suspected HTC, but not for FTC; surgery followed by I-131 therapy may provide an alternative approach to lymph node surgery for PTC and HTC. For the other neck compartments, the ATA guidelines suggest that functional compartmental en-bloc dissection is favored over selective dissection (berry picking) when malignant lymph nodes are found in the lateral neck (compartments II to IV) and posterior compartment (level V) on preoperative ultrasonography or at the time of surgery. This surgery should not be done empirically when lymph node metastases are not present.[110] Patients with cervical lymph node metastasis, those with primary tumor invading beyond the thyroid capsule, and women older than 60 years appear to benefit most from modified radical neck dissection.[220] The NCCN guidelines[109,110] advise neck compartmental lymph node surgery only when lymph node biopsy is positive. Lymph node surgery is discussed in detail in Chapter 9.

Radioactive Iodine (I-131) Therapy

When total or near-total thyroidectomy appears to have successfully removed all visible malignant thyroid tissue, some I-131 uptake usually remains in the thyroid bed.[142] Obliterating this macroscopically normal residual thyroid tissue with I-131 is referred to as thyroid remnant ablation.

Indications for Thyroid I-131 Remnant Ablation

This decision is tightly coupled to the rationale for performing total or near-total thyroidectomy, after which most patients have thyroid bed I-131 uptake.[142] Remnant ablation (RA) should be performed when the patient has a tumor with the potential for recurrence.[142] The ATA thyroid cancer guidelines recommend RA for patients with stage III and IV disease (American Joint Committee on Cancer [AJCC], 6th edition) and all with stage II disease younger than age 45 years and most patients with stage II disease over this age, and selected patients with stage I disease who have multifocal tumor, nodal metastases, extrathyroidal or vascular invasion, or more aggressive histologies. As a practical matter, this amounts to RA for most patients who have undergone total or near-total thyroidectomy.

A large (>2 cm) thyroid remnant not only can obscure I-131 uptake in neck and lung metastases,[221] but also cannot be easily destroyed with I-131,[222] and is best surgically excised. Six to 12 months after RA, if there is no visible I-123 uptake in the thyroid bed, or if visible, the fractional uptake of I-123

is <0.1% and TSH-stimulated serum Tg level is <2 ng/mL, a second RA is unlikely to be necessary.[223]

Thus the goals of I-131 remnant ablation are to destroy residual normal thyroid tissue and occult tumor and to facilitate long-term surveillance with serum Tg measurements. Retrospective studies show a significant reduction in the rates of tumor recurrence[74,224–226] and cancer-specific mortality.[74] The ATA guidelines[110] recommend that the minimum I-131 activity (30 to 200 mCi) necessary to achieve successful RA should be chosen,[227,228] particularly in low-risk patients. The guidelines recommend higher activities of I-131 (100 to 200 mCi) if residual microscopic disease is suspected or documented, or if there is a more aggressive tumor histology (e.g., tall cell, insular, columnar cell PTC). RA can be performed after preparation with recombinant human TSH (rhTSH),[223] which is administered while euthyroid patients continue to take levothyroxine, avoiding symptomatic hypothyroidism that occurs after thyroid hormone withdrawal, which creates symptoms that seriously interfere with daily activities.[229]

Thyroid Hormone Therapy

Thyrotropin (TSH) receptors are expressed in the cell membrane of DTC, and respond to TSH stimulation by increasing the rates of neoplastic cell growth and the expression of several thyroid-specific proteins, including thyroglobulin and the sodium-iodide symporter. As a result, TSH suppression with supraphysiologic doses of levothyroxine (LT$_4$) is commonly used to treat patients with DTC[110] in an effort to decrease the risk of recurrence.[74,230,231] In our studies cancer death rates were 12% without LT$_4$ therapy and 6% following LT$_4$ therapy as the only medical therapy (p <.001).[74] A meta-analysis has suggested an association between LT$_4$ suppression therapy and reduction of major adverse clinical events.[231] Still, the optimal extent of TSH suppression by LT$_4$ remains unknown.[110] One study reported that a continuously suppressed TSH ($\leq$0.05 mIU/L) was associated with a longer relapse-free survival than when serum TSH levels were always $\geq$1 mIU/L and that the degree of TSH suppression was an independent predictor of recurrence.[232] However, in another large study, disease stage, patient age, and I-131 therapy independently predicted tumor progression, but the degree of TSH suppression did not.[230]

The ATA guidelines[110] recommend that, in patients with persistent tumor, the TSH should be maintained below 0.1 mIU/L indefinitely in the absence of specific contraindications such as osteoporosis or heart disease. The guidelines recommend that in patients who are clinically free of disease but who presented with high–risk tumors (e.g., lung metastases that appear to have been cured), the TSH levels should be maintained at 0.1 to 0.5 mIU/L for 5 to 10 years. In patients who are free of disease, especially those at low risk for recurrence, the guidelines recommend that TSH may be kept within the low normal range (0.3 to 2 mIU/L).

Treatment of Distant Metastases

A full discussion of the treatment of distant metastases is beyond the scope of this chapter but is available in the 2006 ATA thyroid cancer guidelines that are available on the ATA Web site at Thyroid.org.[110]

Physicians and surgeons who care for patients before I-131 treatment is given should avoid prescribing iodinated contrast material for radiographic studies, which delays I-131 therapy for 3 to 6 months. Patients with I-131–avid metastatic disease require careful preparation with a 2-week low iodine diet, and often require large cumulative amounts of I-131, ranging up to 500 or 600 mCi, to achieve successful destruction of metastatic tumors that concentrate the isotope. Larger cumulative amounts of I-131 are not given routinely because this exposes the patient to the risk of developing a variety of secondary tumors, including bladder, breast, parotid, and colon cancer and other solid tumors and myelogenous leukemia, all of which appear years after I-131 therapy.[233]

Ordinarily thyroid hormone withdrawal is necessary to raise the serum TSH to levels sufficient for I-131 therapy, but when withdrawal cannot be done for medical or other reasons, rhTSH may be given to enhance tumor I-131 uptake.[110] The best responses to I-131 occur in children and young adults with diffuse pulmonary metastases that are found at an early stage, generally before the tumors are radiologically apparent except for visualization on the RxWBS. In this case patients are usually rendered disease-free as evidenced by negative RxWBS and other radiologic studies (e.g., 18-fluorodeoxyglucose [^{18}FDG]-PET/CT fusion) and serum Tg levels that fail to rise with TSH stimulation.[76,234]

Medical treatment of macroscopic tumor that does not concentrate I-131 is best determined on an individual basis, but EBRT for such patients over age 45 years is highly effective in controlling local tumor, provided that the metastatic site is amenable to EBRT.[235] Isolated brain or bone metastases may be amenable to surgery, I-131 therapy, or EBRT, depending on the patient's age, the number and location of tumors, and tumor I-131 avidity.[110] For patients with tumors unresponsive or not amenable to these therapeutic modalities, tumor embolization or ethanol ablation may be of benefit in selected cases.[110] Otherwise patients rarely if ever have meaningful responses to standard chemotherapy and should be offered watchful waiting for asymptomatic slow growing tumors or experimental chemotherapy trials, which are an important avenue of hope when standard therapy no longer is an option. Early reports show tumor responses to new tyrosine kinase or angiogenesis inhibitors.

Follow-Up of Patients with Differentiated Thyroid Cancer

Definition of Disease-Free Status

According to the 2006 ATA guidelines,[110] the criteria for absence of persistent tumor are all of the following: no clinical or imaging evidence of tumor (no uptake outside the thyroid bed on the initial RxWBS, or on a recent diagnostic whole-body I-123 scan [DxWBS], and neck ultrasonography), and undetectable serum Tg levels during TSH suppression and stimulation in the absence of interfering antibodies. Still, it is not uncommon to find small neck lymph node metastases by ultrasonography in patients with negative DxWBS I-123 scans and undetectable serum Tg levels that fail to rise with TSH stimulation.[112,236] Also, DxWBS I-123 imaging has little utility prior to I-131 therapy[237] and during follow-up,[236] being largely replaced by neck ultrasonography in both situations.

Serum Thyroglobulin

This protein, which serves as a matrix for the synthesis and storage of thyroid hormones, is normally found in the serum of individuals with an intact thyroid gland and in patients with a large thyroid remnant or persistent DTC. The accuracy of this key test is greatest after TSH stimulation, either after LT$_4$ withdrawal or recombinant human TSH (rhTSH) stimulation,[238] which requires total or near-total thyroidectomy and I-131 remnant ablation. There are, however, serious limitations with Tg measurement, the most important of which is the poor reproducibility of Tg determinations made in different laboratories.[239] Serial Tg determinations must be made in the same laboratory and by the same analytic method;[240] otherwise, it is impossible to interpret changing serum Tg values.

Antithyroglobulin Antibodies

Serum antithyroglobulin antibodies (TgAbs) also interfere with Tg measurement by immunometric assay (IMA). The prevalence of TgAb is approximately 10% in the general population[241] and 25% in patients with DTC.[242] When present in the same serum sample in which Tg is measured, TgAb factitiously lowers Tg values, usually to undetectable levels, if Tg is determined by IMA, which is used by commercial laboratories. There are two ways around this problem. First, a quantitative TgAb level may serve as surrogate for Tg, which over time roughly corresponds to changes in tumor burden, but it may take years for TgAb to disappear as a patient becomes tumor-free.[243] Second, serum Tg may be measured by radioimmunoassay (RIA), which typically undergoes less TgAb interference than does IMA,[244] but unfortunately Tg RIA is performed by few laboratories.[245] The ATA guidelines recommend quantitative serum TgAb measurements in the same specimen undergoing Tg determination.

Heterophile Antibodies

This group of antibodies, which is very common in the general population, also may interfere with Tg measurement by IMA. Unlike TgAb interference, heterophile antibody (HAB) interference usually results in false-positive Tg tests. This has the potential to result in unnecessary I-131 therapy, considering the current trend to treat some thyroid cancer patients empirically with I-131 on the basis of an elevated serum Tg level alone. One study that evaluated the prevalence of HAB interference in a commonly used automated immunoassay found that, after removing HAB from 1106 consecutive specimens with Tg values greater than 1 ng/mL, Tg levels dropped to <1 ng/mL in 32 (3%) specimens, 20 of which fell to <0.1 ng/mL.[248] It is currently unknown whether other IMA Tg assays suffer from similar problems, but it is highly likely that they do. HAB interference should be suspected if Tg results fail to rise and fall with TSH stimulation and suppression and do not fit the clinical picture.

Scanning Studies

18-Fluorodeoxyglucose-PET/CT fusion studies and neck ultrasonography have become the most important imaging follow-up studies for thyroid cancer. Neck ultrasonography has largely replaced DxWBS because of its low sensitivity[113,246] and thyroid stunning, a phenomenon in which amounts of I-131 as small as 2 mCi[247] in DxWBS studies provoke changes in malignant thyroid tissue that reduces therapeutic I-131 uptake on RxWBS.[248] In effect, some of or the entire tumor fails to concentrate I-131.

18-Fluorodeoxyglucose-PET/CT is used to restage thyroid cancer when the I-131 RxWBS is negative in a patient with an elevated serum Tg.[110] Integrating PET and CT scans improves the diagnostic accuracy of the scan by precisely localizing tumor tissue, which is superior to side-by-side interpretation of PET and CT images.[249] One study showed that [18]FDG-PET/CT supplied information that altered or confirmed the management plan in 67% of 33 cases.[250] It had 66% sensitivity in identifying recurrence, a 100% specificity, a 100% a positive predictive value, and a negative predictive value.

18-Fluorodeoxyglucose-PET also estimates prognosis. A study of 400 DTC patients who underwent [18]FDG-PET scanning found by multivariate analysis that only age and [18]FDG-PET uptake were strong predictors of survival. This shows that [18]FDG-PET is a more powerful prognostic tool than clinical and tumor features, and suggests that subsequent therapy should be tailored to match the [18]FDG-PET results.

According to the ATA guidelines,[110] the preferred treatment of metastatic disease, in order of priority, is surgical excision of locoregional disease in potentially curable patients; I-131 therapy, EBRT, and watchful waiting in patients with stable asymptomatic tumor; and experimental therapy chemotherapy trials. Patients with persistent/recurrent tumor confined to the neck should undergo complete ipsilateral or central compartmental dissection of involved compartments while sparing vital structures.

References

1. Mazzaferri EL. An overview of the management of thyroid cancer. In: Mazzaferri EL, Harmer C, Mallick UK, Kendall-Taylor P, eds. Practical Management of Thyroid Cancer: A Multidisciplinary Approach. London: Springer-Verlag, 2006:1–28

2. Davies L, Welch HG. Increasing incidence of thyroid cancer in the United States, 1973–2002. JAMA 2006;295:2164–2167

3. Colonna M, Grosclaude P, Remontet L, et al. Incidence of thyroid cancer in adults recorded by French cancer registries (1978–1997). Eur J Cancer 2002;38:1762–1768

4. Heidenreich WF, Kenigsberg J, Jacob P, et al. Time trends of thyroid cancer incidence in Belarus after the Chernobyl accident. Radiat Res 1999;151:617–625

5. Huszno B, Szybinski Z, Przybylik-Mazurek E, et al. Influence of iodine deficiency and iodine prophylaxis on thyroid cancer histotypes and incidence in endemic goiter area. J Endocrinol Invest 2003;26(2, suppl):71–76

6. Verkooijen HM, Fioretta G, Pache JC, et al. Diagnostic changes as a reason for the increase in papillary thyroid cancer incidence in Geneva, Switzerland. Cancer Causes Control 2003;14:13–17

7. Leenhardt L, Bernier MO, Boin-Pineau MH, et al. Advances in diagnostic practices affect thyroid cancer incidence in France. Eur J Endocrinol 2004;150:133–139

8. Ries LAG, Eisner MP, Kosary CL, et al. SEER Cancer Statistics Review, 1975–2001, National Cancer Institute. Bethesda, MD. http://seer.cancer.gov/csr/1975˜2001/. 2004.

9. Surveillance Epidemiology and End Results (SEER) Program (www.seer.cancer.gov). SEER*Stat Database: Incidence—SEER 9 Regs. Public Use, November 2003 Sub (1973–2001), National Cancer Institute, DCCPS, Surveillance Research Program, Cancer Statistics Branch, released April 2004, based on the November 2003 submission. Natl.Cancer.Ins, 2004

10. Ries LAG, Harkins D, Krapcho D, et al. SEER Cancer Statistics Review, 1997–2003 Based on November 2005 SEER data submission, posted to the SEER Web site, 2006. SEER Surveillance Epidemiology and End Results Cancer Stat Fact Sheets. 6–13–2006.

11. Pinn VW. Sex and gender factors in medical studies: implications for health and clinical practice. JAMA 2003;289:397–400

12. Hundahl SA, Fleming ID, Fremgen AM, Menck HR. A National Cancer Data Base report on 53,856 cases of thyroid carcinoma treated in the US, 1985–1995. Cancer 1998;83:2638–2648

13. Kitamura Y, Shimizu K, Nagahama M, et al. Immediate causes of death in thyroid carcinoma: Clinicopathological analysis of 161 fatal cases. J Clin Endocrinol Metab 1999;84:4043–4049

14. Brunaud L, Zarnegar R, Wada N, et al. Chromosomal aberrations by comparative genomic hybridization in thyroid tumors in patients with familial nonmedullary thyroid cancer. Thyroid 2003;13:621–629

15. Charkes ND. On the prevalence of familial nonmedullary thyroid cancer in multiply affected kindreds. Thyroid 2006;16:181–186

16. Hemminki K, Eng C, Chen B. Familial risks for nonmedullary thyroid cancer. J Clin Endocrinol Metab 2005;90:5747–5753

17. Bevan S, Pal T, Greenberg CR, et al. A comprehensive analysis of MNG1, TCO1, fPTC, PTEN, TSHR, and TRKA in familial nonmedullary thyroid cancer: confirmation of linkage to TCO1. J Clin Endocrinol Metab 2001;86:3701–3704

18. Uchino S, Noguchi S, Kawamoto H, et al. Familial nonmedullary thyroid carcinoma characterized by multifocality and a high recurrence rate in a large study population. World J Surg 2002;26:897–902

19. Lindor NM, Greene MH. The concise handbook of family cancer syndromes. Mayo Familial Cancer Program. J Natl Cancer Inst 1998;90:1039–1071

20. Nagy R, Sweet K, Eng C. Highly penetrant hereditary cancer syndromes. Oncogene 2004;23:6445–6470

21. Cetta F, Montalto G, Gori M, Curia MC, Cama A, Olschwang S. Germline mutations of the APC gene in patients with familial adenomatous polyposis-associated thyroid carcinoma: results from a European cooperative study. J Clin Endocrinol Metab 2000;85:286–292

22. Bell B, Mazzaferri EL. Familial adenomatous polyposis (Gardner's syndrome) and thyroid carcinoma: A case report and review of the literature. Dig Dis Sci 1993;38:185–190

23. Cetta F, Olschwang S, Petracci M, et al. Genetic alterations in thyroid carcinoma associated with familial adenomatous polyposis: clinical implications and suggestions for early detection. World J Surg 1998;22:1231–1236

24. Dahia PLM, Marsh DJ, Zheng ZM, et al. Somatic deletions and mutations in the Cowden disease gene, *PTEN*, in sporadic thyroid tumors. Cancer Res 1997;57:4710–4713

25. Campos FG, Habr-Gama A, Kiss DR, et al. Cowden syndrome: report of two cases and review of clinical presentation and management of a rare colorectal polyposis 2. Curr Surg 2006;63:15–19

26. Stratakis CA, Courcoutsakis NA, Abati A, et al. Thyroid gland abnormalities in patients with the syndrome of spotty skin pigmentation, myxomas, endocrine overactivity, and schwannomas (Carney complex). J Clin Endocrinol Metab 1997;82:2037–2043

27. Krause DS, Van Etten RA. Tyrosine kinases as targets for cancer therapy. N Engl J Med 2005;353:172–187

28. Baselga J. Targeting tyrosine kinases in cancer: the second wave. Science 2006;312:1175–1178

29. Arora A, Scholar EM. Role of tyrosine kinase inhibitors in cancer therapy. J Pharmacol Exp Ther 2005;315:971–979

30. Smanik PA, Furminger TL, Mazzaferri EL, Jhiang SM. Breakpoint characterization of the ret/PTC oncogene in human papillary thyroid carcinoma. Hum Mol Genet 1995;4:2313–2318

31. Grieco M, Santoro M, Berlingieri MT, et al. PTC is a novel rearranged form of the ret proto-oncogene and is frequently detected in vivo in human thyroid papillary carcinomas. Cell 1990;60:557–563

32. Fusco A, Viglietto G, Santoro M. A new mechanism of BRAF activation in human thyroid papillary carcinoma. J Clin Invest 2005;115:20–23

33. Viglietto G, Chiappetta G, Martinez-Tello FJ, et al. RET/PTC oncogene activation is an early event in thyroid carcinogenesis. Oncogene 1995;11:1207–1210

34. Corvi R, Martinez-Alfaro M, Harach HR, Zini M, Papotti M, Romeo G. Frequent RET rearrangements in thyroid papillary microcarcinoma detected by interphase fluorescence in situ hybridization. Lab Invest 2001;81:1639–1645

35. Mizuno T, Kyoizumi S, Suzuki T, Iwamoto KS, Seyama T. Continued expression of a tissue specific activated oncogene in the early steps of radiation-induced human thyroid carcinogenesis. Oncogene 1997;15:1455–1460

36. Nikiforov YE, Koshoffer A, Nikiforova M, Stringer J, Fagin JA. Chromosomal breakpoint positions suggest a direct role for radiation in inducing illegitimate recombination between the ELE1 and RET genes in radiation-induced thyroid carcinomas. Oncogene 1999;18:6330–6334

37. Nikiforova MN, Stringer JR, Blough R, Medvedovic M, Fagin JA, Nikiforov YE. Proximity of chromosomal loci that participate in radiation-induced rearrangements in human cells. Science 2000;290:138–141

38. Jhiang SM, Sagartz JE, Tong Q, et al. Targeted expression of the ret/PTC1 oncogene induces papillary thyroid carcinomas. Endocrinology 1996;137:375–378

39. Powell DJ, Russell J, Nibu K, et al. The *RET/PTC3* oncogene: metastatic solid-type papillary carcinomas in murine thyroids. Cancer Res 1998;58:5523–5528

40. Rabes HM, Demidchik EP, Sidorow JD, et al. Pattern of radiation-induced RET and NTRK1 rearrangements in 191 post-Chernobyl papillary thyroid carcinomas: biological, phenotypic, and clinical implications. Clin Cancer Res 2000;6:1093–1103

41. Fugazzola L, Pilotti S, Pinchera A, et al. Oncogenic rearrangements of the RET proto-oncogene in papillary thyroid carcinomas from children exposed to the Chernobyl nuclear accident. Cancer Res 1995;55:5617–5620

42. Klugbauer S, Lengfelder E, Demidchik EP, Rabes HM. High prevalence of RET rearrangement in thyroid tumors of children from Belarus after the Chernobyl reactor accident. Oncogene 1995;11:2459–2467

43. Nikiforov YE, Rowland JM, Bove KE, Monforte-Munoz H, Fagin JA. Distinct pattern of ret oncogene rearrangements in morphological variants of radiation-induced and sporadic thyroid papillary carcinomas in children. Cancer Res 1997;57:1690–1694

44. Zhu Z, Ciampi R, Nikiforova MN, Gandhi M, Nikiforov YE. Prevalence of RET/PTC rearrangements in thyroid papillary carcinomas: effects of the detection methods and genetic heterogeneity. J Clin Endocrinol Metab 2006;91:3603–3610

45. Cohen Y, Xing M, Mambo E, et al. BRAF mutation in papillary thyroid carcinoma. J Natl Cancer Inst 2003;95:625–627

46. Fukushima T, Suzuki S, Mashiko M, et al. BRAF mutations in papillary carcinomas of the thyroid. Oncogene 2003;22:6455–6457

47. Kimura ET, Nikiforova MN, Zhu Z, Knauf JA, Nikiforov YE, Fagin JA. High prevalence of BRAF mutations in thyroid cancer: genetic evidence for constitutive activation of the RET/PTC-RAS-BRAF signaling pathway in papillary thyroid carcinoma. Cancer Res 2003;63:1454–1457

48. Nikiforova MN, Kimura ET, Gandhi M, et al. BRAF mutations in thyroid tumors are restricted to papillary carcinomas and anaplastic or poorly differentiated carcinomas arising from papillary carcinomas. J Clin Endocrinol Metab 2003;88:5399–5404

49. Xu X, Quiros RM, Gattuso P, Ain KB, Prinz RA. High prevalence of BRAF gene mutation in papillary thyroid carcinomas and thyroid tumor cell lines. Cancer Res 2003;63:4561–4567

50. Xing M, Tufano RP, Tufaro AP, et al. Detection of BRAF mutation on fine needle aspiration biopsy specimens: a new diagnostic tool for papillary thyroid cancer. J Clin Endocrinol Metab 2004;89:2867–2872

51. Xing M, Westra WH, Tufano RP, et al. BRAF mutation predicts a poorer clinical prognosis for papillary thyroid cancer. J Clin Endocrinol Metab 2005;89:2867–2872

52. Xing M. The T1799A BRAF mutation is not a germline mutation in familial nonmedullary thyroid cancer. Clin Endocrinol (Oxf) 2005;63:263–266

53. Kumagai A, Namba H, Saenko VA, et al. Low frequency of BRAFT1796A mutations in childhood thyroid carcinomas. J Clin Endocrinol Metab 2004;89:4280–4284

54. Collins BJ, Schneider AB, Prinz RA, Xu X. Low frequency of BRAF mutations in adult patients with papillary thyroid cancers following childhood radiation exposure. Thyroid 2006;16:61–66

55. Ciampi R, Knauf JA, Kerler R, et al. Oncogenic AKAP9-BRAF fusion is a novel mechanism of MAPK pathway activation in thyroid cancer. J Clin Invest 2005;115:94–101

56. Nikiforova MN, Ciampi R, Salvatore G, et al. Low prevalence of BRAF mutations in radiation-induced thyroid tumors in contrast to sporadic papillary carcinomas. Cancer Lett 2004;209:1–6

57. Vasko V, Hu S, Wu G, et al. High prevalence and possible de novo formation of BRAF mutation in metastasized papillary thyroid cancer in lymph nodes. J Clin Endocrinol Metab 2005;90:5265–5269

58. Xing M, Westra WH, Tufano RP, et al. BRAF mutation predicts a poorer clinical prognosis for papillary thyroid cancer. J Clin Endocrinol Metab 2005;90:6373–6379

59. Namba H, Nakashima M, Hayashi T, et al. Clinical implication of hot spot BRAF mutation, V599E, in papillary thyroid cancers. J Clin Endocrinol Metab 2003;88:4393–4397

60. Kim KH, Kang DW, Kim SH, Seong IO, Kang DY. Mutations of the BRAF gene in papillary thyroid carcinoma in a Korean population. Yonsei Med J 2004;45:818–821

61. Adeniran AJ, Zhu Z, Gandhi M, et al. Correlation between genetic alterations and microscopic features, clinical manifestations, and prognostic characteristics of thyroid papillary carcinomas. Am J Surg Pathol 2006;30:216–222

62. Paloyan E, Lawrence AM. Thyroid neoplasms after radiation therapy for adolescent acne vulgaris. Arch Dermatol 1978;114:53–55

63. Kaplan MM, Garnick MB, Gelber R, et al. Risk factors for thyroid abnormalities after neck irradiation for childhood cancer. Am J Med 1983;74:272–280

64. Mehta MP, Goetowski PG, Kinsella TJ. Radiation induced thyroid neoplasms 1920 to 1987: a vanishing problem. Int J Radiat Oncol Biol Phys 1989;16:1471–1475

65. Hallquist A, Hardell L, Löfroth P-O. External radiotherapy prior to thyroid cancer: a case-control study. Int J Radiat Oncol Biol Phys 1993;27:1085–1089

66. Acharya S, Sarafoglou K, LaQuaglia M, et al. Thyroid neoplasms after therapeutic radiation for malignancies during childhood or adolescence. Cancer 2003;97:2397–2403

67. Kikuchi S, Perrier ND, Ituarte P, Siperstein AE, Duh QY, Clark OH. Latency period of thyroid neoplasia after radiation exposure. Ann Surg 2004;239:536–543

68. Caudill CM, Zhu Z, Ciampi R, Stringer JR, Nikiforov YE. Dose-dependent generation of RET/PTC in human thyroid cells after in vitro exposure to gamma-radiation: a model of carcinogenic chromosomal rearrangement induced by ionizing radiation. J Clin Endocrinol Metab 2005;90:2364–2369

69. Tronko MD, Bogdanova TI, Komissarenko IV, et al. Thyroid carcinoma in children and adolescents in Ukraine after the Chernobyl nuclear accident—statistical data and clinicomorphologic characteristics. Cancer 1999;86:149–156

70. Nikiforov Y, Gnepp DR. Pediatric thyroid cancer after the Chernobyl disaster: pathomorphologic study of 84 cases (1991–1992) from the Republic of Belarus. Cancer 1994;74:748–766

71. Nikiforov Y, Gnepp DR, Fagin JA. Thyroid lesions in children and adolescents after the Chernobyl disaster: implications for the study of radiation tumorigenesis. J Clin Endocrinol Metab 1996;81: 9–14

72. Pacini F, Vorontsova T, Demidchik EP, et al. Post-Chernobyl thyroid carcinoma in Belarus children and adolescents: comparison with naturally occurring thyroid carcinoma in Italy and France. J Clin Endocrinol Metab 1997;82:3563–3569

73. Mazzaferri EL. Thyroid carcinoma: papillary and follicular. In: Mazzaferri EL, Samaan N, eds. Endocrine Tumors. Cambridge: Blackwell Scientific, 1993:278–333

74. Mazzaferri EL, Jhiang SM. Long-term impact of initial surgical and medical therapy on papillary and follicular thyroid cancer. Am J Med 1994;97:418–428

75. Hung W, Sarlis NJ. Current controversies in the management of pediatric patients with well-differentiated non-medullary thyroid cancer: a review. Thyroid 2002;12:683–702

76. Durante C, Haddy N, Baudin E, et al. Long term outcome of 444 patients with distant metastases from papillary and follicular thyroid carcinoma: benefits and limits of radioiodine therapy. J Clin Endocrinol Metab 2006;91:2892–2899

77. Cady B. Staging in thyroid carcinoma. Cancer 1998;83:844–847

78. Miccoli P, Antonelli A, Spinelli C, Ferdeghini M, Fallahi P, Baschieri L. Completion total thyroidectomy in children with thyroid cancer secondary to the Chernobyl accident. Arch Surg 1998;133: 89–93

79. Ohta K, Pang XP, Berg L, Hershman JM. Growth inhibition of new human thyroid carcinoma cell lines by activation of adenylate cyclase through the b-adrenergic receptor. J Clin Endocrinol Metab 1997;82:2633–2638

80. Belfiore A, Russo D, Vigneri R, Filetti S. Graves' disease, thyroid nodules and thyroid cancer. Clin Endocrinol (Oxf) 2001;55:711–718

81. LiVolsi VA. Papillary neoplasms of the thyroid. Pathologic and prognostic features. Am J Clin Pathol 1992;97:426–434

82. Muro-Cacho CA, Ku NN. Tumors of the thyroid gland: histologic and cytologic features—part 1 2. Cancer Control 2000;7:276–287

83. Mazzaferri EL, Kloos RT. Current approaches to primary therapy for papillary and follicular thyroid cancer. J Clin Endocrinol Metab 2001;86:1447–1463

84. Hay ID, Bergstralh EJ, Goellner JR, Ebersold JR, Grant CS. Predicting outcome in papillary thyroid carcinoma: development of a reliable prognostic scoring system in a cohort of 1779 patients surgically treated at one institution during 1940 through 1989. Surgery 1993;114:1050–1058

85. Loh KC, Greenspan FS, Gee L, Miller TR, Yeo PPB. Pathological tumor-node-metastasis (pTNM) staging for papillary and follicular thyroid carcinomas: a retrospective analysis of 700 patients. J Clin Endocrinol Metab 1997;82:3553–3562

86. Siironen P, Louhimo J, Nordling S, et al. Prognostic factors in papillary thyroid cancer: an evaluation of 601 consecutive patients. Tumour Biol 2005;26:57–64

87. Saadi H, Kleidermacher P, Esselstyn C. Conservative management of patients with intrathyroidal well-differentiated follicular thyroid carcinoma. Surgery 2001;130:30–35

88. Sebastian SO, Gonzalez JM, Paricio PP, et al. Papillary thyroid carcinoma: prognostic index for survival including the histological variety. Arch Surg 2000;135:272–277

89. Dobert N, Menzel C, Oeschger S, Grunwald F. Differentiated thyroid carcinoma: the new UICC 6th edition TNM classification system in a retrospective analysis of 169 patients. Thyroid 2004;14:65–70

90. Carrillo JF, Frias-Mendivil M, Ochoa-Carrillo FJ, Ibarra M. Accuracy of fine-needle aspiration biopsy of the thyroid combined with an evaluation of clinical and radiologic factors. Otolaryngol Head Neck Surg 2000;122:917–921

91. Machens A, Holzhausen HJ, Dralle H. The prognostic value of primary tumor size in papillary and follicular thyroid carcinoma. Cancer 2005;103:2269–2273

92. Machens A, Holzhausen HJ, Lautenschlager C, Thanh PN, Dralle H. Enhancement of lymph node metastasis and distant metastasis of thyroid carcinoma. Cancer 2003;98:712–719

93. Jarzab B, Handkiewicz JD, Wloch J, et al. Multivariate analysis of prognostic factors for differentiated thyroid carcinoma in children. Eur J Nucl Med 2000;27:833–841

94. La Quaglia MP, Black T, Holcomb GW, et al. Differentiated thyroid cancer: clinical characteristics, treatment, and outcome in patients under 21 years of age who present with distant metastases.

A report from the Surgical Discipline Committee of the Children's Cancer Group. J Pediatr Surg 2000;35:955–959

95. Witte J, Goretzki PE, Dieken J, Simon D, Roher HD. Importance of lymph node metastases in follicular thyroid cancer. World J Surg 2002;26:1017–1022

96. Watkinson JC, Franklyn JA, Olliff JF. Detection and surgical treatment of cervical lymph nodes in differentiated thyroid cancer. Thyroid 2006;16:187–194

97. Mirallie E, Visset J, Sagan C, Hamy A, Le Bodic MF, Paineau J. Localization of cervical node metastasis of papillary thyroid carcinoma. World J Surg 1999;23:970–973

98. Qubain SW, Nakano S, Baba M, Takao S, Aikou T. Distribution of lymph node micrometastasis in pN0 well-differentiated thyroid carcinoma. Surgery 2002;131:249–256

99. Wada N, Duh QY, Sugino K, et al. Lymph node metastasis from 259 papillary thyroid microcarcinomas: frequency, pattern of occurrence and recurrence, and optimal strategy for neck dissection. Ann Surg 2003;237:399–407

100. Rubello D, Pelizzo MR, Al Nahhas A, et al. The role of sentinel lymph node biopsy in patients with differentiated thyroid carcinoma. Eur J Surg Oncol 2006;32:917–921

101. Pacini F, Molinaro E, Castagna MG, et al. Recombinant human thyrotropin-stimulated serum thyroglobulin combined with neck ultrasonography has the highest sensitivity in monitoring differentiated thyroid carcinoma. J Clin Endocrinol Metab 2003;88:3668–3673

102. Kessler A, Rappaport Y, Blank A, Marmor S, Weiss J, Graif M. Cystic appearance of cervical lymph nodes is characteristic of metastatic papillary thyroid carcinoma. J Clin Ultrasound 2003;31:21–25

103. Wunderbaldinger P, Harisinghani MG, Hahn PF, et al. Cystic lymph node metastases in papillary thyroid carcinoma. AJR Am J Roentgenol 2002;178:693–697

104. Cignarelli M, Ambrosi A, Marino A, et al. Diagnostic utility of thyroglobulin detection in fine-needle aspiration of cervical cystic metastatic lymph nodes from papillary thyroid cancer with negative cytology. Thyroid 2003;13:1163–1167

105. Boi F, Baghino G, Atzeni F, Lai ML, Faa G, Mariotti S. The diagnostic value for differentiated thyroid carcinoma metastases of thyroglobulin (Tg) measurement in washout fluid from fine-needle aspiration biopsy of neck lymph nodes is maintained in the presence of circulating anti-Tg antibodies. J Clin Endocrinol Metab 2006;91:1364–1369

106. Torlontano M, Attard M, Crocetti U, et al. Follow-up of low risk patients with papillary thyroid cancer: role of neck ultrasonography in detecting lymph node metastases. J Clin Endocrinol Metab 2004;89:3402–3407

107. Frasoldati A, Pesenti M, Gallo M, Caroggio A, Salvo D, Valcavi R. Diagnosis of neck recurrences in patients with differentiated thyroid carcinoma. Cancer 2003;97:90–96

108. Kouvaraki MA, Shapiro SE, Fornage BD, et al. Role of preoperative ultrasonography in the surgical management of patients with thyroid cancer. Surgery 2003;134:946–954

109. Sherman S, Angelos P, Ball DW, et al. National Comprehensive Cancer Center Network Thyroid Cancer Guidelines. National Comprehensive Cancer Center Network. 2006.

110. Cooper DS, Doherty GM, Haugen BR, et al. Management guidelines for patients with thyroid nodules and differentiated thyroid cancer. Thyroid 2006;16:109–141

111. Pacini F, Schlumberger M, Dralle H, Elisei R, Smit JW, Wiersinga W. European consensus for the management of patients with differentiated thyroid carcinoma of the follicular epithelium. Eur J Endocrinol 2006;154:787–803

112. Kloos RT, Mazzaferri EL. A single recombinant human thyrotrophin-stimulated serum thyroglobulin measurement predicts differentiated thyroid carcinoma metastases three to five years later. J Clin Endocrinol Metab 2005;90:5047–5057

113. Mazzaferri EL, Robbins RJ, Spencer CA, et al. A consensus report of the role of serum thyroglobulin as a monitoring method for low-risk patients with papillary thyroid carcinoma. J Clin Endocrinol Metab 2003;88:1433–1441

114. Hughes CJ, Shaha AR, Shah JP, Loree TR. Impact of lymph node metastasis in differentiated carcinoma of the thyroid: a matched-pair analysis. Head Neck 1996;18:127–132

115. Podnos YD, Smith D, Wagman LD, Ellenhorn JD. The implication of lymph node metastasis on survival in patients with well-differentiated thyroid cancer. Am Surg 2005;71:731–734

116. Leboulleux S, Rubino C, Baudin E, et al. Prognostic factors for persistent or recurrent disease of papillary thyroid carcinoma with neck lymph node metastases and/or tumor extension beyond the thyroid capsule at initial diagnosis. J Clin Endocrinol Metab 2005;90:5723–5729

117. Yamashita H, Noguchi S, Murakami N, Kawamoto H, Watanabe S. Extracapsular invasion of lymph node metastasis is an indicator of distant metastasis and poor prognosis in patients with thyroid papillary carcinoma. Cancer 1997;80:2268–2272

118. Chow SM, Law SC, Chan JK, Au SK, Yau S, Lau WH. Papillary microcarcinoma of the thyroid—prognostic significance of lymph node metastasis and multifocality. Cancer 2003;98:31–40

119. Bal CS, Padhy AK, Kumar A. Clinical features of differentiated thyroid carcinoma in children and adolescents from a sub-Himalayan iodine-deficient endemic zone. Nucl Med Commun 2001;22:881–887

120. Lopez-Penabad L, Chiu AC, Hoff AO, et al. Prognostic factors in patients with Hurthle cell neoplasms of the thyroid. Cancer 2003;97:1186–1194

121. Schlumberger M, Challeton C, De Vathaire F, Parmentier C. Treatment of distant metastases of differentiated thyroid carcinoma. J Endocrinol Invest 1995;18:170–172

122. Pittas AG, Adler M, Fazzari M, et al. Bone metastases from thyroid carcinoma: clinical characteristics and prognostic variables in one hundred forty-six patients. Thyroid 2000;10:261–268

123. Schlumberger M, Tubiana M, De Vathaire F, et al. Long-term results of treatment of 283 patients with lung and bone metastases from differentiated thyroid carcinoma. J Clin Endocrinol Metab 1986;63:960–967

124. Sisson JC, Giordano TJ, Jamadar DA, et al. 131-I treatment of micronodular pulmonary metastases from papillary thyroid carcinoma. Cancer 1996;78:2184–2192

125. Schlumberger MJ. Diagnostic follow-up of well-differentiated thyroid carcinoma: historical perspective and current status. J Endocrinol Invest 1999;22:3–7

126. Pacini F, Vorontsova T, Molinaro E, et al. Thyroid consequences of the Chernobyl nuclear accident. Acta Paediatr Suppl 1999;88:23–27

127. Sakorafas GH, Giotakis J, Stafyla V. Papillary thyroid microcarcinoma: a surgical perspective. Cancer Treat Rev 2005;31:423–438

128. Bondeson L, Ljungberg O. Occult papillary thyroid carcinoma in the young and the aged. Cancer 1984;53:1790–1792

129. Cohn KH, Backdahl M, Forsslund G, et al. Biologic considerations and operative strategy in papillary thyroid carcinoma: arguments against the routine performance of total thyroidectomy. Surgery 1984;96:957–971

130. Ottino A, Pianzola HM, Castelletto RH. Occult papillary thyroid carcinoma at autopsy in La Plata, Argentina. Cancer 1989;64:547–551

131. Harach HR, Franssila KO, Wasenius VM. Occult papillary carcinoma of the thyroid: a "normal" finding in Finland: a systematic autopsy study. Cancer 1985;56:531–538

132. Lokey JS, Palmer RM, Macfie JA. Unexpected findings during thyroid surgery in a regional community hospital: a 5-year experience of 738 consecutive cases. Am Surg 2005;71:911–913

133. Perez LA, Gupta PK, Mandel SJ, LiVolsi VA, Baloch ZW. Thyroid papillary microcarcinoma. Is it really a pitfall of fine needle aspiration cytology? Acta Cytol 2001;45:341–346

134. Nasir A, Chaudhry AZ, Gillespie J, Kaiser HE. Papillary microcarcinoma of the thyroid: a clinico-pathologic and prognostic review. In Vivo 2000;14:367–376

135. Moosa M, Mazzaferri EL. Occult thyroid carcinoma. Cancer J 1997;10:180–188

136. Baudin E, Travagli JP, Ropers J, et al. Microcarcinoma of the thyroid gland—the Gustave-Roussy Institute Experience. Cancer 1998;83:553–559

137. Pacini F, Elisei R, Capezzone M, et al. Contralateral papillary thyroid cancer is frequent at completion thyroidectomy with no difference in low- and high-risk patients. Thyroid 2001;11:877–881

138. Scheumann GFW, Seeliger H, Musholt TJ, et al. Completion thyroidectomy in 131 patients with differentiated thyroid carcinoma. Eur J Surg 1996;162:677–684

139. Pasieka JL, Thompson NW, McLeod MK, Burney RE, Macha M. The incidence of bilateral well-differentiated thyroid cancer found at completion thyroidectomy. World J Surg 1992;16:711–716

140. Hay ID, Grant CS, Bergstralh EJ, et al. Unilateral total lobectomy: Is it sufficient surgical treatment for patients with AMES low-risk papillary thyroid carcinoma? Surgery 1998;124:958–964

141. Taylor T, Specker B, Robbins J, et al. Outcome after treatment of high-risk papillary and non-Hurthle-cell follicular thyroid carcinoma. Ann Intern Med 1998;129:622–627

142. Mazzaferri EL. Thyroid remnant ^{131}I ablation for papillary and follicular thyroid carcinoma. Thyroid 1997;7:265–271

143. Massin JP, Savoie JC, Garnier H, Guiraudon G, Leger FA, Bacourt F. Pulmonary metastases in differentiated thyroid carcinoma. Study of 58 cases with implications for the primary tumor treatment. Cancer 1984;53:982–992

144. Furlan JC, Bedard Y, Rosen IB. Biologic basis for the treatment of microscopic, occult well-differentiated thyroid cancer. Surgery 2001;130:1050–1054

145. Lupoli G, Vitale G, Caraglia M, et al. Familial papillary thyroid microcarcinoma: a new clinical entity. Lancet 1999;353:637–639

146. Sugg SL, Ezzat S, Rosen IB, Freeman JL, Asa SL. Distinct multiple RET/PTC gene rearrangements in multifocal papillary thyroid neoplasia. J Clin Endocrinol Metab 1998;83:4116–4122

147. Shattuck TM, Westra WH, Ladenson PW, Arnold A. Independent clonal origins of distinct tumor foci in multifocal papillary thyroid carcinoma. N Engl J Med 2005;352:2406–2412

148. Burningham AR, Krishnan J, Davidson BJ, Ringel MD, Burman KD. Papillary and follicular variant of papillary carcinoma of the thyroid: initial presentation and response to therapy. Otolaryngol Head Neck Surg 2005;132:840–844

149. Fadda G, Fiorino MC, Mule A, LiVolsi VA. Macrofollicular encapsulated variant of papillary thyroid carcinoma as a potential pitfall in histologic and cytologic diagnosis. A report of three cases. Acta Cytol 2002;46:555–559

150. LiVolsi VA. Pure versus follicular variant of papillary thyroid carcinoma: clinical features, prognostic factors, treatment, and survival. Cancer 2003;98:1997–1998

151. Baloch ZW, Gupta PK, Yu GH, Sack MJ, LiVolsi VA. Follicular variant of papillary carcinoma—cytologic and histologic correlation. Am J Clin Pathol 1999;111:216–222

152. Zidan J, Karen D, Stein M, Rosenblatt E, Basher W, Kuten A. Pure versus follicular variant of papillary thyroid carcinoma. Cancer 2003;97:1181–1185

153. Moniz S, Catarino AL, Marques AR, Cavaco B, Sobrinho L, Leite V. Clonal origin of non-medullary thyroid tumours assessed by non-random X-chromosome inactivation 7. Eur J Endocrinol 2002;146:27–33

154. Caplan RH, Wester S, Kisken AW. Diffuse sclerosing variant of papillary thyroid carcinoma: case report and review of the literature 3. Endocr Pract 1997;3:287–292

155. Lam AK, Lo CY. Diffuse sclerosing variant of papillary carcinoma of the thyroid: a 35-year comparative study at a single institution 1. Ann Surg Oncol 2006;13:176–181

156. LiVolsi VA. Unusual variants of papillary thyroid carcinoma. In: Mazzaferri EL, Kreisberg RA, Bar RS, eds. Advances in Endocrinology and Metabolism. St. Louis: Mosby-Year Book, 1995:39–54

157. Chow SM, Chan JK, Law SC, et al. Diffuse sclerosing variant of papillary thyroid carcinoma—clinical features and outcome. Eur J Surg Oncol 2003;29:446–449

158. Moreno A, Rodriguez JM, Sola J, Soria T, Parrilla P. Encapsulated papillary neoplasm of the thyroid: Retrospective clinicopathological study with long term follow up. Eur J Surg 1996;162:177–180

159. Schroder S, Bocker W, Dralle H, Kortmann KB, Stern C. The encapsulated papillary carcinoma of the thyroid. A morphologic subtype of the papillary thyroid carcinoma. Cancer 1984;54:90–93

160. Das DK. Age of patients with papillary thyroid carcinoma: is it a key factor in the development of variants? 3. Gerontology 2005;51:149–154

161. Johnson TL, Lloyd RV, Thompson NW, Beierwaltes WH, Sisson JC. Prognostic implications of the tall cell variant of papillary thyroid carcinoma. Am J Surg Pathol 1988;12:22–27

162. Prendiville S, Burman KD, Ringel MD, et al. Tall cell variant: an aggressive form of papillary thyroid carcinoma. Otolaryngol Head Neck Surg 2000;122:352–357

163. Xing M, Westra WH, Tufano RP, et al. BRAF mutation predicts a poorer clinical prognosis for papillary thyroid cancer. J Clin Endocrinol Metab 2005;90:6373–6379

164. Shimizu M, Hirokawa M, Manabe T. Tall cell variant of papillary thyroid carcinoma with foci of columnar cell component. Virchows Arch 1999;434:173–175

165. Jayaram G. Cytology of columnar-cell variant of papillary thyroid carcinoma 9. Diagn Cytopathol 2000;22:227–229

166. Evans HL. Encapsulated columnar-cell neoplasms of the thyroid—a report of four cases suggesting a favorable prognosis. Am J Surg Pathol 1996;20:1205–1211

167. Nikiforov YE, Erickson LA, Nikiforova MN, Caudill CM, Lloyd RV. Solid variant of papillary thyroid carcinoma: incidence, clinical-pathologic characteristics, molecular analysis, and biologic behavior 4. Am J Surg Pathol 2001;25:1478–1484

168. Harness JK, Thompson NW, McLeod MK, Eckhauser FE, Lloyd RV. Follicular carcinoma of the thyroid gland: trends and treatment. Surgery 1984;96:972–980

169. Livolsi VA, Baloch ZW. Follicular neoplasms of the thyroid: view, biases, and experiences. Adv Anat Pathol 2004;11:279–287

170. Muro-Cacho CA, Ku NN. Tumors of the thyroid gland: histologic and cytologic features—parts 1, 2. Cancer Control 2000;7:276–287

171. Weber F, Shen L, Aldred MA, et al. Genetic classification of benign and malignant thyroid follicular neoplasia based on a 3-gene combination. J Clin Endocrinol Metab 2005;90:2512–2521

172. van Heerden JA, Hay ID, Goellner JR, et al. Follicular thyroid carcinoma with capsular invasion alone: A nonthreatening malignancy. Surgery 1992;112:1130–1138

173. Thompson LD, Wieneke JA, Paal E, Frommelt RA, Adair CF, Heffess CS. A clinicopathologic study of minimally invasive follicular carcinoma of the thyroid gland with a review of the English literature 2. Cancer 2001;91:505–524

174. Chao TC, Lin JD, Chen MF. Insular carcinoma: infrequent subtype of thyroid cancer with aggressive clinical course. World J Surg 2004;28:393–396

175. Falvo L, Catania A, D'Andrea V, Grilli P, D'Ercole C, De Antoni E. Prognostic factors of insular versus papillary/follicular thyroid carcinoma. Am Surg 2004;70:461–466

176. Kotiloglu E, Kale G, Senocak ME. Follicular thyroid carcinoma with a predominant insular component in a child: a case report. Tumori 1995;81:296–298

177. Carcangiu ML, Steeper T, Zampi G, Rosai J. Anaplastic thyroid carcinoma. A study of 70 cases. Am J Clin Pathol 1985;83:135–158

178. Jain R, Chaturvedi KU, Khurana N, Aggarwal AK. Insular carcinoma of thyroid—a case report. Indian J Pathol Microbiol 2004;47:420–422

179. Pellegriti G, Giuffrida D, Scollo C, et al. Long-term outcome of patients with insular carcinoma of the thyroid. Cancer 2002;95:2076–2085

180. Lam KY, Lo CY, Chan KW, Wan KY. Insular and anaplastic carcinoma of the thyroid—a 45-year comparative study at a single institution and a review of the significance of p53 and p21. Ann Surg 2000;231:329–338

181. Palestini N, Papotti M, Durando R, Fortunato MA. [Poorly differentiated "insular" carcinoma of the thyroid: long-term survival] Minerva Chir 1993;48:1301–1305

182. Pellegriti G, Giuffrida D, Scollo C, et al. Long-term outcome of patients with insular carcinoma of the thyroid: the insular histotype is an independent predictor of poor prognosis. Cancer 2002;95:2076–2085

183. Herrera MF, Hay ID, Wu PS, et al. Hürthle cell (oxyphilic) papillary thyroid carcinoma: a variant with more aggressive biologic behavior. World J Surg 1992;16:669–674

184. Cheung CC, Ezzat S, Ramyar L, Freeman JL, Asa SL. Molecular basis of Hürthle cell papillary thyroid carcinoma. J Clin Endocrinol Metab 2000;85:878–882

185. Thompson NW, Dunn EL, Batsakis JG, Nishiyama RH. Hürthle cell lesions of the thyroid gland. Surg Gynecol Obstet 1974;139:555–560

186. Sanders LE, Silverman M. Follicular and Hürthle cell carcinoma: predicting outcome and directing therapy. Surgery 1998;124:967–974

187. Hamming JF, Goslings BM, vanSteenis GJ, Claasen H, Hermans J, Velde JH. The value of fine-needle aspiration biopsy in patients with nodular thyroid disease divided into groups of suspicion of malignant neoplasms on clinical grounds. Arch Intern Med 1990;150:113–116

188. Hegedus L. Clinical practice. The thyroid nodule. N Engl J Med 2004;351:1764–1771

189. Mazzaferri EL. Managing small thyroid cancers. JAMA 2006;295:2179–2182

190. Ezzat S, Sarti DA, Cain DR, Braunstein GD. Thyroid incidentalomas. Prevalence by palpation and ultrasonography. Arch Intern Med 1994;154:1838–1840

191. Liebeskind A, Sikora AG, Komisar A, Slavit D, Fried K. Rates of malignancy in incidentally discovered thyroid nodules evaluated with sonography and fine-needle aspiration. J Ultrasound Med 2005;24:629–634

192. Kang HW, No JH, Chung JH, et al. Prevalence, clinical and ultrasonographic characteristics of thyroid incidentalomas. Thyroid 2004;14:29–33

193. Nam-Goong IS, Kim HY, Gong G, et al. Ultrasonography-guided fine-needle aspiration of thyroid incidentaloma: correlation with pathological findings. Clin Endocrinol (Oxf) 2004;60:21–28

194. Cohen MS, Arslan N, Dehdashti F, et al. Risk of malignancy in thyroid incidentalomas identified by fluorodeoxyglucose-positron emission tomography. Surgery 2001;130:941–946

195. Kim TY, Kim WB, Ryu JS, Gong G, Hong SJ, Shong YK. 18F-fluorodeoxyglucose uptake in thyroid from positron emission tomogram (PET) for evaluation in cancer patients: high prevalence of malignancy in thyroid PET incidentaloma. Laryngoscope 2005;115:1074–1078

196. Kim EK, Park CS, Chung WY, et al. New sonographic criteria for recommending fine-needle aspiration biopsy of nonpalpable solid nodules of the thyroid. AJR Am J Roentgenol 2002;178:687–691

197. Kang HW, No JH, Chung JH, et al. Prevalence, clinical and ultrasonographic characteristics of thyroid incidentalomas. Thyroid 2004;14:29–33

198. Nam-Goong IS, Kim HY, Gong G, et al. Ultrasonography-guided fine-needle aspiration of thyroid incidentaloma: correlation with pathological findings. Clin Endocrinol (Oxf) 2004;60:21–28

199. Mazzaferri EL. Management of a solitary thyroid nodule. N Engl J Med 1993;328:553–559

200. Hundahl SA, Cady B, Cunningham MP, et al. Initial results from a prospective cohort study of 5583 cases of thyroid carcinoma treated in the United States during 1996. U.S. and German Thyroid Cancer Study Group. An American College of Surgeons Commission on Cancer Patient Care Evaluation study. Cancer 2000;89:202–217

201. Cooper DS, Doherty GM, Haugen BR, et al. Management guidelines for patients with thyroid nodules and differentiated thyroid cancer. Thyroid 2006;16:109–142

202. Belfiore A, La Rosa GL, LaPorta GA, et al. Cancer risk in patients with cold thyroid nodules: Relevance of iodine intake, sex, age and multinodularity. Am J Med 1992;93:363–369

203. Yang GC, Liebeskind D, Messina AV. Should cytopathologists stop reporting follicular neoplasms on fine-needle aspiration of the thyroid? Cancer 2003;99:69–74

204. Baloch ZW, LiVolsi VA. Fine-needle aspiration of thyroid nodules: past, present, and future. Endocr Pract 2004;10:234–241

205. Ceresini G, Corcione L, Morganti S, et al. Ultrasound-guided fine-needle capillary biopsy of thyroid nodules, coupled with on-site cytologic review, improves results. Thyroid 2004;14:385–389

206. Yang GC, Liebeskind D, Messina AV. Ultrasound-guided fine-needle aspiration of the thyroid assessed by Ultrafast Papanicolaou stain: data from 1135 biopsies with a two- to six-year follow-up. Thyroid 2001;11:581–589

207. Papini E, Guglielmi R, Bianchini A, et al. Risk of malignancy in nonpalpable thyroid nodules: predictive value of ultrasound and color-Doppler features. J Clin Endocrinol Metab 2002;87:1941–1946

208. Gorges R, Eising EG, Fotescu D, et al. Diagnostic value of high-resolution B-mode and power-mode sonography in the follow-up of thyroid cancer. Eur J Ultrasound 2003;16:191–206

209. Cooper DS, Doherty GM, Haugen BR, et al. Management guidelines for patients with thyroid nodules and differentiated thyroid cancer. Thyroid 2006;16:109–142

210. Alexander EK, Hurwitz S, Heering JP, et al. Natural history of benign solid and cystic thyroid nodules. Ann Intern Med 2003;138:315–318

211. Cooper DS, Doherty GM, Haugen BR, et al. Management guidelines for patients with thyroid nodules and differentiated thyroid cancer. Thyroid 2006;16:109–142

212. Xing M, Westra WH, Tufano RP, et al. BRAF mutation predicts a poorer clinical prognosis for papillary thyroid cancer. J Clin Endocrinol Metab 2005;90:6373–6379

213. Cooper DS, Doherty GM, Haugen BR, et al. Management guidelines for patients with thyroid nodules and differentiated thyroid cancer. Thyroid 2006;16:109–142

214. Elisei R, Bottici V, Luchetti F, et al. Impact of routine measurement of serum calcitonin on the diagnosis and outcome of medullary thyroid cancer: experience in 10,864 patients with nodular thyroid disorders. J Clin Endocrinol Metab 2004;89:163–168

215. Bonnema SJ, Bennedbaek FN, Ladenson PW, Hegedus L. Management of the nontoxic multinodular goiter: a North American survey. J Clin Endocrinol Metab 2002;87:112–117

216. Yeh MW, Demircan O, Ituarte P, Clark OH. False-negative fine-needle aspiration cytology results delay treatment and adversely affect outcome in patients with thyroid carcinoma. Thyroid 2004;14:207–215

217. Cooper DS, Doherty GM, Haugen BR, et al. Management guidelines for patients with thyroid nodules and differentiated thyroid cancer. Thyroid 2006;16:109–142

218. Mazzaferri EL. NCCN thyroid carcinoma practice guidelines. Oncology 1999;13(suppl 11A); NCCN Proceedings http://www.nccn.org/physician'gls/f guidelines.html:391–442

219. Scheumann GFW, Gimm O, Wegener G, Hundeshagen H, Dralle H. Prognostic significance and surgical management of locoregional lymph node metastases in papillary thyroid cancer. World J Surg 1994;18:559–568

220. Noguchi S, Murakami N, Yamashita H, Toda M, Kawamoto H. Papillary thyroid carcinoma—modified radical neck dissection improves prognosis. Arch Surg 1998;133:276–280

221. Vassilopoulou-Sellin R, Goepfert H, Raney B, Schultz PN. Differentiated thyroid cancer in children and adolescents: clinical outcome and mortality after long-term follow-up. Head Neck 1998;20:549–555

222. Maxon HR, Thomas SR, Hertzberg VS, et al. Relation between effective radiation dose and outcome of radioiodine therapy for thyroid cancer. N Engl J Med 1983;309:937–941

223. Pacini F, Ladenson PW, Schlumberger M, et al. Radioiodine ablation of thyroid remnants after preparation with recombinant human thyrotropin in differentiated thyroid carcinoma: results of an international, randomized, controlled study. J Clin Endocrinol Metab 2006;91:926–932

224. DeGroot LJ, Kaplan EL, McCormick M, Straus FH. Natural history, treatment, and course of papillary thyroid carcinoma. J Clin Endocrinol Metab 1990;71:414–424

225. Samaan NA, Schultz PN, Hickey RC, Haynie TP, Johnston DA, Ordonez NG. Well-differentiated thyroid carcinoma and the results of various modalities of treatment. A retrospective review of 1599 patients. J Clin Endocrinol Metab 1992;75:714–720

226. Verburg FA, de Keizer B, Lips CJ, Zelissen PM, de Klerk JM. Prognostic significance of successful ablation with radioiodine of differentiated thyroid cancer patients. Eur J Endocrinol 2005;152:33–37

227. Bal C, Padhy AK, Jana S, Pant GS, Basu AK. Prospective randomized clinical trial to evaluate the optimal dose of remnant ablation in patients with differentiated thyroid carcinoma. Cancer 1996;77:2574–2580

228. Bal CS, Kumar A, Pant GS. Radioiodine dose for remnant ablation in differentiated thyroid carcinoma: a randomized clinical trial in 509 patients. J Clin Endocrinol Metab 2004;89:1666–1673

229. Schroeder PR, Haugen BR, Pacini F, et al. A comparison of short-term changes in health-related quality of life in thyroid carcinoma patients undergoing diagnostic evaluation with recombinant human thyrotropin compared with thyroid hormone withdrawal. J Clin Endocrinol Metab 2006;91:878–884

230. Cooper DS, Specker B, Ho M, et al. Thyrotropin suppression and disease progression in patients with differentiated thyroid cancer: results from the National Thyroid Cancer Treatment Cooperative Registry. Thyroid 1998;8:737–744

231. McGriff NJ, Csako G, Gourgiotis L, Lori CG, Pucino F, Sarlis NJ. Effects of thyroid hormone suppression therapy on adverse clinical outcomes in thyroid cancer. Ann Med 2002;34:554–564

232. Pujol P, Daures JP, Nsakala N, Baldet L, Bringer J, Jaffiol C. Degree of thyrotropin suppression as a prognostic determinant in differentiated thyroid cancer. J Clin Endocrinol Metab 1996;81:4318–4323

233. Rubino C, Adjadj E, Guerin S, et al. Long-term risk of second malignant neoplasms after neuroblastoma in childhood: role of treatment. Int J Cancer 2003;107:791–796

234. Bal CS, Kumar A, Chandra P, Dwivedi SN, Mukhopadhyaya S. Is chest x-ray or high-resolution computed tomography scan of the chest sufficient investigation to detect pulmonary metastasis in pediatric differentiated thyroid cancer? Thyroid 2004;14:217–225

235. Meadows KM, Amdur RJ, Morris CG, Villaret DB, Mazzaferri EL, Mendenhall WM. External beam radiotherapy for differentiated thyroid cancer. Am J Otolaryngol 2006;27:24–28

236. Torlontano M, Crocetti U, D'Aloiso L, et al. Serum thyroglobulin and 131I whole body scan after recombinant human TSH stimulation in the follow-up of low-risk patients with differentiated thyroid cancer. Eur J Endocrinol 2003;148:19–24

237. Salvatori M, Perotti G, Rufini V, Maussier ML, Dottorini M. Are there disadvantages in administering 131I ablation therapy in patients with differentiated thyroid carcinoma without a preablative diagnostic 131I whole-body scan? Clin Endocrinol (Oxf) 2004;61:704–710

238. Eustatia-Rutten CF, Smit JW, Romijn JA, et al. Diagnostic value of serum thyroglobulin measurements in the follow-up of differentiated thyroid carcinoma, a structured meta-analysis. Clin Endocrinol (Oxf) 2004;61:61–74

239. Spencer CA, Bergoglio LM, Kazarosyan M, Fatemi S, LoPresti JS. Clinical impact of thyroglobulin (Tg) and Tg autoantibody method differences on the management of patients with differentiated thyroid carcinomas. J Clin Endocrinol Metab 2005;90:5566–5575

240. Cooper DS, Doherty GM, Haugen BR, et al. Management Guidelines for patients with thyroid nodules and differentiated thyroid cancer. Thyroid 2006;16:109–142

241. Hollowell JG, Staehling NW, Flanders WD, et al. Serum TSH, T, and thyroid antibodies in the United States population (1988 to 1994): National Health and Nutrition Examination Survey (NHANES III). J Clin Endocrinol Metab 2002;87:489–499

242. Spencer CA, LoPresti JS, Fatemi S, Nicoloff JT. Detection of residual and recurrent differentiated thyroid carcinoma by serum thyroglobulin measurement. Thyroid 1999;9:435–441

243. Chiovato L, Latrofa F, Braverman LE, et al. Disappearance of humoral thyroid autoimmunity after complete removal of thyroid antigens. Ann Intern Med 2003;139(5 pt 1):346–351

244. Spencer CA, Takeuchi M, Kazarosyan M, et al. Serum thyroglobulin autoantibodies: prevalence, influence on serum thyroglobulin measurement, and prognostic significance in patients with differentiated thyroid carcinoma. J Clin Endocrinol Metab 1998;83:1121–1127

245. Preissner CM, O'Kane DJ, Singh RJ, Morris JC, Grebe SK. Phantoms in the assay tube: heterophile antibody interferences in serum

thyroglobulin assays. J Clin Endocrinol Metab 2003;88:3069–3074

246. Mazzaferri EL, Kloos RT. Is diagnostic iodine-131 scanning with recombinant human TSH (rhTSH) useful in the follow-up of differentiated thyroid cancer after thyroid ablation? J Clin Endocrinol Metab 2002;87:1490–1498

247. Lassmann M, Luster M, Hanscheid H, Reiners C. Impact of (131)I diagnostic activities on the biokinetics of thyroid remnants. J Nucl Med 2004;45:619–625

248. Morris LF, Waxman AD, Braunstein GD. Thyroid stunning. Thyroid 2003;13:333–340

249. Palmedo H, Bucerius J, Joe A, et al. Integrated PET/CT in differentiated thyroid cancer: diagnostic accuracy and impact on patient management. J Nucl Med 2006;47:616–624

250. Nahas Z, Goldenberg D, Fakhry C, et al. The role of positron emission tomography/computed tomography in the management of recurrent papillary thyroid carcinoma. Laryngoscope 2005;115:237–243

11 Management of Medullary and Anaplastic Thyroid Cancer

Lisa A. Orloff and David W. Eisele

Medullary Thyroid Cancer

Epidemiology

Medullary thyroid cancer (MTC) is an entity distinct from well-differentiated follicular cell–derived thyroid cancers. The existence of this distinct thyroid neoplasm was first described by Hazard, Hawk and Crile[1] in 1959, but the characterization of the cell of origin, the parafollicular C cell, and its hormone product calcitonin, only unfolded over the following decade.[2] Subsequent recognition of the occasional association of MTC with other endocrine neoplasms led to the definition of the multiple endocrine neoplasia (MEN) syndromes.[3] All MTCs secrete calcitonin, and the ability to measure and detect elevated serum calcitonin levels was the first revolution in the early diagnosis of, and surveillance for, MTC. The availability of genetic testing for *ret* proto-oncogene mutations over the past 10 years has further enhanced the screening for MTC, and thus its treatment and outcomes.

Medullary thyroid cancer makes up approximately 10% of all thyroid cancers, of which approximately 75% are sporadic (nonfamilial) and 25% are familial and associated with identifiable genetic mutations,[4] as further discussed below.

Medullary thyroid cancer is derived from the thyroid C cell, which is of neural crest origin and which produces the hormone calcitonin. Embryologically, the C cells originate in the ultimobranchial body and the fourth branchial pouch, and migrate to the upper two thirds of each thyroid lobe. C cells account for only approximately 0.1% of the normal thyroid mass, and their presence and action seem to be dispensable. Following total thyroidectomy, there appears to be no appreciable functional deficit relating to the absence of calcitonin. Calcitonin is a polypeptide hormone whose effect is to decrease serum calcium, but in humans, calcium homeostasis is controlled mainly by parathyroid hormone (PTH).[5] C-cell hyperplasia is associated with MTC, particularly familial MTC, and tumors in familial MTC are typically bilateral and multifocal.[6-8]

Medullary thyroid cancer is usually a slow-growing malignancy with an indolent clinical course. However, regional lymph node metastases are frequently present at the time of diagnosis, necessitating a fairly aggressive initial surgical treatment regimen. The central neck nodes (levels VI and VII) are the nodal basins that are most often involved, followed by nodes in the ipsilateral neck, and then the contralateral neck, levels II to V. Hematogenous spread to liver, lungs, and bone occurs variably, and may be difficult to detect on imaging studies due to a fine miliary pattern. Persistent or recurrent hypercalcitoninemia following initial surgery motivates the search for local, regional, and distant metastases.

Most patients with sporadic MTC present with a palpable thyroid nodule, and up to 75% of these patients harbor cervical lymph node metastases. Only 15% of patients have evidence of distant metastases at presentation. Local symptoms, which are present in only approximately 15% of patients, include dysphagia, dyspnea, and hoarseness.

Fine-needle aspiration (FNA) is typically diagnostic for MTC, particularly if calcitonin immunohistochemical staining is performed (**Fig. 11.1**). Cytologically, MTC cells are uniform polygonal cells with finely granular eosinophilic cytoplasm and central nuclei. A distinctive but not ubiquitous feature of MTC is the presence of amyloid, consisting of calcitonin and procalcitonin molecules. In addition to

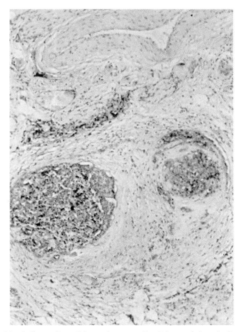

Fig. 11.1 Medullary thyroid carcinoma. Positive calcitonin immunohistochemical staining on histologic section.

immunohistochemical positivity for calcitonin, most MTC cells stain positive for carcinoembryonic antigen (CEA) and negative for thyroglobulin.

In addition to the cytologic diagnosis, basal and stimulated serum calcitonin levels are important diagnostic and prognostic markers. The normal range for calcitonin is generally below 10 pg/mL. Basal levels >10 pg/mL are typically seen in sporadic MTC. Stimulated levels, measured before and at 1, 2, 3, 5, and 10 minutes after injection of calcium gluconate, pentagastrin, or a combination of both, are diagnostic for MTC if they increase to more than 100 pg/mL, even in the absence of a detectable thyroid mass. Stimulated calcitonin measurements are most useful in the screening and diagnosis of family members with familial forms of MTC. Preoperative calcitonin levels correlate with tumor size and have prognostic significance. Calcitonin levels greater than 10,000 pg/mL are associated with a poor prognosis and a remote likelihood of biochemical cure. Serum CEA levels are also useful in the evaluation and surveillance of MTC, with high levels being associated with aggressive disease and indicative of disease progression.[9,10]

Medullary thyroid cancer does not concentrate iodine, and it appears as a cold nodule on thyroid scintigraphy. Computed tomography (CT) scanning may reveal characteristic calcifications within a thyroid mass or masses, as well as extrathyroidal disease (**Fig. 11.2**). Limited success has been reported with other nuclear scans, including iodine-131 (I-131)-metaiodobenzylguanidine (MIBG scan), radiolabeled anti-CEA antibody, anticalcitonin antibody, or somatostatin receptor scintigraphy for the detection of metastatic disease. The most sensitive nonsurgical method for localizing occult metastases is regional venous sampling with pentagastrin stimulation of calcitonin release. The most sensitive

method for the detection of liver metastases is diagnostic laparoscopy with liver inspection for characteristic lesions that may be missed on imaging studies.

Familial cases of MTC occur as part of the MEN syndromes. These include MEN-2A (MTC, pheochromocytoma, and hyperparathyroidism); MEN-2B (MTC, pheochromocytoma, mucosal ganglioneuromatosis, and Marfanoid habitus); and familial medullary thyroid carcinoma (FMTC), which is characterized by MTC alone. These syndromes all show an autosomal dominant inheritance pattern, related to mutations in the *ret* proto-oncogene located on chromosome 10 (region 10q11.12). MEN-2A is caused by mutations at extracellular cysteine residues, MEN-2B is usually associated with a methionine to threonine mutation at codon 918 in the tyrosine kinase catalytic domain, and FMTC carries the same mutations as MEN-2A plus less common mutations in the intracellular portion of the protein.[4]

Due to the significant likelihood of a familial basis, as well as the existence of effective early surgical therapy, all patients diagnosed with MTC should undergo genetic screening for germline *ret* mutations. The 2001 MEN consensus guidelines recommended that analysis for the classic MEN-2A mutations in *ret* exons 10 and 11 be followed with direct sequencing of exons 13, 14, 15, and 16, where other clinically significant *ret* mutations can be located.[11] In addition, the diagnosis of pheochromocytoma should be ruled out in all cases of MTC prior to surgery, either with a negative genetic screen or by measuring plasma metanephrines or urine catecholamines.

The aggressiveness and clinical course of MTC varies widely across familial syndromes. In general, MTC as part of the MEN-2B syndrome is the most aggressive, with invasive carcinoma often present before the age of 1 year, and

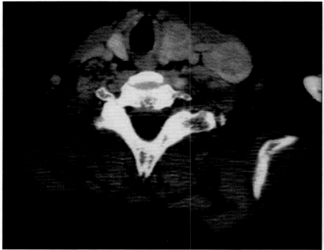
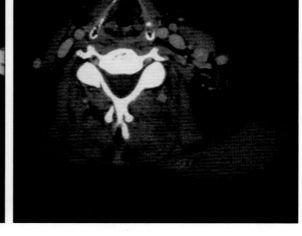

A   B

Fig. 11.2 (**A**) Medullary thyroid carcinoma, axial computed tomography (CT) scan at level of thyroid, demonstrating primary tumor in left thyroid lobe and metastatic disease in level IV cervical nodes. (**B**) CT scan of same patient showing additional metastatic disease in level III cervical nodes.

lymph node metastases by the age of 2 years.[12,13] The next most aggressive is MTC as part of the MEN-2A syndrome or codon 611, 618, 620, or 634 mutations, with invasive carcinoma usually occurring by the age of 2 years and lymph node metastases by the age of 5 years.[14,15] The least aggressive form of MTC is FMTC or codon 609, 768, 790, 791, 804, or 891 mutations, where the carcinoma is usually identifiable in the patient's second or third decade of life.

Because of the variability in the observed aggressiveness of MTC, the timing of treatment is also variable. Early prophylactic thyroidectomy can be curative or preventative in almost all MEN-2 patients, so genetic testing for all at-risk members of known kindreds should be performed soon after birth. Furthermore, all at-risk family members of new index patients should undergo genetic testing. Patients with MEN-2 *ret* mutations should undergo meticulous surgical removal of all thyroid tissue, because MTC in the setting of MEN-2 variants is almost always multifocal and bilateral, and all remaining C cells are at risk for developing future malignancy. Early thyroidectomy has been shown to improve outcomes in patients with MEN-2 syndromes,[16,17] and treatment failures can be attributed to operations performed after biochemical evidence (hypercalcitoninemia) of MTC. Prior to the availability of genetic testing, provocative calcitonin screening (using calcium and pentagastrin stimulation) of at risk family members[16,18] was the standard. With the arrival of *ret* mutation testing, earlier, more effective, and well-tolerated intervention can be offered in the form of total thyroidectomy, even in infancy, prior to the spread of disease; *ret* mutations are stratified according to risk of early and aggressive MTC, and recommendations for the timing of surgery are guided by these risk groups.

The highest risk of early and aggressive MTC is level 3, which includes the MEN-2B mutations in codons 883, 918, and 922. Thyroidectomy and central neck dissection are recommended within the first 6 months of life, and preferably within the first month. Mutations classified as level 2 include those at codons 634, 620, 618, and 611, and thyroidectomy with or without central node dissection is recommended before the age of 5 years. The lowest risk for aggressive MTC, level 1, includes *ret* mutations at codons 609, 768, 790, 791, 804, and 891. The recommendations for this group are less clear, with some experts favoring thyroidectomy at 5 years, others at 10 years, and still others on the basis of stimulated calcitonin levels.

Several additional *ret* mutations have been associated with FMTC, including a R912P mutation,[19] codon 630,[20] and a 9-base-pair duplication in exon 8.[21] Although there is limited clinical information regarding these mutations, they are thought to carry a lower risk than level 1 mutations.

Treatment

The treatment of MTC is surgical because these tumors do not take up radioactive iodine and are not radiosensitive or chemosensitive. The surgical strategy for this malignancy is influenced by several factors: (1) the clinical course of MTC is typically more aggressive than that of well-differentiated thyroid cancer (WDTC), with higher recurrence and mortality rates, especially in young patients; (2) MTC is multicentric in 90% of hereditary cases and 20% of sporadic cases; (3) nodal metastases are present in more than 70% of patients with palpable primary tumors; and (4) the ability to measure calcitonin levels postoperatively provides feedback on the adequacy of surgical resection.

For preventive surgery of hereditary MTC, total thyroidectomy is the minimal operation that should be performed. For individuals with mutations in risk levels 2 or 3, the risk of future recurrence and the need for subsequent reoperation is lowest when total thyroidectomy and central node dissection are performed as the initial surgical approach.

For patients with palpable or sporadic MTC, total thyroidectomy and a central neck dissection are the minimum recommended components of surgery (**Fig. 11.3**). However, given evidence that metastases are present in 80% of central nodes, 75% of ipsilateral jugular nodes (levels II, III, and IV), and in 47% of contralateral jugular nodes[22] in patients with palpable MTC, a lateral selective neck dissection is also appropriate. The incidence of nodal metastases correlates with the size of the primary lesion; only 11% of patients with primary tumors smaller than 1 cm have positive nodes, compared with 60% of patients with tumors larger than 2 cm.[23] A thorough selective neck dissection with removal of all nodal tissue confers improved recurrence and survival rates compared with node "plucking,"[24] especially because intraoperative assessment of nodes has been found to have only a 64% sensitivity and 71% specificity.[22] Given the fact that there is no effective adjuvant therapy for MTC, completeness of surgical resection of disease is of paramount importance. Thus

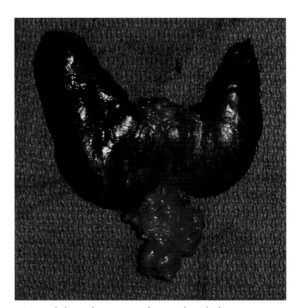

Fig. 11.3 Total thyroidectomy and central neck dissection specimen, medullary carcinoma.

total thyroidectomy, central node dissection, and unilateral or bilateral selective neck dissection (levels II to V) based on preoperative assessment are appropriate.

The strategy for managing the parathyroid glands in the surgical treatment of MTC is somewhat controversial. Parathyroid gland identification and preservation in situ with an intact blood supply is a more traditional approach. However, many experts believe that a more complete thyroidectomy and central neck dissection, extending from the level of the hyoid bone superiorly to the innominate vessels inferiorly, can be achieved only when complete parathyroidectomy with autotransplantation is performed.[25] Parathyroid autotransplantation into the ipsilateral sternocleidomastoid muscle is generally accepted, except in cases of MEN-2A, where subsequent hyperparathyroidism may arise. In these patients, transplantation to the nondominant forearm is preferred so that parathyroidectomy can be facilitated should future or recurrent hyperparathyroidism occur.[4]

Postoperative surveillance of MTC involves serial serum calcitonin measurements. The initial postoperative calcitonin level is a gross indicator of degree of success in eradicating the tumor, and the term *biochemical cure* refers to MTC patients with normal or undetectable serum calcitonin levels.

Unlike the biochemical cure achieved in most patients with hereditary MTC associated with MEN-2A and FMTC, in whom the diagnosis is made and treatment rendered based on genetic screening or detection of hypercalcitoninemia, more than 50% of patients with sporadic MTC or in whom the diagnosis is made when palpable tumor is present harbor persistent disease and elevated serum calcitonin levels after surgery.[6,26] Nevertheless, the clinical course in these patients is typically indolent, and patients with elevated serum calcitonin levels may remain otherwise asymptomatic for years.[27]

If a neck mass is detected by physical examination or by imaging such as ultrasound or CT scanning, then a formalized neck dissection should be performed if not done previously. Distant metastatic disease should also be ruled out by CT or MRI scanning of the chest and abdomen, as well as by diagnostic laparoscopy, which can detect fine liver metastases that may be missed with imaging studies.[28] Even in the setting of previous neck dissection, reoperation and "microdissection" of the neck for recurrent MTC can result in a significant reduction or normalization of calcitonin levels.[29–33] Whereas patients with highly invasive primary tumors are not as likely to benefit from reoperation, a majority of patients with recurrence in the neck may derive long-term survival benefit and avoidance of complications of disease through reoperation in the neck.

For patients with recurrent or metastatic disease who are not surgical candidates, the options of chemotherapy and radiation therapy exist but have not been extensively studied, due to lack of encouraging results. Traditional agents such as doxorubicin, cisplatin, vindesine, dacarbazine, 5- fluorouracil, and streptozocin, used alone or in combination, have produced rare partial responses.[34–37] Anecdotal use of interferon-α has also yielded partial responses in some patients.[38]

Targeted therapies hold promise, and clinical trials using anticarcinoembryonic antigen monoclonal antibody (MAb) combined with autologous hematopoietic stem cell rescue (AHSCR)[39] and immunotherapy with calcitonin-pulsed dendritic cells[40] have shown favorable preliminary results. Somatostatin analogues, although not showing therapeutic effectiveness, have been found to provide symptomatic relief of diarrhea and flushing associated with hypercalcitoninemia.[41,42] In vitro studies using tyrosine kinase inhibitors have been very encouraging,[43,44] and clinical trials are underway to test this targeted form of therapy.

Adjuvant radiation therapy has not been convincingly shown to provide significant benefit in controlling neck disease,[45,46] but it does appear to have palliative benefit in controlling painful bony metastases.[4] The toxicity, the lack of evidence of a calcitonin response, and the added difficulty of any future surgery have deterred the routine use of adjuvant radiation therapy for MTC.

Outcomes

Survival rates from MTC have increased dramatically over the past 20 years, mainly due to early intervention in familial cases detected by genetic screening. Whereas survival rates at 5 and 10 years were only 48% and 12%, respectively, in the 1970s, more recent series report survival rates as high as 90% and 80%, respectively.[23] MTC in MEN-2A and FMTC have a more favorable prognosis, whereas the more aggressive MTC in MEN-2B and sporadic MTC carry a less favorable prognosis.

Favorable prognostic factors, in addition to the genetic mutations mentioned above, include a smaller primary tumor size, young age, female gender, and tumor confined to the thyroid gland. Multivariate analysis of nearly 900 patients with MTC diagnosed between 1952 and 1996 revealed that age and stage were independent predictors of survival.[14]

Nondetectable postoperative calcitonin levels are associated with a 98% survival rate at 10 years, whereas even patients with persistent hypercalcitoninemia have survival rates of 80% and 70% at 5 and 10 years, respectively.

Anaplastic Thyroid Cancer

Unlike its well-differentiated counterparts, anaplastic thyroid cancer (ATC) is one of the most lethal of all human malignancies.[47–50] The median survival from the time of diagnosis of ATC is 4 to 12 months.[47,48,51–61] Death typically occurs due to airway obstruction by tumor, despite tracheotomy. Local progression is rapid, and cervical lymph node as well as distant metastases are present in more than 50% of patients at the time of diagnosis.[47,58] ATC is classified as stage IV thyroid cancer by the American Joint Committee on Cancer (AJCC) regardless of tumor size or detection of metastases.[62] ATC accounts for less than 2% of all thyroid cancers, but more than half of the annual deaths from thyroid cancer in the United States.[63] Only since the 1980s have immunohistochemical techniques been available that enable differentiation of ATC from other aggressive thyroid malignancies such as MTC and lymphoma.[54,64] More recently still, multicenter trials have evaluated single modality (chemotherapy) and combination therapies (including radiation therapy) in the treatment and palliation of ATC.

Epidemiology

No specific causative agent essential for anaplastic tumor development has been identified. It has generally become accepted that the development of ATC is part of the natural history of untreated WDTC.[65] Nevertheless, the etiology of anaplastic "transformation" of thyroid tumors remains unclear. There is clinical evidence to suggest that radiation exposure may play a causative role, and that the radiation effect is partially exerted through hypofunction of the thyroid gland, leading to increased TSH stimulation.[66,67] However, contrary evidence has demonstrated that growth of ATC is independent of TSH function.[68] Furthermore, only a small percentage of patients with ATC have a history of radiation exposure.[47–50,55] What is even less clear is whether the coexistence of WDTC has a favorable or a harmful influence on the development of ATC.

Despite an increase in the incidence of WDTC in recent years, the incidence of ATC has been declining. The predominant reason is likely the aggressive resection of WDTC and, therefore, the elimination of the risk of dedifferentiation of WDTC into ATC.[48,69] An additional factor in the decline of ATC may be the increase in worldwide iodine prophylaxis, as ATC is twice as common in areas with endemic goiter.[48,54,70,71] The reported rates of WDTC found in association with ATC range from 23 to 90%.[47–50,57,61,72,73] It has been said that foci of WDTC are found in every specimen of ATC if the search is sufficiently thorough.[74] Inability to find evidence of WDTC within ATC may be attributed to inadequate tissue sectioning or to the invasion of ATC with obscuration of any remaining WDTC cells.[49]

The cell of origin for ATC does appear to be the thyroid follicular cell, whether via WDTC or not.[75] Ultrastructural studies confirm epithelial differentiation,[76] and molecular and genetic techniques suggest that the loss or mutation of the tumor suppressor gene *p53* can be responsible for the transformation of WDTC cells to ATC.[77,78] Furthermore, restoration of *p53* expression in in vitro ATC cell lines has been shown to be associated with reversal of some aspects of the anaplastic transformation, including restoration of chemosensitivity and radiosensitivity, inhibition of cellular proliferation, restoration of response to TSH, and reexpression of thyroid peroxidase.[79–82]

On the other hand, it appears that thyroid tumors with *ret/ptc* oncogene activation tend not to undergo progression to ATC.[83] Genes that do appear to play a role in anaplastic transformation and are under investigation include *cyclin D1*,[84] *β-catenin*,[85] *met*,[86] c-*myc*,[87] *bcl-2*,[88] *Nm23*,[89] and *ras*.[90] The DNA content of thyroid tumors can also be of prognostic significance, and tumors containing both WDTC and ATC components can exhibit an aneuploid DNA content.[91] However, in some studies ATCs were aneuploid whereas their coexisting WDTC components were diploid.[92] These varied findings suggest that ATC may arise via anaplastic transformation of a preexisting WDTC, but may also arise from de novo genetic alterations.

Anaplastic thyroid cancer occurs in older individuals, often with a long-standing history of a thyroid mass or presumed goiter; 90% of patients are older than 50 years at the time of diagnosis,[58] and the peak incidence is in the sixth to seventh decade of life.[47,48,54,63,70,93] Women outnumber men by up to 3:1 or more.[47–49,58,93] A rapidly enlarging mass is the most common presenting symptom in 97% of patients.[63] Typically, the mass is firm and fixed. Symptoms related to mechanical compression, including dysphagia, dyspnea, stridor, hoarseness, and neck pain are also common. Pain and rapid growth may in part be attributed to hemorrhage into the mass, but tumor doubling alone can lead to increased volume that is apparent over a period of days. Direct invasion of local structures including muscle, trachea, esophagus, laryngeal nerves, and larynx occur in up to 70% of patients,[94] and direct extension through the skin is not uncommon. Approximately 50% of patients have evidence of distant metastatic disease at the time of presentation, and 70% develop distant metastases at some point,[63] most commonly to lung, bone, or brain.[47,54,63,95]

The important prognostic factors that help predict survival and response to treatment remain unclear. Patient age, gender, tumor size, tumor extent, leukocytosis, local symptoms, coexisting goiter or WDTC, surgical resection, and multimodality therapy have all been reported to influence survival.[47,52,54,57,63,72] However, a more recent review of the National Cancer Institute's Surveillance, Epidemiology, and End Results (SEER) database for ATC has identified only patient age at diagnosis (less than 60 years) and the presence of intrathyroidal ATC as independent predictors of lower cause-specific mortality.[96]

The microscopic pathology of ATC can be varied. Three main varieties include spindle cell, giant cell, and squamoid, but the patterns may be mixed, and the prognosis is similar for all patterns. Four additional rare variants of ATC include insular carcinoma, pure squamous cell carcinoma, carcinosarcoma, and paucicellular ATC. Insular carcinoma was only fully characterized in 1984,[49] and is considered a dedifferentiated form of WDTC that is intermediate in the anaplastic transformation process.[51,77,97–99] The important distinction is between ATC and lymphoma or poorly differentiated medullary carcinoma, whose treatment and prognosis are quite different, and whose detection is facilitated by immunohistochemical staining. For example, staining for calcitonin, neuron-specific enolase, and chromagranin

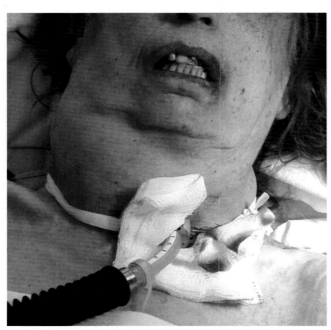

Fig. 11.4 Anaplastic thyroid carcinoma (ATC). Large fixed neck mass, airway obstruction, palliative tracheotomy. (Courtesy of El-Sayed, MD, and J. Biller, MD.)

favors MTC, whereas positive staining for vimentin, keratin, desmin, and α_1-chymotrypsin and negative staining for thyroglobulin favors ATC.[47,49,100–104] The diagnosis of ATC can be made by fine-needle aspiration (FNA) with 90% accuracy.[69,70,105]

Treatment

The treatment of patients with ATC is not standardized. For patients with inoperable or metastatic disease at presentation, treatment is generally palliative, and surgery may be limited to tracheotomy for impending airway obstruction (**Fig. 11.4**). Even tracheotomy in this setting can be technically difficult or even impossible, and is associated with significant morbidity and a high incidence of postoperative healing problems.[106]

Surgery

The role of surgical resection for ATC is limited, and is reserved for patients with localized primary tumors and no evidence of metastatic disease. In this small minority of patients, the aim of surgery is complete macroscopic resection.[107] Complete resection with clear margins has been shown in some but not all studies to confer a survival benefit compared with leaving residual disease postoperatively.[52,57,108] To have a meaningful impact, surgery is followed by adjuvant treatment consisting of concurrent chemotherapy and radiotherapy (RT),[108,109] although in some instances initial treatment with RT and chemotherapy may enhance operability.[53,110]

Radiation Therapy

Because most patients with ATC ultimately die from uncontrolled locoregional disease, therapy directed at prolonging locoregional control can improve short-term survival as well as quality of life.[111] RT is therefore used directly for palliation as well as for preoperative or postoperative adjuvant therapy. The timing, the dose administered, and the pattern of delivery of RT are all important considerations. Current protocols utilize doses between 30 and 60 Gy. Several studies have shown that doses of 46 Gy achieve greater success compared with doses below 30 Gy.[55,57,110] Hyperfractionation can improve control of the rapid doubling volumes of ATC,[52,56,110] permitting higher doses over a shorter time with less toxicity. Complications of RT including pharyngoesophagitis, tracheitis, skin changes, and myelopathy (especially when daily doses exceed 3 Gy).

Chemotherapy

Anaplastic thyroid cancer should be regarded as a systemic disease, and therefore chemotherapy is an important component of any treatment regimen, even though responses to chemotherapy have been limited. Chemotherapy may have its most valuable impact in promoting radiosensitivity to enhance local control. Nevertheless, chemotherapy for ATC has evolved from monotherapy with doxorubicin[112] to combination therapy that adds bleomycin, cyclophosphamide, 5-fluorouracil, cisplatin, mitoxantrone, or paclitaxel.[113–116] In vitro studies have shown that ATC cell lines express increased multidrug resistance-associated protein (MRP),[117,118] which expels chemotherapy agents out of cells, thus apparently conferring resistance to almost all known chemotherapy agents.

Combination Therapy

The individual limitations and failures of each modality have prompted the use of multimodality regimens in the management of ATC. Several studies have demonstrated better results following multimodality therapy compared with monotherapy.[47,52,53,55,56,110,119] Controversy still exists as to whether chemotherapy is best administered prior to or following surgery. Preoperative chemoradiation may improve resectability, but also may result in delay of surgery and can further lead to a higher rate of surgical complications. Regardless of the sequence of treatment, multimodality regimens have been associated with survival rates as high as 10% at 2 years and 5 years.[53,54] Still, most remissions are only transient or apparent only as long as chemotherapy is continued, and median survival from ATC is still in the range of 6 months.[107]

Outcomes and Novel Therapies

The unifying theme of all major studies involving ATC is the consistently dismal outcome regardless of treatment strategy. Multimodality regimens have become the norm, and surgery has evolved from tracheotomy alone to attempts at complete resection whenever possible, albeit in a select subset of patients presenting with localized ATC. The best outcomes may be in those patients treated for WDTC who are found to have an incidental component of ATC. Multidrug chemotherapy, and hyperfractionated RT, both in the preoperative and postoperative settings, may produce marginal improvements in outcome, but newer, novel approaches to treating this lethal disease are needed.

The chemoresistance of ATC cells appears to be bypassed by the chemotherapy agent paclitaxel.[120] Combination therapy using paclitaxel and manumycin (a farnesyl protein transferase inhibitor)[121–123] appears to be synergistic and to inhibit angiogenesis and enhance apoptosis. A new vascular targeting agent, combretastatin A4,[124–126] selectively disrupts the newly formed blood vessels that supply tumors, while being devoid of cytotoxic effects.[124] Anecdotal reports of the efficacy of combretastatin A4 in ATC are emerging.[125,126] Alternatively, attempts to undo the dedifferentiation of thyroid carcinomas using gene therapy with a sodium iodine symporter may enable the application of radioactive iodine to ATC.[127,128] In vitro application of oncolytic herpes simplex viruses to ATC cell lines causes significant cytotoxicity and tumor regression.[129]

References

1. Hazard JB, Hawk WA, Crile G. Medullary (solid) carcinoma of the thyroid: a clinicopathological entity. J Clin Endocrinol Metab 1959;19:152–161
2. Brunt LM, Wells SA Jr. Advances in the diagnosis and treatment of medullary thyroid carcinoma. Surg Clin North Am 1987;67:263–279
3. Sahay U. Bilateral phaeochromocytoma associated with carcinoma of the thyroid. Br Med J 1987;67(2):263–279
4. Quayle FJ, Moley JF. Medullary thyroid carcinoma: including MEN 2A and MEN 2B syndromes. J Surg Oncol 2005;89:122–129
5. Mihai R, Farndon JR. Medullary carcinoma of the thyroid. In: Randolph GW, ed. Surgery of the Thyroid and Parathyroid Glands. Philadelphia: Elsevier Science, 2003:232–243
6. Block MA, Jackson CE, Greenawald KA, et al. Clinical characteristics distinguishing hereditary from sporadic medullary thyroid carcinoma. Treatment implications. Arch Surg 1980;115:142–148
7. Graze K, Spiler IJ, Tashjian AH, et al. Natural history of familial medullary thyroid carcinoma: Effect of a program for early diagnosis. N Engl J Med 1978;299:980–985
8. Wolfe HJ, Melvin KE, Cervi-Skinner SJ, et al. C-cell hyperplasia preceding medullary thyroid carcinoma. N Engl J Med 1973;289:437–441
9. Leboulleux S, Baudin E, Travagli JP, Schlumberger M. Medullary thyroid carcinoma. Clin Endocrinol (Oxf) 2004;61:299–310
10. Juweid M, Sharkey RM, Swayne LC, Goldenberg DV. Improved selection of patients for reoperation for medullary thyroid cancer by imaging with radiolabeled anticarcinoembryonic antigen antibodies. Surgery 1997;122:1156–1165
11. Brandi ML, Gagel RF, Angeli A, et al. Guidelines for diagnosis and therapy of MEN type 1 and type 2. J Clin Endocrinol Metab 2001;86:5658–5671
12. Skinner MA, DeBenedetti MK, Moley JF, et al. Medullary thyroid carcinoma in children with multiple endocrine neoplasia types 2A and 2B. J Pediatr Surg 1996;31:177–181, discussion 181–182
13. Samaan NA, Draznin MB, Halpin RE, et al. Multiple endocrine syndrome type IIb in early childhood. Cancer 1991;68:1832–1834
14. Modigliani E, Cohen R, Campos JM, et al. Prognostic factors for survival and for biochemical cure in medullary thyroid carcinoma: results in 899 patients. The GETC Study Group. Groupe d'etude des tumeurs a calcitonine. Clin Endocrinol (Oxf) 1998;48:265–273
15. Gill JR, Reyes-Mugica M, Iyengar S, et al. Early presentation of metastatic medullary carcinoma in multiple endocrine neoplasia, type IIA: implications for therapy. J Pediatr 1996;129:459–464
16. Gagel RF, Tashjian AH, Cummings T, et al. The clinical outcome of prospective screening for multiple endocrine neoplasia type 2a. An 18-year experience. N Engl J Med 1988;318:478–484
17. Niccoli-Sire P, Murat A, Baudin E, et al. Early or prophylactic thyroidectomy in MEN 2/FMTC gene carriers: results in 71 thyroidectomized patients. The French Calcitonin Tumours Study Group (GETC). Eur J Endocrinol 1999;141:468–474
18. Wells SA, Dilley WG, Farndon JA, et al. Early diagnosis and treatment of medullary thyroid carcinoma. Arch Intern Med 1985;145:1248–1252
19. Jimenez C, Dang GT, Schultz PN, et al. A novel point mutation of the RET protooncogene involving the second intracellular tyrosine kinase domain in a family with medullary thyroid carcinoma. J Clin Endocrinol Metab 2004;89:3521–3526
20. Komminoth P, Kunz EK, Matias-Guiu X, et al. Analysis of RET protooncogene point mutations distinguishes heritable from nonheritable medullary thyroid carcinomas. Cancer 1995;76:479–489
21. Pigny P, Bauters C, Wemeau JL, et al. A novel 9-base pair duplication in RET exon 8 in familial medullary thyroid carcinoma. J Clin Endocrinol Metab 1999;84:1700–1704
22. Moley JF, DeBenedetti MK. Patterns of nodal metastases in palpable medullary thyroid carcinoma: Recommendations for extent of node dissection. Ann Surg 1999;229:880–887, discussion 887–888
23. Duh QY, Sancho JJ, Greenspan FS, et al. Medullary thyroid carcinoma. The need for early diagnosis and total thyroidectomy. Arch Surg 1989;124:1206–1210
24. Dralle H, Damm I, Scheumann GF, et al. Compartment-oriented microdissection of regional lymph nodes in medullary thyroid carcinoma. Surg Today 1994;24:112–121
25. Herfarth KK, Bartsch D, Doherty GM, et al. Surgical management of hyperparathyroidism in patients with multiple endocrine neoplasia type 2A. Surgery 1996;120:966–973, discussion 973–974
26. Stepanas AV, Samaan NA, Hill CS, et al. Medullary thyroid carcinoma: importance of serial serum calcitonin measurement. Cancer 1979;43:825–837
27. van Heerden JA, Grant CS, Gharib H, Hay ID, Ilstrup DM. Long-term course of patients with persistent hypercalcitoninemia after apparent curative primary surgery for medullary thyroid carcinoma. Ann Surg 1990;212:395–400
28. Tung WS, Vesely TM, Moley JF. Laparoscopic detection of hepatic metastases in patients with residual or recurrent medullary thyroid cancer. Surgery 1995;118:1024–1029
29. Block MA, Jackson CE, Tashjian AH. Management of occult medullary thyroid carcinoma: Evidenced only by serum calcitonin level elevations after apparently adequate neck operations. Arch Surg 1978;113:368–372
30. Dralle H. Lymph node dissection and medullary thyroid carcinoma. Br J Surg 2002;89:1073–1075
31. Buhr HJ, Kallinowski F, Raue F, et al. Microsurgical neck dissection

for occultly metastasizing medullary thyroid carcinoma. Three-year results. Cancer 1993;72:3685–3693

32. Moley JF, Wells SA, Dilley WG. Reoperation for recurrent or persistent medullary thyroid cancer. Surgery 1993;114:1090–1095

33. Moley JF, Dilley W, DeBenedetti M. Improved results of cervical reoperation for medullary thyroid carcinoma. Ann Surg 1997;225:734–743

34. Husain M, Alsever RN, Lock JP, et al. Failure of medullary carcinoma of the thyroid to respond to doxorubicin therapy. Horm Res 1978;9:22–25

35. Scherubl H, Raue F, Ziegler R. Combination chemotherapy of advanced medullary and differentiated thyroid cancer. Phase II study. J Cancer Res Clin Oncol 1990;116:21–23

36. Orlandi F, Caraci P, Berruti A, et al. Chemotherapy with dacarbazine and 5-fluorouracil in advanced medullary thyroid cancer. Ann Oncol 1994;5:763–765

37. Schlumberger M, Abdoulmoumene N, Delisle MJ, et al. Treatment of advanced medullary thyroid cancer with an alternating combination of 5 fu-streptozocin and 5 fu-dacarbazine. Br J Cancer 1995;71:363–365

38. Grohn P, Kumpulainen E, Jakobsson M. Response of medullary thyroid cancer to low-dose alpha-interferon therapy. Acta Oncol 1990;29:950–951

39. Juweid ME, Hajjar G, Stein R, et al. Initial experience with high-dose radioimmunotherapy of metastatic medullary thyroid cancer using 131I-MN-14 F(ab)2 anti-carcinoembryonic antigen MAb and AHSCR. [comment] J Nucl Med 2000;41:93–103

40. Schott M, Feldkamp J, Klucken M, et al. Calcitonin-specific antitumor immunity in medullary thyroid carcinoma following dendritic cell vaccination. Cancer Immunol Immunother 2002;51:663–668

41. Mahler C, Verhelst J, de Longueville M, Harris A. Long-term treatment of metastatic medullary thyroid carcinoma with the somatostatin analogue octreotide. Clin Endocrinol (Oxf) 1990;33:261–269

42. Vitale G, Tagliaferri P, Caraglia M, et al. Slow release lanreotide in combination with interferon-alpha2b in the treatment of symptomatic advanced medullary thyroid carcinoma. J Clin Endocrinol Metab 2000;85:983–988

43. Cohen MS, Hussain HB, Moley JF. Inhibition of medullary thyroid carcinoma cell proliferation and RET phosphorylation by tyrosine kinase inhibitors. Surgery 2002;132:960–966

44. Carlomagno F, Vitagliano D, Guida T, et al. ZD6474, an orally available inhibitor of KDR tyrosine kinase activity, efficiently blocks oncogenic RET kinases. Cancer Res 2002;62:7284–7290

45. Brierley JD, Tsang RW. External radiation therapy in the treatment of thyroid malignancy. Endocrinol Metab Clin North Am 1996;25:141–157

46. Nguyen TD, Chassard JL, Lagarde P, et al. Results of postoperative radiation therapy in medullary carcinoma of the thyroid: A retrospective study by the French Federation of Cancer Institutes—The Radiotherapy Cooperative Group. Radiother Oncol 1992;23:1–5

47. Venkatesh YS, Ordonez NG, Schultz PN, Hickey RC, Goepfert H, Samaan NA. Anaplastic carcinoma of the thyroid: a clinicopathologic study of 121 cases. Cancer 1990;66:321–330

48. DeMeter JG, De Jong SA, Lawrence AM, Paloyan E. Anaplastic thyroid carcinoma: risk factors and outcome. Surgery 1991;110:956–963

49. Carcangiu ML, Steeper T, Zampi G, Rosai J. Anaplastic thyroid carcinoma: a study of 70 cases. Am J Clin Pathol 1985;83:135–158

50. Passler C, Scheuba C, Prager G, et al. Anaplastic (undifferentiated) thyroid carcinoma (ATC). Langenbecks Arch Surg 1999;384:284–293

51. Spires JR, Schwartz MR, Miller RH. Anaplastic thyroid carcinoma:

association with differentiated thyroid cancer. Arch Otolaryngol Head Neck Surg 1988;114:40–44

52. Haigh PI, Ituarte PH, Wu HS, et al. Completely resected anaplastic thyroid carcinoma combined with adjuvant chemotherapy and irradiation is associated with prolonged survival. Cancer 2001;91:2335–2342

53. Nilsson O, Lindberg J, Zedenius J. Anaplastic giant cell carcinoma of the thyroid gland: treatment and survival over a 25 year period. World J Surg 1998;22:725–730

54. Tan RK, Finley RK, Driscoll D, Bakamjian V, Hicks WL, Shedd DP. Anaplastic carcinoma of the thyroid: a 24 year experience. Head Neck 1995;17:41–48

55. Junor EJ, Paul J, Reed NS. Anaplastic thyroid carcinoma: 91 patients treated by surgery and radiotherapy. Eur J Surg Oncol 1992;18:83–88

56. Tennvall J, Lundell G, Hallquist A, Wahlberg P, Wallin G, Tibblin S. Combined doxorubicin, hyperfractionated radiotherapy and surgery in anaplastic thyroid carcinoma: a report of two protocols. Cancer 1994;74:1348–1354

57. Kobayashi T, Asakawa H, Umeshita K, et al. Treatment of 37 patients with anaplastic carcinoma of the thyroid. Head Neck 1996;18:36–41

58. Are C, Shaha AR. Anaplastic thyroid carcinoma: biology, pathogenesis, prognostic factors, and treatment approaches. Ann Surg Oncol 2006;13:453–464

59. Mitchell G, Huddart R, Harmer C. Phase II evaluation of high dose accelerated radiotherapy for anaplastic thyroid carcinoma. Radiother Oncol 1999;50:33–38

60. Tennvall J, Tallroth E, el Hassan A, et al. Anaplastic thyroid carcinoma. Doxorubicin, hyperfractionated radiotherapy and surgery. Acta Oncol 1990;29:1025–1028

61. Voutilainen PE, Multanen M, Haapiainen RK, Leppaniemi AK, Sivula AH. Anaplastic thyroid carcinoma survival. World J Surg 1999;23:975–979

62. Greene FL, Page DL, Fleming ID, et al, eds. Thyroid. AJCC Cancer Staging Manual, 6th ed. New York: Springer-Verlag, 2002:77

63. McIver B, Hay ID, Giuffrida D, et al. Anaplastic thyroid carcinoma: a 50 year experience at a single institution. Surgery 2001;130:1028–1034

64. Holting T, Moller P, Tschahargane C, Meybier H, Buhr H, Herfarth C. Immunohistochemical reclassification of anaplastic carcinoma reveals small and giant cell lymphoma. World J Surg 1990;14:291–295

65. Wiseman SM, Loree TR, Rigual NR, et al. Anaplastic transformation of thyroid cancer: review of clinical, pathologic, and molecular evidence provides new insights into disease biology and future therapy. Head Neck 2003;25:662–670

66. Mooradian AD, Allam CK, Khalil MF, Salti I, Salem PA. Anaplastic transformation of thyroid cancer: report of two cases and review of the literature. J Surg Oncol 1983;23:95–98

67. Getaz EP, Shimaoka K. Anaplastic carcinoma of the thyroid in a population irradiated for Hodgkin disease, 1910–1960. J Surg Oncol 1979;12:181–189

68. Abe Y, Ichikawa Y, Muraki T, Ito K, Homma M. Thyrotropin (TSH) receptor and adenylate cyclase activity in human thyroid tumors: absence of high affinity receptor and loss of TSH responsiveness in undifferentiated thyroid carcinoma. J Clin Endocrinol Metab 1981;52:23–28

69. Ain KB. Anaplastic thyroid carcinoma: a therapeutic challenge. Semin Surg Oncol 1999;16:64–69

70. Ain KB. Anaplastic thyroid carcinoma: behaviour, biology and therapeutic approaches. Thyroid 1998;8:715–726

71. Bakiri F, Djemli FK, Mokrane LA, Djidel FK. The relative roles of en-

demic goiter and socio economic development status in the prognosis of thyroid carcinoma. Cancer 1998;82:1146–1153

72. Sugitani I, Kasai N, Fujimoto Y, Yanagisawa A. Prognostic factors and therapeutic strategies for anaplastic carcinoma of the thyroid. World J Surg 2001;25:617–622

73. Lu WT, Lin JD, Huang HS, et al. Does surgery improve the survival of patients with anaplastic carcinoma of the thyroid. Otolaryngol Head Neck Surg 1998;118:728–731

74. Nishiyama RH, Dunn EL, Thompson NW. Anaplastic spindle-cell and giant cell tumours of the thyroid gland. Cancer 1972;30:113–127

75. Dumitriu L, Stefaneanu L, Tasca C. The anaplastic transformation of differentiated thyroid carcinoma. Rev Roum Med Endocrinol 1984;22:91–96

76. Newland JR, Mackay B, Hill CS, Hickey RC. Anaplastic thyroid carcinoma: an ultrastructural study of 10 cases. Ultrastruct Pathol 1981;2:121–129

77. Lam KY, Lo CY, Chan KW, Wan KY. Insular and anaplastic thyroid carcinoma of the thyroid: a 45 year comparative study at a single institution and a review of the significance of p53 and p21. Ann Surg 2000;231:329–338

78. Ito T, Seyama T, Mizuno T, et al. Unique association of p53 mutations with undifferentiated but not with differentiated carcinomas of the thyroid gland. Cancer Res 1992;52:1369–1371

79. Blagosklonny MV, Giannakakou P, Wojtowicz M, et al. Effects of p53-expressing adenovirus on the chemosensitivity and differentiation of anaplastic thyroid cancer cells. J Clin Endocrinol Metab 1998;83:2516–2522

80. Moretti F, Farsetti A, Soddu S, et al. p53 re expression inhibits proliferation and restores differentiation of human thyroid anaplastic carcinoma cells. Oncogene 1997;14:729–740

81. Stoler DL, Datta RV, Charles MA, et al. Genomic instability measurement in the diagnosis of thyroid neoplasms. Head Neck 2002;24:290–295

82. Fagin JA, Tang SH, Zeki K, Di Lauro R, Fusco A, Gonsky R. Re expression of thyroid peroxidase in a derivative of an undifferentiated thyroid carcinoma cell line by introduction of wild type p53. Cancer Res 1996;56:765–771

83. Tallini G, Santoro M, Helie M, et al. RET/PCT oncogene activation defines a subset of papillary thyroid carcinomas lacking evidence of progression to poorly differentiated or undifferentiated tumor phenotypes. Clin Cancer Res 1998;4:287–294

84. Wang S, Lloyd RV, Hutzler MJ, Safran MS, Parwardhan NA, Khan A. The role of cell cycle regulatory protein, cyclin D1, in the progression of thyroid cancer. Mod Pathol 2000;13:882–887

85. Garcia-Rostan G, Tallini G, Herrero A, Aquila TGD, Carcangiu ML, Rimm DL. Frequent mutation and nuclear localization of β-catenin in anaplastic thyroid carcinoma. Cancer Res 1999;59:1811–1815

86. Bergstrom JD, Hermansson A, de Diaz Stahl T, Heldin NE. Non-autocrine, constitutive activation of Met in human anaplastic thyroid carcinoma cells in culture. Br J Cancer 1999;80:650–656

87. Hoang-Vu C, Dralle H, Scheumann G, et al. Gene expression of differentiation- and dedifferentiation markers in normal and malignant human thyroid tissues. Exp Clin Endocrinol 1992;100:51–56

88. Pilotti S, Collini P, Rilke F, Cattoretti G, Del Bo R, Pierotti MA. Bcl-2 protein expression in carcinomas originating from the follicular epithelium of the thyroid gland. J Pathol 1994;172:337–342

89. Zou M, Shi Y, Al-Sedairy S, Farid NR. High levels of Nm23 gene expression in advanced stage of thyroid carcinomas. Br J Cancer 1993;68:385–388

90. Stringer BM, Rowson JM, Parkar MH, et al. Detection of the H-

RAS oncogene in human thyroid anaplastic carcinomas. Experientia 1989;45:372–376

91. Galera-Davidson H, Bibbo M, Dytch HED, Gonzalez-Campora R, Fernandez A, Wied GL. Nuclear DNA in anaplastic thyroid carcinoma with a differentiated component. Histopathology 1987;11:715–722

92. Wallin G, Backdahl M, Tallroth-Ekman E, Lundell G, Auer G, Lowhagen T. Co-existent anaplastic and well differentiated thyroid carcinomas: a nuclear DNA study. Eur J Surg Oncol 1989;15:43–48

93. Gilliland FD, Hunt WC, Morris DM, Key CR. Prognostic factors for thyroid carcinoma. A population based study of 15,698 cases from the Surveillance, Epidemiology and End Results (SEER) program 1973–91. Cancer 1997;79:564–573

94. Giuffrida D, Gharib D. Anaplastic thyroid carcinoma: current diagnosis and treatment. Ann Oncol 2000;11:1083–1089

95. Besic N, Auersperg M, Us-Krasovec M, Golouh R, Frkovic-Grazio S, Vodnik A. Effects of primary treatment on survival in anaplastic thyroid carcinoma. Eur J Surg Oncol 2001;27:260–264

96. Kebebew E, Greenspan FS, Clark OH, Woeber KA, McMillan A. Anaplastic thyroid carcinoma. Treatment outcome and prognostic factors. Cancer 2005;103:1330–1335

97. Rodriguez JM, Pinero A, Ortiz S, et al. Clinical and histological differences in anaplastic thyroid carcinoma. Eur J Surg 2000;166:34–38

98. Saunders CA, Nayar R. Anaplastic spindle-cell squamous carcinoma arising in association with tall cell papillary cancer of the thyroid: a potential pitfall. Diagn Cytopathol 1999;21:413–418

99. Moreno Egea A, Rodriguez Gonzalez JM, Sola Perez J, et al. Prognostic value of the tall cell variety of papillary cancer of the thyroid. Eur J Surg Oncol 1993;19:517–521

100. Pasieka JL. Anaplastic thyroid cancer. Curr Opin Oncol 2003;15:78–83

101. Ordonez NG, El-Naggar AK, Hickey RC, Samaan NA. Anaplastic thyroid carcinoma: immunocytochemical study of 32 cases. Am J Clin Pathol 1991;96:15–24

102. LiVolsi VA, Brooks JJ, Arendash-Durand B. Anaplastic thyroid tumours: immunohistology. Am J Clin Pathol 1987;87:434–442

103. Shvero J, Gal R, Avidor I, Hadar T, Kessler E. Anaplastic thyroid carcinoma: a clinical, histologic and immunohistochemical study. Cancer 1988;62:319–325

104. Austin JR, El-Naggar AK, Goepfort H. Thyroid cancers II: medullary, anaplastic, lymphoma, sarcoma, squamous cell. Otolaryngol Clin North Am 1996;29:611–627

105. Us-Krasovec M, Golouh R, Auersperg M. Anaplastic carcinoma in fine needle aspirates. Acta Cytol 1996;40:953–958

106. Holting T, Meybier H, Buhr H. Status of tracheotomy in treatment of the respiratory emergency in anaplastic thyroid cancer. (in German) Wien Klin Wochenschr 1990;102:264–266

107. Veness MJ, Porter GS, Morgan GJ. Anaplastic thyroid carcinoma: dismal outcome despite current treatment approach. ANZ J Surg 2004;74:559–562

108. Pierie JP, Muzikansky A, Gaz RD, Faquin WC, Ott MJ. The effect of surgery and radiotherapy on outcome of anaplastic thyroid carcinoma. Ann Surg Oncol 2002;9:57–64

109. Heron DE, Karimpour S, Grigsby PW. Anaplastic thyroid carcinoma: comparison of conventional radiotherapy and hyperfractionation chemoradiotherapy in two groups. Am J Clin Oncol 2002;25:442–446

110. Tennvall J, Lundell G, Wahlberg P, et al. Anaplastic thyroid carcinoma: three protocols combining doxorubicin, hyperfractionated radiotherapy and surgery. Br J Cancer 2002;86:1848–1853

111. Levendag PC, De Porre PM, van Putten WL. Anaplastic carcinoma of the thyroid gland treated by radiation therapy. Int J Radiat Oncol Biol Phys 1993;26:125–128

112. Poster DS, Bruno S, Penta J, Pina K, Catane R. Current status of chemotherapy in the treatment of advanced carcinoma of the thyroid gland. Cancer Clin Trials 1981;4:301–307

113. Shimaoka K, Schoenffeld DA, DeWys WD, Creech RH, DeConti R. A randomized trial of doxorubicin versus doxorubicin plus cisplatin in patients with advanced thyroid carcinoma. Cancer 1985;56:2155–2160

114. Williams SD, Birch R, Einhorn LH. Phase II evaluation of doxorubicin plus cisplatin in advanced thyroid cancer: a Southeastern Cancer Study Group trial. Cancer Treat Rep 1986;70:405–407

115. Asakawa H, Koboyashi T, Komoije Y, et al. Chemosensitivity of anaplastic thyroid carcinoma and poorly differentiated thyroid carcinoma. Anticancer Res 1997;17:2757–2762

116. De Besi P, Busnardo B, Toso S, et al. Combined chemotherapy with bleomycin, Adriamycin, and platinum in advanced thyroid carcinoma. J Endocrinol Invest 1991;14:475–480

117. Satake S, Sugawara I, Watanabe M, Takami H. Lack of point mutation of human DNA topoisomerase II in multidrug-resistant anaplastic thyroid carcinoma cell lines. Cancer Lett 1997;116:33–39

118. Lehnert M. Clinical multidrug resistance in cancer: a multifactorial problem. Eur J Cancer 1996;32A:912–920

119. Tennvall J, Lundell G, Hallquist A, Wahlberg P, Wallin G, Tibblin S. Combined doxorubicin, hyperfractionated radiotherapy and surgery in anaplastic thyroid carcinoma. Report on two protocols. The Swedish Anaplastic Thyroid Cancer Group. Cancer 1994;74(4):1348–1349.

120. Ain KB, Egorin MJ, DeSimone PA. Treatment of anaplastic thyroid carcinoma with paclitaxel: phase II trial using ninety six hour infusion. Thyroid 2000;7:587–594

121. Yeung SC, Xu G, Pan J, Christgen M, Bamiagis A. Manumycin enhances the cytotoxic effect of paclitaxel on anaplastic thyroid carcinoma cells. Cancer Res 2000;60:650–656

122. Xu G, Pan J, Martin C, Yeung SJ. Angiogenesis inhibition in the in vivo antineoplastic effect of manumycin and paclitaxel against anaplastic thyroid carcinoma. J Clin Endocrinol Metab 2001;86:1769–1777

123. Pan J, Xu G, Yeung SJ. Cytochrome c release is upstream to activation of caspase-9, caspase-8 and caspase-3 in the enhanced apoptosis of anaplastic thyroid cancer cells induced by manumycin and paclitaxel. J Clin Endocrinol Metab 2001;86:4731–4740

124. Dowlati A, Cooney M, Robertson K, et al. A phase I pharmacokinetic and translational study of the novel vascular targeting agent combretastatin a-4 phosphate on a single dose intravenous schedule in patients with advanced cancer. Cancer Res 2002;62:3408–3416

125. Randal J. Antiangiogenesis drugs target specific cancers, mechanisms. J Natl Cancer Inst 2000;92:520–522

126. Dziba JM, Marcinek R, Venkataraman GM, Robinson JA, Ain KB. Combretastatin A4 phosphate has primary antineoplastic activity against human anaplastic thyroid carcinoma cell lines and xenograft tumours. Thyroid 2002;12:1063–1070

127. Venkataraman GM, Yatin M, Marcinek R, Ain KB. Restoration of iodine uptake in dedifferentiated thyroid carcinoma: relationship to human Na +/I- symported gene methylation status. J Clin Endocrinol Metab 1999;84:2449–2457

128. Spitzweg C, Harrington KJ, Pinke LA, Vile RG, Morris JC. The sodium iodide symporter and its potential in cancer therapy. J Clin Endocrinol Metab 2001;86:3327–3335

129. Yu Z, Eisenberg DP, Singh B, Shah JP, Fong Y, Wong RJ. Treatment of aggressive thyroid cancer with an oncolytic herpes virus. Int J Cancer 2004;112:525–532

12 Surgical Management of Thyroid Cancer

Michael E. Kupferman and Randal S. Weber

Perhaps no other issue in head and neck surgery provokes such fierce debate as that of the optimal surgical management of thyroid cancer. Due to the lack of prospective randomized trials, sufficient long-term patient follow-up, and an overall favorable prognosis, decision making in thyroid surgery rests largely on individual surgeon preference and treatment philosophy. Much of our understanding of the biology and outcomes in this disease stems from large single-institution retrospective reviews. The limited objective data that are available makes individualized treatment decisions difficult. The evaluation, staging, and medical treatment of thyroid cancer are discussed in other chapters in this text. This chapter focuses on the surgical controversies and provides the practitioner with a framework for the appropriate operative management of patients with thyroid cancer.

Extent of Initial Surgery

Despite the overwhelming consensus among endocrinologists for total thyroidectomy as the standard of care in patients with well-differentiated thyroid cancer, debate persists today among surgeons over the extent of resection necessary for this disease.[1,2] In framing this controversy, it is helpful to stratify patients based on their prognosis and likelihood of local recurrence (**Table 12.1**). Patients who are

categorized as low risk tend to be young and have small lesions that do not harbor any adverse pathologic features; conversely, high-risk patients tend to be older and have biologically aggressive tumors.[3] Although reductionist in nature, this stratification integrates many prognostic factors, allowing for careful and thoughtful therapeutic decision making.

There is general agreement that patients in the high-risk group are at risk of developing local recurrences, nodal metastasis, and systemic disease, and thus should be treated in a comprehensive fashion.[1,4] This multimodality approach includes total thyroidectomy, radioactive iodine ablation, and thyroid suppression therapy. Paratracheal node dissection is performed when there are suspicious nodes noted on preoperative imaging or at operative setting. Retrospective studies support this approach, which results in decreased locoregional recurrence and improved survival.[5]

Much of the controversy surrounding the surgical management of well-differentiated thyroid cancer revolves around the decision to perform a total thyroidectomy or a unilateral lobectomy in patients with low-risk tumors.[6,7] It has been argued that small foci of well-differentiated thyroid cancer (WDTC) may be effectively treated with thyroid lobectomy alone, with frequent monitoring of the remaining lobe utilizing ultrasonography. With this treatment paradigm, local recurrences are infrequent. A matched-pair analysis of a large cohort of patients treated at a single institution demonstrated no survival benefit for total thyroidectomy when compared with thyroid lobectomy.[8] The likelihood of regional metastasis was also similar between both groups. In addition, proponents of this philosophy point to the attendant risks of hypoparathyroidism and recurrent laryngeal nerve injury as justification for a less-than-total thyroidectomy.

However, most surgeons and endocrinologists advocate the complete removal of all thyroid tissue in all patients with thyroid carcinoma. There are several compelling arguments for adhering to the practice of total thyroidectomy, even for low-risk patients. This practice is based on the biology of this complex disease, oncologic control, and the need for intensive posttreatment monitoring. First and foremost, the majority of large patient studies confirm the primacy of total thyroidectomy as the initial procedure of choice for patients with WDTC. This has been borne out by multiple retrospective reviews from several high-volume thyroid practices.[5,7]

Another issue is the scenario of occult thyroid carcinoma found after a unilateral lobectomy. When diagnosed

Table 12.1 Prognostic Factors in Well-Differentiated Thyroid Cancer

Low Risk	High Risk
Patient variables	
Age 15–45	Age <15 or >45
Female	Male
No family history	Family history of thyroid cancer
Tumor variables	
Tumor <4 cm	≥4 cm
Unilateral disease	Multifocal or bilateral disease
No extrathyroidal extension	Extrathyroidal extension
No vascular invasion	Vascular invasion
No lymphatic metastasis	Cervical or mediastinal metastasis
Iodine-avid tumors	Aggressive histologic subtypes: Hürthle cell, tall cell, columnar cell, diffuse sclerosis, insular
Absence of distant metastasis	Distant metastasis

with a unilateral focus of thyroid carcinoma, a substantial number of patients harbor carcinoma in the contralateral gland.[9] Multifocal disease in papillary thyroid carcinoma is not an uncommon occurrence. Although the clinical significance of this finding is unknown, surveillance of a residual thyroid lobe is fraught with psychological and oncologic implications, and necessitates frequent radiographic studies, without the benefit of radioactive iodine scanning or serum thyroglobulin monitoring.

Another argument for performing a total thyroidectomy for all patients with thyroid carcinoma is the impact of residual thyroid tissue on the implementation of adjuvant treatments.[10] Postsurgical radioactive iodine scanning, in conjunction with serum thyroglobulin levels, is effective at identifying tumor recurrences in the thyroid bed and regional metastasis.[11] Neither of these noninvasive tests can be utilized for patients who have residual thyroid tissue in the native thyroid bed. Additionally, lower doses of radioactive iodine are needed in athyroid patients, compared with those with residual tissue.[10] Furthermore, the sonographic detection of central compartment metastases is facilitated by complete surgical extirpation of all thyroid tissue.

Total Thyroidectomy for Thyroid Carcinoma

Intraoperative management of thyroid carcinoma is not dissimilar from that of benign disease; however, certain technical details warrant mentioning. Adherence to these surgical principles facilitates consistent and safe thyroid surgery, with satisfactory oncologic results (**Fig. 12.1**).

An extraglandular dissection of the thyroid parenchyma is required because one of the primary predictors of patient prognosis in WDTC is extracapsular disease outside of the thyroid gland. Positive identification of the recurrent laryngeal nerve (RLN) in the tracheoesophageal groove is required, and meticulous microdissection is needed to avoid postoperative paralysis or paresis. As the thyroid gland typically is densely adherent to the trachea at the Berry ligament, the surgeon should thoroughly dissect this area to avoid leaving thyroid tissue in situ (**Fig. 12.2**). Palpation of the central compartment lymph nodes is done after the gland is removed; any suspicion of cervical metastasis warrants a level VI neck dissection.[12]

In summary, the overwhelming evidence and experience points to total thyroidectomy as the optimal initial surgical modality for patients with WDTCs, a practice advocated by the endocrinologists. Deviation from this paradigm should be considered only in a small group of patients being treated by an experienced multidisciplinary team.

Management of Laryngotracheal Involvement

Although WDTC has a favorable long-term prognosis, locally invasive tumors pose therapeutic challenges that contribute

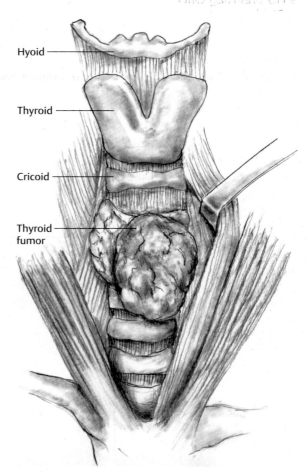

Fig. 12.1 Artist's depiction of a large carcinoma of the left lobe.

to significant morbidity and mortality in patients. Patients with extrathyroidal disease have a high risk of locoregional recurrence and poor prognosis. In fact, almost 50% of all thyroid cancer–related deaths result from uncontrolled local disease.[13] At the time of death, 80% of patients with differentiated thyroid cancer have local recurrence. Locally invasive thyroid cancer, with extension to the neck musculature, laryngotracheal complex, and esophagus, occurs in approximately 5 to 15% of all patients. Therefore, complete tumor extirpation is required to prevent the dreaded sequelae of massive hemoptysis, airway compromise, and pharyngoesophageal obstruction.[14] The management of invasive thyroid cancer is complex, requiring a thorough understanding of tumor behavior, expertise in complex resections and reconstructions of the visceral organs of the neck, and the need for anatomic and functional preservation of structures vital to voice and swallowing.

Pathology

Papillary thyroid carcinoma (PTC) is the most common form of thyroid cancer, and accounts for the majority of invasive lesions in most published series. In a review of patients treated at the Mayo Clinic, McCaffrey et al[15] found that

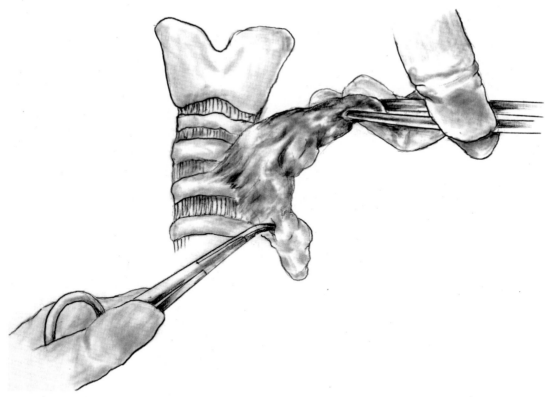

Fig. 12.2 Artist's rendering of the surgical dissection, demonstrating thyroid gland and associated carcinoma adherent to the trachea wall at the Berry ligament.

89% of invasive thyroid cancers were PTCs. Despite its indolent behavior, PTC has a predilection for local and regional spread, and approximately 15% of patients have extraglandular spread pathologically. Tall cell and insular carcinomas, which are variants of PTC, display extrathyroidal extension in 35 to 50% of cases.[16] The surgeon should be mindful of the propensity for extrathyroidal extension when managing patients who harbor these pathologic variants, as they may require more extensive resections.

The propensity for follicular carcinoma to involve cervicovisceral structures is variable, and has accounted for 5 to 40% of invasive thyroid cancers. Although these tumors are known to spread distantly to the lung, brain, and bone, 20% of patients with follicular thyroid cancer (FTC) presented with widely invasive lesions.[15,17,18] Hürthle cell carcinoma, a variant of follicular carcinoma, is a particularly aggressive subtype with a propensity for regional metastasis and local recurrences.[19] Patients with sporadic and familial forms of medullary thyroid carcinoma can develop laryngotracheal invasion; 44% of patients treated at a single institution with invasive thyroid cancer had medullary thyroid cancer (MTC).[20] Although anaplastic thyroid cancer (ATC) often is not responsive to standard therapeutic modalities, some patients undergo extensive extirpations, often requiring the removal of adjacent structures. However, the overall 1-year survival for ATC remains approximately 10% and has not improved with the advent of multimodality treatment approaches.

Presentation

Although most patients with locally invasive thyroid malignancies have symptoms that are attributable to the site of involvement, early invasion may not be evident on preoperative clinical examination. Evidence of local extension is often identified intraoperatively, and the surgeon must be comfortable with surgical management of the central compartment viscera to provide the patient with an oncologically appropriate resection. Conservatism under these circumstances results in uncontrolled locoregional disease.

After taking into account strap muscle invasion, the recurrent laryngeal nerve is the cervical structure most commonly involved by thyroid cancer.[21] It is not uncommon for patients to complain of vocal fatigue, hoarseness, and an inability to alter pitch and volume. However, young patients may accommodate to long-standing paralyses with contralateral vocal cord hyperfunction and with the recruitment of false vocal cord adduction. Preoperative fiberoptic laryngoscopy is necessary to assess vocal cord function, as vocal cord weakness or paralysis, with concomitant vocal cord atrophy, may indicate tumor extension to the tracheoesophageal groove, or involvement of the cricothyroid joint, the anatomic site at which the nerve enters the larynx to innervate the intrinsic phonatory musculature. The presence of vocal fold fasciculations and tremor in the setting of recurrent thyroid cancer is an ominous sign, and suggests frank perineural involvement. Videostroboscopy should be utilized to document presurgical laryngeal dysfunction and may be beneficial in monitoring laryngeal function postoperatively. If the presurgical evaluation suggests that the recurrent laryngeal nerve may need to be resected, the surgeon should counsel the patient on potential functional outcomes and surgical options for future vocal rehabilitation. It must be emphasized, however, that the decision to resect a recurrent laryngeal nerve is often made intraoperatively, and should be performed based on the judgment of the operating surgeon. In the setting of recurrent disease with a preexisting vocal cord paralysis, injury to the remaining functioning nerve results in emergent airway obstruction and necessitates the placement of a tracheotomy.

Despite its anatomic proximity to the thyroid gland, the trachea is rarely involved with aggressive thyroid cancer (**Fig. 12.3**). Patients with early invasion of the trachea may be asymptomatic. Symptoms related to tracheal invasion may be subtle, such as chronic cough, globus sensation, or audible wheezing. When hemoptysis, dysphagia, stridor, or dyspnea are evident, it suggests a more invasive lesion, and the patient may require emergent surgical management of the airway.[22] In certain patients, office bronchoscopy may be performed after topically anesthetizing the vocal cords to evaluate the status of the tracheal lumen. Photo documentation and biopsy, if possible, should be undertaken when bronchoscopy is performed.

Invasion into the laryngeal skeleton usually occurs via direct extension through the laryngeal cartilages or via the paraglottic space at the posterior free margin of the thyroid cartilage. Tumor may then progress superiorly to enter the supraglottis or inferiorly into the pyriform sinus or glottis.[15]

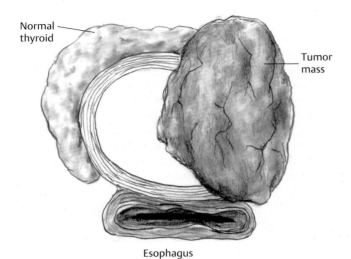

Normal thyroid

Tumor mass

Esophagus

Fig. 12.3 Cross section of an invasive thyroid malignancy involving the tracheal wall, lumen, and recurrent laryngeal nerve.

Alternatively, thyroid carcinoma may enter the larynx via the cricothyroid joint, following the anatomic pathway of the recurrent laryngeal nerve. Complaints of hoarseness or globus sensation are suggestive of laryngeal framework invasion. Some of the subtle findings on the physical examination that suggest laryngeal invasion include submucosal fullness, rotation of the hemilarynx, and restriction of vocal cord mobility. In more advanced disease, thyroid cancer directly invades the laryngeal lumen and results in airway obstruction, necessitating immediate surgical intervention for airway control.

Diagnostic Studies

Any patients suspected of having laryngotracheal involvement with invasive thyroid cancer should undergo axial imaging to evaluate the extent of disease. For uncomplicated thyroid carcinoma, ultrasonography is the study of choice, and is useful in assessing the extent of nodal disease. However, it has limited utility in evaluating soft tissue involvement. This is primarily due to the operator-dependence of ultrasonographic techniques, the air–cartilage interface, and the rigidity of the trachea. Despite this, certain institutions have utilized ultrasonography with great success for the evaluation of airway invasion from thyroid cancer.[23]

In general, patients suspected of having extensive soft tissue disease should have anatomic imaging with either computed tomography (CT) with iodinated contrast or magnetic resonance imaging (MRI). CT is advantageous for identifying bony or cartilaginous invasion of the laryngotracheal complex. It is also superior to MRI for the identification of metastatic lymphadenopathy. One innovation in imaging the trachea has been the introduction of four-dimensional (4D) CT scanning, which can precisely delineate the extent of disease. The advantage of this imaging modality is its ability to reduce imaging artifact from respiratory motion.[24] MRI provides superior soft tissue and luminal characterization than CT (**Fig. 12.4**). Additionally, the administration of radioactive iodine must be delayed by 6 weeks after the administration of iodinated contrast agents. Under most circumstances, these studies offer complementary information to the head and neck surgeon in planning the operative resection, and thus are often both performed.

Another technique that has enjoyed some success in the preoperative planning stage is endoscopic ultrasonography, which can detect subtle involvement of the esophageal and tracheal wall. Of utmost importance is the detection of distant metastasis, either by positron emission testing or whole-body CT scanning, as patient management may be altered by the presence of widespread disease. Although a multitude of diagnostic techniques are available to the surgical team, the ideal study is usually based on the surgeon's preference and the experience of the head and neck radiologist.

Any suspected recurrences or soft tissue deposits should be assessed cytologically using fine-needle aspiration,

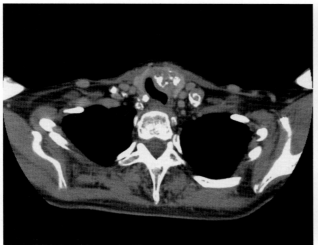

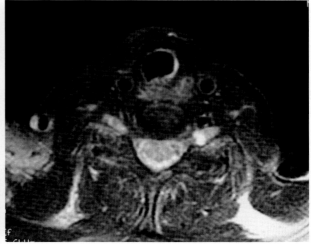

A   B

Fig. 12.4 **(A)** Computed tomography (CT) scan of the neck with iodinated contrast in a patient with a large thyroid cancer with aggressive local invasion of the left trachea. Tracheal ring destruction is evident. **(B)** Magnetic resonance imaging (MRI) of the neck demonstrating intraluminal involvement with thyroid carcinoma.

which may be performed with ultrasound guidance to increase the diagnostic yield. Suspected intraluminal lesions should be biopsied in the operating room under general anesthesia, particularly if there is concern about impending airway compromise.

Operative Management

The issue of extent of resection is one of the many controversial areas in the management of locally invasive thyroid cancers. Historically, authors have stated that total excision of all tumor-bearing tissues to microscopically negative margins is required for the appropriate treatment of aggressive thyroid cancers. More recently, the use of partial, or "shave" resections has been advocated to minimize the morbidity of ablative surgery. Advocates of this approach utilize radioactive iodine ablation or external beam radiation to address residual microscopic disease. Because no survival benefit has been demonstrated for total tumor resection compared with "shave resection" in various retrospective reviews, debate persists.[15,25] It is apparent, based on the biology of the disease, that in the management of locally invasive differentiated thyroid cancer, minimal margins are adequate, in contrast to squamous cell carcinomas of the upper aerodigestive tract. Despite this, there is still no clear consensus on the extent of resection for patients with tumor invading the aerodigestive tract, and thus surgeons must rely on their clinical acumen and experience to make these decisions. One of the guiding principles is the knowledge that the patients with recurrent disease can be expected to enjoy a prolonged life expectancy, and thus any treatment morbidity will have a significant impact on long-term quality of life.

Recurrent Laryngeal Nerve

Despite its intimate relationship with the thyroid gland and the paratracheal nodes, the RLN is rarely invaded by tumor. In most situations, the surgeon can clear the RLN of tumor by carefully skeletonizing the nerve in a superior and inferior direction. Identification and preservation of the RLN can be facilitated by intraoperative neurologic monitoring.[26] However, when the tumor or metastatic lymph nodes actually encase the nerve circumferentially, there may be no option other than to sacrifice the nerve. This often occurs in the reoperative setting, when previous microsurgical dissection has exposed the perineurium, allowing for tumor infiltration. Care must be taken in avoiding injury to the contralateral nerve during surgical dissection, as bilateral vocal cord paralysis precipitates acute airway obstruction upon extubation. When both nerves have been sacrificed for oncologic control of disease, a tracheotomy is necessary for maintaining an adequate airway. Postoperatively, the patient with a unilateral vocal cord paralysis may have an adequate voice, as the paralyzed vocal cord is initially in a median and inferior position. Gradually, lateralization of the cord ensues, with subsequent diminution in voice quality. Surgical rehabilitation with a medialization thyroplasty, in conjunction with an arytenoid adduction, can restore adequate voice quality.

Larynx

Difficult management decisions arise when thyroid cancer extends superiorly to enter the laryngeal skeleton, either directly though the cricothyroid membrane or into the paraglottic space. It is imperative to determine the extent of the involvement of the cricoid cartilage because this dictates the extent of resection and the potential need for a laryngectomy. Some surgeons recommend a shave resection of the cartilage for anterior cricoid invasion, but there is higher risk of recurrence when this is performed.[27] Up to one third of the cricoid can be resected without the need for a cartilage graft; the defect can be usually be reconstructed using a myoperiosteal flap, based upon the sternocleidomastoid. If resection of the anterior one third to one half of the cartilage is performed, cartilage graft harvested from rib can be interpositioned into the defect to prevent postoperative stenosis. The costal perichondrium must be preserved and placed intraluminally to provide a bed for remucosalization.[28] More invasive subglottic extension necessitates a total laryngectomy for oncologic control, although some authors advocate a cricotracheal resection and primary thyrotracheal anastomosis, with preservation of the arytenoids and vocal cords, under these circumstances. Similar to the surgical approach for subglottic stenosis, a thin portion of cricoid cartilage, upon which the arytenoids sit, may be preserved and sutured directly to the remnant trachea. The experience of the surgeon and the extent of disease should dictate the extent of resection and reconstruction that the patient requires.

When the thyroid cartilage has a small focus of invasion, without paraglottic or preepiglottic space invasion, the outer perichondrium and cartilage may be resected, with preservation of the inner perichondrium. The approach can be curative in selected situations. Ipsilateral laryngeal involvement can be managed with a vertical hemilaryngectomy, if the surgeon is assured of the ability to obtain negative margins. Preoperative imaging and intraoperative laryngoscopy are critical for accurate assessment of the extent of laryngeal resection necessary. When thyroid cancer invades the anterior commissure or both hemilarynges, a total laryngectomy is indicated for complete tumor eradication.

Trachea

Tracheal invasion is often identified during the preoperative evaluation, but previously unrecognized foci of tracheal invasion may be encountered during the course of surgical resection. Invasion of the trachea with thyroid cancer occurs via the intercartilaginous spaces or directly through the cartilaginous rings. In both instances, full-thickness resection of the tracheal wall is necessary for complete tumor extirpation (**Fig. 12.5**). Shave resection is an option when the tumor is adherent but has not invaded the tracheal cartilage or lumen. Some advocate a shave resection of the tracheal ring perichondrium, but this technique does not allow for proper pathologic evaluation of the specimen margins. We therefore recommend complete tumor resection under these circumstances.

The presence of localized invasion of the trachea with thyroid carcinoma can be effectively managed with a window resection of the involved tracheal cartilage and intercartilaginous space. To minimize potential postoperative tracheomalacia and stenosis, a regional myofascial flap, based on the sternocleidomastoid muscle, can be effectively rotated into the defect for repair. Placement of a temporary

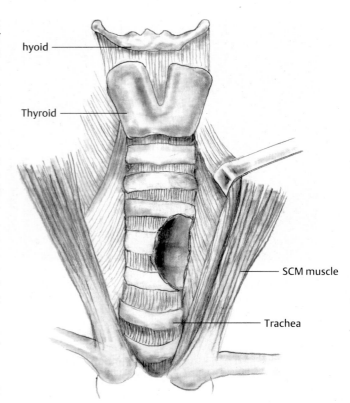

Fig. 12.5 The margins of the resection after removal of the involved tracheal rings. SCM, sternocleidomastoid.

Labels in figure: hyoid, Thyroid, SCM muscle, Trachea

tracheostomy may be necessary to maintain an adequate airway in the perioperative setting. Larger anterior wall defects that involve up to six tracheal rings should be reconstructed with rib cartilage, ensuring that that the grafted perichondrium is placed intraluminally to prevent postoperative granulation. The use of a temporary tracheal stent, with or without free mucosal grafts, has been advocated to ensure the success of the reconstruction, without excessive granulation and cicatrix formation.

When greater than 50% of the tracheal circumference or more than six tracheal rings are invaded by tumor, total resection of the involved segment with primary anastomosis must be performed (**Figs. 12.6** and **12.7**). Meticulous surgical technique, using interrupted submucosal sutures, is necessary to prevent postoperative granulation tissue and scar formation, which will render the reconstruction nonfunctional (**Figs. 12.8** to **12.10**). Close collaboration with the anesthesiology team is critical for maintenance of the airway during reconstruction. Closure can be facilitated by mediastinal dissection of the anterior tracheal wall down to the carina. Care must be taken to avoid devascularizing the trachea with lateral dissection. An additional 5 cm of length can be obtained with a suprahyoid release, at the expense of increased risk of postoperative aspiration (**Fig. 12.11**). Tracheal resection can usually be performed without the need for a tracheostomy tube, but one should not hesitate to place one, out of concern for the reconstruction, if needed for pulmonary toilet or

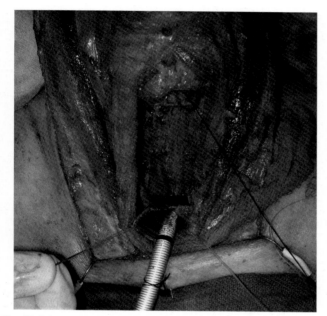

Fig. 12.6 Intraoperative view of a partial tracheal resection for invasive thyroid carcinoma.

airway control. The decision to extubate the patient at the end of the procedure should take into consideration the skills and experience of the surgical and anesthesiology teams. Postoperatively, these patients are at an increased risk of aspiration, infection, obstruction, and fistula formation.

Alternatively, there has been recent interest in the use of vascularized free tissue transfer techniques for the reconstruction of large circumferential tracheal defects. This approach is particularly useful in the reoperative setting, when scarring and previous resections may limit the ability to perform and end-to-end anastomosis.[29] The pliable radial forearm free flap can be tubed around a flexible tracheal stent, or may be used as an epithelial lining for an external tracheal scaffold. Disadvantages of this approach include absence of a mucosal lining, pooling of secretions, mucus plugging, and the risk of infection. The long-term outcome of this reconstructive approach remains to be seen.

Occasionally, patients with thyroid cancer may present with unresectable airway disease. Palliative stenting with endotracheal resection is often necessary to establish the airway and bypass the obstructing lesion. Repeated endoscopic ablative procedures, with either laser or cold techniques, are indicated for comfort measures and can temporarily relieve the chronic dyspnea and obstruction. The addition of tracheal

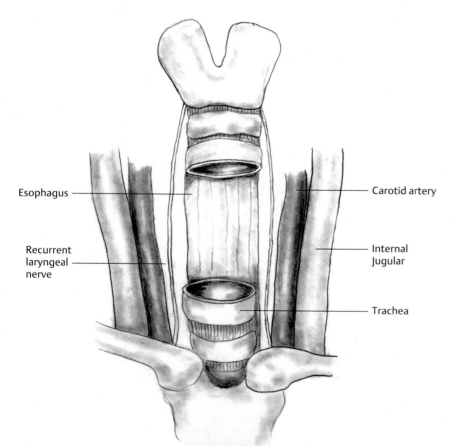

Esophagus

Recurrent laryngeal nerve

Carotid artery

Internal Jugular

Trachea

Fig. 12.7 To ensure an adequate end-to-end anastomosis, tracheal rings that are involved with tumor are completely resected. Note the intact party wall, and preserved recurrent laryngeal nerves. Bilateral paratracheal node dissections have also been performed.

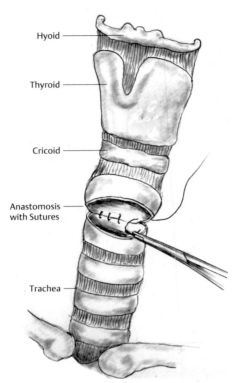

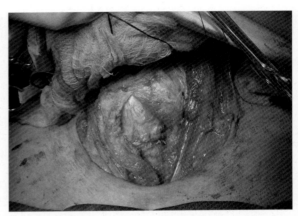

Fig. 12.9 Intraoperative view of the end-to-end tracheal anastomosis.

Fig. 12.8 Reconstruction of the trachea after a full-thickness resection of multiple tracheal rings. The posterior wall of the trachea is closed using interrupted sutures. The lateral tracheal walls are closed using submucosally placed absorbable sutures, with the knots tied extraluminally.

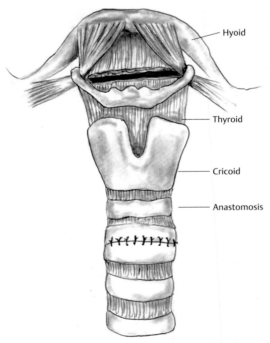

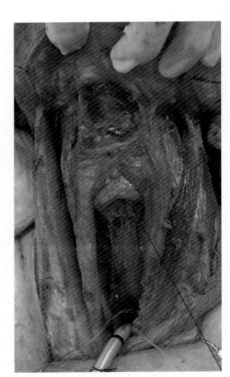

Fig. 12.10 Completed tracheal reconstruction, with end-to-end anastomosis. Note the suprahyoid release, which was necessary for a tension-free closure. The mylohyoid musculature is dissected from the hyoid bone, allowing the laryngotracheal complex to descend approximately 5 cm.

Fig. 12.11 Intraoperative view of the resection and the suprahyoid release.

stenting or a Montgomery T-tube can provide further symptom control to this group of patients.

A lack of uniformity in reporting results in the literature makes it difficult to provide concrete survival statistics for patients with locally aggressive thyroid cancer. Nonetheless, it is clear that invasion of the aerodigestive tract portends a high rate of local recurrence, distant metastasis, and poor survival. McCaffrey[30] recently determined that among patients with locally invasive thyroid tumors, those with either laryngeal or tracheal involvement had a decrement in overall survival. Among patients in whom complete resection is possible, a 5-year survival benefit between 60% and 80% is possible.[15,17,31–33] This decreases when gross tumor extirpation is not possible.

Internal Jugular Vein/Carotid Artery

It is uncommon for vascular invasion with thyroid cancer to incur physical symptoms, unless gross invasion of the internal or common carotid arteries is present (**Fig. 12.12**). Carotid encasement may present with mental status changes and neurologic insults, which suggest stenosis or thrombosis. Resection of the internal jugular vein can be safely performed

when necessary.[34] When tumor involves the carotid artery, reconstruction is necessary.

Surgical Management of Pharyngoesophageal Invasion

Posterior extension of thyroid carcinoma to involve the hypopharynx and cervical esophagus is rare and may be difficult to distinguish from extrinsic tumor compression. Patients may complain only of dysphagia, but, with more aggressive disease, hematemesis and esophageal obstruction may ensue. In most instances, the tumor invades the muscular wall; however, transmural or intraluminal extension is rare.[35] Esophagoscopy or barium swallow should be performed when there is concern that tumor has spread to the esophagus.

When thyroid cancer invades the esophagus, extensive resection and reconstruction is often necessary. Cervical esophagectomy is a morbid procedure, necessitating reconstruction with a tubed radial forearm or jejunal free tissue transfer for small defects. However, in most situations, only the muscular wall is invaded, allowing for preservation of the mucosa and submucosa.[14] The defect can then be reinforced

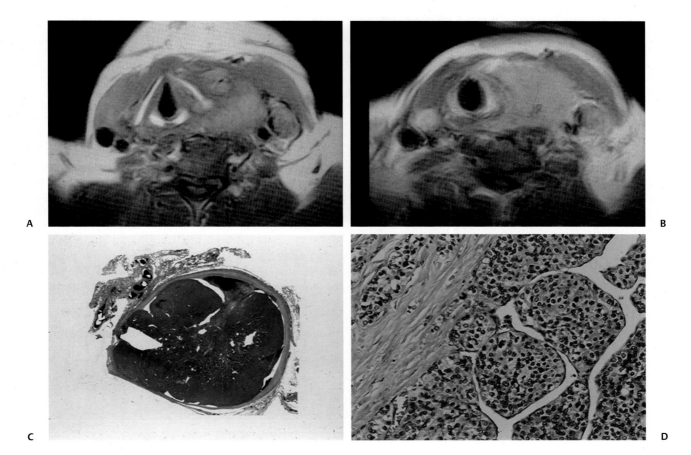

Fig. 12.12 (A,B) T1-weighted MRI of the neck in a patient with a left thyroid carcinoma, demonstrating occlusion of the internal jugular vein with intramural thrombus. (**C**) Low-power photomicrograph of the resected internal jugular vein, with complete obliteration of the vessel lumen with tumor. (**D**) High-power view demonstrating invasion of the vessel wall by tumor.

with a pedicled muscle flap interposed between the esophagus and the trachea and carotid sheath. When the distal anastomosis extends below the thoracic inlet, total esophagectomy with gastric pull-up is required for adequate local control. These procedures pose high risks of morbidity and mortality to the patient, and the patient's general medical fitness and overall survival must be taken into account. Regardless of the treatment plan, ensuring adequate nutritional intake with placement of an enteral feeding tube, either via gastrostomy or jejunostomy, should not be neglected.

The Role of Radioactive Iodine Therapy

It is becoming increasingly clear that adjuvant treatments are necessary after definitive surgical resection for the management of well-differentiated thyroid cancer. Retrospective reviews suggest that postoperative radioactive iodine (RAI) ablation decreases the risk of local recurrences, regional metastasis, and distant spread. Further, combined therapy, utilizing surgery, RAI, and thyroid suppression, has been shown to improve overall survival from this disease.[3] Other indications for the use of iodine 131 (I-131) include therapeutic management of pulmonary metastasis, ablation of thyroid remnants, and the treatment of cervical recurrences.[10] In general, RAI is effective for lesions less than 1 cm in size; when I-131 treatment fails, or when lesions enlarge, surgical resection is indicated.

Radioactive iodine is effective in ablating microscopic cervical disease after thyroidectomy, and for residual thyroid tissue that persists after surgical resection. The rationale for this multimodality treatment paradigm rests on the need for biochemical monitoring with thyroglobulin, the transformative potential of residual thyroid tissue, and the risk of recurrences from microscopic nests of tumor.[10] With an improvement in overall survival as the primary goal, I-131 is an effective adjuvant treatment in the postoperative setting, although this is controversital.[5,36]

Complications of I-131 therapy are minor, and are limited to xerostomia and transient gonadal failure. Rarely, patients may develop leukemia, usually when radioactive dosages exceed 500 mCi. In summary, RAI is an effective modality in the treatment armamentarium for thyroid carcinoma, particularly in the postoperative and recurrent settings.

External Beam Radiation Therapy

Patients with locally advanced thyroid cancer should receive additional therapy to control microscopic disease, prevent locoregional recurrences, and reduce the risk of distant metastases. Options include radioactive iodine therapy and external beam radiation (EBRT). Certainly, all patients with iodine-avid invasive thyroid cancers should be treated with I-131 and suppressive exogenous thyroxine.[37] There are scant data in the literature on the use of EBRT for the management of WDTC. A recent retrospective review at a single institution demonstrated that patients with microscopic margins who had received EBRT had improvement in locoregional control, compared with patients with grossly positive disease.[38] Others have shown that for patients with microscopic disease, EBRT improved locoregional control of disease.[37] Although limited, these data suggest that EBRT may be beneficial in a small group of patients. Those patients with WDTC who may benefit from post-operative irradiation include those with previously resected tumors but with persistent microscopic disease, regional metastases with poor pathologic features, unresectable cervical disease, and aggressive histologic subtypes, such as tall cell variant and Hürthle cell carcinomas. Although no prospective studies have been undertaken, EBRT is felt to be beneficial for patients with extrathyroidal extension of tumor, as they have a high risk of recurrence in the thyroid bed. Further, patients who have involved microscopic margins on final pathologic analysis may also benefit from external beam radiation.[39] As no clear consensus exists regarding the appropriate indications for EBRT in these patients, therapeutic planning is at the discretion of the multidisciplinary team.

Conclusion

The management of thyroid cancer is complex, with little agreement in the literature over the extent of treatment necessary. This is primarily due to the lack of prospective studies and the good prognosis these patients enjoy. Despite the infrequent incidence of locally aggressive thyroid cancers, careful attention to presenting signs and symptoms should alert the surgeon to the presence of upper aerodigestive tract involvement. Thorough evaluation with imaging and endoscopy is warranted to determine the extent of disease and helps guide the surgeon in determining the extent of resection needed. The primary goals of treatment should be (1) complete tumor eradication and (2) minimization of patient morbidity. Adjuvant therapies, including radioactive iodine and external beam radiation, should be considered in all management strategies to maximize local control and minimize distant metastasis.

References

1. American Association of Clinical Endocrinologists and American College of Endocrinology. Medical/surgical guidelines for clinical practice: management of thyroid carcinoma. Endocr Pract 2001;7:202–220

2. Kouvaraki MA, Shapiro SE, Lee JE, Evans DB, Perrier ND. Surgical management of thyroid carcinoma. J Natl Compr Canc Netw 2005;3:458–466

3. Mazzaferri EL, Kloos RT. Clinical review 128: current approaches to

primary therapy for papillary and follicular thyroid cancer. J Clin Endocrinol Metab 2001;86:1447–1463

4. Shaha AR. Implications of prognostic factors and risk groups in the management of differentiated thyroid cancer. Laryngoscope 2004;114:393–402

5. Mazzaferri EL, Jhiang SM. Long-term impact of initial surgical and medical therapy on papillary and follicular thyroid cancer. Am J Med 1994;97:418–428

6. Shaha AR, Shah JP, Loree TR. Low-risk differentiated thyroid cancer: the need for selective treatment. Ann Surg Oncol 1997;4:328–333

7. Hay ID, Grant CS, Bergstralh EJ, Thompson GB, van Heerden JA, Goellner JR. Unilateral total lobectomy: is it sufficient surgical treatment for patients with AMES low-risk papillary thyroid carcinoma? Surgery 1998;124:958–964 discussion 964–956

8. Shah JP, Loree TR, Dharker D, Strong EW. Lobectomy versus total thyroidectomy for differentiated carcinoma of the thyroid: a matched-pair analysis. Am J Surg 1993;166:331–335

9. Kupferman ME, Mandel SJ, DiDonato L, Wolf P, Weber RS. Safety of completion thyroidectomy following unilateral lobectomy for well-differentiated thyroid cancer. Laryngoscope 2002;112(7 pt 1):1209–1212

10. Robbins RJ, Schlumberger MJ. The evolving role of (131)I for the treatment of differentiated thyroid carcinoma. J Nucl Med 2005;46(suppl 1):28S–37S

11. Mazzaferri EL, Robbins RJ, Spencer CA, et al. A consensus report of the role of serum thyroglobulin as a monitoring method for low-risk patients with papillary thyroid carcinoma. J Clin Endocrinol Metab 2003;88:1433–1441

12. Delbridge L. Total thyroidectomy: the evolution of surgical technique. ANZ J Surg 2003;73:761–768

13. Tollefsen HR, Decosse JJ, Hutter RV. Papillary carcinoma of the thyroid. A clinical and pathological study of 70 fatal cases. Cancer 1964;17:1035–1044

14. Hammoud ZT, Mathisen DJ. Surgical management of thyroid carcinoma invading the trachea. Chest Surg Clin N Am 2003;13:359–367

15. McCaffrey TV, Bergstralh EJ, Hay ID. Locally invasive papillary thyroid carcinoma: 1940–1990. Head Neck 1994;16:165–172

16. McConahey WM, Hay ID, Woolner LB, van Heerden JA, Taylor WF. Papillary thyroid cancer treated at the Mayo Clinic, 1946 through 1970: initial manifestations, pathologic findings, therapy, and outcome. Mayo Clin Proc 1986;61:978–996

17. Kowalski LP, Filho JG. Results of the treatment of locally invasive thyroid carcinoma. Head Neck 2002;24:340–344

18. D'Avanzo A, Treseler P, Ituarte PH, et al. Follicular thyroid carcinoma: histology and prognosis. Cancer 2004;100:1123–1129

19. Lopez-Penabad L, Chiu AC, Hoff AO, et al. Prognostic factors in patients with Hurthle cell neoplasms of the thyroid. Cancer 2003;97:1186–1194

20. Machens A, Hinze R, Dralle H. Surgery on the cervicovisceral axis for invasive thyroid cancer. Langenbecks Arch Surg 2001;386:318–323

21. Breaux GP, Guillamondegui OM. Treatment of locally invasive carcinoma of the thyroid: how radical? Am J Surg 1980;140:514–517

22. Grillo HC, Suen HC, Mathisen DJ, Wain JC. Resectional management of thyroid carcinoma invading the airway. Ann Thorac Surg 1992;54:3–9, discussion 9–10

23. Yamamura N, Fukushima S, Nakao K, et al. Relation between ultrasonographic and histologic findings of tracheal invasion by differentiated thyroid cancer. World J Surg 2002;26:1071–1073

24. Rietzel E, Chen GTY, Choi NC, Willet CG. Four-dimensional image-based treatment planning: target volume segmentation and dose calculation in the presence of respiratory motion. Int J Radiat Oncol Biol Phys 2005;61:1535–1550

25. Czaja JM, McCaffrey TV. The surgical management of laryngotracheal invasion by well-differentiated papillary thyroid carcinoma. Arch Otolaryngol Head Neck Surg 1997;123:484–490

26. Kim MK, Mandel SH, Baloch Z, et al. Morbidity following central compartment reoperation for recurrent or persistent thyroid cancer. Arch Otolaryngol Head Neck Surg 2004;130:1214–1216

27. Park CS, Suh KW, Min JS. Cartilage-shaving procedure for the control of tracheal cartilage invasion by thyroid carcinoma. Head Neck 1993;15:289–291

28. Friedman M. Surgical management of thyroid carcinoma with laryngotracheal invasion. Otolaryngol Clin North Am 1990;23:495–507

29. Beldholm BR, Wilson MK, Gallagher RM, Caminer D, King MJ, Glanville A. Reconstruction of the trachea with a tubed radial forearm free flap. J Thorac Cardiovasc Surg 2003;126:545–550

30. McCaffrey JC. Aerodigestive tract invasion by well-differentiated thyroid carcinoma: diagnosis, management, prognosis, and biology. Laryngoscope 2006;116:1–11

31. Bayles SW, Kingdom TT, Carlson GW. Management of thyroid carcinoma invading the aerodigestive tract. Laryngoscope 1998;108:1402–1407

32. Kasperbauer JL. Locally advanced thyroid carcinoma. Ann Otol Rhinol Laryngol 2004;113:749–753

33. Ballantyne AJ. Resections of the upper aerodigestive tract for locally invasive thyroid cancer. Am J Surg 1994;168:636–639

34. Leong JL, Yuen HW, LiVolsi VA, et al. Insular carcinoma of the thyroid with jugular vein invasion. Head Neck 2004;26:642–646

35. Gillenwater AM, Goepfert H. Surgical management of laryngotracheal and esophageal involvement by locally advanced thyroid cancer. Semin Surg Oncol 1999;16:19–29

36. Hay ID, McConahey WM, Goellner JR. Managing patients with papillary thyroid carcinoma: insights gained from the Mayo Clinic's experience of treating 2,512 consecutive patients during 1940 through 2000. Trans Am Clin Climatol Assoc 2002;113:241–260

37. Tsang RW, Brierley JD, Simpson WJ, Panzarella T, Gospodarowicz MK, Sutcliffe SB. The effects of surgery, radioiodine, and external radiation therapy on the clinical outcome of patients with differentiated thyroid carcinoma. Cancer 1998;82:375–388

38. Meadows KM, Amdur RJ, Morris CG, Villaret DB, Mazzaferri EL, Mendenhall WM. External beam radiotherapy for differentiated thyroid cancer. Am J Otolaryngol 2006;27:24–28

39. Brierley JD, Tsang RW. External-beam radiation therapy in the treatment of differentiated thyroid cancer. Semin Surg Oncol 1999;16:42–49

13 Management of the Neck in Thyroid Cancer

Stephen Y. Lai and Jonas T. Johnson

The incidence of cervical metastases in thyroid cancer patients is quite high, especially in papillary and medullary thyroid carcinoma.[1-4] Many patients with papillary thyroid carcinoma may initially present with a solitary neck mass. In the pediatric population, lymph node metastasis can occur in as many as 80% of cases.[5,6] The size of the primary lesion is a poor predictor of regional metastasis, leading to questions related to the preoperative assessment and intraoperative treatment of cervical lymph nodes.

The management of regional metastasis in patients with well-differentiated thyroid cancer has evolved from the selective removal of involved cervical lymph nodes ("berry-picking") to more comprehensive neck dissection. General guidelines have been developed regarding the extent of dissection needed in patients with palpable and histologically demonstrated lymph node metastases. Questions still remain regarding the necessity and effectiveness of elective dissection of cervical lymph nodes.

The difficulty with resolving such issues is related to the nature of thyroid cancer. The overall incidence of well-differentiated thyroid cancer is relatively low. The generally indolent course of thyroid cancer results in a need for large patient cohorts and prolonged follow-up periods of at least 10 years to detect clinically significant differences related to clinical interventions. Such studies become impractical to undertake and complete. Additionally, in most available studies, lymph node metastases appear to have a comparatively small impact on patient survival.

Prognostic Significance of Lymph Node Metastasis

Although the presence of regional metastasis in other head and neck cancers decreases 5-year survival by nearly 50%, the impact of cervical lymph node metastasis on patient survival is less clear with well-differentiated thyroid cancer. Many early studies suggested that regional metastases had no adverse effect on the survival of patients with papillary carcinoma.[7-11] However, these studies had some variability in their initial treatment of cervical disease, may not have adequately controlled for patient age in the survival analysis, and lacked sufficient follow-up time. A landmark study of 1355 patients by Mazzaferri and Jhiang[12] with follow-up of 10 to 30 years demonstrated a statistically significant increase in the 30-year cancer-specific mortality rate in patients with cervical metastases (10%), as compared with those without metastases (6%).

The current general consensus is that cervical metastases increase the risk of local recurrence and cancer-specific mortality in older patients (>45 years old).[13] Children and adolescents appear to do well regardless of the extent of disease at diagnosis or the presence of regional/distant metastases or recurrent disease.[5,14] Bilateral or mediastinal metastases are especially concerning. Additionally, extracapsular invasion or fixation to cervical structures are significant for worse patient outcome.[12,15]

Lymph Node Drainage and Pattern of Metastasis

Lymphatic drainage from the thyroid gland appears to follow three main routes[16] (**Fig. 13.1**). The inferior medial aspect of the thyroid lobe drains via the inferior thyroid veins to the primary echelon nodes located in the pretracheal, prelaryngeal (Delphian), paratracheal (level VI), and lower jugular (level IV) regions (**Fig. 13.2**). Secondary drainage leads to the nodes of the anterior-superior mediastinum (level VII). Within the lateral portion of the gland, lymphatic drainage follows the middle thyroid vein to the upper, middle, and lower jugular lymph nodes (levels II to IV). Superior thyroid and isthmus lymphatic drainage is directed to the prelaryngeal and midjugular nodes (level III).

Although the lymphatic drainage of the thyroid gland appears to be quite orderly, regional metastatic spread of thyroid carcinoma is less predictable. In one study of papillary thyroid cancer, patients were treated with total thyroidectomy and bilateral modified radical neck dissection (MRND).[17] This study did not demonstrate any correlation between the location of the primary tumor within the thyroid with the site of lymph node metastases.

Regional metastasis usually involves the paratracheal nodes regardless of the primary tumor location in the thyroid gland.[1,18] Involvement of the paratracheal lymph nodes does not appear to predict involvement of lateral cervical lymph nodes, suggesting that "skip" lesions to levels II to V are quite common.[7] Papillary carcinoma metastases to the jugular chain of lymph nodes are quite common: level II (30%), level III (45%), level IV (52%), and level V (33%).[1,6] In several studies, 9 to 18% of patients with normal paratracheal nodes had metastases present in the lateral neck.[17,19] Thus

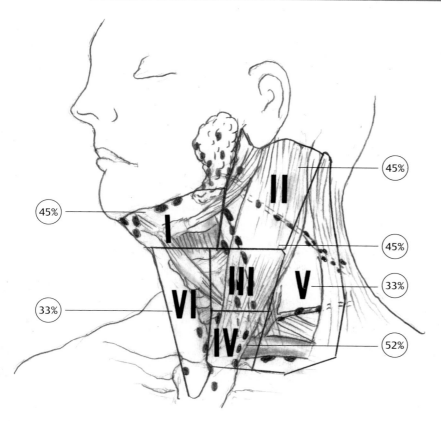

Fig. 13.1 Standard anatomic classification of the cervical lymphatics. The percentages noted with the anatomic levels indicate the frequency of disease found at a specific level when cervical metastases are present (I through VI).

the presence of metastatic disease in the paratracheal region (level VI) is not predictive of disease in the other regions of the neck.

In patients with unilateral papillary thyroid cancer, bilateral or contralateral (unilateral) metastases can be demonstrated in 24% of patients.[20] The risk of contralateral jugular node metastasis appears to be higher when metastases are present in the contralateral paratracheal nodes (38%). The risk of bilateral nodal involvement is even higher in patients with extensive cancer involvement in the thyroid gland, extension of disease into the isthmus, and recurrent tumors.

Risk Factors

Several clinical features have been associated with metastasis of thyroid cancer to the cervical lymph nodes. The association between tumor size and the risk of lymph node metastasis is not clear. Large tumors may occur without metastasis, whereas microscopic lesions may present with extensive bilateral cervical involvement. Examination of a large patient cohort at the Mayo Clinic did not reveal any correlation between tumor size and the development of lymph node metastases.[21] In thyroid cancer patients who have extrathyroidal extension or vascular invasion, the incidence of lymph node metastasis is higher.[21,22] In this situation, males seem to be at particular risk.[23]

Papillary carcinoma has an incidence of clinically detectable lymph node metastasis that ranges from 30 to

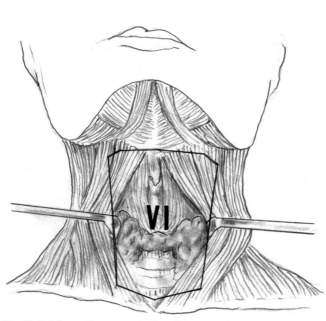

Fig. 13.2 Schematic representation of the central compartment. A central compartment neck dissection refers to the removal of lymph nodes surrounding the midline structures of the anterior neck. These lymph nodes include the precricoid (Delphian), pretracheal, paratracheal, and perithyroidal nodes.

90%.[1,2] A palpable cervical lymph node is a common presenting feature in approximately 20% of patients with thyroid papillary microcarcinoma (<10 mm).[24] The incidence of subclinical regional metastasis is similarly high.[19,25] Interestingly, the risk of developing lymph node metastases from the follicular variant of papillary carcinoma is lower than from the pure papillary variant.[26]

Metastasis of medullary thyroid carcinoma is similarly high, with rates ranging from 50 to 81%.[3,4] In contrast, follicular thyroid carcinomas are associated with lymph node metastases in only 12 to 30% of patients.[2,27] Hürthle cell carcinomas, a subtype of follicular carcinoma, demonstrate a similar rate of regional metastasis in 10 to 21% of patients, but are associated with a higher risk of distant metastases.[28,29]

Assessment of the Neck in Thyroid Cancer Patients

When a patient with thyroid cancer presents initially with a solitary neck mass, evaluation begins with a fine-needle aspiration biopsy (FNAB) to confirm the diagnosis of metastatic thyroid cancer. Subsequent evaluation includes imaging of the thyroid by ultrasound to identify the location of the primary lesion, and imaging of the neck in an attempt to characterize additional disease burden that may be unilateral or bilateral.

In considering the assessment of the neck in patients with thyroid cancer, two additional scenarios need to be considered: preoperative evaluation of the clinically negative neck (N0) and follow-up surveillance in patients after initial treatment for thyroid cancer. In addition to serum thyroglobulin level and whole-body radioiodine scan, cervical ultrasound examination has been used for monitoring patients for recurrent differentiated thyroid cancer.[30] Recent studies of cervical ultrasound examination have demonstrated that clinical "recurrence" in the cervical lymph nodes may have been persistent or residual disease.[31,32] These findings suggest that preoperative cervical ultrasonography may have identified metastatic disease and potentially prevented the subsequent "recurrence" and need for additional treatment. The detection of nonpalpable lymph nodes in the preoperative ultrasound examination could allow for cervical node dissection in the initial surgical treatment of patients with thyroid cancer. Additionally, in low-risk patients, cervical ultrasound examination may replace whole-body radioiodine scan.[32] Ultrasound examination is more sensitive for detecting cervical recurrence, and confirmation can be obtained with an ultrasound-guided FNAB.

Other imaging modalities have been examined for use in the preoperative assessment of cervical lymph nodes. Technetium-99m (Tc-99m) methoxyisobutyl isonitrile (MIBI) scans have been examined for the ability to detect nodal metastases following thyroidectomy.[33] Similarly, investigators have examined the utility of fluorodeoxyglucose positron emission tomography (FDG-PET).[34] FDG-PET may be useful in the posttreatment monitoring, especially

in patients who have elevated serum thyroglobulin and a negative whole-body iodine-131 (I-131) scan.[35] Although preliminary studies have been interesting, neither imaging modality is presently consistent enough to be useful in the preoperative assessment of the clinically N0 neck in thyroid cancer patients.

Some surgeons have promoted the sampling of cervical lymph nodes intraoperatively to guide management of the neck. A few studies have demonstrated the ability to detect sentinel lymph nodes in thyroid cancer patients.[36–38] However, these studies did not include any additional neck dissection so that the false-negative rate of this technique could not be determined. Thus the utility of sentinel lymph node biopsy in thyroid cancer remains uncertain.

Lymph node dissection from the pretracheal and paratracheal regions is often performed in papillary thyroid cancer patients, especially when the patient fits high-risk criteria, including age greater than 45 years and large (>4 cm) or locally invasive primary tumors.[20,39,40] Some surgeons advocate frozen section analysis of this specimen to determine treatment of the lateral neck.[41–43] Although these nodes represent the first echelon of lymphatic drainage, the presence of metastatic disease within these lymph nodes is not predictive of metastatic disease to the lateral compartment of the neck (levels II to V). Several studies have demonstrated that in up to 18% of thyroid cancer patients, metastatic disease can be present in the lateral neck even when the paratracheal lymph nodes are disease-free.[17,19] These findings raise serious question as to the reliability of paratracheal node sampling in determining treatment of the lateral neck.

Management of the Clinically Negative Neck (N0)

There is currently no clear role for elective nodal dissection in follicular thyroid carcinoma, which tends to spread through hematogenous routes. In patients with papillary carcinoma or medullary carcinoma, the indications for elective nodal dissection remain to be clearly defined. Management of the paratracheal (level VI) and upper mediastinal (level VII) regions is more subject to debate than management of the lateral neck compartment (levels II to V).[44] Elective dissection of the pretracheal and ipsilateral paratracheal lymph nodes is typically performed in these patients, especially those with high-risk factors. Patients who have cancer involving the isthmus or both lobes of the thyroid gland or those who have suspected disease present by palpation or visual inspection in the pretracheal or paratracheal regions will have concurrent pretracheal and bilateral paratracheal (central compartment) lymph node dissection with a total thyroidectomy or completion thyroid lobectomy. Nodal disease within the lateral neck tends to grow quite large without involvement of the internal jugular vein, sternocleidomastoid muscle, or the spinal accessory nerve (cranial nerve [CN] XI). Within the central compartment, metastases tend to be more invasive and can involve the recurrent laryngeal nerve (RLN), trachea, or esophagus at a relatively early stage.[41] Elective removal may prevent recurrence in a lymph node and reduce the likelihood of injury to the RLN and parathyroid glands, which would be at risk in a reoperative setting.

Central Compartment Dissection

Central compartment dissection should include the prelaryngeal (Delphian) lymph nodes and bilateral paratracheal and upper mediastinal lymph nodes. The dissection is performed through the standard low-collar incision made for the thyroidectomy. Following removal of the thyroid gland or completion thyroid lobectomy, the jugular vein and the common carotid artery are retracted laterally (**Fig. 13.3**). The fatty areolar tissue between the carotid laterally and the trachea and esophagus medially is dissected and divided between clamps as low as possible in the neck. Special attention is given on the left side to avoid injury to the thoracic duct. The lymph node–containing tissue in the paratracheal and upper mediastinal regions is elevated superiorly and medially over the trachea to include the prelaryngeal lymph nodes. The lymphatic tissue should be removed en bloc from

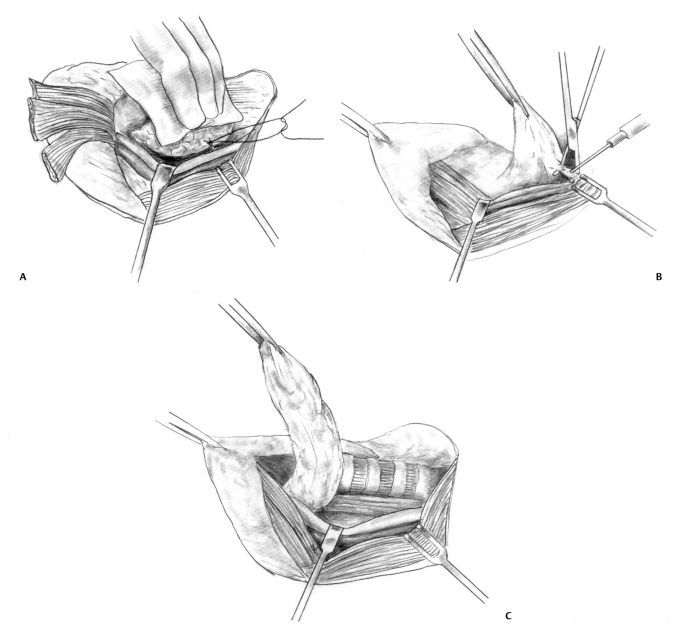

Fig. 13.3 Central compartment lymph node dissection. (**A,B**) Retraction of the internal jugular vein and the common carotid artery permits access to the fibroadipose tissue between the great vessels laterally and the trachea and esophagus medially. The specimen is divided as low in the neck as possible. (**C**) Upon completion, the lymph nodes have been removed from the central compartment that is bounded by the hyoid bone, suprasternal notch, and the carotid arteries.

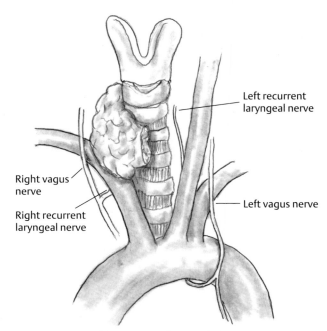

Right vagus nerve

Right recurrent laryngeal nerve

Left recurrent laryngeal nerve

Left vagus nerve

Fig. 13.4 Location of the recurrent laryngeal nerves. During dissection of the central compartment, the recurrent laryngeal nerve may be more easily identified deep to the common carotid artery than in a thyroid bed with postoperative scarring.

the level of the cricoid to the innominate artery. The RLN, inferior thyroid artery, and parathyroid glands should be clearly identified. In cases of repeat surgery, the RLN can be difficult to identify in the thyroid bed due to postsurgical scarring. Dissection in the paratracheal region may facilitate identification of the RLN as it passes deep to the common carotid artery and into the thoracic cavity (**Fig. 13.4**).

Preservation of the parathyroid glands can be difficult when performing bilateral central compartment lymph node dissection. Efforts should be made during the dissection to identify and preserve the ascending branch of the inferior thyroid artery that supplies the superior parathyroid gland, especially on the contralateral side when there is a primary unilateral thyroid lesion. If the vascular supply to the parathyroid is compromised, the gland should be biopsied and verified by frozen tissue analysis. The parathyroid gland should be minced into small pieces and placed within a pocket in the sternocleidomastoid muscle.

The decision to perform a central compartment dissection needs to balance the possible consequences of disease recurrence in this region with the potential morbidity related to RLN injury or hypoparathyroidism. A retrospective comparison of patients who were treated with a total thyroidectomy alone or with a central compartment dissection demonstrated that the nodal dissection did not increase the risk of RLN paresis, but did increase the risk of transient and permanent hypoparathyroidism.[40] Given these risks, the presence of papillary thyroid cancer alone does not justify routine central compartment dissection in all of these patients.

Lateral Compartment Dissection

The role of elective cervical node dissection has been more clearly established for medullary thyroid carcinoma. Given the frequency of microscopic spread and the lack of radioiodine uptake, elective central compartment lymph node dissection is commonly performed.[45] When these patients present with palpable anterior cervical lymphadenopathy, bilateral central compartment dissection is performed with the total thyroidectomy and the lateral cervical nodes are carefully inspected. An ipsilateral comprehensive neck dissection should be considered. Removal of the contralateral neck lymph nodes should be considered when the primary lesion is 2 cm or greater because bilateral neck dissection may improve regional control.[3]

Currently, there is no clear evidence that would support elective cervical neck dissection for patients with papillary or follicular thyroid carcinoma. As previously described, there is no predictable pattern for cervical node metastasis. The involvement of multiple cervical levels and skip lesions is present in at least one third of patients with papillary carcinoma.[17,46,47] Thus any elective procedure with the intent to remove all nodal metastases and decrease the likelihood of recurrence would require comprehensive dissection of levels II through VII.

In Japan, some surgeons advocate performing an elective modified radical neck dissection in patients with papillary thyroid carcinomas larger than 1 cm. The basis of this practice appears to be several retrospective studies that demonstrated improved patient survival when patients with papillary thyroid cancer were treated with thyroidectomy and comprehensive neck dissection (levels II through VI), rather than selective node plucking or "berry picking."[47,48] The authors of these studies analyzed the survival of patients with and without palpable metastases (N+ and N0), but did not stratify the data accordingly. Thus the findings may not directly support the more common use of elective modified radical neck dissection.

Most surgeons do not currently support elective lateral neck dissection in patients with well-differentiated thyroid cancer. The biologic significance of subclinical cervical metastases remains unclear. Elective neck dissection in papillary thyroid cancer patients has demonstrated the presence of microscopic disease in up to 90% of cervical lymph nodes.[25,39,49] However, the development of recurrent disease in a similar cohort of patients who do not have elective neck dissections is only 7 to 15%.[42,50,51] Additionally, the effect of nodal dissection on overall survival is not clear. Thus performing a neck dissection once regional metastases are detected does not seem to affect patient prognosis.[41,52,53]

Management of the Clinically Positive Neck (N+)

Selective cervical lymph node excision or "berry-picking" is not appropriate in thyroid cancer patients with regional

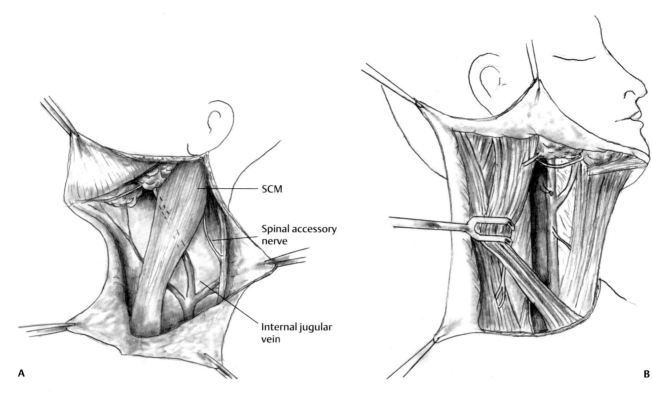

A

B

Fig. 13.5 Comprehensive functional neck dissection. (**A,B**) The removal of cervical lymphatics from levels II through VII is advocated in patients with metastatic well-differentiated thyroid carcinoma. The spinal accessory nerve (cranial nerve [CN] XI), internal jugular vein, and sternocleidomastoid (SCM) muscle are typically preserved.

metastases. The presence of clinically palpable disease in a single cervical lymph node is strongly suggestive of additional ipsilateral metastatic disease.[17,54] With the limited removal of a single metastatic node, patients are at unnecessary risk for disease recurrence and the need for repeat surgery. Although some surgeons have suggested dissection limited to an involved level of the neck, this approach also seems inadequate given the likelihood of multilevel nodal involvement and skip metastases.

When palpable lateral cervical nodes are present and metastatic disease is confirmed by fine-needle aspiration cytology (FNAC), a comprehensive functional neck dissection, including levels II through VII, should be performed with preservation of the spinal accessory nerve (CN XI), the internal jugular vein, and the sternocleidomastoid muscle[55–57] (**Fig. 13.5**). If enlarged lymph nodes are not clinically identified in the preoperative assessment and are encountered intraoperatively, the suspicious nodes are examined by frozen section analysis and a comprehensive functional neck dissection is performed when metastatic disease is verified (**Fig. 13.6**). The submandibular and submental nodes (level I) are rarely involved and should only be dissected when there is clinically positive disease in this region.[58,59] The incidence of contralateral subclinical metastasis is less than 20%.[60] Therefore, elective neck dissection of the contralateral neck is not advocated.

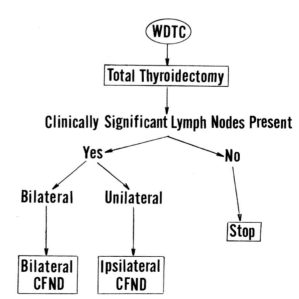

Fig. 13.6 Algorithm for the management of lymph node metastases from well-differentiated thyroid carcinoma (WDTC). Clinically significant lymph nodes may be identified during the preoperative or intraoperative assessment. *Abbreviation:* CFND, comprehensive functional neck dissection (levels II to VII).

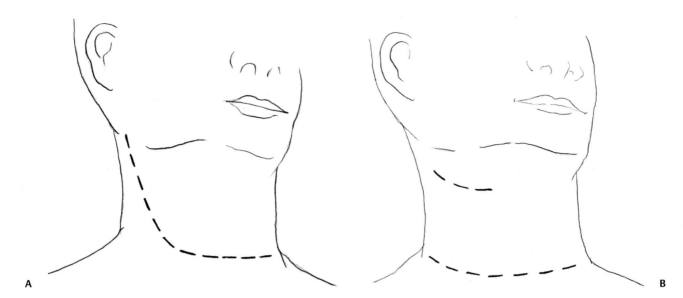

Fig. 13.7 Commonly employed incisions for thyroidectomy and concurrent neck dissection. (**A**) A thyroidectomy incision is extended in a hockey-stick fashion. (**B**) A modified MacFee incision. The thyroidec- tomy incision is extended laterally to the anterior border of the trapez- ius. A smaller, upper incision provides adequate exposure to the upper neck.

The authors typically extend a utility apron flap from the original thyroidectomy incision to perform the comprehensive functional neck dissection (**Fig. 13.7**). Raising the cervical flap above the mastoid tip provides excellent exposure of the lateral neck. Other surgeons advocate an extended transverse cervical incision for cosmetic considerations. In this instance, a smaller, parallel incision, 2 to 3 cm below the angle of the mandible provides adequate exposure for the dissection of the upper jugular and upper posterior triangle regions (modified MacFee incision) (**Fig. 13.7**). Careful inspection and dissection should be performed along the spinal accessory nerve (CN XI), as this is a common site of metastatic thyroid disease.[61] Although metastases in the cervical lymph nodes can grow quite large without local invasion, a more extensive modified radical neck dissection and possibly even a radical neck dissection is required in the setting of gross extension of primary or metastatic disease involving vital neck structures.

In patients with medullary thyroid cancer, lymph node metastasis can be present in up to 81% of cases.[3] Palpable cervical disease necessitates both central compartment dissection (VI) and bilateral comprehensive neck dissection (II–V). Given the higher likelihood of disease-specific death in this form of thyroid cancer, there is no controversy in this clinical situation, and we employ a utility apron incision from mastoid tip to mastoid tip to ensure complete lateral neck exposure. A retrospective study revealed a 10-year survival rate of 67% for patients treated with neck dissection versus 43% for those who were not.[50]

Safety and Efficacy of Neck Dissection

Although morbidity following a comprehensive functional neck dissection can include temporary or permanent hypocalcemia, RLN paresis, spinal accessory nerve (CN XI) paresis, and chyle leak, several studies suggest that central compartment and lateral neck dissection can be performed with minimal permanent morbidity.[20,62,63] The most concerning permanent complications were RLN injury and hypoparathyroidism. Thus surgeons need to balance the risks of this surgery with the potential benefits with respect to locoregional control and survival.

Although many surgeons agree that formal neck dissection is more appropriate in the treatment of metastatic thyroid disease than "berry picking" of individual cervical lymph nodes, the efficacy of such treatment remains unclear, especially with respect to disease-free survival. Assessing the efficacy of surgical treatment in this setting is quite difficult given the mixed findings regarding the impact of lymph node metastases on patient survival.[10,12,21] Additionally, the potential survival benefit may be small enough that the size and length of a definitive clinical study to demonstrate such a clinical benefit would be prohibitive.

Nevertheless, treatment of the neck does improve locoregional control and facilitate disease surveillance.[39,64] The removal of clinically palpable disease may permit more effective eradication of microscopic disease when the thyroid cancer cells are I-131 avid. Additionally, serum thyroglobulin levels are more predictive of disease recurrence when gross regional metastases have been removed.

Adjuvant Therapy

The recent management guidelines published by the American Thyroid Association advocate surgical excision as the most appropriate management of patients with locoregional disease either at initial presentation or subsequent recurrence.[65] The preferred hierarchy of treatment following surgical excision included I-131 treatment; external beam radiation; watchful waiting in patients with stable, asymptomatic disease; and experimental chemotherapy trials.

I-131 therapy can be effective for subclinical or microscopic metastases, but does not appear to be as effective against palpable clinically apparent disease. A small series of patients with metastatic papillary carcinoma were treated nonoperatively with I-131.[66] Unfortunately, 47% developed recurrent tumor and 36% died of disease. The enthusiasm for I-131 therapy must also be tempered by the observation that only 72% of recurrences and metastases from differentiated thyroid carcinoma are I-131 avid.[67] Additionally, only 68% of those patients with I-131–avid metastases had complete resolution of disease following radioiodine ablation therapy. However, the combination of surgery and I-131 therapy does appear to lower the overall incidence of recurrent lymph node metastasis.

External beam radiation therapy (EBRT) does not appear to be especially effective as a primary treatment of clinically palpable metastases. Few studies have been performed and thyroid carcinomas tend to be slow growing and thus more resistant to radiation treatment. EBRT may have a limited role as an adjuvant treatment. Following incomplete surgery, treatment of patients with at least 50 Gy resulted in lower locoregional recurrence as compared with surgery alone.[60,68] However, the uncertain effectiveness of EBRT on well-differentiated thyroid carcinomas has led the American Thyroid Association to suggest that experimental chemotherapy trials may be utilized prior to EBRT for locoregional disease.[65]

Unfortunately, a subset of patients presents with well-differentiated thyroid carcinoma that exhibits very aggressive invasive and metastatic behavior. Single-agent doxorubicin or paclitaxel may demonstrate temporary partial response, but durable responses are uncommon.[70] Combination chemotherapy does not demonstrate increased response, but is associated with increased toxicity.[70] It is hoped that continuing research may identify potential inhibitors to the *ret/ptc* oncogene or other molecular targets that can improve upon the effectiveness of our current therapies.

References

1. Noguchi S, Noguchi A, Murakami N. Papillary carcinoma of the thyroid. I. Developing pattern of metastasis. Cancer 1970;26:1053–1060

2. Shaha AR, Shah JP, Loree TR. Patterns of nodal and distant metastasis based on histologic varieties in differentiated carcinoma of the thyroid. Am J Surg 1996;172:692–694

3. Moley JF, DeBenedetti MK. Patterns of nodal metastases in palpable medullary thyroid carcinoma: recommendations for extent of node dissection. Ann Surg 1999;229:880–887

4. Ellenhorn JD, Shah JP, Brennan MF. Impact of therapeutic regional lymph node dissection for medullary carcinoma of the thyroid gland. Surgery 1993;114:1078–1081

5. Goepfert H, Dichtel WJ, Samaan NA. Thyroid cancer in children and teenagers. Arch Otolaryngol 1984;110:72–75

6. Frankenthaler RA, Sellin RV, Cangir A, et al. Lymph node metastasis from papillary-follicular thyroid carcinoma in young patients. Am J Surg 1990;160:341–343

7. Noguchi M, Yamada H, Ohta N, et al. Regional lymph node metastases in well-differentiated thyroid carcinoma. Int Surg 1987;72:100–103

8. Rossi RL, Cady B, Silverman ML, et al. Current results of conservative surgery for differentiated thyroid carcinoma. World J Surg 1986;10:612–622

9. Farrar WB, Cooperman M, James AG. Surgical management of papillary and follicular carcinoma of the thyroid. Ann Surg 1980;192:701–704

10. Shah JP, Loree TR, Dharker D, et al. Prognostic factors in differentiated carcinoma of the thyroid gland. Am J Surg 1992;164:658–661

11. Simpson WJ, McKinney SE, Carruthers JS, et al. Papillary and follicular thyroid cancer. Prognostic factors in 1,578 patients. Am J Med 1987;83:479–488

12. Mazzaferri EL, Jhiang SM. Long-term impact of initial surgical and medical therapy on papillary and follicular thyroid cancer. Am J Med 1994;97:418–428

13. Schelfhout LJ, Creutzberg CL, Hamming JF, et al. Multivariate analysis of survival in differentiated thyroid cancer: the prognostic significance of the age factor. Eur J Cancer Clin Oncol 1988;24:331–337

14. Vassilopoulou-Sellin R, Goepfert H, Raney B, et al. Differentiated thyroid cancer in children and adolescents: clinical outcome and mortality after long-term follow-up. Head Neck 1998;20:549–555

15. Yamashita H, Noguchi S, Murakami N, et al. Extracapsular invasion of lymph node metastasis is an indicator of distant metastasis and poor prognosis in patients with thyroid papillary carcinoma. Cancer 1997;80:2268–2272

16. Mansberger AR, Wei JP. Surgical embryology and anatomy of the thyroid and parathyroid glands. Surg Clin North Am 1993;73:727–746

17. Mirallie E, Visset J, Sagan C, et al. Localization of cervical node metastasis of papillary thyroid carcinoma. World J Surg 1999;23:970–973

18. Sisson GA, Feldman DE. The management of thyroid carcinoma metastatic to the neck and mediastinum. Otolaryngol Clin North Am 1980;13:119–126

19. Ozaki O, Ito K, Kobayashi K, et al. Modified neck dissection for patients with nonadvanced, differentiated carcinoma of the thyroid. World J Surg 1988;12:825–829

20. Noguchi M, Kinami S, Kinoshita K, et al. Risk of bilateral cervical lymph node metastases in papillary thyroid cancer. J Surg Oncol 1993;52:155–159

21. McConahey WM, Hay ID, Woolner LB, et al. Papillary thyroid cancer treated at the Mayo Clinic, 1946 through 1970: initial manifestations, pathologic findings, therapy, and outcome. Mayo Clin Proc 1986;61:978–996

22. Mazzaferri EL, Young RL, Oertel JE, et al. Papillary thyroid carcinoma: the impact of therapy in 576 patients. Medicine (Baltimore) 1977;56:171–196

23. Ahuja S, Ernst H, Lenz K. Papillary thyroid carcinoma: occurrence and types of lymph node metastases. J Endocrinol Invest 1991;14:543–549

24. Hay ID, Grant CS, van Heerden JA, et al. Papillary thyroid microcarcinoma: a study of 535 cases observed in a 50-year period. Surgery 1992;112:1139–1146

25. Attie JN, Khafif RA, Steckler RM. Elective neck dissection in papillary carcinoma of the thyroid. Am J Surg 1971;122:464–471

26. Tielens ET, Sherman SI, Hruban RH, et al. Follicular variant of papillary thyroid carcinoma. A clinicopathologic study. Cancer 1994;73:424–431

27. Rao RS, Parikh HK, Deshmane VH, et al. Prognostic factors in follicular carcinoma of the thyroid: a study of 198 cases. Head Neck 1996;18:118–124

28. Goldman ND, Coniglio JU, Falk SA. Thyroid cancers. I. Papillary, follicular, and Hürthle cell. Otolaryngol Clin North Am 1996;29:593–609

29. Tollefsen HR, Shah JP, Huvos AG. Hürthle cell carcinoma of the thyroid. Am J Surg 1975;130:390–394

30. Duh QY. What's new in general surgery: endocrine surgery. J Am Coll Surg 2005;201:746–753

31. Kouvaraki MA, Lee JE, Shapiro SE, et al. Preventable reoperations for persistent and recurrent papillary thyroid carcinoma. Surgery 2004;136:1183–1191

32. Torlontano M, Attard M, Crocetti U, et al. Follow-up of low risk patients with papillary thyroid cancer: role of neck ultrasonography in detecting lymph node metastases. J Clin Endocrinol Metab 2004;89:3402–3407

33. Rubello D, Mazzarotto R, Casara D. The role of technetium-99m methoxyisobutylisonitrile scintigraphy in the planning of therapy and follow-up of patients with differentiated thyroid carcinoma after surgery. Eur J Nucl Med 2000;27:431–440

34. Alnafisi NS, Driedger AA, Coates G, et al. FDG PET of recurrent or metastatic 131I-negative papillary thyroid carcinoma. J Nucl Med 2000;41:1010–1015

35. Watkinson JC, Franklyn JA, Olliff JF. Detection and surgical treatment of cervical lymph nodes in differentiated thyroid cancer. Thyroid 2006;16:187–194

36. Kelemen PR, Van Herle AJ, Giuliano AE. Sentinel lymphadenectomy in thyroid malignant neoplasms. Arch Surg 1998;133:288–292

37. Gallowitsch HJ, Mikosch P, Kresnik E, et al. Lymphoscintigraphy and gamma probe-guided surgery in papillary thyroid carcinoma: the sentinel lymph node concept in thyroid carcinoma. Clin Nucl Med 1999;24:744–746

38. Rettenbacher L, Sungler P, Gmeiner D, et al. Detecting the sentinel lymph node in patients with differentiated thyroid carcinoma. Eur J Nucl Med 2000;27:1399–1401

39. Scheumann GF, Gimm O, Wegener G, et al. Prognostic significance and surgical management of locoregional lymph node metastases in papillary thyroid cancer. World J Surg 1994;18:559–567

40. Henry JF, Gramatica L, Denizot A, et al. Morbidity of prophylactic lymph node dissection in the central neck area in patients with papillary thyroid carcinoma. Langenbecks Arch Surg 1998;383:167–169

41. Attie JN. Modified neck dissection in treatment of thyroid cancer: a safe procedure. Eur J Cancer Clin Oncol 1988;24:315–324

42. McHenry CR, Rosen IB, Walfish PG. Prospective management of nodal metastases in differentiated thyroid cancer. Am J Surg 1991;162:353–356

43. King WW, Li AK. What is the optimal treatment of nodal metastases in differentiated thyroid cancer? Aust N Z J Surg 1994;64:815–817

44. Hutter RV, Frazell EL, Foote FW. Elective radical neck dissection: an assessment of its use in the management of papillary thyroid cancer. CA Cancer J Clin 1970;20:87–93

45. Block MA. Surgical treatment of medullary carcinoma of the thyroid. Otolaryngol Clin North Am 1990;23:453–473

46. Ducci M, Appetecchia M, Marzetti M. Neck dissection for surgical treatment of lymph node metastasis in papillary thyroid carcinoma. J Exp Clin Cancer Res 1997;16:333–335

47. Noguchi M, Kumaki T, Taniya T, et al. Impact of neck dissection on survival in well-differentiated thyroid cancer: a multivariate analysis of 218 cases. Int Surg 1990;75:220–224

48. Noguchi S, Murakami N, Yamashita H, et al. Papillary thyroid carcinoma: modified radical neck dissection improves prognosis. Arch Surg 1998;133:276–280

49. Frazell EL, Foote FW. Papillary thyroid carcinoma: pathological findings in cases with and without clinical evidence of cervical node involvement. Cancer 1955;8:1164–1166

50. Block MA. Management of carcinoma of the thyroid. Ann Surg 1977;185:133–144

51. McGregor GI, Luoma A, Jackson SM. Lymph node metastases from well-differentiated thyroid cancer. A clinical review. Am J Surg 1985;149:610–612

52. Cunningham MP, Duda RB, Recant W, et al. Survival discriminants for differentiated thyroid cancer. Am J Surg 1990;160:344–347

53. Grebe SK, Hay ID. Thyroid cancer nodal metastases: biologic significance and therapeutic considerations. Surg Oncol Clin N Am 1996;5:43–63

54. Kupferman ME, Patterson M, Mandel SJ, et al. Patterns of lateral neck metastasis in papillary thyroid carcinoma. Arch Otolaryngol Head Neck Surg 2004;130:857–860

55. Hamming JF, van de Velde CJ, Fleuren GJ, et al. Differentiated thyroid cancer: a stage adapted approach to the treatment of regional lymph node metastases. Eur J Cancer Clin Oncol 1988;24:325–330

56. Demeure MJ, Clark OH. Surgery in the treatment of thyroid cancer. Endocrinol Metab Clin North Am 1990;19:663–683

57. Shaha AR. Management of the neck in thyroid cancer. Otolaryngol Clin North Am 1998;31:823–831

58. Marchetta FC, Sako K, Matsuura H. Modified neck dissection for carcinoma of the thyroid gland. Am J Surg 1970;120:452–455

59. Noguchi M, Hashimoto T, Ohyama S, et al. Indications for bilateral neck dissection in well-differentiated carcinoma of the thyroid. Jpn J Surg 1987;17:439–444

60. Tubiana M, Haddad E, Schlumberger M, et al. External radiotherapy in thyroid cancers. Cancer 1985;55:2062–2071

61. Pingpank JF, Sasson AR, Hanlon AL, et al. Tumor above the spinal accessory nerve in papillary thyroid cancer that involves lateral neck nodes: a common occurrence. Arch Otolaryngol Head Neck Surg 2002;128:1275–1278

62. Cheah WK, Arici C, Ituarte PH, et al. Complications of neck dissection for thyroid cancer. World J Surg 2002;26:1013–1016

63. Kupferman ME, Patterson DM, Mandel SJ, et al. Safety of modified radical neck dissection for differentiated thyroid carcinoma. Laryngoscope 2004;114:403–406

64. Mazzaferri EL, Jhiang SM. Differentiated thyroid cancer long-term impact of initial therapy. Trans Am Clin Climatol Assoc 1994;106:151–168

65. Cooper DS, Doherty GM, Haugen BR, et al. Management guidelines for patients with thyroid nodules and differentiated thyroid cancer. Thyroid 2006;16:109–142

66. Wilson SM, Bock GE. Carcinoma of the thyroid metastatic to lymph nodes of the neck. Arch Surg 1971;102:285–291

67. Maxon HR, Smith HS. Radioiodine-131 in the diagnosis and treatment of metastatic well differentiated thyroid cancer. Endocrinol Metab Clin North Am 1990;19:685–718

68. Wu XL, Hu YH, Li QH, et al. Value of postoperative radiotherapy for thyroid cancer. Head Neck Surg 1987;10:107–112

69. Gottlieb JA, Hill CS, Ibanez ML, et al. Chemotherapy of thyroid cancer. An evaluation of experience with 37 patients. Cancer 1972;30:848–853

70. Haugen BR. Management of the patient with progressive radioiodine non-responsive disease. Semin Surg Oncol 1999;16:34–41

14 Molecular Advances in the Diagnosis and Treatment of Thyroid Cancer

Kepal N. Patel and Bhuvanesh Singh

The thyroid gland is composed of two distinct cell types: the follicular cell and the parafollicular, or C, cell. Follicular cells compose most of the epithelium and are responsible for iodine uptake and thyroid hormone synthesis. C cells are scattered intrafollicular or parafollicular cells that are dedicated to the production of the calcium-regulating hormone calcitonin. Cancers of thyroid gland origin are the most common endocrine malignancies and account for the majority of endocrine cancer-related deaths each year.[1,2] The incidence of thyroid cancer has steadily increased over the past few decades. More than 90% of thyroid carcinomas are derived from follicular cells. A minority of cancers referred to as medullary thyroid carcinoma (MTC) are of C-cell origin. Most thyroid carcinomas can be effectively managed by surgical resection with or without radioactive iodine ablation. However, a subset of these tumors can behave aggressively, leading to significant morbidity and mortality. During the past decade our knowledge of the genetics and molecular pathways involved in oncogenesis has increased dramatically. Several molecular abnormalities have been identified that participate in the transformation of thyroid follicular and parafollicular cells. This chapter focuses on the abnormalities that underlie the initiation and progression of thyroid cancer, and develops a framework for understanding the transformed phenotype.

Thyroid Cancer of Follicular Cell Origin

Thyroid cancers derived from thyroid follicular epithelial cells (thyrocytes) are broadly classified as well-differentiated (WDTC), poorly differentiated (PDTC), and undifferentiated or anaplastic (ATC). WDTC such as papillary and follicular thyroid cancer behave in an indolent manner and usually have an excellent prognosis. By contrast, ATC is highly aggressive and usually rapidly fatal. PDTC is morphologically and behaviorally intermediate between WDTC and ATC. Accumulating evidence indicates that thyrocyte-derived thyroid carcinomas constitute a biologic continuum progressing from the highly curable WDTC to the often incurable ATC.[3,4] PDTC and aggressive variants of WDTC, such as tall cell and columnar cell, frequently serve as intermediates in this progression model.[5,6] Clinical, epidemiologic, and pathologic evidence supports the concept of stepwise progression and dedifferentiation.[7] For example, the gradual loss of papillary and follicular growth patterns and the

simultaneous increase in a solid growth pattern, with increased mitoses, necrosis, and nuclear pleomorphism, are often observed in aggressive thyroid carcinomas.[8,9] A majority of these tumors exhibit residual foci of differentiated thyroid carcinoma.

The true incidence of histologic dedifferentiation is difficult to assess. Metastatic or recurrent thyroid cancer is often not surgically managed; therefore, the functional and histologic dedifferentiation of a well-differentiated, low-risk neoplasm evolving into a high-risk and potentially lethal malignancy is probably not reported accurately. Furthermore, this transformation can evolve over years or decades, making patient follow-up difficult.

Although observations strongly support a progression concept, little is known regarding the possible mechanisms underlying this process. Because aggressive carcinomas, such as PDTC and ATC, result in significant thyroid cancer-related morbidity and mortality, it is important to identify and appreciate the molecular factors that may play a role in driving the dedifferentiation of WDTC. These factors affecting tumor proliferation, cellular immortalization, and death may serve as potential therapeutic targets. During the past decade we have witnessed an explosion of genetic information, and a large body of information has been generated on the molecular alterations involved in the pathogenesis of thyroid carcinoma. Thyrocyte growth requires the combined effects of hormones, such as thyroid-stimulating hormone (TSH), growth factor signaling factors (insulin-like growth factor, epidermal growth factor), cytokines, and other mitogens. Activation of signaling pathways such as the mitogen-activated protein kinase (MAPK) pathway seems to play a crucial role in thyrocyte transformation. It is therefore fitting that genetic alterations and mutations in factors that regulate thyrocyte growth and differentiation play a prominent role in the pathogenesis of thyroid neoplasia (**Fig. 14.1**).

Receptor Tyrosine Kinases

ret/ptc

The *ret* (*re*arranged during *t*ransfection) proto-oncogene is a 21-exon gene located on the proximal long arm of chromosome 10 (10q11.2) that encodes a tyrosine kinase receptor. *ret* was the first activated receptor tyrosine kinase to be identified in thyroid cancer. It consists of an extracellular domain with a ligand-binding site, a transmembrane domain, and an intracellular tyrosine kinase domain. *ret* is activated by

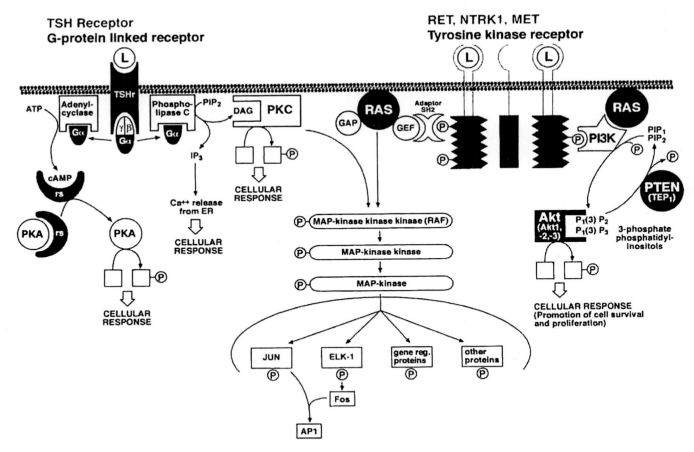

Fig. 14.1 Many of the molecular alterations associated with thyroid tumors involve common signaling pathways. ATP, adenosine triphosphate; cAMP, cyclic adenosine monophosphate; DAG, diacylglycerol; Ga, a-subunit of stimulatory G-protein; GAP, GTPase-activating protein; GEF, guanine nucleotide exchange factor; IP3, inositol triphosphate; L, ligand; PI3K, phosphatidylinositol 3-kinase; PKA, protein kinase A; PKC, protein kinase C; PLPN, phosphatidylinositol n-phosphate; TSH, thyroid-stimulating hormone; TSHr, TSH receptor protein. Used with permission from Tallini G. Molecular pathobiology of thyroid neoplasms. Endocr Pathol 2202;13:271–288.

interaction with a multicomponent complex that includes a soluble ligand family, the glial-derived neurotrophic factors (GDNF), and also a family of cell surface bound co-receptors, the GDNF family receptor α (GFR-α).[10] Ligand binding results in receptor dimerization leading to autophosphorylation of the protein on the tyrosine residues, activating several signaling pathways, including extracellular regulated kinase (ERK, also known as MAPK 1 and 3), phosphatidylinositol 3-kinase (PI3K), MAPK p38, and C-JUN kinase (JNK, also known as MAPK 8) (**Fig. 14.1**).[11,12] *ret* is normally expressed in the developing central and peripheral nervous system and is required for renal organogenesis and enteric neurogenesis.[13] It is not normally expressed in the thyroid follicular cell.[14] Rearrangements of the *ret* gene, known as *ret/ptc* rearrangements, occur in papillary thyroid carcinoma (PTC). The unique spatial proximity of translocation-prone gene loci, which may be preferentially occurring in thyrocytes in their mitotic interphase, favors *ret* gene rearrangements.[15,16] This may help explain why *ret* rearrangements are specific for thyroid tumors.[17,18] Although more than 10 rearrangements have been described, *ret/ptc1*, *ret/ptc2*, and *ret/ptc3* account

for most of the rearrangements found in PTC.[19,20] In each of these rearrangements, the upstream (5′) component of a "housekeeping" (or ubiquitously expressed) gene drives the expression of the tyrosine kinase domain of *ret* (**Table 14.1**). Expression of the RET/PTC chimeric proteins is facilitated by the heterologous promoters provided by the fused genes and results in constitutive, ligand-independent activation of RET receptor tyrosine kinase in papillary cancer cells.[21–23]

Table 14.1 Summary of the Common *ret/ptc* Rearrangements and Their Resulting Chimeric Products

ret/ptc Rearrangements	Chimeric Product
ret/ptc1	10q paracentric inversion; H4 (ubiquitously expressed gene of unknown origin)
ret/ptc2	t(10;17)(q11.2;q23); regulatory subunit of cAMP-dependent protein kinase A
ret/ptc3	Intrachromosomal rearrangements; *ELEI*, a gene of unknown function

In the adult population, the *ret* rearrangements have been found in 2.6% to 34% of PTC (**Table 14.2**).[24–33] However, in the pediatric population, *ret* rearrangements, specifically *ret/ptc1* and *ret/ptc3,* have been found in up to 80% of the cases.[34,35] Initial studies showed that this was especially true in cancers in children exposed to radiation after the Chernobyl nuclear accident or to external irradiation for treatment of benign diseases of the head and neck.[28,36–38] Recent reviews show that the *ret/ptc* rearrangements occur commonly in pediatric PTC regardless of radiation history. It is therefore probably an event associated with young age, although individuals of young age are particularly susceptible to development of PTC after radiation exposure.[39]

The role of *ret* rearrangements in the development of PTC has been demonstrated convincingly in transgenic mice with targeted overexpression of *ret/ptc1* and *ret/ptc3.* These mice develop thyroid tumors with microscopic features recapitulating those of human papillary carcinomas.[30,40,41]

There is evidence to support the belief that *ret/ptc* rearrangements represent early genetic changes leading to the development of PTC.[32,42] Several studies have shown that *ret/ptc* rearrangements are associated with PTC that lacks evidence of progression to PDTC or ATC.[17,43] A study by Santoro et al[44] showed that less than 10% of PDTCs were positive for *ret/ptc* rearrangements. They concluded that PTCs with *ret/ptc* rearrangements have a relatively low potential for progression to PDTC or ATC. The low prevalence of expression of *ret* rearrangements in PDTC and ATC supports a minor role for the fusion proteins in tumor progression. However, the suggestion that *ret/ptc* rearrangements predict indolent behavior must be interpreted with caution.

The recent success in the treatment of chronic myelogenous leukemia with imatinib mesylate, an inhibitor of constitutively activated Abelson (ABL) tyrosine kinase, has generated considerable interest in developing therapeutic protein kinase inhibitors. Recently, compounds have been identified that exhibit significant inhibitory activity on RET kinase.[45] This new class of drugs may prove to be clinically beneficial for patients with RET-induced thyroid carcinomas.

Table 14.2 Prevalence of Specific Genetic Alterations in Various Types of Thyroid Carcinoma Reported in the Literature

	Papillary	Follicular	Poorly Differentiated	Anaplastic
BRAF	39%	0%	13%	14%
RAS	15%	35%	35%	53%
ret/ptc	28%	0%	9%	0%
PAX8-PPARγ	1%	34%	0%	0%
P53	5%	7%	24%	59%
β-catenin	0%	0%	16%	66%

NTRK1

The neurotrophic receptor tyrosine kinase *NTRK1* (also known as *TRK* and *TRKA*) gene is located on chromosome 1q22 and encodes the receptor for nerve growth factor. It was the second identified subject of chromosomal rearrangement in thyroid tumorigenesis. *NTRK1* expression is typically restricted to neurons of the sensory spinal and cranial ganglia of neural-crest origin, and regulates neuronal growth and survival.[11] The activated receptor initiates several signal transduction cascades, including ERK, PI3K, and the phospholipase-Cγ (PLCγ) pathways.[46]

Similar to *ret, NTRK1* undergoes oncogenic activation by chromosomal rearrangements that fuse the *NTRK1*-tyrosine kinase domain to the 5′-terminal region of heterologous genes. The resulting chimeric protein exhibits constitutively active tyrosine kinase activity. Several NTRK1 chimeric proteins have been described in thyroid cancer (TRK, TRK-T1, TRK-T2, TRK-T3).[47–49] Similar to *ret/ptc,* the *NTRK1* oncogenes appear restricted to PTC but are found with a lower prevalence (approximately 10%) than that reported for *ret/ptc.* The prevalence of *NTRK1* rearrangements is approximately 3% in post-Chernobyl PTCs.[50,51]

met Proto-Oncogene

The *met* gene encodes a transmembrane protein acting as the receptor for hepatocyte growth factor/scatter factor (HGF/SF). HGF/SF is a powerful mitogen for epithelial cells, including thyroid follicular cells.[52] It induces a variety of tissue-specific changes, causing epithelial cell dissociation, migration, invasion, growth, and polarity. Increased expression of *met* is thought to be due to transcriptional or posttranscriptional regulation. Papillary thyroid cancers typically express very high levels of the MET protein.[53–56] Papillary thyroid cancer cells overexpressing *met* may have acquired an HGF/SF-dependent invasive phenotype. Furthermore, *ret* and *ras* have been shown to induce *met* overexpression in primary thyroid cell cultures, suggesting that *met* may modulate their tumorigenic effects.[57] Although some studies have shown that increased *met* expression in PTC is associated with advanced stage and poor prognosis,[55,58] others have found decreased *met* expression in aggressive PTC, PDTC, and ATC.[56,59] The clinicopathologic significance of *met* overexpression in thyroid carcinoma is still unclear.

Signal Transduction Proteins

RAS

Three *ras* genes, *H-ras, K-ras,* and *N-ras,* synthesize a family of 21-kd proteins that play an important role in tumorigenesis.[60] The RAS proteins exist in two different forms: an inactive form that is bound to guanosine diphosphate (GDP), and an active form that exhibits guanosine triphosphatase (GTPase) activity. Their function is to convey signals originating from tyrosine kinase membrane receptors to a cascade of mitogen-activated protein kinases (MAPKs). This activates the transcription of target genes involved in cell proliferation, survival, and apoptosis (**Fig. 14.1**).[60] Oncogenic *ras* activation results from point mutations, affecting the GTP-binding domain (codons 12 or 13) in exon 1 or the GTPase domain (codon 61) in exon 2, which fix the protein in the activated state and thus result in chronic stimulation of downstream targets, genomic instability, additional mutations, and malignant transformation.[61]

The *ras* mutations are among the most common mutations found in transformed cells. Mutations in all three cellular *ras* genes have been identified in benign and malignant thyroid tumors. They seem to be common in follicular carcinoma, PDTC, and ATC and occur less frequently in PTC (**Table 14.2**).[62–68] Interestingly, the frequency of *ras* mutations in the follicular variant of PTC (FVPTC) is high (33%). This is similar to the frequency seen in follicular carcinomas.[69,70] These findings suggest that the FVPTC may occupy an intermediate position between follicular tumors and classic PTC.

The role of oncogenic *ras* in thyroid tumor progression is unclear. Some studies have shown a similar prevalence of *ras* mutations in benign and malignant thyroid neoplasms, suggesting that *ras* activation may represent an early event.[62,71] Other studies have shown that *ras* mutations, specifically mutations at codon 61 of *N-ras*, are involved with tumor progression and aggressive clinical behavior.[68,72–77] Transgenic mice with thyroid-specific mutant *ras* expression develop thyroid hyperplasia and carcinoma.[78] A study by Garcia-Rostan et al[77] demonstrated that the presence of *ras* mutations predicted a poor outcome for WDTC independent of tumor stage. Furthermore, they found that PDTC and ATC often harbor multiple *ras* mutations. These mutations probably represent an intermediate event in the progression of thyroid carcinoma.

BRAF

The most recent and major development in the field of thyroid cancer genetics has been the identification of the BRAF-activating point mutation as the most common molecular defect in PTC.[39] There are three isoforms of the serine-threonine kinase RAF in mammalian cells: ARAF, BRAF, and CRAF or RAF-1. CRAF is expressed ubiquitously, whereas BRAF is expressed predominantly in hematopoietic cells, neurons, and testes.[79] BRAF is also the predominant isoform in thyroid follicular cells.[39]

As with *ret/ptc* rearrangements and *ras* mutations, most of the genetic alterations in thyroid cancer exert their oncogenic effect at least partially through the activation of the MAPK pathway. The RAF isoforms activate MAPK/extracellular signal-regulated kinase (ERK) kinase (MEK) cascade (**Fig. 14.1**).[80] This is a key component in the MAPK pathway, which activates the transcription of target genes involved in cell proliferation, survival, and apoptosis.[80] When constitutively activated, the MAPK pathway leads to

tumorigenesis.[81] Among the three forms of RAF kinases, BRAF, with its gene located on chromosome 7, is the most potent activator of the MAPK pathway.[82,83]

The BRAF-activating point mutation in thyroid cancer is almost exclusively a thymine-to-adenine transversion at position 1799 (T1799A) in exon 15. This leads to a valine-to-glutamate substitution at residue 600 (V600E) and subsequent constitutive activation of the BRAF kinase.[84,85] The initial discovery of *BRAF* mutations indicated a high prevalence of this event in malignant melanoma, colorectal carcinoma, and ovarian carcinoma.[85] Studies have reported a prevalence of *BRAF* mutation in 29% to 83% of PTC, making it the most common oncogene identified in sporadic forms of PTC (**Table 14.2**).[39,86–94]

In all the studies published to date, *BRAF* mutation (V600E) has been found only in PTC, PDTC, and ATC.[39] It is not seen in follicular carcinoma or benign thyroid neoplasms. Some studies have shown *BRAF* mutation in follicular adenomas and follicular variant of PTC; however, the mutation is not V600E.[87,95,96] The high frequency and specificity of *BRAF* mutation suggest that this mutation may play a fundamental role in the initiation of PTC tumorigenesis. PTCs with *BRAF* mutation have distinct phenotypic and biologic properties. They seem to behave more aggressively and carry a poorer prognosis.[93] The tall cell variant, an aggressive variant of PTC, usually harbors the *BRAF* mutation.[39,69,89] PTCs with *BRAF* mutation present more commonly at an advanced stage, usually with extrathyroidal extension. Some authors suggest that this may reflect the age of the patient and not the presence of a *BRAF* mutation.[96] However, others have shown that PTC with *BRAF* mutation displays an increased incidence of locoregional recurrence and a decreased response of the recurrent tumor to radioactive iodine.[89,91,97,98] The *BRAF* mutation has also been found in approximately 15% of PDTC and ATC.[89,91] The *BRAF* mutation–positive ATC is likely derived from *BRAF* mutation-positive PTC, as suggested by the coexistence of PTC and ATC in the same tumor, both of which harbored the *BRAF* mutation.[39,89,93,99,100] Further studies have shown that a subset of papillary microcarcinomas harbor the *BRAF* mutation, indicating that this oncogene may be activated during tumor initiation.[89] These data suggest that *BRAF* mutation may be a tumor-initiating early event in PTC and thus is associated with tumor dedifferentiation.

An elegant study by Knauf et al[101] provides the most convincing evidence to support a role of *BRAF* mutation in the initiation and progression of PTC. The study showed that transgenic mice with thyroid specific expression of mutated BRAF developed PTC that transitioned to PDTC. These findings provide molecular evidence for the stepwise progression of PTC to PDTC and ATC.

Recently a new mechanism of BRAF activation has been identified. It involves inversion of chromosome 7q, leading to an in-frame fusion between *BRAF* and the *AKAP9* gene.[102] This activating rearrangement generates a constitutively active oncoprotein. This fusion is rarely found in sporadic

PTC and is more common in PTC associated with radiation exposure.[103]

Because both *ras* and *BRAF* mutations activate the MAPK pathway, it is interesting to note that *BRAF* mutations appear to be a marker for papillary thyroid carcinomas, whereas *ras* mutations are more often found in follicular thyroid carcinomas (FTC) or FVPTC. This suggests that the RAS and BRAF oncoproteins can activate distinct sets of downstream effectors. *BRAF* mutations, *ras* mutations, and *ret/ptc* rearrangements all appear to be mutually exclusive in PTC.[69,86,87]

Phosphatidylinositol 3-kinase (PI3K)/AKT/*PTEN*

PI3K/AKT signaling results in cell growth and inhibition of apoptosis that is mediated by phosphorylation of downstream targets by the serine threonine kinase AKT. The PI3K/AKT pathway is negatively regulated by *PTEN* but activated by *ras* and *ret/ptc* (**Fig. 14.1**). Mutations of the tumor suppressor gene *PTEN* have been identified in up to 25% of sporadic follicular adenomas and carcinomas but rarely in PTC.[104-106] Germline *PTEN* gene mutations have been identified in patients with Cowden syndrome, which is an autosomal dominant condition characterized by multiple hamartomas of skin, intestines, breast, and thyroid. Thyroid nodules or thyroiditis are present in 60 to 70% of patients, while thyroid cancer (usually FTC) develops in 10% of cases.[107] *PTEN*+/– transgenic mice have been shown to develop thyroid tumors.[108]

Nuclear Receptors and Cell Cycle Regulation

PAX8-PPARγ

The *PAX8* gene encodes a transcription factor essential for the genesis of thyroid follicular cell lineages and regulation of thyroid specific gene expression. The peroxisome proliferator-activated receptor γ (*PPARγ*) is a member of the nuclear hormone receptor superfamily that includes thyroid hormone, retinoic acid, and androgen and estrogen receptors.[52] The *PAX8-PPARγ* rearrangement leads to in-frame fusion of exon 7, 8, or 9 of *PAX8* on 2q13 with exon 1 of *PPARγ* on 3p25.[109] The exact mechanism by which this rearrangement imparts a carcinogenic phenotype is not fully understood. It appears as though the PAX8-PPARγ chimeric protein inactivates the wild-type PPARγ which is a putative tumor suppressor.[109,110]

As with *RAS* mutations, *PAX8-PPARγ* rearrangement has also been shown to be involved in the development of FTC. The *PAX8-PPARγ* rearrangement is found in FTC where it occurs in approximately 33% of all tumors (**Table 14.2**).[7,111-115] The rearrangement has also been shown to occur in follicular adenomas and is not specific for carcinoma.[111] The presence of a *PAX8-PPARγ* rearrangement in FVPTC is controversial and it has not been detected in PDTC and ATC. The role of this rearrangement in the progression and dedifferentiation of FTC to PDTC and ATC has not been well defined.

Cyclin D1

Cell-cycle regulators govern growth activity. Progression factors (cyclin D1, cyclin E1, cyclin-dependent kinases [CDKs], and E2Fs) and competitor factors (retinoblastoma protein RB, p16[INK4A], p21[CIP1], p27[KIP1], and p53) regulate the transition from G1 to S phase. Overexpression of cyclin D1 has been documented in PTC and FTC. Expression of cyclin D1 and cyclin E1 is observed in approximately 30% and 76% of papillary thyroid carcinomas, respectively.[116-120] Furthermore, cyclin D1 overexpression correlates with metastatic spread in PTC, and significant overexpression of cyclin D1 is observed in ATC.[121-123] Gene amplification has not been identified as a cause of cyclin D1 overexpression; therefore, upregulation of transcription or a posttranscriptional mechanism is likely.[121]

p53

The *p53* gene encodes a nuclear transcription factor that plays a central role in the regulation of cell cycle, DNA repair, and apoptosis.[124] As the policeman of the genome, *p53* is overexpressed after cellular exposure to DNA-damaging agents and causes transient cell cycle arrest, presumably to allow for DNA repair.[125] However, if the damage is severe, it initiates apoptosis to prevent replication of the flawed cell.[7] Cells with impaired *p53* function are likely to accumulate genetic damage and are at a selective advantage for clonal expansion. Alterations in the *p53* tumor suppressor gene by inactivating point mutations, usually involving exons 5 to 8, or by deletion result in progressive genome destabilization, additional mutations, and propagation of malignant clones. This represents the most frequent genetic damage in human cancer, usually occurring as a late tumorigenic event.[52]

Among thyroid tumors, *p53* mutations are generally restricted to PDTC and ATC.[126,127] Point mutations of *p53* occur in approximately 60% of ATC and in 25% of PDTC (**Table 14.2**).[126-132] Moreover, in tumors with both well-differentiated and anaplastic components, *p53* mutations were present only in the anaplastic component.[126,130,133] These findings are consistent with the hypothesis that *p53* inactivation likely serves as a second hit, triggering tumor dedifferentiation and progression to PDTC and ATC.

Experimental studies have shown that loss of *p53* results in progressive dedifferentiation of thyroid tumors. Transgenic mice with thyroid-specific *ret/ptc* rearrangements developed PTC, but when crossed with *p53* –/– mice, the progeny succumbed to rapidly growing PDTC and ATC.[134,135] Conversely, the recovery of wild-type *p53* in cultured ATC cells resulted in the reexpression of thyroid-specific genes and the recovered ability to respond to thyroid-stimulating hormone.[136,137] It is unlikely that *p53* mutation is an initiating event in PDTC or ATC; it is likely a late event that contributes to the evolution of the transformed phenotype.

Cell Surface Adhesion Molecules

Cadherins

Cadherins belong to a family of single transmembrane calcium-dependent cell–cell adhesion proteins.[11] There are three classic cadherins: neuronal (N)-, placental (P)-, and epithelial (E)-cadherin. E-cadherin is highly expressed in normal thyroid and benign adenomas. It is required for normal epithelial differentiation and function. It serves to suppress tumor spread and invasion. Expression of E-cadherin is maintained in some well-differentiated minimally invasive thyroid carcinomas. However, in widely invasive, recurrent, or metastatic thyroid carcinomas, expression of E-cadherin is low or absent. Expression of E-cadherin in ATC is extremely low.[138–140] The expression of E-cadherin is thought to be regulated by gene promoter methylation.[141]

β-catenin

β-catenin, a cytoplasmic protein encoded by the *CTNNB1* gene, plays an important role in E-cadherin–mediated cell–cell adhesion. It is also an integral intermediate in the wingless (Wnt) signaling pathway.[142] Point mutations in exon 3 of the gene stabilize the protein and make it insensitive to its degradation by the adenomatous polyposis coli (APC) multiprotein complex. This results in the accumulation of β-catenin and the constitutive activation of target gene expression. β-catenin upregulates the transcriptional activity of cyclin D1, *C-myc*, *C-jun*, and other genes.

Point mutations in exon 3 have been reported in up to 25% of PDTC and 66% of ATC, but not in WDTC (**Table 14.2**).[143,144] The data suggest that the role of β-catenin mutations in thyroid carcinoma probably represents a late event in the tumor progression model, likely to trigger directly the process of dedifferentiation.

Fibronectin

Fibronectin is an extracellular matrix protein that regulates cell adhesion, migration, invasion, and metastasis. Fibronectin expression is upregulated in WDTC compared with normal thyroid tissue.[145,146] By contrast, reduced fibronectin expression is documented in transformed cell lines and at the periphery of invasive WDTC.[147] The tumor suppressor *PTEN* has been shown to increase fibronectin-mediated cell adhesion.[148]

CD44

CD44 is a polymorphic family of integral membrane proteoglycans and glycoproteins involved in cell–cell adhesion, cell–matrix adhesion, cell migration, and tumor metastasis. Multiple different CD44 isoforms exist as a result of alternative messenger RNA (mRNA) splicing. Variant CD44 molecules are expressed widely throughout the body on epithelial cells in a tissue-specific pattern.[149,150] Significant levels of CD44 protein are expressed on the plasma membranes of papillary thyroid cancer cells.[151] Papillary thyroid carcinomas exhibit specific patterns of aberrant CD44 mRNA splicing. These aberrations are postulated to affect the function of CD44 protein molecules and might regulate PTC growth patterns and metastatic potential.[152,153]

DNA Methylation

Epigenetic alterations, changes around a gene that alter the gene expression without affecting the nucleotide sequence, play a fundamental role in the regulation of human gene expression.[154] Two epigenetic mechanisms commonly used by cells to regulate gene expression are DNA methylation and histone modifications. During DNA methylation a methyl group is added to the cytosine residue in a CpG dinucleotide. CpG sites are regions of DNA where a cytosine nucleotide occurs next to a guanine nucleotide in the linear sequence of bases along its length. Gene promoter methylation, particularly near a transcription start site, usually results in silencing of the gene.[155,156]

Aberrant methylation and hence inappropriate silencing of tumor suppressor genes are common in thyroid tumors. Examples of these genes include *PTEN*, *RASSF1A*, tissue inhibitor of metalloproteinase-3 (*TIMP3*), *SLC5A8*, death-associated protein kinase (*DAPK*), and retinoic acid receptor β2 (*RARβ2*). These tumor suppressor genes have well-established functions. It is therefore conceivable that silencing of these genes through methylation has serious consequences and plays an important role in thyroid tumorigenesis.[157–161]

Other Molecular Factors

Angiogenic Factors

The vascular endothelial growth factor (VEGF) plays a critical role in angiogenesis. Increased expression of VEGF has been reported in thyroid carcinomas.[162–164] Overexpression of VEGF in PTC correlates with the density of lymphatics and lymph-node metastasis.[165] Increased expression of VEGF might contribute to the papillary morphogenesis of PTC.[166] Abrogation of VEGF activity with an anti-VEGF monoclonal antibody inhibits the growth of ATC and PTC xenografts in nude mice.[167,168]

Growth Factors

Several growth factors have been described in thyroid neoplasms. These include transforming growth factor-α (TGF-α), epidermal growth factor (EGF), insulin-like growth factor I (IGF-I), and fibroblast growth factors 1 and 2 (FGF-1, FGF-2). They have been shown to stimulate thyroid cell proliferation and are overexpressed in benign and malignant thyroid neoplasms.[169] Growth factor overexpression is likely to be a secondary, not a primary, event in thyroid cancer pathogenesis.

Thyroid-Stimulating Hormone Receptor and G Proteins

Activating mutations of the thyroid-stimulating hormone (TSH) receptor have been described in toxic hyperfunctioning (hot) adenomas.[170] It is well known that these adenomas rarely exhibit malignant behavior, which holds to the idea that activation of the adenylate cyclase pathway maintains the differentiated thyrocyte phenotype. Activating mutations in the TSH receptor are quite rare in differentiated and PDTC. Only a few cases have been reported.[171]

When TSH binds to its membrane receptor, a conformational change occurs in the TSH receptor allowing it to bind trimeric G proteins. This results in dissociation of the Gsα-subunit from the G-protein complex, allowing Gsα to stimulate adenylate cyclase to produce cyclic adenosine monophosphate (cAMP). The cAMP exerts its downstream effects by activating cAMP-dependent protein kinase A (PKA), which catalyzes the transfer of phosphate groups from adenosine triphosphate (ATP) to specific serine or threonine residues of selected proteins (**Fig. 14.1**). The oncogene *gsp* encodes the Gsα subunit, and is commonly mutated in hyperfunctioning adenomas.[170] Activating *gsp* mutations have been occasionally described in thyroid cancers. However, this is rare, and it is likely that *gsp* must be activated in concert with another oncogene to promote cancer formation.

Genomic Instability

Thyroid cancers accumulate several alterations at the genomic level. Chromosome instability has been identified in follicular adenomas and carcinomas. These tumors are frequently aneuploid with a high prevalence of loss of heterozygosity (LOH) involving multiple chromosomal regions. Papillary thyroid carcinomas show less frequent LOH.[172,173] This contrasting pattern of chromosome instability indicates that these two distinct types of thyroid cancer occur through discrete molecular pathways. It has been proposed that genomic instability plays a crucial role in the progression of thyroid cancer.[174] Certain genetic aberrations (MAPK activation, *p53* inactivation) appear to render rapidly dividing cells more susceptible to further genetic damage. As additional mutations are acquired, cells may attain a growth advantage. They may evade apoptosis and continue to proliferate and accumulate more genetic damage. This multiple-hit theory predicts a multistep process of clonal evolution of thyroid neoplasms (**Fig. 14.2**).

Genetic Syndromes Associated with Nonmedullary Thyroid Carcinoma

The prevalence of thyroid cancer is increased in certain genetic syndromes. Included in this group are Cowden syndrome, Gardner syndrome, familial adenomatous polyposis (FAP), and familial papillary thyroid cancer syndromes (**Table 14.3**).[175–178]

Table 14.3

Malignant neoplasms of follicular cell origin
- Genetic syndromes associated with papillary thyroid carcinoma
  - Familial adenomatous polyposis and Gardner syndrome
  - Peutz-Jeghers syndrome
- Genetic syndromes associated with follicular thyroid carcinoma
  - Cowden syndrome
- Familial nonmedullary thyroid carcinoma (FNMTC)
  - FNMTC1
  - Oxyphilic variant
  - MNG1 (multinodular goiter)

Malignant neoplasms of C-cell origin
- Multiple endocrine neoplasia type II (MEN-II)
  - *ret* proto-oncogene
    - MEN-IIA
      - Medullary thyroid carcinoma (100%)
      - Pheochromocytoma (50%)
      - Parathyroid neoplasia (15%)
    - MEN-IIA with cutaneous lichen amyloidosis
    - MEN-IIA with Hirschsprung's disease
    - MEN-IIB
      - Medullary thyroid carcinoma (100%)
      - Pheochromocytoma (50%)
      - Marfanoid habitus (~100%)
      - Intestinal ganglioneuromatosis and mucosal neuromas (~100%)
- Familial non-MEN medullary thyroid carcinoma
  - *ret* proto-oncogene

Cowden syndrome is an autosomal dominant disorder resulting from a germline mutation of the *PTEN* gene. The mucocutaneous manifestations include trichilemmomas, oral papillomas, and acral and palmoplantar keratoses. Affected patients have an increased incidence of endometrial and thyroid carcinomas. The lifetime risk of thyroid cancer approaches 10%, and most are of follicular type.

Thyroid tumors associated with FAP are clinically detectable in 2% of patients. These tumors are often a cribriform variant of PTC.[179]

Medullary Thyroid Carcinoma

Medullary thyroid carcinomas (MTC) arise from the parafollicular, or C, cells of the thyroid. These tumors are uncommon and account for approximately 15% of all thyroid malignancies. Approximately 80% of medullary thyroid carcinomas are sporadic, whereas the remainder appear to be familial.[10]

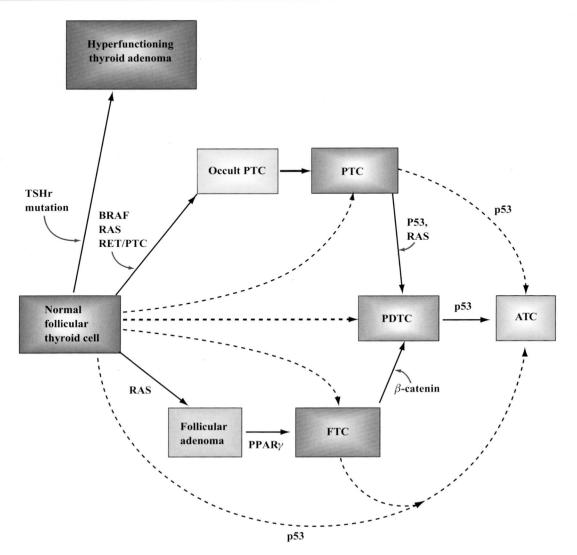

Fig. 14.2 Interactions between genomic instability and genetic alterations promotes progression from well differentiated to undifferentiated thyroid carcinoma. Distinct pathways proposed for neoplastic proliferation of thyroid follicular cells, including hyper-functioning follicular thyroid adenoma (tumors that are almost always benign without a propensity for progression).

The tumors in patients with sporadic MTC may vary considerably in size but are usually unilateral, unlike familial MTC tumors, which are frequently bilateral and multicentric. The tumors in patients with sporadic MTC sometimes arise from a somatic *ret* mutation in a single cell, in contrast to familial MTC, which almost always results from a germline *ret* mutation that affects all cells.[180]

Familial MTC is an autosomal dominant disorder that occurs in three recognized forms: familial non-MEN medullary thyroid carcinoma (FMTC), MTC associated with multiple endocrine neoplasia type IIA syndrome (MEN-IIA), and MTC associated with MEN-IIB syndrome. The genetic predisposition to develop a familial MTC is conferred by a point mutation in the germline DNA that encodes the *ret* oncogene.[181] These mutations serve to constitutively activate the tyrosine kinase function of the *ret* gene product and predispose to the

development of C-cell hyperplasia and multifocal MTC. Several inherited *ret* mutations have been described in the three inherited medullary thyroid carcinoma syndromes. These mutations demonstrate different mechanisms of oncogenic activation. In MEN-IIA, 98% of the mutations are found in the extracellular domain and are involved in changing a cysteine residue to a noncysteine residue. The cysteine residues normally form intramolecular disulfide bonds. When one is mutated, the other forms an intermolecular bond with another mutant *ret* receptor, causing constitutive dimerization and activation of the receptor.[182–184] Alternatively, in MEN-IIB, 95 to 98% of patients demonstrate a point mutation in the kinase domain of *ret* that changes a methionine to a threonine. This mutation activates the tyrosine kinase activity, but the ligand is still required for full activation of the receptor.[185] These differing mechanisms to activate the

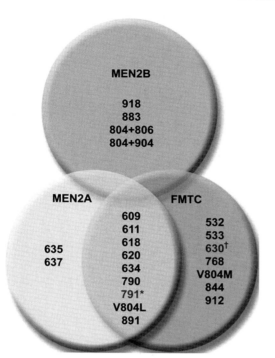

Fig. 14.3 Correlation of specific *ret* codon mutations with the phenotypic expression of hereditary medullary thyroid cancer (MTC). *Development of pheochromocytoma has not been reported. †Distinction between MEN-IIA and FMTC cannot be made. Used with permission from Kouvaraki MA, et al. RET proto-oncogene: a review and update of genotype-phenotype correlations in hereditary medullary thyroid cancer and associated endocrine tumors. Thyroid 2005;15:531–544.

ret oncogene may explain some phenotypic variations between MEN-IIA and MEN-IIB, perhaps by causing the phosphorylation of different tyrosine residues and the subsequent activation of different downstream signaling pathways. Known *ret* mutations in familial MTC and their biologic aggressiveness are summarized in **Fig. 14.3** and **Fig. 14.4**.[186]

New Molecular Targeted Therapies in Thyroid Cancer

Thyroid cancer serves as a good model for targeted therapies. The retained expression and function of the TSH receptor and sodium-iodide symporter (NIS) in most thyroid cells have enabled the successful use of TSH suppressive doses of levothyroxine and radioiodine. These targeted treatments, along with surgery, have led to long-term survival rates for patients with early-stage thyroid cancers that approach 98% at 20 years.[187] However, this excellent prognosis is not shared by individuals with aggressive thyroid cancers, which dedifferentiate and lose expression and function of the TSH receptor and NIS, such as PDTC or ATC. These tumors have increased rates of recurrence and metastasis, and do not respond well to traditional nontargeted cytotoxic chemotherapeutic agents. Using recently gained knowledge of critical pathways involved in thyroid cancer initiation and progres-

sion, RET, RAS/RAF/MAPK, and novel targeted therapies are being designed for patients with aggressive thyroid malignancies.

VEGF Receptor, EGF Receptor, and RET Pathway Inhibitors

ZD6474

ZD6474 is a novel oral heteroaromatic-substituted anilinoquinazoline that acts as a potent and reversible inhibitor of ATP binding to VEGF receptor (VEGFR) type 2.[188] This blocks VEGF signaling. ZD6474 also inhibits EGFR tyrosine kinase activity. ZD6474 has also demonstrated potent inhibition of ligand-dependent RET receptor and selective inhibition of RET-dependent thyroid tumor cell growth in vitro,[189,190] providing a potential treatment option for subgroups of patients with PTC and familial MTC. It has been found to effectively block phosphorylation and signaling of *ret/ptc3* and RET/MEN-IIB proteins. A possible advantage of ZD6474 in RET-associated tumors is that it has the potential to act both as an antiangiogenic drug and as an anticancer drug. The simultaneous assault on both endothelial (VEGFR pathway) and neoplastic cells (RET and EGFR pathways) may offer a mechanism to circumvent the development of resistance. ZD6474 is currently being investigated in phase II trials.[191]

AMG706

AMG706 is a potent oral multikinase inhibitor that targets VEGF, platelet-derived growth factor (PDGF), and KIT and RET receptors, and has antiangiogenic and antitumor activity. In a preclinical study, AMG706 produced a statistically significant reduction in vascular blood flow in human tumor xenografts.[192] A phase II study of AMG706 in advanced thyroid cancer is ongoing.

PTK787/ZK2225854

PTK787/ZK2225854 (vatalanib) is an orally active protein kinase inhibitor that potently and selectively blocks the VEGF/VEGFR system. Vatalanib has been studied in preclinical models of human ATC and FTC xenografts that were implanted into nude mice. After 4 weeks of treatment with vatalanib, a 41.4% reduction in tumor volume was seen, with a significant decrease in angiogenesis.[193]

ZD1839 (Gefitinib)

In preclinical studies, EGF has been shown to stimulate thyrocyte proliferation, and to enhance the migration and invasiveness of PTC.[194] Studies have also shown that EGF receptor (EGFR) is universally expressed in ATC cell lines.[195] Sufficient data suggest that EGFR plays a role in determining the malignant potential of ATC.

ZD1839 is a synthetic anilinoquinazoline, orally active EGFR inhibitor, which is highly selective, with minimal activity against other tyrosine kinases. Gefitinib blocks

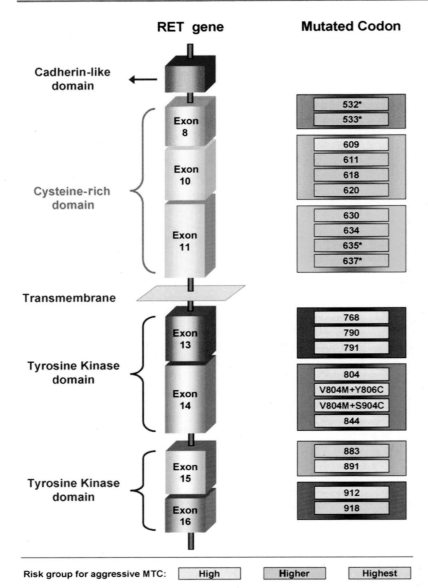

Fig. 14.4 Schematic diagram of the *ret* gene and reported codons responsible for three levels of biologic aggressiveness of MTC. Used with permission from Kouvaraki MA, et al. RET proto-oncogene: a review and update of genotype-phenotype correlations in hereditary medullary thyroid cancer and associated endocrine tumors. Thyroid 2005;15:531–544.

EGF-stimulated EGFR autophosphorylation and EGFR-mediated downstream signal transduction.[196] Gefitinib is now approved in the United States as single-agent treatment for non–small-cell lung cancer.[197]

Gefitinib was found to inhibit EGFR phosphorylation in vitro and in vivo, and to reduce the growth of subcutaneous ATC xenografts in a nude mouse model.[198] In another study, marked growth inhibition of ATC xenografts was found in gefitinib-treated mice. These results point to gefitinib as a potential molecular targeted therapeutic agent for aggressive thyroid cancer.

Cetuximab

Cetuximab is a human-murine chimeric monoclonal antibody to EGFR. It was recently approved by the Food and Drug Administration (FDA) for use in patients with head and neck squamous cell carcinoma. When combined with irinotecan, it has been shown to potentiate antiproliferative and proapoptotic effects in mouse ATC models. The combination of these two agents resulted in a 93% in vivo inhibition of tumor growth.[199] This combination was more effective and less toxic in the orthotopic ATC xenografts than doxorubicin, which is used frequently for the treatment of ATC.[199]

AEE788

AEE788 is a dual inhibitor of EGFR and VEGFR. Recent studies have demonstrated its efficacy in inhibiting the proliferation and inducing apoptosis of ATC cells, both in vitro and in vivo.[200]

PP1 and PP2

PP1 and PP2 are pyrazolopyrimidines with strong activity toward RET kinase.[201] They are small molecule tyrosine kinase inhibitors that are effective in blocking *ret/ptc* signaling and in abolishing its tumorigenic effects in experimental animals.[201,202]

BRAF/MEK Inhibitors

After identification of *BRAF* mutations as the most common genetic alteration in PTC, efforts have focused on the development of BRAF inhibitors. They would be valuable because of the well-proven role of mutant *BRAF* in tumor dedifferentiation, recurrence, and resistance to radioiodine therapy.[103] Furthermore, because BRAF shares a common MAPK pathway with RET and RAS, BRAF inhibitors may be effective in tumors with RAS or RET alterations. This prediction remains to be proven in the clinical setting.

BAY 43–9006 (Sorafenib)

Among BRAF inhibitors, sorafenib has been the first molecule to undergo clinical development. This compound is a potent competitive inhibitor of ATP binding in the catalytic domain of wild-type and mutant BRAF. By binding with the kinase domain of BRAF, sorafenib locks the kinase in an inactive state, inhibiting BRAF-stimulated DNA synthesis and cell proliferation and inducing apoptosis.[203] Sorafenib has also been shown to exert an antiangiogenic effect by targeting the receptor tyrosine kinases VEGFR-2 and PDGFR and their associated signaling cascades.[204] Sorafenib has been found to inhibit the BRAF signaling and growth of all thyroid cell lines carrying the *BRAF* mutation.[205] It also retarded the growth of ATC cell line xenografts in nude mice.[205] Sorafenib cytostatic effect has also been found in cells carrying the activated forms of *ret*, including *ret/ptc3*.[206] A huge phase I program with sorafenib has been performed, and a phase II trial in thyroid carcinoma is planned.

CI-1040

Additional therapeutic targets along the MAPK kinase pathway are located downstream of BRAF. In a recent study, MEK inhibitor CI-1040 was found to abrogate tumor growth in BRAF mutant xenografts derived from various tumor types.[207] Binding of CI-1040 in the hydrophobic binding pocket of MEKs induces a conformational change in unphosphorylated MEK that locks it into a closed but catalytically inactive form. The therapeutic activity of CI-1040 in thyroid cancer is under investigation.

Imatinib Mesylate

Imatinib mesylate is a tyrosine kinase inhibitor that selectively suppresses the activity of ABL, PDGFR, and c-KIT. It has induced growth inhibition in p53-defective or mutant ATC cell lines.[208,209] This effect is mediated by inhibition of c-ABL kinase, a ubiquitous nonreceptor tyrosine kinase. An ongoing phase II trial is being conducted to test the effect of imatinib in patients with ATC.

Histone Deacetylase (HDAC) Inhibitors

For normal gene transcription to occur, the tightly compacted chromatin must relax to facilitate the binding of transcription factors. Chromatin relaxation is associated with histone acetylation by histone acetyltransferases. Histone deacetylation by HDACs, which are recruited by oncogenes, prevents chromatin relaxation, thereby blocking transcription. HDAC inhibitors can increase acetylation of histones and various other proteins, and can induce programmed cell death in transformed cells, which makes them promising anticancer agents.[210]

Depsipeptide is a HDAC inhibitor that induces expression of a specific subset of genes linked to inhibition of cell growth and induction of differentiation.[211] It has demonstrated potent cytotoxic activity against human tumor xenografts and a phase I trial has been completed.[212] A phase II study for patients with recurrent or metastatic thyroid cancer that has not responded to radioiodine is ongoing.

A class of novel synthetic hybrid polar compounds includes hydroxamic acid–based suberoylanilide hydroxamic acid (SAHA), which causes accumulation of acetylated histones in cultured cells and induces differentiation or apoptosis of transformed cells in culture.[213] Tumor cells are much more sensitive to SAHA than normal cells. SAHA seems to be active even against tumors with *p53* mutations. Early phase I trial results confirm the biologic activity of SAHA.[214,215]

PPARγ Expression Ligands

The ligands for PPARγ include naturally occurring prostaglandins and thiazolidinediones, a class of antidiabetic drugs.[216] Studies have shown that PPARγ-expressing thyroid cancer cells respond favorably, with decreased growth and increased apoptosis, when treated with a PPARγ ligand. PPARγ seems to predict the response to ligand treatment.

Efforts targeted at inhibiting activated pathways may lead to development of novel therapies for thyroid cancer. This could substantially change the outcome of patients with aggressive, refractory, or metastatic disease.

References

1. Sarlis NJ, Benvenga S. Molecular signaling in thyroid cancer. Cancer Treat Res 2004;122:237–264
2. Sarlis NJ. Expression patterns of cellular growth-controlling genes in non-medullary thyroid cancer: basic aspects. Rev Endocr Metab Disord 2000;1:183–196
3. Venkatesh YS, Ordonez NG, Schultz PN, et al. Anaplastic

carcinoma of the thyroid. A clinicopathologic study of 121 cases. Cancer 1990;66:321–330

4. Carcangiu ML, Steeper T, Zampi G, Rosai J. Anaplastic thyroid carcinoma. A study of 70 cases. Am J Clin Pathol 1985;83:135–158

5. Carcangiu ML, Zampi G, Rosai J. Poorly differentiated ("insular") thyroid carcinoma. A reinterpretation of Langhans' "wuchernde" Struma. Am J Surg Pathol 1984;8:655–668

6. Sakamoto A, Kasai N, Sugano H. Poorly differentiated carcinoma of the thyroid. A clinicopathologic entity for a high-risk group of papillary and follicular carcinomas. Cancer 1983;52:1849–1855

7. Nikiforov YE. Genetic alterations involved in the transition from well-differentiated to poorly differentiated and anaplastic thyroid carcinomas. Endocr Pathol 2004;15:319–327

8. Rosai J, Saxen EA, Woolner L. Undifferentiated and poorly differentiated carcinoma. Semin Diagn Pathol 1985;2:123–136

9. Hunt JL, Tometsko M, LiVolsi VA, et al. Molecular evidence of anaplastic transformation in coexisting well-differentiated and anaplastic carcinomas of the thyroid. Am J Surg Pathol 2003;27:1559–1564

10. DeLellis RA. Pathology and genetics of thyroid carcinoma. J Surg Oncol 2006;94:662–669

11. Kondo T, Ezzat S, Asa SL. Pathogenetic mechanisms in thyroid follicular-cell neoplasia. Nat Rev Cancer 2006;6:292–306

12. Airaksinen MS, Saarma M. The GDNF family: signalling, biological functions and therapeutic value. Nat Rev Neurosci 2002;3:383–394

13. Neumann S, Schuchardt K, Reske A, et al. Lack of correlation for sodium iodide symporter mRNA and protein expression and analysis of sodium iodide symporter promoter methylation in benign cold thyroid nodules. Thyroid 2004;14:99–111

14. Viglietto G, Chiappetta G, Martinez-Tello FJ, et al. RET/PTC oncogene activation is an early event in thyroid carcinogenesis. Oncogene 1995;11:1207–1210

15. Nikiforova MN, Stringer JR, Blough R, et al. Proximity of chromosomal loci that participate in radiation-induced rearrangements in human cells. Science 2000;290:138–141

16. Roccato E, Bressan P, Sabatella G, et al. Proximity of TPR and NTRK1 rearranging loci in human thyrocytes. Cancer Res 2005;65:2572–2576

17. Santoro M, Carlomagno F, Hay ID, et al. Ret oncogene activation in human thyroid neoplasms is restricted to the papillary cancer subtype. J Clin Invest 1992;89:1517–1522

18. Santoro M, Sabino N, Ishizaka Y, et al. Involvement of RET oncogene in human tumours: specificity of RET activation to thyroid tumours. Br J Cancer 1993;68:460–464

19. Santoro M, Thomas GA, Vecchio G, et al. Gene rearrangement and Chernobyl related thyroid cancers. Br J Cancer 2000;82:315–322

20. Vecchio G, Santoro M. Oncogenes and thyroid cancer. Clin Chem Lab Med 2000;38:113–116

21. Moretti F, Nanni S, Pontecorvi A. Molecular pathogenesis of thyroid nodules and cancer. Best Pract Res Clin Endocrinol Metab 2000;14:517–539

22. Learoyd DL, Messina M, Zedenius J, et al. RET/PTC and RET tyrosine kinase expression in adult papillary thyroid carcinomas. J Clin Endocrinol Metab 1998;83:3631–3635

23. De Vita G, Zannini M, Cirafici AM, et al. Expression of the RET/PTC1 oncogene impairs the activity of TTF-1 and Pax-8 thyroid transcription factors. Cell Growth Differ 1998;9:97–103

24. Ishizaka Y, Kobayashi S, Ushijima T, et al. Detection of retTPC/PTC transcripts in thyroid adenomas and adenomatous goiter by an RT-PCR method. Oncogene 1991;6:1667–1672

25. Jhiang SM, Caruso DR, Gilmore E, et al. Detection of the PTC/retTPC oncogene in human thyroid cancers. Oncogene 1992;7:1331–1337

26. Sugg SL, Zheng L, Rosen IB, et al. ret/PTC-1, -2, and -3 oncogene rearrangements in human thyroid carcinomas: implications for metastatic potential? J Clin Endocrinol Metab 1996;81:3360–3365

27. Delvincourt C, Patey M, Flament JB, et al. Ret and trk proto-oncogene activation in thyroid papillary carcinomas in French patients from the Champagne-Ardenne region. Clin Biochem 1996;29:267–271

28. Bounacer A, Wicker R, Caillou B, et al. High prevalence of activating ret proto-oncogene rearrangements, in thyroid tumors from patients who had received external radiation. Oncogene 1997;15:1263–1273

29. Bongarzone I, Butti MG, Coronelli S, et al. Frequent activation of ret protooncogene by fusion with a new activating gene in papillary thyroid carcinomas. Cancer Res 1994;54:2979–2985

30. Santoro M, Chiappetta G, Cerrato A, et al. Development of thyroid papillary carcinomas secondary to tissue-specific expression of the RET/PTC1 oncogene in transgenic mice. Oncogene 1996;12:1821–1826

31. Cheung CC, Carydis B, Ezzat S, Bedard YC, Asa SL. Analysis of ret/PTC gene rearrangements refines the fine needle aspiration diagnosis of thyroid cancer. J Clin Endocrinol Metab 2001;86:2187–2190

32. Nikiforov YE. RET/PTC rearrangement in thyroid tumors. Endocr Pathol 2002;13:3–16

33. Fagin JA. Perspective: lessons learned from molecular genetic studies of thyroid cancer–insights into pathogenesis and tumor-specific therapeutic targets. Endocrinology 2002;143:2025–2028

34. Bongarzone I, Fugazzola L, Vigneri P, et al. Age-related activation of the tyrosine kinase receptor protooncogenes RET and NTRK1 in papillary thyroid carcinoma. J Clin Endocrinol Metab 1996;81:2006–2009

35. Nikiforov YE, Rowland JM, Bove KE, Monforte-Munoz H, Fagin JA. Distinct pattern of ret oncogene rearrangements in morphological variants of radiation-induced and sporadic thyroid papillary carcinomas in children. Cancer Res 1997;57:1690–1694

36. Klugbauer S, Demidchik EP, Lengfelder E, Rabes HM. A new form of RET rearrangement in thyroid carcinomas of children after the Chernobyl reactor accident. Oncogene 1996;13:1099–1102

37. Klugbauer S, Demidchik EP, Lengfelder E, Rabes HM. High prevalence of RET rearrangement in thyroid tumors of children from Belarus after the Chernobyl reactor accident. Oncogene 1995;11:2459–2467

38. Fugazzola L, Pilotti S, Pinchera A, et al. Oncogenic rearrangements of the RET proto-oncogene in papillary thyroid carcinomas from children exposed to the Chernobyl nuclear accident. Cancer Res 1995;55:5617–5620

39. Xing M. BRAF mutation in thyroid cancer. Endocr Relat Cancer 2005;12:245–262

40. Jhiang SM, Sagartz JE, Tong Q, et al. Targeted expression of the ret/PTC1 oncogene induces papillary thyroid carcinomas. Endocrinology 1996;137:375–378

41. Powell DJ, Russell J, Nibu K, et al. The RET/PTC3 oncogene: metastatic solid-type papillary carcinomas in murine thyroids. Cancer Res 1998;58:5523–5528

42. Tallini G, Asa SL. RET oncogene activation in papillary carcinoma. Adv Anat Pathol 2001;8:345–354

43. Tallini G, Santoro M, Helie M, et al. RET/PTC oncogene activation defines a subset of papillary thyroid carcinomas lacking evidence of progression to poorly differentiated or undifferentiated tumor phenotypes. Clin Cancer Res 1998;4:287–294

44. Santoro M, Papotti M, Chiappetta G, et al. RET activation and clinicopathologic features in poorly differentiated thyroid tumors. J Clin Endocrinol Metab 2002;87:370–379

45. Lanzi C, Cassinelli G, Pensa T, et al. Inhibition of transforming activity of the ret/ptc1 oncoprotein by a 2-indolinone derivative. Int J Cancer 2000;85:384–390
46. Miller FD, Kaplan DR. On Trk for retrograde signaling. Neuron 2001;32:767–770
47. Greco A, Roccato E, Pierotti MA. TRK oncogenes in papillary thyroid carcinoma. Cancer Treat Res 2004;122:207–219
48. Bongarzone I, Vigneri P, Mariani L, et al. RET/NTRK1 rearrangements in thyroid gland tumors of the papillary carcinoma family: correlation with clinicopathological features. Clin Cancer Res 1998;4:223–228
49. Pierotti MA. Chromosomal rearrangements in thyroid carcinomas: a recombination or death dilemma. Cancer Lett 2001;166:1–7
50. Beimfohr C, Klugbauer S, Demidchik EP, et al. NTRK1 rearrangement in papillary thyroid carcinomas of children after the Chernobyl reactor accident. Int J Cancer 1999;80:842–847
51. Rabes HM, Demidchik EP, Sidorow JD, et al. Pattern of radiation-induced RET and NTRK1 rearrangements in 191 post-Chernobyl papillary thyroid carcinomas: biological, phenotypic, and clinical implications. Clin Cancer Res 2000;6:1093–1103
52. Tallini G. Molecular pathobiology of thyroid neoplasms. Endocr Pathol 2002;13:271–288
53. Di Renzo MF, Narsimhan RP, Olivero M, et al. Expression of the Met/HGF receptor in normal and neoplastic human tissues. Oncogene 1991;6:1997–2003
54. Di Renzo MF, Olivero M, Ferro S, et al. Overexpression of the c-MET/HGF receptor gene in human thyroid carcinomas. Oncogene 1992;7:2549–2553
55. Di Renzo MF, Olivero M, Serini G, et al. Overexpression of the c-MET/HGF receptor in human thyroid carcinomas derived from the follicular epithelium. J Endocrinol Invest 1995;18:134–139
56. Ruco LP, Ranalli T, Marzullo A, et al. Expression of Met protein in thyroid tumours. J Pathol 1996;180:266–270
57. Ivan M, Bond JA, Prat M, et al. Activated ras and ret oncogenes induce over-expression of c-met (hepatocyte growth factor receptor) in human thyroid epithelial cells. Oncogene 1997;14:2417–2423
58. Chen BK, Ohtsuki Y, Furihata M, et al. Overexpression of c-Met protein in human thyroid tumors correlated with lymph node metastasis and clinicopathologic stage. Pathol Res Pract 1999;195:427–433
59. Belfiore A, Gangemi P, Costantino A, et al. Negative/low expression of the Met/hepatocyte growth factor receptor identifies papillary thyroid carcinomas with high risk of distant metastases. J Clin Endocrinol Metab 1997;82:2322–2328
60. Barbacid M. ras genes. Annu Rev Biochem 1987;56:779–827
61. Finney RE, Bishop JM. Predisposition to neoplastic transformation caused by gene replacement of H-ras1. Science 1993;260:1524–1527
62. Lemoine NR, Mayall ES, Wyllie FS, et al. High frequency of ras oncogene activation in all stages of human thyroid tumorigenesis. Oncogene 1989;4:159–164
63. Namba H, Gutman RA, Matsuo K, et al. H-ras protooncogene mutations in human thyroid neoplasms. J Clin Endocrinol Metab 1990;71:223–229
64. Suarez HG, du Villard JA, Severino M, et al. Presence of mutations in all three ras genes in human thyroid tumors. Oncogene 1990;5:565–570
65. Karga H, Lee JK, Vickery AL, et al. Ras oncogene mutations in benign and malignant thyroid neoplasms. J Clin Endocrinol Metab 1991;73:832–836
66. Manenti G, Pilotti S, Re FC, Della Porta G, Pierotti MA. Selective activation of ras oncogenes in follicular and undifferentiated thyroid carcinomas. Eur J Cancer 1994;30A:987–993
67. Meinkoth JL. Biology of Ras in thyroid cells. Cancer Treat Res 2004;122:131–148
68. Vasko V, Ferrand M, Di Cristofaro J, et al. Specific pattern of RAS oncogene mutations in follicular thyroid tumors. J Clin Endocrinol Metab 2003;88:2745–2752
69. Adeniran AJ, Zhu Z, Gandhi M, et al. Correlation between genetic alterations and microscopic features, clinical manifestations, and prognostic characteristics of thyroid papillary carcinomas. Am J Surg Pathol 2006;30:216–222
70. Di Cristofaro J, Marcy M, Vasko V, et al. Molecular genetic study comparing follicular variant versus classic papillary thyroid carcinomas: association of N-ras mutation in codon 61 with follicular variant. Hum Pathol 2006;37:824–830
71. Namba H, Rubin SA, Fagin JA. Point mutations of ras oncogenes are an early event in thyroid tumorigenesis. Mol Endocrinol 1990;4:1474–1479
72. Basolo F, Pisaturo F, Pollina LE, et al. N-ras mutation in poorly differentiated thyroid carcinomas: correlation with bone metastases and inverse correlation to thyroglobulin expression. Thyroid 2000;10:19–23
73. Motoi N, Sakamoto A, Yamochi T, et al. Role of ras mutation in the progression of thyroid carcinoma of follicular epithelial origin. Pathol Res Pract 2000;196:1–7
74. Hara H, Fulton N, Yashiro T, et al. N-ras mutation: an independent prognostic factor for aggressiveness of papillary thyroid carcinoma. Surgery 1994;116:1010–1016
75. Ezzat S, Zheng L, Kolenda J, et al. Prevalence of activating ras mutations in morphologically characterized thyroid nodules. Thyroid 1996;6:409–416
76. Esapa CT, Johnson SJ, Kendall-Taylor P, Lennard TW, Harris PE. Prevalence of Ras mutations in thyroid neoplasia. Clin Endocrinol (Oxf) 1999;50:529–535
77. Garcia-Rostan G, Zhao H, Camp RL, et al. ras mutations are associated with aggressive tumor phenotypes and poor prognosis in thyroid cancer. J Clin Oncol 2003;21:3226–3235
78. Rochefort P, Caillou B, Michiels FM, et al. Thyroid pathologies in transgenic mice expressing a human activated Ras gene driven by a thyroglobulin promoter. Oncogene 1996;12:111–118
79. Daum G, Eisenmann-Tappe I, Fries HW, Troppmair J, Rapp UR. The ins and outs of Raf kinases. Trends Biochem Sci 1994;19:474–480
80. Chang F, Steelman LS, Lee JT, et al. Signal transduction mediated by the Ras/Raf/MEK/ERK pathway from cytokine receptors to transcription factors: potential targeting for therapeutic intervention. Leukemia 2003;17:1263–1293
81. Peyssonnaux C, Eychene A. The Raf/MEK/ERK pathway: new concepts of activation. Biol Cell 2001;93:53–62
82. Mercer KE, Pritchard CA. Raf proteins and cancer: B-Raf is identified as a mutational target. Biochim Biophys Acta 2003;1653:25–40
83. Sithanandam G, Druck T, Cannizzaro LA, et al. B-raf and a B-raf pseudogene are located on 7q in man. Oncogene 1992;7:795–799
84. Kumar R, Angelini S, Czene K, et al. BRAF mutations in metastatic melanoma: a possible association with clinical outcome. Clin Cancer Res 2003;9:3362–3368
85. Davies H, Bignell GR, Cox C, et al. Mutations of the BRAF gene in human cancer. Nature 2002;417:949–954
86. Kimura ET, Nikiforova MN, Zhu Z, et al. High prevalence of BRAF mutations in thyroid cancer: genetic evidence for constitutive activation of the RET/PTC-RAS-BRAF signaling pathway in papillary thyroid carcinoma. Cancer Res 2003;63:1454–1457
87. Soares P, Trovisco V, Rocha AS, et al. BRAF mutations and RET/PTC rearrangements are alternative events in the etiopathogenesis of PTC. Oncogene 2003;22:4578–4580
88. Trovisco V, Vieira de Castro I, Soares P, et al. BRAF mutations are

associated with some histological types of papillary thyroid carcinoma. J Pathol 2004;202:247–251

89. Nikiforova MN, Kimura ET, Gandhi M, et al. BRAF mutations in thyroid tumors are restricted to papillary carcinomas and anaplastic or poorly differentiated carcinomas arising from papillary carcinomas. J Clin Endocrinol Metab 2003;88:5399–5404

90. Fukushima T, Suzuki S, Mashiko M, et al. BRAF mutations in papillary carcinomas of the thyroid. Oncogene 2003;22:6455–6457

91. Namba H, Nakashima M, Hayashi T, et al. Clinical implication of hot spot BRAF mutation, V599E, in papillary thyroid cancers. J Clin Endocrinol Metab 2003;88:4393–4397

92. Xu X, Quiros RM, Gattuso P, Ain KB, Prinz RA. High prevalence of BRAF gene mutation in papillary thyroid carcinomas and thyroid tumor cell lines. Cancer Res 2003;63:4561–4567

93. Cohen Y, Xing M, Mambo E, et al. BRAF mutation in papillary thyroid carcinoma. J Natl Cancer Inst 2003;95:625–627

94. Kim KH, Kang DW, Kim SH, et al. Mutations of the BRAF gene in papillary thyroid carcinoma in a Korean population. Yonsei Med J 2004;45:818–821

95. Lima J, Trovisco V, Soares P, et al. BRAF mutations are not a major event in post-Chernobyl childhood thyroid carcinomas. J Clin Endocrinol Metab 2004;89:4267–4271

96. Trovisco V, Soares P, Preto A, et al. Type and prevalence of BRAF mutations are closely associated with papillary thyroid carcinoma histotype and patients' age but not with tumour aggressiveness. Virchows Arch 2005;446:589–595

97. Xing M, Westra WH, Tufano RP, et al. BRAF mutation predicts a poorer clinical prognosis for papillary thyroid cancer. J Clin Endocrinol Metab 2005;90:6373–6379

98. Vasko V, Hu S, Wu G, et al. High prevalence and possible de novo formation of BRAF mutation in metastasized papillary thyroid cancer in lymph nodes. J Clin Endocrinol Metab 2005;90:5265–5269

99. Begum S, Rosenbaum E, Henrique R, et al. BRAF mutations in anaplastic thyroid carcinoma: implications for tumor origin, diagnosis and treatment. Mod Pathol 2004;17:1359–1363

100. Cohen Y, Rosenbaum E, Clark DP, et al. Mutational analysis of BRAF in fine needle aspiration biopsies of the thyroid: a potential application for the preoperative assessment of thyroid nodules. Clin Cancer Res 2004;10:2761–2765

101. Knauf JA, Ma X, Smith EP, et al. Targeted expression of BRAFV600E in thyroid cells of transgenic mice results in papillary thyroid cancers that undergo dedifferentiation. Cancer Res 2005;65:4238–4245

102. Ciampi R, Knauf JA, Kerler R, et al. Oncogenic AKAP9-BRAF fusion is a novel mechanism of MAPK pathway activation in thyroid cancer. J Clin Invest 2005;115:94–101

103. Ciampi R, Nikiforov YE. RET/PTC rearrangements and BRAF mutations in thyroid tumorigenesis. Endocrinology 2007;148:936–941

104. Halachmi N, Halachmi S, Evron E, et al. Somatic mutations of the PTEN tumor suppressor gene in sporadic follicular thyroid tumors. Genes Chromosomes Cancer 1998;23:239–243

105. Dahia PL, Marsh DJ, Zheng Z, et al. Somatic deletions and mutations in the Cowden disease gene, PTEN, in sporadic thyroid tumors. Cancer Res 1997;57:4710–4713

106. Bruni P, Boccia A, Baldassarre G, et al. PTEN expression is reduced in a subset of sporadic thyroid carcinomas: evidence that PTEN-growth suppressing activity in thyroid cancer cells mediated by p27kip1. Oncogene 2000;19:3146–3155

107. Longy M, Lacombe D. Cowden disease. Report of a family and review. Ann Genet 1996;39:35–42

108. Di Cristofano A, Pesce B, Cordon-Cardo C, Pandolfi PP. Pten is essential for embryonic development and tumour suppression. Nat Genet 1998;19:348–355

109. Kroll TG, Sarraf P, Pecciarini L, et al. PAX8-PPARgamma1 fusion oncogene in human thyroid carcinoma. [corrected] Science 2000;289:1357–1360

110. Ying H, Suzuki H, Zhao L, Willingham MC, Meltzer P, Cheng SY. Mutant thyroid hormone receptor beta represses the expression and transcriptional activity of peroxisome proliferator-activated receptor gamma during thyroid carcinogenesis. Cancer Res 2003;63:5274–5280

111. Marques AR, Espadinha C, Catarino AL, et al. Expression of PAX8-PPAR gamma 1 rearrangements in both follicular thyroid carcinomas and adenomas. J Clin Endocrinol Metab 2002;87:3947–3952

112. Nikiforova MN, Biddinger PW, Caudill CM, Kroll TG, Nikiforov YE. PAX8-PPARgamma rearrangement in thyroid tumors: RT-PCR and immunohistochemical analyses. Am J Surg Pathol 2002;26:1016–1023

113. Cheung L, Messina M, Gill A, et al. Detection of the PAX8-PPAR gamma fusion oncogene in both follicular thyroid carcinomas and adenomas. J Clin Endocrinol Metab 2003;88:354–357

114. Dwight T, Thoppe SR, Foukakis T, et al. Involvement of the PAX8/peroxisome proliferator-activated receptor gamma rearrangement in follicular thyroid tumors. J Clin Endocrinol Metab 2003;88:4440–4445

115. Castro P, Rebocho AP, Soares RJ, et al. PAX8-PPARgamma rearrangement is frequently detected in the follicular variant of papillary thyroid carcinoma. J Clin Endocrinol Metab 2006;91:213–220

116. Basolo F, Caligo MA, Pinchera A, et al. Cyclin D1 overexpression in thyroid carcinomas: relation with clinico-pathological parameters, retinoblastoma gene product, and Ki67 labeling index. Thyroid 2000;10:741–746

117. Lazzereschi D, Sambuco L, Carnovale Scalzo C, et al. Cyclin D1 and Cyclin E expression in malignant thyroid cells and in human thyroid carcinomas. Int J Cancer 1998;76:806–811

118. Zou M, Shi Y, Farid NR, al-Sedairy ST. Inverse association between cyclin D1 overexpression and retinoblastoma gene mutation in thyroid carcinomas. Endocrine 1998;8:61–64

119. Saiz AD, Olvera M, Rezk S, et al. Immunohistochemical expression of cyclin D1, E2F-1, and Ki-67 in benign and malignant thyroid lesions. J Pathol 2002;198:157–162

120. Brzezinski J, Migodzinski A, Gosek A, Tazbir J, Dedecjus M. Cyclin E expression in papillary thyroid carcinoma: relation to staging. Int J Cancer 2004;109:102–105

121. Khoo ML, Ezzat S, Freeman JL, Asa SL. Cyclin D1 protein expression predicts metastatic behavior in thyroid papillary microcarcinomas but is not associated with gene amplification. J Clin Endocrinol Metab 2002;87:1810–1813

122. Khoo ML, Beasley NJ, Ezzat S, Freeman JL, Asa SL. Overexpression of cyclin D1 and underexpression of p27 predict lymph node metastases in papillary thyroid carcinoma. J Clin Endocrinol Metab 2002;87:1814–1818

123. Wang S, Lloyd RV, Hutzler MJ, et al. The role of cell cycle regulatory protein, cyclin D1, in the progression of thyroid cancer. Mod Pathol 2000;13:882–887

124. Farid NR, Shi Y, Zou M. Molecular basis of thyroid cancer. Endocr Rev 1994;15:202–232

125. Segev DL, Umbricht C, Zeiger MA. Molecular pathogenesis of thyroid cancer. Surg Oncol 2003;12:69–90

126. Donghi R, Longoni A, Pilotti S, et al. Gene p53 mutations are restricted to poorly differentiated and undifferentiated carcinomas of the thyroid gland. J Clin Invest 1993;91:1753–1760

127. Dobashi Y, Sugimura H, Sakamoto A, et al. Stepwise participation of p53 gene mutation during dedifferentiation of human thyroid carcinomas. Diagn Mol Pathol 1994;3:9–14

128. Fagin JA, Matsuo K, Karmaker A, Chen DL, Tang SH, Koeffler HP. High

prevalence of mutations of the p53 gene in poorly differentiated human thyroid carcinomas. J Clin Invest 1993;91:179–184

129. Nakamura T, Yana I, Kobayashi T, et al. p53 gene mutations associated with anaplastic transformation of human thyroid carcinomas. Jpn J Cancer Res 1992;83:1293–1298

130. Ito T, Seyama T, Mizuno T, et al. Genetic alterations in thyroid tumor progression: association with p53 gene mutations. Jpn J Cancer Res 1993;84:526–531

131. Ho YS, Tseng SC, Chin TY, Hsieh LL, Lin JD. p53 gene mutation in thyroid carcinoma. Cancer Lett 1996;103:57–63

132. Takeuchi Y, Daa T, Kashima K, Yokoyama S, Nakayama I, Noguchi S. Mutations of p53 in thyroid carcinoma with an insular component. Thyroid 1999;9:377–381

133. Matias-Guiu X, Villanueva A, Cuatrecasas M, et al. p53 in a thyroid follicular carcinoma with foci of poorly differentiated and anaplastic carcinoma. Pathol Res Pract 1996;192:1242–1249 discussion 1250–1251

134. La Perle KM, Jhiang SM, Capen CC. Loss of p53 promotes anaplasia and local invasion in ret/PTC1-induced thyroid carcinomas. Am J Pathol 2000;157:671–677

135. Powell DJ, Russell JP, Li G, et al. Altered gene expression in immunogenic poorly differentiated thyroid carcinomas from RET/PTC3p53−/− mice. Oncogene 2001;20:3235–3246

136. Moretti F, Farsetti A, Soddu S, et al. p53 re-expression inhibits proliferation and restores differentiation of human thyroid anaplastic carcinoma cells. Oncogene 1997;14:729–740

137. Fagin JA, Tang SH, Zeki K, Di Lauro R, Fusco A, Gonsky R. Reexpression of thyroid peroxidase in a derivative of an undifferentiated thyroid carcinoma cell line by introduction of wild-type p53. Cancer Res 1996;56:765–771

138. Brabant G, Hoang-Vu C, Cetin Y, et al. E-cadherin: a differentiation marker in thyroid malignancies. Cancer Res 1993;53:4987–4993

139. Scheumman GF, Hoang-Vu C, Cetin Y, et al. Clinical significance of E-cadherin as a prognostic marker in thyroid carcinomas. J Clin Endocrinol Metab 1995;80:2168–2172

140. Kato N, Tsuchiya T, Tamura G, Motoyama T. E-cadherin expression in follicular carcinoma of the thyroid. Pathol Int 2002;52:13–18

141. Soares P, Berx G, van Roy F, Sobrinho-Simoes M. E-cadherin gene alterations are rare events in thyroid tumors. Int J Cancer 1997;70:32–38

142. Abbosh PH, Nephew KP. Multiple signaling pathways converge on beta-catenin in thyroid cancer. Thyroid 2005;15:551–561

143. Garcia-Rostan G, Camp RL, Herrero A, et al. Beta-catenin dysregulation in thyroid neoplasms: down-regulation, aberrant nuclear expression, and CTNNB1 exon 3 mutations are markers for aggressive tumor phenotypes and poor prognosis. Am J Pathol 2001;158:987–996

144. Miyake N, Maeta H, Horie S, et al. Absence of mutations in the beta-catenin and adenomatous polyposis coli genes in papillary and follicular thyroid carcinomas. Pathol Int 2001;51:680–685

145. Huang Y, Prasad M, Lemon WJ, et al. Gene expression in papillary thyroid carcinoma reveals highly consistent profiles. Proc Natl Acad Sci U S A 2001;98:15044–15049

146. Wasenius VM, Hemmer S, Kettunen E, et al. Hepatocyte growth factor receptor, matrix metalloproteinase-11, tissue inhibitor of metalloproteinase-1, and fibronectin are up-regulated in papillary thyroid carcinoma: a cDNA and tissue microarray study. Clin Cancer Res 2003;9:68–75

147. Ryu S, Jimi S, Eura Y, Kato T, Takebayashi S. Strong intracellular and negative peripheral expression of fibronectin in tumor cells contribute to invasion and metastasis in papillary thyroid carcinoma. Cancer Lett 1999;146:103–109

148. Liu W, Asa SL, Ezzat S. 1alpha,25-Dihydroxyvitamin D3 targets PTEN-dependent fibronectin expression to restore thyroid cancer cell adhesiveness. Mol Endocrinol 2005;19:2349–2357

149. Shefelbine SE, Khorana S, Schultz PN, et al. Mutational analysis of the GDNF/RET-GDNFR alpha signaling complex in a kindred with vesicoureteral reflux. Hum Genet 1998;102:474–478

150. Mackay CR, Terpe HJ, Stauder R, et al. Expression and modulation of CD44 variant isoforms in humans. J Cell Biol 1994;124:71–82

151. Figge J, del Rosario AD, Gerasimov G, et al. Preferential expression of the cell adhesion molecule CD44 in papillary thyroid carcinoma. Exp Mol Pathol 1994;61:203–211

152. Ermak G, Jennings T, Robinson L, Ross JS, Figge J. Restricted patterns of CD44 variant exon expression in human papillary carcinoma. Cancer Res 1996;56:1037–1042

153. Ermak G, Gerasimov G, Troshina K, et al. Deregulated alternative splicing of CD44 messenger RNA transcripts in neoplastic and nonneoplastic lesions of the human thyroid. Cancer Res 1995;55:4594–4598

154. Xing M. Gene methylation in thyroid tumorigenesis. Endocrinology 2007;148:948–953

155. Bird A. DNA methylation patterns and epigenetic memory. Genes Dev 2002;16:6–21

156. Yoo CB, Jones PA. Epigenetic therapy of cancer: past, present and future. Nat Rev Drug Discov 2006;5:37–50

157. Alvarez-Nunez F, Bussaglia E, Mauricio D, et al. PTEN promoter methylation in sporadic thyroid carcinomas. Thyroid 2006;16:17–23

158. Schagdarsurengin U, Gimm O, Hoang-Vu C, et al. Frequent epigenetic silencing of the CpG island promoter of RASSF1A in thyroid carcinoma. Cancer Res 2002;62:3698–3701

159. Xing M, Cohen Y, Mambo E, et al. Early occurrence of RASSF1A hypermethylation and its mutual exclusion with BRAF mutation in thyroid tumorigenesis. Cancer Res 2004;64:1664–1668

160. Hoque MO, Rosenbaum E, Westra WH, et al. Quantitative assessment of promoter methylation profiles in thyroid neoplasms. J Clin Endocrinol Metab 2005;90:4011–4018

161. Hu S, Liu D, Tufano RP, et al. Association of aberrant methylation of tumor suppressor genes with tumor aggressiveness and BRAF mutation in papillary thyroid cancer. Int J Cancer 2006;119:2322–2329

162. Soh EY, Duh QY, Sobhi SA, et al. Vascular endothelial growth factor expression is higher in differentiated thyroid cancer than in normal or benign thyroid. J Clin Endocrinol Metab 1997;82:3741–3747

163. Klein M, Picard E, Vignaud JM, et al. Vascular endothelial growth factor gene and protein: strong expression in thyroiditis and thyroid carcinoma. J Endocrinol 1999;161:41–49

164. Bunone G, Vigneri P, Mariani L, et al. Expression of angiogenesis stimulators and inhibitors in human thyroid tumors and correlation with clinical pathological features. Am J Pathol 1999;155:1967–1976

165. Yasuoka H, Nakamura Y, Zuo H, et al. VEGF-D expression and lymph vessels play an important role for lymph node metastasis in papillary thyroid carcinoma. Mod Pathol 2005;18:1127–1133

166. Katoh R, Miyagi E, Kawaoi A, et al. Expression of vascular endothelial growth factor (VEGF) in human thyroid neoplasms. Hum Pathol 1999;30:891–897

167. Bauer AJ, Patel A, Terrell R, et al. Systemic administration of vascular endothelial growth factor monoclonal antibody reduces the growth of papillary thyroid carcinoma in a nude mouse model. Ann Clin Lab Sci 2003;33:192–199

168. Bauer AJ, Terrell R, Doniparthi NK, et al. Vascular endothelial growth factor monoclonal antibody inhibits growth of anaplastic thyroid cancer xenografts in nude mice. Thyroid 2002;12:953–961

169. Vella V, Sciacca L, Pandini G, et al. The IGF system in thyroid cancer: new concepts. Mol Pathol 2001;54:121–124

170. Russo D, Arturi F, Chiefari E, Filetti S. Genetic alterations in thyroid hyperfunctioning adenomas. J Clin Endocrinol Metab 1995;80:1347–1351

171. Russo D, Tumino S, Arturi F, et al. Detection of an activating mutation of the thyrotropin receptor in a case of an autonomously hyperfunctioning thyroid insular carcinoma. J Clin Endocrinol Metab 1997;82:735–738

172. Belge G, Roque L, Soares J, et al. Cytogenetic investigations of 340 thyroid hyperplasias and adenomas revealing correlations between cytogenetic findings and histology. Cancer Genet Cytogenet 1998;101:42–48

173. Castro P, Eknaes M, Teixera MR, et al. Adenomas and follicular carcinomas of the thyroid display two major patterns of chromosomal changes. J Pathol 2005;206:305–311

174. Sobrinho-Simoes M, Preto A, Rocha AS, et al. Molecular pathology of well-differentiated thyroid carcinomas. Virchows Arch 2005;447:787–793

175. Plail RO, Bussey HJ, Glazer G, et al. Adenomatous polyposis: an association with carcinoma of the thyroid. Br J Surg 1987;74:377–380

176. Lote K, Andersen K, Nordal E, Brennhovd IO. Familial occurrence of papillary thyroid carcinoma. Cancer 1980;46:1291–1297

177. Liaw D, Marsh DJ, Li J, et al. Germline mutations of the PTEN gene in Cowden disease, an inherited breast and thyroid cancer syndrome. Nat Genet 1997;16:64–67

178. Malchoff CD, Malchoff DM. The genetics of hereditary nonmedullary thyroid carcinoma. J Clin Endocrinol Metab 2002;87:2455–2459

179. Cameselle-Teijeiro J, Chan JK. Cribriform-morular variant of papillary carcinoma: a distinctive variant representing the sporadic counterpart of familial adenomatous polyposis-associated thyroid carcinoma? Mod Pathol 1999;12:400–411

180. Wohllk N, Cote GJ, Bugalho MM, et al. Relevance of RET proto-oncogene mutations in sporadic medullary thyroid carcinoma. J Clin Endocrinol Metab 1996;81:3740–3745

181. Fialkowski EA, Moley JF. Current approaches to medullary thyroid carcinoma, sporadic and familial. J Surg Oncol 2006;94:737–747

182. Asai N, Iwashitra T, Murakami H, et al. Mechanism of activation of the ret proto-oncogene by multiple endocrine neoplasia 2A mutations. Mol Cell Biol 1995;15:1613–1619

183. Borrello MG, Smith DP, Pasini B, et al. RET activation by germline MEN2A and MEN2B mutations. . Oncogene 1995;11:2419–2427

184. Santoro M, Carlomagno F, Romano A, et al. Activation of RET as a dominant transforming gene by germline mutations of MEN2A and MEN2B. Science 1995;267:381–383

185. Ichihara M, Murakumo Y, Takahashi M. RET and neuroendocrine tumors. Cancer Lett 2004;204:197–211

186. Kouvaraki MA, Shapiro SE, Perrier ND, et al. RET proto-oncogene: a review and update of genotype-phenotype correlations in hereditary medullary thyroid cancer and associated endocrine tumors. Thyroid 2005;15:531–544

187. Hundahl SA, Fleming ID, Fremgen AM, Menck HR. A National Cancer Data Base report on 53,856 cases of thyroid carcinoma treated in the U.S., 1985–1995. [see comments] Cancer 1998;83:2638–2648

188. Brekken RA, Overholser JP, Stastny VA, et al. Selective inhibition of vascular endothelial growth factor (VEGF) receptor 2 (KDR/Flk-1) activity by a monoclonal anti-VEGF antibody blocks tumor growth in mice. Cancer Res 2000;60:5117–5124

189. Carlomagno F, Vitagliano D, Guida T, et al. ZD6474, an orally available inhibitor of KDR tyrosine kinase activity, efficiently blocks oncogenic RET kinases. Cancer Res 2002;62:7284–7290

190. Carlomagno F, Guida T, Anaganti S, et al. Disease associated mutations at valine 804 in the RET receptor tyrosine kinase confer resistance to selective kinase inhibitors. Oncogene 2004;23:6056–6063

191. Holden SN, Eckhardt SG, Basser R, et al. Clinical evaluation of ZD6474, an orally active inhibitor of VEGF and EGF receptor signaling, in patients with solid, malignant tumors. Ann Oncol 2005;16:1391–1397

192. Milano A, Chiafalo MG, Basile M, et al. New molecular targeted therapies in thyroid cancer. Anticancer Drugs 2006;17:869–879

193. Schoenberger J, Grimm D, Kossmehl P, et al. Effects of PTK787/ZK222584, a tyrosine kinase inhibitor, on the growth of a poorly differentiated thyroid carcinoma: an animal study. Endocrinology 2004;145:1031–1038

194. Bechtner G, Schopohl D, Rafferzeder M, et al. Stimulation of thyroid cell proliferation by epidermal growth factor is different from cell growth induced by thyrotropin or insulin-like growth factor I. Eur J Endocrinol 1996;134:639–648

195. Nobuhara Y, Onoda N, Yamashita Y, et al. Efficacy of epidermal growth factor receptor-targeted molecular therapy in anaplastic thyroid cancer cell lines. Br J Cancer 2005;92:1110–1116

196. Wakeling AE, Guy SP, Woodburn JR, et al. ZD1839 (Iressa): an orally active inhibitor of epidermal growth factor signaling with potential for cancer therapy. Cancer Res 2002;62:5749–5754

197. Kris MG, Natale RB, Herbst RS, et al. Efficacy of gefitinib, an inhibitor of the epidermal growth factor receptor tyrosine kinase, in symptomatic patients with non-small cell lung cancer: a randomized trial. JAMA 2003;290:2149–2158

198. Schiff BA, McMurphy AB, Jasser SA, et al. Epidermal growth factor receptor (EGFR) is overexpressed in anaplastic thyroid cancer, and the EGFR inhibitor gefitinib inhibits the growth of anaplastic thyroid cancer. Clin Cancer Res 2004;10:8594–8602

199. Kim S, Prichard CN, Younes MN, et al. Cetuximab and irinotecan interact synergistically to inhibit the growth of orthotopic anaplastic thyroid carcinoma xenografts in nude mice. Clin Cancer Res 2006;12:600–607

200. Kim S, Schiff BA, Orhan G, et al. Targeted molecular therapy of anaplastic thyroid carcinoma with AEE788. Mol Cancer Ther 2005;4:632–640

201. Carlomagno F, Vitagliano D, Guida T, et al. The kinase inhibitor PP1 blocks tumorigenesis induced by RET oncogenes. Cancer Res 2002;62:1077–1082

202. Carlomagno F, Vitagliano D, Guida T, et al. Efficient inhibition of RET/papillary thyroid carcinoma oncogenic kinases by 4-amino-5-(4-chloro-phenyl)-7-(t-butyl)pyrazolo[3,4-d]pyrimidine(PP2). J Clin Endocrinol Metab 2003;88:1897–1902

203. Karasarides M, Chiloeches A, Hayward R, et al. B-RAF is a therapeutic target in melanoma. Oncogene 2004;23:6292–6298

204. Wilhelm SM, Carter C, Tang L, et al. BAY 43-9006 exhibits broad spectrum oral antitumor activity and targets the RAF/MEK/ERK pathway and receptor tyrosine kinases involved in tumor progression and angiogenesis. Cancer Res 2004;64:7099–7109

205. Salvatore G, De Falco V, Salerno P, et al. BRAF is a therapeutic target in aggressive thyroid carcinoma. Clin Cancer Res 2006;12:1623–1629

206. Carlomagno F, Anaganti S, Guida T, et al. BAY 43-9006 inhibition of oncogenic RET mutants. J Natl Cancer Inst 2006;98:326–334

207. Solit DB, Garraway LA, Pratilas CA, et al. BRAF mutation predicts sensitivity to MEK inhibition. Nature 2006;439:358–362

208. Podtcheko A, Ohtsuru A, Namba H, et al. Inhibition of ABL tyrosine kinase potentiates radiation-induced terminal growth arrest in anaplastic thyroid cancer cells. Radiat Res 2006;165:35–42

209. Podtcheko A, Ohtsuru A, Tsuda S, et al. The selective tyrosine kinase inhibitor, STI571, inhibits growth of anaplastic thyroid cancer cells. J Clin Endocrinol Metab 2003;88:1889–1896

210. Shao Y, Gao Z, Marks PA, Jiang X. Apoptotic and autophagic cell death induced by histone deacetylase inhibitors. Proc Natl Acad Sci U S A 2004;101:18030–18035

211. Della Ragione F, Criniti V, Della Pietra V, et al. Genes modulated by histone acetylation as new effectors of butyrate activity. FEBS Lett 2001;499:199–204

212. Ueda H, Nakajima H, Hori Y, Goto T, Okuhara M. Action of FR901228, a novel antitumor bicyclic depsipeptide produced by Chromobacterium violaceum no. 968, on Ha-ras transformed NIH3T3 cells. Biosci Biotechnol Biochem 1994;58:1579–1583

213. Glick RD, Swendeman SL, Coffey DC, et al. Hybrid polar histone deacetylase inhibitor induces apoptosis and CD95/CD95 ligand expression in human neuroblastoma. Cancer Res 1999;59:4392–4399

214. Kelly WK, O'Connor OA, Krug LM, et al. Phase I study of an oral histone deacetylase inhibitor, suberoylanilide hydroxamic acid, in patients with advanced cancer. J Clin Oncol 2005;23:3923–3931

215. Kelly WK, Richon VM, O'Connor O, et al. Phase I clinical trial of histone deacetylase inhibitor: suberoylanilide hydroxamic acid administered intravenously. Clin Cancer Res 2003;9(10 pt 1):3578–3588

216. Kersten S, Desvergne B, Wahli W. Roles of PPARs in health and disease. Nature 2000;405:421–424

IV Parathyroid Diseases

15 Imaging of the Parathyroid Glands

Brett M. Clarke and Brendan C. Stack Jr.

Hyperparathyroidism is a disease of calcium dysregulation throughout the body. Estimates from population-based data (1983–1992) suggest the United States incidence of primary hyperparathyroidism is approximately 20 per 100,000. Hyperparathyroidism affects predominately women 55 to 75 years of age, with a prevalence of 1 per 1000.[1] Up to 97% of primary hyperparathyroidism results from single-adenoma disease, with the remaining cases resulting from four-gland hyperplasia (up to 10%), multiple adenomas (<3%), and carcinoma (<1%).[2,3] Once a symptomatic disease, morbid hyperparathyroidism is largely historical. With the development of screening serum calcium assays in the 1970s, a new asymptomatic or significantly less symptomatic hyperparathyroidism patient has emerged. "Asymptomatic" means the absence of traditional signs and symptoms of severe hypercalcemia such as psychosis or mental derangement, saber shins, bone pain, nephrolithiasis, and renal failure. Some of the known signs and symptoms of mild hypercalcemia include nephrolithiasis, vague constitutional complaints, memory loss, depression, lethargy, constipation, sleep abnormalities, muscle atrophy, hyperreflexia, abnormal gait, tongue fasciculation, and bone pain. Most patients present simply with an elevated serum calcium level. Despite being asymptomatic during preoperative evaluation, patients often report postoperative retrospective amelioration of unreported preoperative signs and symptoms of hypercalcemia.

With so many asymptomatic hyperparathyroid patients, management of these patients has been debated. Traditionally symptomatic patients underwent bilateral neck exploration with biopsy of the parathyroid glands and excision of identifiable adenomas. Traditional bilateral neck exploration has maintained a greater than 96% cure rate.[4,5] Such an extensive and potentially morbid procedure, however, seemed radical for patients with "asymptomatic" disease. In 1991, the National Institutes of Health (NIH) consensus guidelines for the management of asymptomatic hyperparathyroidism were released in an effort to ease the decision-making process. These guidelines were revised in 2002.[6] Despite these guidelines, there has been continued reluctance on the part of the endocrinology community to refer asymptomatic patients for parathyroidectomy due to the extensive nature of traditional bilateral neck exploration. In an era of improved parathyroid imaging and minimal access parathyroid surgery, this referral reluctance has diminished somewhat.

Since hyperparathyroidism was first described in the 1930s, parathyroid imaging methods have been evolving.[7,8] For example, early attempts to visualize the parathyroid glands involved anatomic displacement on barium swallow.[9] This technique was still used as recently as 1997.[10] Low sensitivity and specificity has hampered the utility of many such techniques. With the introduction of radioactive tracers near the end of World War II, advances in nuclear medicine made possible physiologic evaluation of the parathyroid glands. Localization of hyperfunctional glands has led to the development of directed surgery and ultimately minimally invasive parathyroidectomy (MIP).[2,11,12] Although the popularity and indeed the technique of minimally invasive parathyroid surgery continue to evolve, MIP requires the use of preoperative localization studies. This chapter focuses on the various localizing techniques that can be used to assist focused MIP surgery.

Localization Techniques

Nuclear Medicine

Nuclear medicine techniques for imaging abnormal parathyroid glands have evolved clinically over the past 70 years. With the relatively new focus on localization rather than diagnosis, the sensitivity and specificity of a particular technique have been markedly emphasized. An ideal study is both sensitive and specific; several factors combine to influence sensitivity and specificity. Some of these factors include patient factors (cooperation, specimen size), physiologic factors (radioactive tracer uptake quantity, washout characteristics, parathyroid specificity), dosimetry (what dose produces the best images), imaging technique (camera position, collimator shape), and postcapture image processing (computed image production). Patient factors are most variable.

Radioactive Tracers

Several tracers have been used unsuccessfully including Co-57-cyanocobalamine and Se-75-selenomethionine in the early 1960s.[9,13] Uptake of these tracers was sufficiently poor as to produce marginal image quality and drive parathyroid scintigraphy out of use. Then, in the late 1970s thallium 201 (Tl-201) was incidentally noted to have parathyroid adenoma uptake.[13] Tl-201 parathyroid avidity was targeted using a subtraction technique.[14] Tl-201 is taken up by thyroid and parathyroid tissue alike in a nonspecific fashion. When evaluated against technetium-99m (Tc-99m)-pertechnetate chloride, which had thyroid tissue-specific uptake, computerized subtraction of the Tl-201 and Tc-99m-pertechnetate images could be performed to identify parathyroid

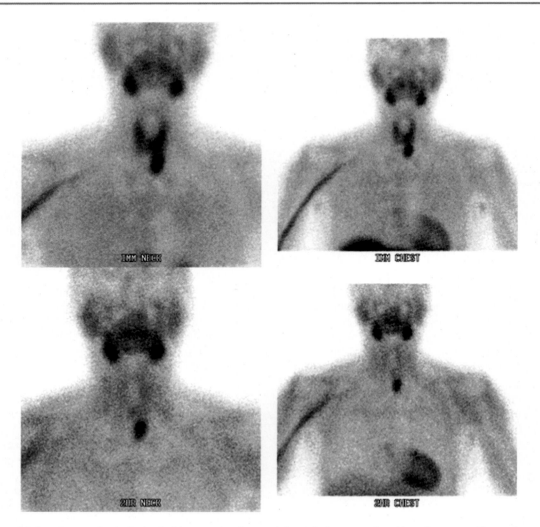

Fig. 15.1 Sestamibi. Four images in clockwise fashion starting from the upper left corner: Immediate neck view, immediate chest view, 2-hour chest view, and 2-hour neck view. This is a classic-appearing left inferior parathyroid adenoma. The adenoma is seen clearly on the immediate view, thus making a delayed view unnecessary.

adenomas. For adenomas 500 mg or larger (at least 10 times normal size), this technique localized quite well. Despite this success, Tl-201 has suboptimal physical properties for imaging with a gamma camera. Specifically, the energy of its radiation is lower than ideal and there is a relatively high radiation dose to the patient.[15]

Technetium-99m-sestamibi was first discovered to have persistent uptake in parathyroid tissue during myocardial perfusion studies.[16,17] Technetium-99m-sestamibi is taken up by thyroid and parathyroid glands alike (**Fig. 15.1**). However, in contrast to precursor radiotracers such as Tl-201, sestamibi washout time from parathyroid glands is longer than the thyroid tissue, remaining in the richer mitochondrial tissues.[18,19] This time differential has proven useful to search for parathyroid adenomas with a single agent, which is approximately 80% sensitive (range, 50–90%) on planar studies.[2,20,21] The broad sensitivity range for sestamibi may stem from various interinstitutional imaging techniques as well as patient factors. Sestamibi has been reported to iden-

tify adenomas ranging from 64 mg to over 8000 mg (normal is 40–50 mg), while at the same time missing adenomas weighing 300 mg on average.[22] False-negative results on sestamibi have been attributed to small glands (less than 100 mg); parathyroid hyperplasia, which has poorer parathyroid-tracer uptake; and adenomatous properties, such as higher concentration of clear cells or the presence of a multidrug-resistance gene.[3,23–28] False-positive studies commonly result from overlying thyroid pathology.[29] Dual isotope studies with sestamibi and low-dose Tc-99m-pertechnetate or iodine 123 have been advocated to improve study sensitivity.[20,30,31]

Technetium-99m-tetrofosmin, also a myocardial perfusion agent, has been tested for parathyroid uptake. Although parathyroid tetrofosmin uptake is avid, tetrofosmin tends to clear from parathyroid tissue at a rate faster than sestamibi.[32,33] Despite this, Gallowitsch et al[32] and Ishibashi et al[34] produced sensitivities comparable to those for sestamibi. Ishibashi et al demonstrated 100%

sensitivity and specificity of both sestamibi and tetrofosmin for adenoma. Hyperplasia results were similar. Gallowitsch et al, using less tetrofosmin (24 mCi versus 10 mCi), found that tetrofosmin had delayed clearance from parathyroid tissue similar to sestamibi on early images. Delayed studies several hours after injection, however, showed greater washout, thereby decreasing sensitivity to 62%. They compensated for lower sensitivity on planar images with the addition of single photon emission computed tomography SPECT (discussed below). The use of SPECT with tetrofosmin increased sensitivity for parathyroid adenoma to 94% with a specificity of 85%. Gallowitsch et al suggested tetrofosmin as a sensitive alternative to sestamibi if the use of such is required based on institutional availability of tetrofosmin.

Nuclear Imaging Techniques

Fundamental imaging requires a radioactive source and a camera. More advanced imaging techniques involve multiple camera positions and computer image compilation. A detailed discussion of nuclear medicine imaging is beyond the scope of this chapter; interested readers should consult a nuclear medicine imaging text. But briefly, handheld probes that lacked spatial orientation with respect to the anatomic site were the first detection instruments. These gave way to rectilinear scanners, which were very simply collimated probe arrays. Gamma scintillation cameras displaced rectilinear scanners. The gamma camera offered more imaging flexibility and the capability of doing computed tomography.

A gamma camera consists of a collimator (lens equivalent), a layer of sodium iodide crystals positioned under photomultiplier tubes, a position computer, and an output monitor/recording device. Random x-rays or gamma rays filter through the collimator and strike the NaI crystals, causing a release of photon energy. Photons are captured in the photomultiplier tubes where they displace electrons. Electrons then convey a signal to a position computer, which then relays information to the output device (see Thrall and Ziessman[35]). The collimator acts as an attenuation plate allowing only correctly positioned radioactive waves to contact the NaI crystals to produce an image (similar to a polarizing lens). Four fundamental collimators exist for the gamma camera: parallel, pinhole, converging, and diverging. The pinhole collimator, most commonly used for parathyroid imaging, collects radiation from a small source and then inverts and magnifies the image like a pinhole camera. It can be positioned to collect oblique views in addition to anteroposterior (AP) views, which improve localization accuracy over the AP view obtained with a parallel collimator.[36–38] The Norman technique (discussed below) achieves high localization accuracy without the use of a pinhole collimator.[39]

The use of Tl-201 for parathyroid imaging required the development of an image subtraction technique to digitally remove the thyroid gland.[14] Subtraction imaging was often performed with iodine 123 or Tc-99m-pertechnetate.[40] Soon Tc-99m-pertechnetate gained favor over I-123 for its shorter

peak emission time, and therefore shorter imaging time. This technique was the first to have good accuracy at localization, but it introduced multiple variables that made reproducibility difficult. Some of these variables included dual tracer dosing, tracer administration sequence, mobility restraints of patients, and computer evaluation.[21] Patient immobility was paramount, and attaining it was challenging, with imaging lasting as long as 30 minutes even with pertechnetate in place of I-123.[13] Indeed, Price,[41] in his review, suggested that the most common cause of a false-positive study was patient movement. Despite these challenges, adenoma sensitivity ranged from 35 to 80%, with hyperplasia sensitivity ranging from 37 to 43%.[41–46] With the complexity required for subtraction imaging (double isotope imaging), a simpler single agent was desired.

After O'Doherty et al[17] demonstrated only marginally impressive results with subtraction sestamibi, Taillefer et al[21] reported the dual- (or double) phase technique. The novelty of the dual-phase technique lay in the absence of subtraction imaging. Taillefer et al exploited the late parathyroid washout characteristics of sestamibi and demonstrated early and late imaging as a form of thyroid subtraction. "Early" imaging typically occurs 5 to 15 minutes after injection of radiotracer. Late imaging occurs 2 to 3 hours after injection, which is adequate time for thyroid washout to occur. Several studies suggest that early imaging is most accurate because late imaging is subject to unpredictable washout of the parathyroid glands.[21,34,37] This dual-phase technique has proven useful with Tc-99m-tetrofosmin tracer as well.[34] Again the Norman technique, emphasized here for its reported success at reliably localizing parathyroid adenomas for radioguided minimally invasive surgery and for use on patients reported as having "negative" scans, also suggests that early imaging is best.[39] Several key points make the Norman technique successful: (1) the patient is placed in the standard parathyroid operative position (neck extended with a shoulder roll); (2) the gamma camera is placed as close to the patient as possible; (3) parallel collimation is used; (4) left and right oblique anterior views are captured by moving the camera 31 degrees off midline (not by turning the patient's head); (5) intravenous (IV) sestamibi, 20 mCi, is given; and (6) early images are captured in 5 to 10 minutes. Late images may be acquired at no later than 2.5 hours, though they are seldom obtained.

Single photo emission computed tomography (SPECT) has found utility by increasing sestamibi sensitivity (**Fig. 15.2**). In contrast to traditional planar imaging as described above with a fixed position gamma camera, SPECT involves using a mobile camera to collect images at multiple angles around the patient. The multiple images are then compiled by a computer and displayed as a 3D image (similar to positron emission tomography [PET] scan images seen commonly today). Sfakianakis et al[47] saw high sensitivity with SPECT, though a comparison to planar films is not reported. Moka et al[48] reported an 87 to 95% sensitivity with subtraction sestamibi/SPECT and three-dimensional (3D) imaging rendering; adenoma size positively correlated with localization.

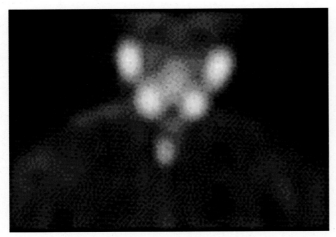

Fig. 15.2 Single photon emission computed tomography (SPECT). A frozen anteroposterior imaging from a rotating SPECT exam demonstrating a right inferior parathyroid. Courtesy of James Norman, MD.

Interestingly, of 92 patients, no hyperplastic glands were identified. Slater and Gleeson[49] found an increase in sensitivity from 62 to 73% with SPECT over low-dose (16 mCi) planar sestamibi. SPECT adds improved sensitivity for ectopic lesions.[50,51] Gayed et al[52] determined that SPECT/CT added no clinical benefit to SPECT alone. Some authors feel that SPECT adds unnecessary cost for small incremental sensitivity gains if planar films are performed correctly.[3,39,53] Given the published variability of technique with planar sestamibi imaging, SPECT may prove itself to be an equalizer across institutions. Continued improvement in imaging accuracy will lead to improved minimally invasive parathyroid surgeries.

Ultrasound

High-resolution ultrasound facilitates anatomic evaluation of parathyroid glands (**Fig. 15.3**). Normal parathyroid glands are not detectable with any imaging modality due to small size and structural patterns similar to adjacent thyroid tissue. However, when biochemical evidence of hyperparathyroidism exists, high-frequency ultrasound can localize associated parathyroid disease.

Ultrasound Technique

The patient is positioned as in an examination of the thyroid gland. The neck is hyperextended with a bolster between the shoulders. A high-frequency probe is used. Typical locations within the thyroid bed and paratracheal tissues are carefully searched for parathyroid tissue. The superior gland is usually found posterior to the middle third of the thyroid. The inferior gland usually lies near the inferior tip of the thyroid. One percent to 3% of glands are found in ectopic locations including the thyroid parenchyma, the carotid sheath, and the mediastinum. Maximum rotation of the neck away from the side being examined and swallowing by the patient may bring an enlarged gland into view.[54] Intrathyroidal adenomas are usually hypoechoic but can be distinguished accurately from thyroid nodules by fine-needle aspiration (FNA) biopsy. As many as 13% of people have more than four parathyroid glands,[55] suggesting that a thorough and systematic examination is required. For high resolution, a 10-MHz or higher transducer probe is recommended.[56] It is more challenging to examine patients with obese necks, which at times requires the use of a 5-MHz transducer.[57] The lower the transducer frequency, the lower the image resolution and sensitivity of examination.[58]

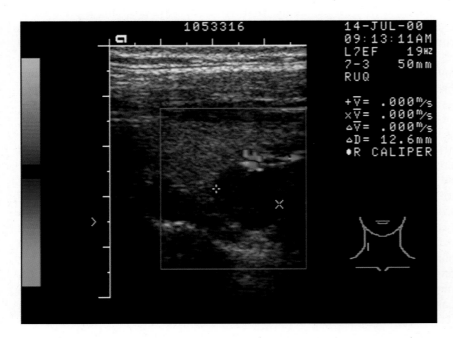

Fig. 15.3 Ultrasound. This is a right upper quadrant, hypoechoic lesion underneath the thyroid with a rim of color flow Doppler activity. This is a classic finding for a parathyroid adenoma. Courtesy of Jon Meilstrup, MD.

On ultrasound, a typical parathyroid adenoma appears as an oval mass, with a homogeneous texture and low echogenicity. The low echogenicity is a result of the uniform hypercellularity of the adenoma. Most adenomas are solid, though some may be cystic.[55] A more elongated and tubular appearance may develop as well.[59] Color flow Doppler may reveal a peripheral vascular arc around a portion of the gland. Patients with primary parathyroid hyperplasia may not have enlarged glands, or one gland may be larger, leading to the incorrect conclusion that an adenoma is present. The sensitivity of ultrasonography in these instances is less than 50%.[60] In patients with four-gland hyperplasia secondary to renal failure, all four glands may be enlarged and even similar in size.[60] False-positive findings are caused by thyroid nodules, lymph nodes, esophagus, longus coli muscle, and perithyroidal veins (oval on transverse views).[55] Indeed, distinguishing between a posterior thyroid nodule and parathyroid gland can be challenging. Meilstrup[59] recommends looking for a separating plane of tissue. According to Hopkins and Reading,[57] false-negative findings are related to three factors: (1) adenoma size, (2) thyroid pathology obscuring visualization, and (3) ectopic location. Sonographer skill obviously also plays an important role in localization.[61] In most instances adjusting transducer positioning provides additional clues to the identity of anatomic structures. In instances where identity remains in doubt, ultrasound-guided FNA may be of utility.[57,62] At some institutions parathyroid aspirates are obtained and tested for parathyroid hormone (PTH) for further confirmation, but this may complicate later surgery.[62,63]

Ultrasound Utility

Low-cost, high-availability, front-line provider reimbursement and ease of examination drive the utility of ultrasound preoperative localization. Ultrasound has traditionally been the least expensive parathyroid localizing study.[46,58] Unfortunately, inherent variability regarding ultrasound examination leads to a wide range of sensitivity (27–95%).[3,34,58,61,64–67] Differences in sonographer skill and static versus dynamic image interpretation are chiefly responsible for this variability. High-resolution ultrasound is at least as effective as sestamibi for localizing multiple gland disease.[3] Retroesophageal, retrotracheal, and mediastinal adenomas can produce false-negative ultrasound evaluations.[60,64] Some have suggested performing nuclear medicine studies in addition to ultrasound to increase the sensitivity of localization.[61,66,67]

Ultrasound-guided FNA of suspicious masses not only identifies parathyroid tissue but also identifies adenomatous or hyperplastic thyroid disease.[68] In persistent or recurrent hyperparathyroidism, the reported sensitivity of ultrasound ranges from 36 to 63%.[69,70] Ultrasound augmented by FNA and PTH assay can lead to a specificity approaching 100%.[71,72] Ultrasound offers the additional benefit of surveillance for synchronous thyroid disease, in particular cancer that has occurred in up to 6% of cases presenting with primary hyperparathyroidism (HPT).[73]

Ultrasound-guided parathyroid ablation is an option for patients too ill to undergo surgery or those patients who refuse surgery.[63] The technique, as described by Lewis et al,[63] requires ultrasound-guided fine-needle injection of pure ethanol into the adenoma. The needle is re-sited and the injection repeated until the entire adenoma is hypoechoic and there is a drop in serum PTH and calcium levels. Recurrence of hypercalcemia is common on follow-up several years later, requiring repeated injections of ethanol. The major risk of this procedure is recurrent laryngeal nerve dysfunction (temporary or permanent) from alcohol diffusion. A literature review by Bennedbaek et al[74] revealed a 15% rate of temporary dysphonia and a 1% rate of permanent dysphonia after ethanol ablation. This compares to a roughly 8 to 10% temporary dysphonia rate and a 0 to 4% permanent dysphonia rate with a traditional neck exploration,[44,75] and minimally invasive and unilateral surgery dysphonia rates are 0.04 to 1% (reoperated), respectively.[76,77] Ultrasound-guided laser ablation may be a future alternative to ethanol injection.[78]

Other Imaging Techniques

Various other imaging techniques have been used to localize parathyroid adenomas and hyperplasia. Because of their consistently low sensitivity and specificity in addition to their higher cost, these techniques are considered second line and reserved for failed localization attempts with sestamibi, ultrasound, and surgery. Each of these following techniques as well as those previously discussed may provide complementary information when used sequentially to evaluate for ectopic adenomata.[79]

Computed tomography may isolate large adenomas or larger hyperplastic glands[80] (**Fig. 15.4**). Besides exposing the patient to ionizing radiation, CT is also limited by swallowing and shoulder artifact.[80] Despite these limitations, CT sensitivity ranges from 46 to 87% for parathyroid adenomas, and may be particularly useful for ectopic glands.[80] In addition, CT has found increased sensitivity when combined with SPECT[52,81–83] or PET,[84] especially for ectopic glands.

Magnetic resonance imaging (MRI) can be useful for parathyroid imaging (**Fig. 15.5**). Sensitivity for localizing parathyroid adenomas ranges from 65 to 92%[80,85] for primary cases. Sensitivity decreases in patients requiring reoperation because of prior neck surgery.[86] Hyperfunctioning parathyroid glands on MRI tend to be isointense to low signal intensity on T1-weighted images, high signal intensity on T2-weighted images, with intense enhancement after intravenous gadolinium administration. T1 signal intensity may match that of T2 intensity in cystic or hemorrhagic lesions. Lower signal intensity may be seen on both T1 and T2 in fibrotic, older, hemorrhagic, and degenerated lesions.[80] Limitations of the use of MRI include cost and patient tolerance of the close confines and the exam duration.[80]

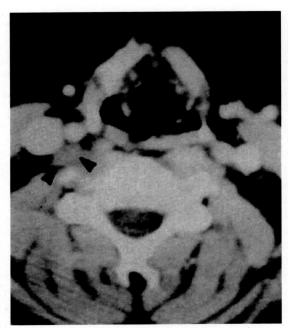

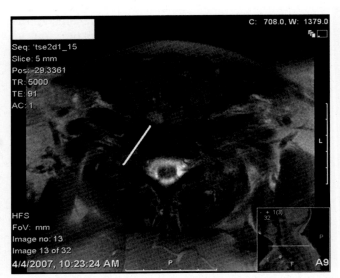

Fig. 15.5 Magnetic resonance imaging (MRI). T2 axial, fat-suppressed MRI scan demonstrating a posterior, right-sided parathyroid adenoma between the right carotid sheath and the esophagus.

Fig. 15.4 Computed tomography (CT). Although this dated CT has localized an adenoma, CT is not considered a reliable method to localize parathyroid adenomas, even with technical enhancement to modern CT machines. Used with permission from Doppman JL, Shawker TH, Krudy AG, et al. Parathymic parathyroid: CT, US, and angiographic findings. Radiology 1985;157:419–423.

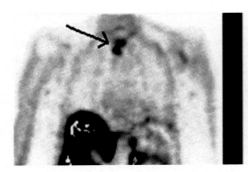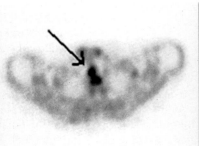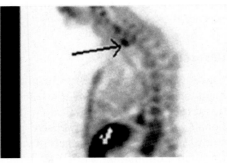

Fig. 15.6 Positron emission tomography (PET). Recurrent primary HPT with retroesophageal adenoma. PET 10 minutes postinjection of 900 MBq[11]C-methionine revealed focal tracer accumulation (*arrows*) suggestive of adenomatous–hyperplastic parathyroid tissue. Used with permission from Otto D, Boerner AA, Hofmann M, et al. Pre-operative localization of hyperfunctional parathyroid tissue with 11C-methionine PET. Eur J Nucl Med Mol Imaging 2004;31:1405–1412.

Positron emission tomography (PET) thus far has been of limited use for parathyroid localization (**Fig. 15.6**). Both fluorodeoxyglucose (FDG) and ^{11}C-methionine PET have demonstrated a fairly high sensitivity and specificity for localizing parathyroid glands.[87–90] Sensitivity for localizing hyperplastic glands appears to be higher with ^{11}C-methionine PET than standard sestamibi or ultrasound.[91] As cost decreases and availability increases, the use of PET alone or in combination with CT or other modalities may increase as this modality holds promise for improved preoperative localization of parathyroid disease.

Historically, venous sampling was used more commonly as a localizing modality.[92] In contrast to the aforementioned noninvasive localizing techniques, venous sampling requires femoral venipuncture and canalization of perithyroidal veins under fluoroscopic guidance. Sampled blood is then analyzed for parathyroid hormone levels. These levels are then compared with those of other sites sampled. Though time intensive, costly, and invasive, its sensitivity for localization falls into the range of other localizing modalities (39 to 93%). This modality of localization has demonstrated usefulness in select cases such as reoperative necks when done by an experienced radiologist.[93–96]

Conclusion

As surgical options have changed, parathyroid imaging options have expanded in an attempt to provide better preoperative localization. Sestamibi continues to be the most sensitive and specific for localizing parathyroid adenomata. Sestamibi has decreased sensitivity for localizing hyperplastic glands. Ultrasound with or without fine-needle aspiration, CT, and MRI all have similar sensitivities and specificities for adenoma localization. PET scanning is relatively unstudied as a localization tool, and may provide an option for increased localization of hyperplastic glands as well as adenomas. Combinations of these modalities may provide improved localization results, especially with ectopic glands, but also at an increased cost.

References

1. Melton LJ. The epidemiology of primary hyperparathyroidism in North America. J Bone Miner Res 2002;17(suppl 2):N12–N17
2. Denham DW, Norman J. Cost-effectiveness of preoperative sestamibi scan for primary hyperparathyroidism is dependent solely upon the surgeon's choice of operative procedure. J Am Coll Surg 1998;186:293–305
3. Ruda JM, Hollenbeak CS, Stack BC. A systematic review of the diagnosis and treatment of primary hyperparathyroidism from 1995 to 2003. Otolaryngol Head Neck Surg 2005;132:359–372
4. Snell SB, Gaar EE, Stevens SP, et al. Parathyroid cancer, a continued diagnostic and therapeutic dilemma: report of four cases and review of the literature. Am Surg 2003;69:711–716
5. Low RA, Katz AD. Parathyroidectomy via bilateral cervical exploration: a retrospective review of 866 cases. Head Neck 1998;20:583–587
6. Bilezikian JP, Potts JT, Fuleihan Gel H, et al. Summary statement from a workshop on asymptomatic primary hyperparathyroidism: a perspective for the 21st century. J Clin Endocrinol Metab 2002;87:5353–5361
7. Albright F, Bauer W, Claflin D, et al. Studies in parathyroid physiology: III. The effect of phosphate ingestion in clinical hyperparathyroidism. J Clin Invest 1932;11:411–435
8. Albright A. Hyperparathyroidism. Some early patients. Arch Intern Med 1970;126:558–559, passim
9. Potchen EJ. Parathyroid imaging–current status and future prospects. J Nucl Med 1992;33:1807–1809
10. Vazquez-Quintana E. Parathyroid carcinoma: diagnosis and management. Am Surg 1997;63:954–957
11. Irvin GL, Prudhomme DL, Deriso GT, et al. A new approach to parathyroidectomy. Ann Surg 1994;219:574–579 discussion 79–81
12. Lee WJ, Ruda J, Stack BC. Minimally invasive radioguided parathyroidectomy using intraoperative sestamibi localization. Otolaryngol Clin North Am 2004;37:789–798 ix.
13. Price D, Okerlund MD. Parathyroid gland. In: Early PJ, Sodee DB, eds. Principles and Practice of Nuclear Medicine, 2nd ed. St. Louis: Mosby, 1995:641–651
14. Ferlin G, Conte N, Borsato N, et al. Parathyroid scintigraphy with 131Cs and 201Tl. J Nucl Med Allied Sci 1981;25:119–123
15. Geatti O, Shapiro B, Orsolon PG, et al. Localization of parathyroid enlargement: experience with technetium-99m methoxyisobutylisonitrile and thallium-201 scintigraphy, ultrasonography and computed tomography. Eur J Nucl Med 1994;21:17–22
16. Coakley AJ, Kettle AG, Wells CP, et al. 99Tcm sestamibi—a new agent for parathyroid imaging. Nucl Med Commun 1989;10:791–794
17. O'Doherty MJ, Kettle AG, Wells P, et al. Parathyroid imaging with technetium-99m-sestamibi: preoperative localization and tissue uptake studies. J Nucl Med 1992;33:313–318
18. Chiu ML, Kronauge JF, Piwnica-Worms D. Effect of mitochondrial and plasma membrane potentials on accumulation of hexakis (2-methoxyisobutylisonitrile) technetium(I) in cultured mouse fibroblasts. J Nucl Med 1990;31:1646–1653
19. Piwnica-Worms D, Holman BL. Noncardiac applications of hexakis(alkylisonitrile) technetium-99m complexes. J Nucl Med 1990;31:1166–1167
20. Chen CC, Holder LE, Scovill WA, et al. Comparison of parathyroid imaging with technetium-99m-pertechnetate/sestamibi subtraction, double-phase technetium-99m-sestamibi and technetium-99m-sestamibi SPECT. J Nucl Med 1997;38:834–839
21. Taillefer R, Boucher Y, Potvin C, et al. Detection and localization of parathyroid adenomas in patients with hyperparathyroidism using a single radionuclide imaging procedure with technetium-99m-sestamibi (double-phase study). J Nucl Med 1992;33:1801–1807
22. Takami H, Satake S, Nakamura K, et al. Technetium 99m sestamibi scan is the useful procedure to locate parathyroid adenomas before surgery. Am J Surg 1996;172:93
23. Westreich RW, Brandwein M, Mechanick JI, et al. Preoperative parathyroid localization: correlating false-negative technetium 99m sestamibi scans with parathyroid disease. Laryngoscope 2003;113:567–572
24. Yamaguchi S, Yachiku S, Hashimoto H, et al. Relation between technetium 99m-methoxyisobutylisonitrile accumulation and multidrug resistance protein in the parathyroid glands. World J Surg 2002;26:29–34
25. Kao A, Shiau Y-C, Tsai S-C, et al. Technetium-99m methoxyisobutylisonitrile imaging for parathyroid adenoma: relationship to P-glycoprotein or multidrug resistance-related protein expression. Eur J Nucl Med Mol Imaging 2002;29:1012–1015
26. Mehta NY, Ruda JM, Kapadia S, et al. Relationship of technetium Tc 99m sestamibi scans to histopathological features of hyperfunctioning parathyroid tissue. Arch Otolaryngol Head Neck Surg 2005;131:493–498
27. Pons F, Torregrosa JV, Fuster D. Biological factors influencing parathyroid localization. Nucl Med Commun 2003;24:121–124
28. Arbab AS, Koizumi K, Hemmi A, et al. Tc-99m-MIBI scintigraphy for detecting parathyroid adenoma and hyperplasia. Ann Nucl Med 1997;11:45–49
29. McBiles M, Lambert AT, Cote MG, et al. Sestamibi parathyroid imaging. Semin Nucl Med 1995;25:221–234
30. Leslie WD, Dupont JO, Bybel B, et al. Parathyroid 99mTc-sestamibi scintigraphy: dual-tracer subtraction is superior to double-phase washout. Eur J Nucl Med Mol Imaging 2002;29:1566–1570
31. Neumann DR, Esselstyn CB, Go RT, et al. Comparison of double-phase 99mTc-sestamibi with 123I–99mTc-sestamibi subtraction SPECT in hyperparathyroidism. AJR Am J Roentgenol 1997;169:1671–1674
32. Gallowitsch HJ, Mikosch P, Kresnik E, et al. Technetium 99m tetrofosmin parathyroid imaging. Results with double-phase study and SPECT in primary and secondary hyperparathyroidism. Invest Radiol 1997;32:459–465
33. Fjeld JG, Erichsen K, Pfeffer PF, et al. Technetium-99m-tetrofosmin for parathyroid scintigraphy: a comparison with sestamibi. J Nucl Med 1997;38:831–834
34. Ishibashi M, Nishida H, Hiromatsu Y, et al. Comparison of technetium-99m-MIBI, technetium-99m-tetrofosmin, ultrasound

and MRI for localization of abnormal parathyroid glands. J Nucl Med 1998;39:320–324

35. Thrall JH, Ziessman HA. Nuclear Medicine: The Requisites, 2nd ed. St Louis: Mosby, 2001:16–32, 363–387

36. Arveschoug AK, Bertelsen H, Vammen B. Presurgical localization of abnormal parathyroid glands using a single injection of Tc-99m sestamibi: comparison of high-resolution parallel-hole and pinhole collimators, and interobserver and intraobserver variation. Clin Nucl Med 2002;27:249–254

37. Arveschoug AK, Bertelsen H, Vammen B, et al. Preoperative dual-phase parathyroid imaging with tc-99m-sestamibi: accuracy and reproducibility of the pinhole collimator with and without oblique images. Clin Nucl Med 2007;32:9–12

38. Ho Shon IA, Bernard EJ, Roach PJ, Delbridge LW. The value of oblique pinhole images in pre-operative localisation with 99mTc-MIBI for primary hyperparathyroidism. Eur J Nucl Med 2001;28:736–742

39. Norman J. The sestamibi scan—technical details. http://www.parathyroidcom/Sestamibi-Technicalhtm 2007.

40. O'Doherty MJ, Kettle AG. Parathyroid imaging: preoperative localization. Nucl Med Commun 2003;24:125–131

41. Price DC. Radioisotopic evaluation of the thyroid and parathyroids. Radiol Clin North Am 1993;31:991–1015

42. Okerlund MD, Sheldon K, Corpuz S, et al. A new method with high sensitivity and specificity for localization of abnormal parathyroid glands. Ann Surg 1984;200:381–388

43. Sandrock D, Merino MJ, Norton JA, et al. Parathyroid imaging by Tc/Tl scintigraphy. Eur J Nucl Med 1990;16:607–613

44. Miller DL. Pre-operative localization and interventional treatment of parathyroid tumors: when and how? World J Surg 1991;15:706–715

45. Fine EJ. Parathyroid imaging: its current status and future role. Semin Nucl Med 1987;17:350–359

46. Clark OH, Duh QY. Primary hyperparathyroidism. A surgical perspective. Endocrinol Metab Clin North Am 1989;18:701–714

47. Sfakianakis GN, Irvin GL, Foss J, et al. Efficient parathyroidectomy guided by SPECT-MIBI and hormonal measurements. J Nucl Med 1996;37:798–804

48. Moka D, Voth E, Dietlein M, et al. Technetium 99m-MIBI-SPECT: a highly sensitive diagnostic tool for localization of parathyroid adenomas. Surgery 2000;128:29–35

49. Slater A, Gleeson FV. Increased sensitivity and confidence of SPECT over planar imaging in dual-phase sestamibi for parathyroid adenoma detection. Clin Nucl Med 2005;30:1–3

50. Teigen EL, Kilgore EJ, Cowan RJ, et al. Technetium-99m-sestamibi SPECT localization of mediastinal parathyroid adenoma. J Nucl Med 1996;37:1535–1537

51. Billotey C, Sarfati E, Aurengo A, et al. Advantages of SPECT in technetium-99m-sestamibi parathyroid scintigraphy. J Nucl Med 1996;37:1773–1778

52. Gayed IW, Kim EE, Broussard WF, et al. The value of 99mTc-sestamibi SPECT/CT over conventional SPECT in the evaluation of parathyroid adenomas or hyperplasia. J Nucl Med 2005;46:248–252

53. Norman JG, Jaffray CE, Chheda H. The false-positive parathyroid sestamibi: a real or perceived problem and a case for radioguided parathyroidectomy. Ann Surg 2000;231:31–37

54. Barraclough BM, Barraclough BH. Ultrasound of the Thyroid and Parathyroid Glands. World J Surg 2000;24:158–165

55. Hopkins CR, Reading CC. Thyroid, parathyroid and other glands. In: McGahan JP, Goldberg BB, eds. Diagnostic Ultrasound: A Logical Approach. Philadelphia: Lippincott-Raven, 1998:1087–1114

56. Kamaya A, Quon A, Jeffrey RB. Sonography of the abnormal parathyroid gland. Ultrasound Q 2006;22:253–262

57. Hopkins CR, Reading CC. Thyroid and parathyroid imaging. Semin Ultrasound CT MR 1995;16:279–295

58. Koslin DB, Adams J, Andersen P, et al. Preoperative evaluation of patients with primary hyperparathyroidism: role of high-resolution ultrasound. Laryngoscope 1997;107:1249–1253

59. Meilstrup JW. Ultrasound examination of the parathyroid glands. Otolaryngol Clin North Am 2004;37:763–778 ix.

60. Gooding GA. Sonography of the thyroid and parathyroid. Radiol Clin North Am 1993;31:967–989

61. Burkey SH, Snyder WH, Nwariaku F, et al. Directed parathyroidectomy: feasibility and performance in 100 consecutive patients with primary hyperparathyroidism. Arch Surg 2003;138:604–609

62. Sacks BA, Pallotta JA, Cole A, et al. Diagnosis of parathyroid adenomas: efficacy of measuring parathormone levels in needle aspirates of cervical masses. AJR Am J Roentgenol 1994;163:1223–1226

63. Lewis BD, Charboneau JW, Reading CC. Ultrasound-guided biopsy and ablation in the neck. Ultrasound Q 2002;18:3–12

64. Gooding GA, Clark OH, Stark DD, et al. Parathyroid aspiration biopsy under ultrasound guidance in the postoperative hyperparathyroid patient. Radiology 1985;155:193–196

65. Lane MJ, Desser TS, Weigel RJ, et al. Use of color and power Doppler sonography to identify feeding arteries associated with parathyroid adenomas. AJR Am J Roentgenol 1998;171:819–823

66. Lumachi F, Ermani M, Basso S, et al. Localization of parathyroid tumours in the minimally invasive era: which technique should be chosen? Population-based analysis of 253 patients undergoing parathyroidectomy and factors affecting parathyroid gland detection. Endocr Relat Cancer 2001;8:63–69

67. Purcell GP, Dirbas FM, Jeffrey RB, et al. Parathyroid localization with high-resolution ultrasound and technetium Tc 99m sestamibi. Arch Surg 1999;134:824–830

68. Tseng FY, Hsiao YL, Chang TC. Ultrasound-guided fine needle aspiration cytology of parathyroid lesions. A review of 72 cases. Acta Cytol 2002;46:1029–1036

69. Weinberger MS, Robbins KT. Diagnostic localization studies for primary hyperparathyroidism. A suggested algorithm. Arch Otolaryngol Head Neck Surg 1994;120:1187–1189

70. Rodriquez JM, Tezelman S, Siperstein AE, et al. Localization procedures in patients with persistent or recurrent hyperparathyroidism. Arch Surg 1994;129:870–875

71. Kairaluoma MV, Kellosalo J, Makarainen H, et al. Parathyroid re-exploration in patients with primary hyperparathyroidism. Ann Chir Gynaecol 1994;83:202–206

72. Miller DL, Doppman JL, Shawker TH, et al. Localization of parathyroid adenomas in patients who have undergone surgery. Part I. Noninvasive imaging methods. Radiology 1987;162:133–137

73. Beus KS, Stack BC. Synchronous thyroid pathology in patients presenting with primary hyperparathyroidism. Am J Otolaryngol 2004;25:308–312

74. Bennedbaek FN, Karstrup S, Hegedus L. Percutaneous ethanol injection therapy in the treatment of thyroid and parathyroid diseases. Eur J Endocrinol 1997;136:240–250

75. Moley JF, Lairmore TC, Doherty GM, et al. Preservation of the recurrent laryngeal nerves in thyroid and parathyroid reoperations. Surgery 1999;126:673–679

76. Jacobson SR, van Heerden JA, Farley DR, et al. Focused cervical exploration for primary hyperparathyroidism without intraoperative parathyroid hormone monitoring or use of the gamma probe. World J Surg 2004;28:1127–1131

77. Norman J. Parathyroid surgery cure rates. http://www.parathyroidcom/surgery'cure'rateshtm 2007.

78. Bennedbaek FN, Karstrup S, Hegedus L. Ultrasound guided laser ablation of a parathyroid adenoma. Br J Radiol 2001;74:905–907

79. Yusim A, Aspelund G, Ahrens W, et al. Intrathyroidal parathyroid adenoma. Thyroid 2006;16:619–620

80. Ahuja AT, Wong KT, Ching ASC, et al. Imaging for primary hyperparathyroidism–what beginners should know. Clin Radiol 2004;59:967–976
81. Krausz Y, Bettman L, Guralnik L, et al. Technetium-99m-MIBI SPECT/CT in primary hyperparathyroidism. World J Surg 2006;30:76–83
82. Roach PJ, Schembri GP, Ho Shon IA, et al. SPECT/CT imaging using a spiral CT scanner for anatomical localization: Impact on diagnostic accuracy and reporter confidence in clinical practice. Nucl Med Commun 2006;27:977–987
83. Serra A, Bolasco P, Satta L, et al. Role of SPECT/CT in the preoperative assessment of hyperparathyroid patients. Radiol Med (Torino) 2006;111:999–1008
84. Beggs AD, Hain SF. Use of co-registered 11C-methionine PET and computed tomography for the localisation of parathyroid adenomas. Eur J Nucl Med Mol Imaging 2003;30:1602
85. Saeed S, Yao M, Philip B, et al. Localizing hyperfunctioning parathyroid tissue: MRI or nuclear study or both? Clin Imaging 2006;30:257–265
86. Udelsman R, Donovan PI. Remedial parathyroid surgery: changing trends in 130 consecutive cases. Ann Surg 2006;244:471–479
87. Beggs AD, Hain SF. Localization of parathyroid adenomas using 11C-methionine positron emission tomography. Nucl Med Commun 2005;26:133–136
88. Hellman P, Ahlstrom H, Bergstrom M, et al. Positron emission tomography with 11C-methionine in hyperparathyroidism. Surgery 1994;116:974–981
89. Neumann DR, Esselstyn CB, MacIntyre WJ, et al. Comparison of FDG-PET and sestamibi-SPECT in primary hyperparathyroidism. J Nucl Med 1996;37:1809–1815
90. Sundin A, Johansson C, Hellman P, et al. PET and Parathyroid L-[carbon-11]methionine accumulation in hyperparathyroidism. J Nucl Med 1996;37:1766–1770
91. Otto D, Boerner AA, Hofmann M, et al. Pre-operative localization of hyperfunctional parathyroid tissue with 11C-methionine PET. Eur J Nucl Med Mol Imaging 2004;31:1405–1412
92. Reitz RE, Pollard JJ, Wang CA, et al. Localization of parathyroid adenomas by selective venous catheterization and radioimmunoassay. N Engl J Med 1969;281:348–351
93. Nilsson BE, Tisell LE, Jansson S, et al. Parathyroid localization by catheterization of large cervical and mediastinal veins to determine serum concentrations of intact parathyroid hormone. World J Surg 1994;18:605–610 discussion 10–1
94. Jaskowiak N, Norton JA, Alexander HR, et al. A prospective trial evaluating a standard approach to reoperation for missed parathyroid adenoma. Ann Surg 1996;224:308–320 discussion 20–1
95. Mariette C, Pellissier L, Combemale F, et al. Reoperation for persistent or recurrent primary hyperparathyroidism. Langenbecks Arch Surg 1998;383:174–179
96. Reidel MA, Schilling T, Graf S, et al. Localization of hyperfunctioning parathyroid glands by selective venous sampling in reoperation for primary or secondary hyperparathyroidism. Surgery 2006;140:907–913

16 Pathophysiology of the Parathyroid Glands

Jason A. Smith and Brendan C. Stack

The parathyroid glands are four glands located on the posterior aspect of the thyroid. The parathyroids are small (less than 50 mg) and produce only one hormone, which is known as parathyroid hormone (PTH) or parathormone. PTH functions to maintain calcium homeostasis by acting on the renal tubule, calcium stores in the skeletal system, and indirectly on the gastrointestinal tract through activation of vitamin D. These glands and their function appear to be simple at first glance; however, clinicians involved in the treatment of patients with parathyroid disorders quickly realize that the pathophysiology involved can be quite complex. To accurately diagnose and adequately manage patients with parathyroid diseases, one must have a thorough understanding of the pathophysiology involved. This chapter reviews the pathologic processes that occur with the parathyroids.

Hyperparathyroidism

The most common derangement in parathyroid function is the excess production of parathyroid hormone, which is called hyperparathyroidism. Hyperparathyroidism was described simultaneously in Europe and the United States in the 1920s.[1] Patients initially presented with significant renal and skeletal manifestations including nephrolithiasis, renal failure, osteoporosis, and pathologic fractures. With our increased understanding of this disease process, and with the addition of calcium to routine metabolic panels, the clinical presentation has changed drastically. Most patients diagnosed with hyperparathyroidism currently are asymptomatic. Although this early detection is an accomplishment of modern medicine, the treatment of asymptomatic patients presents a therapeutic dilemma. Hyperparathyroidism is defined as primary, secondary, or tertiary based on the etiology and associated manifestations. Primary hyperparathyroidism implies inappropriately elevated levels of PTH when compared with the serum calcium. In the physiologic state, hypercalcemia reduces the PTH level by negative feedback acting through calcium-sensing receptors on the parathyroid glands. Secondary hyperparathyroidism is an elevated PTH level due to another cause. The most common disease process leading to chronic secondary hyperparathyroidism is vitamin D defficiency or chronic renal failure. Tertiary hyperparathyroidism occurs in glands affected by secondary hyperparathyroidism that have been stimulated to the extent that the glands become autonomous, and are no longer governed by the normal feedback mechanisms. Even if the underlying pathology is corrected, the hyperparathyroidism persists. The classic example of tertiary hyperparathyroidism is a patient who has secondary hyperparathyroidism due to chronic renal failure, undergoes a renal transplant, and the hyperparathyroidism persists.

Primary Hyperparathyroidism

Pathology

Primary hyperparathyroidism (PHPT) is hypercalcemia secondary to excess PTH production from a dysfunctional gland or glands, and is the most common cause of hypercalcemia in the ambulatory setting. Primary hyperparathyroidism affects roughly 1% of the adult population, and the incidence increases significantly with age. Women are affected at least twice as often as men.[2-4] PHPT can be attributable to a single adenoma (80–88% of cases), four-gland hyperplasia (8–10%), double adenomas (4–6%), and rarely parathyroid carcinoma (<1%) (**Figs. 16.1** and **16.2**).[5-8]

Genetic alterations have been shown to contribute to the development of primary hyperparathyroidism. Two specific genetic mutations have been demonstrated in nonfamilial parathyroid adenomas.[1,9] Decreased expression of the multiple endocrine neoplasia type I (MEN-I) tumor suppression gene has been found in up to 20% of these adenomas. Activation of the cyclin D1/*PRAD1* oncogene results in overproduction of cyclin D1 and is found in up to 40% of adenomas. Parathyroid adenomas with these genetic alterations are hypercellular and have calcium-sensing receptors that do not function properly.

The calcium-sensing receptor (CaSR) plays an important role in calcium homeostasis. This receptor is found in abundance on the surface of the normal parathyroid gland in addition to many other locations in the body including the renal tubule, bone marrow, osteoclasts, breast tissue, parafollicular cells in the thyroid, and G cells in the gastric mucosa. Adenomatous cells have a decreased concentration of calcium-sensing receptors compared with normal cells, and have altered set points, which allow for inappropriate production of parathormone despite normal or high serum calcium levels.[10]

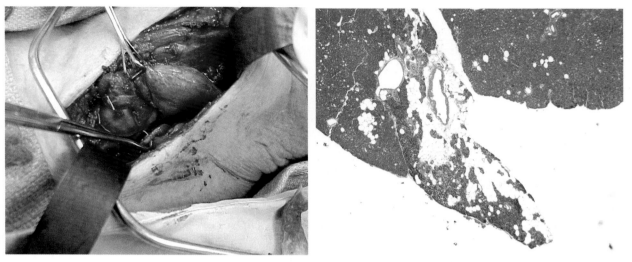

Fig. 16.1 (**A**) Parathyroid adenoma in vivo. An anterior Babcock retracts the thyroid gland anteriorly, and a posterior Babcock retracts the parathyroid adenoma. (**B**) Histology of parathyroid adenoma surrounding a remnant of normal parathyroid tissue (bottom).

Clinical Manifestations

The clinical spectrum of PHPT involves multiple organ systems. Renal manifestations are the most common, and occur in 20 to 25% of these patients. Nephrolithiasis accounts for virtually all of kidney related complications. Parathyroid hormone increases renal calcium absorption, renal phosphorus excretion, and activity of 1α-hydroxylase. 1α-Hydroxylase converts vitamin D to its active form, which increases intestinal absorption of calcium. The excess of filtered calcium compared with that absorbed leads to hypercalciuria and the predisposition to calcium stones. Hyperparathyroidism also leads to a decrease in the glomerular filtration rate and a mild metabolic acidosis. Nephrocalcinosis

is a rare complication of hyperparathyroidism and is diffuse calcification of the renal tubular system and parenchyma, which can be seen on a plain radiograph.[1]

Skeletal manifestations of PHPT are second in incidence only to renal complications. Osteitis fibrosis cystica, Brown tumors, and fractures were common presenting entities with hyperparathyroidism in the past. With earlier detection, these have often been replaced by osteopenia or generalized bone demineralization and bone pain. The osteopenia associated with PHPT continues to carry a fracture rate that is greater than normative controls. In the current form of the disease, this generalized bone loss cannot be visualized well on plain radiographs, but is identifiable early in the process with bone densitometry. The dexascan is used to assess bone

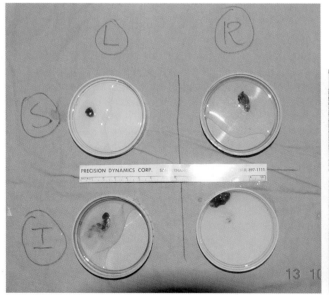

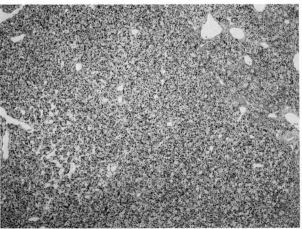

Fig. 16.2 (**A**) Gross specimen of four-gland hyperplasia. (**B**) Histology of hyperplastic parathyroid.

density, and this density is typically reported for the lumbar spine, femoral neck, and distal radius. Hyperparathyroidism decreases bone density in cortical bone more than trabecular bone, and therefore the distal radius is often the most affected. The bone density is reported as a T-score, which gives the density as a standard deviation from normal, and a T-score of –2.5 is often used as an indication for surgical intervention on the parathyroids.[2]

Gastrointestinal symptoms are less specific, but are part of the clinical picture of HPT. Pancreatitis, peptic ulcer disease, constipation, nausea, and emesis have all been described. Peptic ulcer disease is most commonly reported, although no clear mechanism has been demonstrated.

There are several symptoms associated with HPT; they are nonspecific and include depression, impaired cognition, fatigue, malaise, sleep disorders, and irritability. Although these symptoms are difficult to characterize, they stress the importance of obtaining a thorough neuropsychiatric history since these symptoms have been shown to improve after correction of the underlying hyperparathyroidism.[2, 11-13]

Evaluation

Primary hyperparathyroidism can be diagnosed with precision with a serum calcium level, serum parathyroid hormone level, 24-hour urinary calcium and creatinine, and an adequate patient history. If the serum albumin levels are normal, total serum calcium is preferred and more reliable than ionized calcium.[14] The newer assays that measure intact, biologically active PTH are preferred when compared with the older methods of measuring fragments of the PTH molecule. An elevated serum calcium level in the presence of elevated levels of parathyroid hormone is virtually diagnostic for primary hyperparathyroidism. There are a few exceptions that need to be considered. Thiazide diuretics and lithium excess can produce laboratory findings similar to primary hyperparathyroidism and should be investigated in the patient history. Twenty-four-hour calcium and creatinine excretion is important in the evaluation of hyperparathyroidism. These laboratory results can rule out the possibility of a rare condition known as familial hypocalciuric hypercalcemia (FHH); see discussion later in the chapter. Urinary calcium and creatinine excretion can also help with determining prognosis, as total 24-hour calcium excretion in excess of 400 mg/24 hours is associated with an increase in renal complications and is another surgical indication.[2]

All patients who are diagnosed with primary hyperparathyroidism by laboratory data warrant a dexascan to assess bone mineral density. This will determine the degree of secondary osteopenia and risk of impending fracture. Conversely, any patients who have nephrolithiasis with calcium stones, pathologic fractures, or significant osteoporosis should be worked up for hyperparathyroidism with a serum calcium and PTH level to rule out hyperparathyroidism as a cause.

Management

The typical clinical presentation of PHPT has changed dramatically since its description in the 1920s. When this condition was first described, patients often presented with the classic "renal stones, painful bones, abdominal groans, psychic moans, and fatigue overtones."[15] Early in the 19th century, patients often presented with severe bone disease, renal sequela, and even neurologic changes and coma. As previously mentioned, with increased understanding of PHPT and the addition of calcium to routine metabolic panels, patients are being identified much earlier in their clinical course. It is estimated that only 30 to 40% of contemporary patients with PHPT present with significant symptoms.[2] Many argue that a larger number of patients are actually symptomatic but present with nonspecific symptoms including depression, fatigue, bone pain, or anorexia. This debate aside, 60 to 70% of patients who present with primary hyperparathyroidism are asymptomatic or have only nonspecific symptoms. This leaves practitioners with the therapeutic dilemma of which asymptomatic patients warrant treatment.

This dilemma has been the topic of recent meetings and recommendations from the National Institutes of Health (NIH) as well as the American Association of Clinical Endocrinologists and American Association of Endocrine Surgeons. It has been commonly accepted that patients presenting with classic symptoms of hyperparathyroidism including fracture, nephrolithiasis, and neuromuscular complaints warrant treatment. Recent reports have indicated that asymptomatic hyperparathyroid patients have a long-term increase in cardiovascular disease and malignancy.[2] Furthermore, 23 to 62% of patients who present without symptoms become symptomatic within 10 years of presentation.[2] For these reasons, in 2002 an NIH consensus panel met and modified its first consensus guidelines and recommended treatment for asymptomatic patients if any of the following apply[1]: serum calcium is >1.0 mg/dL above the normal range,[2] urinary calcium is >400 mg/24 hour,[3] age <50,[4] there is a 30% decrease in creatinine clearance as compared with normal age-matched controls,[5] the patient cannot participate in follow-up,[6] severe psychoneurologic disorder,[7] or other complications of PHPT including nephrocalcinosis or osteoporosis (T-score < –2.5 standard deviation [SD] at lumbar spine, hip, or wrist) (**Table 16.1**).

An in-depth discussion of all the surgical and medical treatment options can be found in other chapters, so current treatment options and recommendations are only briefly addressed here. There are no long-term studies demonstrating the efficacy of medical management or observation in these patients. Several medications target the effects of hyperparathyroidism without treating the underlying problem. Bisphosphonates have been shown to increase bone mineral density in patients with hyperparathyroidism, with no significant effect on PTH levels.[16] Similarly, estrogen replacement can stabilize bone loss in postmenopausal women with PHPT.[17] Furosemide can help to reduce calcium

Table 16.1 Indications for Parathyroidectomy in Asymptomatic Patients According to 2002 National Institutes of Health (NIH) Guidelines

Parameter	Indication
Serum calcium	>1.0 mg/dL above normal range
24-hour urinary calcium	>400 mg/24 hours
Age	<50 years old
Creatinine clearance	30% less than age-matched control
Osteoporosis	T score <−2.5 standard deviation (SD) (forearm)
Neuropsychiatric	Severe psychoneurologic disorder
Compliance	Poor compliance
Renal complications	Nephrocalcinosis

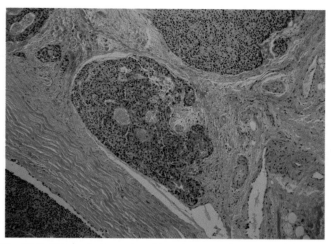

Fig. 16.3 Histology of parathyroid carcinoma with invasion of the capsule.

levels acutely. Calcimimetic medications are an intriguing class of medications that target the problem in hyperparathyroidism. With their mimetic activity these medications negatively feed back on the calcium sensing receptors of the parathyroids and can reduce parathormone production. One of these medications, cinacalcet, has been shown to reduce PTH levels and normalize serum calcium in a recent report.[18] If patients with PHPT are managed medically, they require clinical follow-up, biannual serum calcium levels, annual serum creatinine levels, and annual bone densitometry, and they incur the cost of chronic pharmacotherapy.[1]

The cost of follow-up after several years of medical management for primary hyperparathyroidism has been shown to exceed the costs of successful surgical management.[19] Surgical management has been reported to be 95 to 98% curative with complication rates of 1 to 2% in experienced hands. It is for these reasons that the recent position statement from endocrinologists and endocrine surgeons recommended surgical intervention in patients who meet the above criteria for treatment. Calcimimetics have promising initial results, but long-term data are needed before an adequate comparison can be made with the gold standard of parathyroidectomy.[2]

Parathyroid Carcinoma

Another cause of primary hyperparathyroidism that warrants discussion is parathyroid carcinoma (PTC) (**Fig. 16.3**). This is a rare condition that accounts for less than 1% of primary hyperparathyroidism on presentation. It affects men and women equally, and the average age of presentation is 55. One problem with this malignancy is that the diagnosis is rarely apparent upon initial presentation because the symptoms are the same as benign causes of hyperparathyroidism. Consistent findings in parathyroid carcinoma are preoperative calcium and parathormone levels much higher

than those typically found with benign disease.[20] The calcium levels for PTC are often >14.0 mg/dL, and parathyroid hormone levels are commonly three to four times normal. The tumor itself is usually larger than the typical adenoma, on average measuring 2 to 6 cm in diameter. A palpable neck mass is present in up to one half of patients found to have PTC, which is not characteristic of benign disease. Cervical lymphadenopathy is found in one third of patients presenting with PTC and should also raise suspicion. Patients with parathyroid carcinoma are also more commonly symptomatic. In contrast to reports of 30 to 40% of patients with primary hyperparathyroidism who present with symptoms, in one series eight of nine patients who were found to have parathyroid carcinoma intraoperatively had symptoms at presentation.[20]

Intraoperative findings that are consistent with parathyroid carcinoma include adherence to or invasion of surrounding structures (thyroid lobe or strap muscles), fibrosis, nodularity, induration, and gray color instead of the typical tan adenoma. Careful attention to these characteristics are important during surgery as the treatment of choice for parathyroid carcinoma is wide surgical excision, because adjuvant treatments such as external beam radiation and chemotherapy have not been shown to improve survival. Intraoperative frozen pathology is not reliable, making careful intraoperative examination paramount. Surgical excision should include en bloc excision of the tumor including the ipsilateral thyroid lobe and straps if involved.[21]

Parathyroid carcinoma carries a poor prognosis, with the 5-year survival reported as low as 50%. Interestingly, these patients usually die as a result of their uncontrolled hypercalcemia as opposed to local or metastatic disease. Fraker[22] reported a local and regional recurrence rate of 36% and 14%, respectively, after surgical resection. This recurrence can be determined by monitoring serum calcium, parathyroid hormone, and carcinoembryonic antigen (CEA), with an increase being an ominous sign of recurrence.

Secondary Hyperparathyroidism

Any disorder that results in hypocalcemia or vitamin D deficiency will elevate PTH levels and can serve as a secondary cause of hyperparathyroidism. Classically this condition is caused by chronic renal failure, and the resulting alterations in vitamin D, phosphorus, and calcium. Chronic renal failure results in decreased levels of 1,25-dihydroxyvitamin D, hyperphosphatemia, and hypocalcemia. As renal function declines, there is loss of available 1α-hydroxylase, resulting in a decrease in active vitamin D (1,25-dihydroxyvitamin D) levels. This occurs when the glomerular filtration rate (GFR) drops below 60 mL/min. Significant increases in the PTH level develop later in the progression, when the GFR drops to 30 mL/min, and significant hyperphosphatemia occurs with a GFR of 20 ml/min or lower.[1,23] The elevation in phosphorus levels and hypocalcemia that develops from decreased vitamin D acts to further increase the level of parathyroid hormone. Early in the disease process, the elevated PTH is appropriate and serves to increase phosphate excretion and calcium absorption in the kidney and counterbalances the metabolic derangement. However, as renal disease progresses and the filtered fraction of phosphate decreases, the ability of PTH to increase phosphate excretion is saturated and the phosphate released from bone as a result of elevated PTH exacerbates the hyperphosphatemia.[24]

Over time, chronic stimulation leads to hyperplasia of the parathyroid glands. Histologic studies from resected glands of patients with secondary hyperparathyroidism show nodular and diffuse hyperplasia.[23] Decreased expression of the CaSR have been demonstrated in both types of hyperplasia, but is more evident in areas of nodular hyperplasia.[25–27] This decreased expression of the CaSR results in decreased negative feedback, and explains why PTH levels remain elevated when calcium levels are normal or elevated.

Historical symptoms of secondary hyperparathyroidism, or renal osteodystrophy, include spontaneous fractures, bone pain, radiographic bone lesions, and extraskeletal calcifications. However, as with primary hyperparathyroidism, patients now often present prior to the onset of any significant symptoms.[15] Calciphylaxis, coronary artery calcification, and psychoneurologic disorders are more serious manifestations seen in secondary hyperparathyroidism. Calciphylaxis and coronary artery calcification have been shown to be associated with elevated calcium-phosphorus product. A product over 70 has been correlated with an increased risk of developing these deadly complications.[28]

There are no specific tests that definitively diagnose a patient with secondary hyperparathyroidism. This is a diagnosis based on the clinical picture and metabolic derangements. The presence of hypocalcemia and elevated PTH is diagnostic of secondary hyperparathyroidism. When phosphorus levels are also elevated, this points to chronic renal failure as the etiology. If phosphorus levels are low, other anomalies such as vitamin D deficiency should be considered. This is rapidly becoming recognized as an increasing cause for secondary hyperparathyroidism with decreasing sun exposure and an aging population.

Prevention is truly the best treatment of hyperparathyroidism in chronic renal failure. This is accomplished by aggressive phosphorus management early in the progression of renal failure and adequate replacement of vitamin D. Low phosphorus diets and the use of phosphorus-binding drugs that prevent enteral absorption can decrease the hyperphosphatemia. Phosphorus binders containing aluminum are currently avoided because they can be toxic to bones. The current recommendation is the use of calcium containing phosphorus binders as long as the calcium × phosphorus product is less than 55 mg^2/mL^2. If the product exceeds 55, or if serum calcium is elevated over 10.2 mg/dl, alternatives such as sevelamer are recommended since they have no calcium or aluminum.[29] This recommendation is an attempt to keep the calcium × phosphorus product less than 70 mg^2/mL^2, at all costs, because coronary artery calcification and calciphylaxis have been shown to occur at these levels. Vitamin D or its analogues can be given to reduce PTH levels. Vitamin D can act on the parathyroid to reduce PTH, but can have the undesired effect of elevating calcium and phosphate. Therefore, vitamin D formulations (e.g., calcitriol) are only recommended when phosphorus is less than 6 mg/mL. Newer vitamin D analogues are available that can reduce PTH without the undesired effects. Patients taking one such analogue, paricalcitol, experienced fewer episodes of hypercalcemia and a more rapid reduction in PTH as compared with patients taking calcitriol.[30] Calcimimetic medications such as cinacalcet have promise because they can negatively feed back on the parathyroid glands but do not have the consequences of calcium supplementation. Long-term trials with these calcimimetics are needed before their clinical utility will be ascertained.

The indications for surgical intervention in secondary hyperparathyroidism are not as clear as those for primary disease. There are no NIH guidelines dictating surgical intervention. Currently accepted indications for surgery include failure of medical management, calcium × phosphorus products persistently over 70 despite medical intervention, serum calcium over 11 mg/dL, elevated or rapidly rising serum PTH, severe bone disease, or severe pruritus (**Table 16.2**).[15] Surgery for correction of secondary hyperparathyroidism involves subtotal parathyroidectomy with excision of three or three-and-one-half glands, or total

Table 16.2 Relative Surgical Indications for Secondary Hyperparathyroidism

Failure of medical management
Serum calcium >11.0
Rapidly rising PTH (or PTH >1000)
Severe bone disease
Severe pruritus

parathyroidectomy where all four glands are excised and one of the glands is autotransplanted in the sternocleido-mastoid muscle in the neck or in the brachioradialis muscle in the forearm.

Tertiary Hyperparathyroidism

The definition of tertiary hyperparathyroidism is not straightforward. Tertiary HPT results from progression of secondary HPT and is less prevalent. In tertiary HPT, PTH, calcium, and phosphorus levels are elevated. It is rare for this condition to occur outside of chronic renal failure. The distinction between secondary HPT and tertiary HPT is that, in tertiary HPT, the glands have become autonomous. This manifests by continuation of the electrolyte derangements despite correction of the underlying renal condition. For example, if a patient with chronic renal failure and hyperparathyroidism undergoes a renal transplant and continues to have hyperparathyroidism, this would be classified as tertiary HPT. The indications for prevention and treatment are similar to those listed above for secondary HPT.

Familial Hypocalciuric Hypercalcemia (FHH)

There are many causes of hypercalcemia that must be differentiated from primary hyperparathyroidism. This task is usually not difficult because other causes of hypercalcemia cause a compensatory suppression of PTH by negative feedback. This is in contrast to the elevated PTH seen despite hypercalcemia in primary hyperparathyroidism. One clinical condition where PTH can also be elevated in the presence of hypercalcemia, leading to a diagnostic dilemma, is familial hypocalciuric hypercalcemia. FHH is an autosomal dominant condition caused by a defect in the CaSR located on both the parathyroid glands and renal tubule. The CaSR has been mapped to chromosome 3q21-q24, and multiple inactivating mutations have been described.[31] This inactivation of the CaSR requires a higher serum calcium to act on the parathyroids to suppress PTH, which increases the set point allowing hypercalcemia in the presence of normal to slightly elevated PTH levels. In the renal tubule, the defect in the CaSR leads to increased calcium and magnesium reabsorption.[32,33] The net result is hypercalcemia, hypocalciuria, and frequently hypermagnesemia. Patients are rarely symptomatic, which is in stark contrast to primary hyperparathyroidism, in which 30 to 40% of patients present with symptoms. The distinction between these two disorders is made with family history and laboratory findings. Genetic testing for FHH has recently become available. A family history of hypercalcemia should raise the suspicion of this autosomal dominant condition, especially if there is a family history of hypercalcemia that did not improve after parathyroidectomy for presumed hyperparathyroidism. PTH levels are typically normal to mildly elevated in FHH as opposed to primary hyperparathyroidism, in which they are more

significantly elevated, but the true laboratory distinction between these two disease processes is made with urinary electrolyte studies. Twenty-four-hour urine collection for creatinine and calcium can confirm the diagnosis of FHH. In FHH 75% of patients have 24-hour calcium excretion levels of less than 100 mg, whereas patients with primary hyperparathyroidism usually have excretions in excess of 200 mg in 24 hours. The calcium creatinine clearance ratio is less than 0.01 in a majority of patients with FHH and greater than 0.02 in most patients with primary hyperparathyroidism.[34,35] The distinction between these conditions is not difficult if urine studies are performed. However, many patients have undergone surgical intervention with no benefit because they were incorrectly identified as having primary hyperparathyroidism. This underscores the importance of routine use of the 24-hour urine collection for calcium and creatinine to exclude FHH patients from parathyroid surgery.

Multiple Endocrine Neoplasia (MEN) Syndromes

Multiple endocrine neoplasia syndromes are characterized by the presence of functional tumors of endocrine organs that produce hormones that lead to the characteristic symptoms. The current classification divides the syndromes into MEN-I (Wermer syndrome), MEN-IIA (Sipple syndrome), and MEN-IIB (also known as MEN-III). These syndromes are inherited in an autosomal dominant manner. Hyperparathyroidism plays a significant role in MEN-I and MEN-IIA, but is not part of the spectrum of disease with MEN-IIB.

Multiple Endocrine Neoplasia Type I

MEN-I is a disease with a genetic predisposition for tumors of the parathyroids, pancreatic islet cells, and anterior pituitary. This syndrome is also known to include duodenal tumors, adrenal adenomas, thyroid adenomas, carcinoid tumors, and lipomas (**Table 16.3**). Parathyroid tumor development in MEN-I occurs decades earlier than in the sporadic forms and the gastrointestinal tumors have an increased malignant potential.[36]

Table 16.3 Clinical Presentation of Multiple Endocrine Neoplasia Type I (MEN-I)

Clinical Manifestation	Prevalence (MEN-I)
Primary hyperparathyroidism	90–100%
Pancreatic islet cell tumors	33%
Pituitary adenomas	20%
Thymic carcinoids	5%

Less common findings: angiofibromas, collagenomas, lipomas, spinal ependymomas, thyroid adenomas, adrenocortical adenomas

Primary hyperparathyroidism is the most consistent feature of MEN-I, and has been reported to affect 90 to 100% of these patients by the age of 40, making it also the earliest feature. It is estimated that up to 2% of primary hyperparathyroidism is attributable to MEN-I.[36] As is the case with sporadic primary hyperparathyroidism, most patients are asymptomatic. Symptoms common to MEN-I–associated primary hyperparathyroidism are the same as seen in the sporadic forms.[37] The diagnosis for PHPT in MEN-I is the same as nonsyndromic cases.

Although the presenting symptoms and diagnostic criteria are the same for PHPT in MEN-I as they are for sporadic cases of PHPT, there are significant differences in the patient populations. For example, hyperparathyroidism develops much earlier in patients with MEN-I than it does in the general population. PHPT is almost universal in patients with MEN-I by the age of 40, and annual screening with serum calcium and PTH is recommended to begin at 8 years of age.[38] This is 20 years sooner than the average presentation of PHPT in other patients. The female predominance seen in nonfamilial hyperparathyroidism is not seen in MEN-I–associated hyperparathyroidism, which has an even male-to-female ratio. Perhaps the most important distinction between PHPT found in MEN-I patients and sporadic PHPT is that multiple gland involvement is characteristic of PHPT in MEN-I patients, where 80 to 85% of nonsyndromic PHPT is caused by a single parathyroid adenoma.[38,39]

The multiple gland involvement found in these patients necessitates a therapeutic approach that differs from the approach taken to other patients with PHPT. Patients with sporadic primary hyperparathyroidism who meet the NIH criteria for surgery can undergo surgery directed only at the affected gland or glands assuming adequate preoperative localization. However, the multiple gland hyperplasia seen in the parathyroids of MEN-I patients necessitates a more aggressive approach. Although some parathyroid glands may appear grossly normal during neck exploration of these patients, it is felt that these glands are not histologically normal but represent asymmetric hyperplasia.[35,38] This explains the increased failure rate found in MEN-I patients who undergo surgical intervention for hyperparathyroidism. It is reported that roughly 50% of these patients will have recurrent hyperparathyroidism 10 to 12 years after surgical correction.[40,41] There are two surgical options commonly employed in these patients. The first consists of a bilateral neck exploration with subtotal parathyroidectomy and thymectomy leaving a 20- to 50-mg remnant of vascularized parathyroid tissue in situ. The thymectomy is added due to the increased incidence of supernumerary parathyroid glands found in MEN-I, and if the subtotal approach is used, it is advisable to leave a surgical clip at the site of the remnant parathyroid for reference if future neck explorations for recurrent hyperparathyroidism are required. The second option employed is a total parathyroidectomy combined with thymectomy and autotransplantation of a portion of the resected parathyroid tissue into either the sternocleidomastoid muscle in the

neck or the brachioradialis muscle in the forearm. There is no consensus regarding which of these two approaches is more appropriate.[42–46] Due to the high failure rate of surgical intervention and the known pathogenesis involving multiple gland hyperplasia, selective parathyroidectomy resecting only grossly involved glands is not recommended. Due to the surgical intent of bilateral exploration with exposure of all parathyroid tissue, preoperative localization studies are not necessary for initial surgical intervention. Studies have shown technetium-99m-sestamibi, single photon emission computed tomography (SPECT), and positron emission tomography (PET) with ^{11}C-methionine to be of benefit in selected patients undergoing reoperation for recurrent hyperparathyroidism.[37,47,48] Intraoperative PTH measurements have become popular and useful in determining adequate resection in sporadic cases of HPT especially when caused by a single adenoma. Recent reports advocate the use of the intraoperative PTH assay for reexploration and for total parathyroidectomy.[49,50] The decline in PTH is not as abrupt as that seen after the resection of an offending adenoma, and more experience with this assay in MEN-I patients is required.

Although this chapter focuses on parathyroid diseases, a discussion of MEN-I without mention of its other manifestations would be incomplete. Pituitary adenomas are another common finding in these patients. Most studies report a 20% incidence of clinically evident pituitary adenomas in MEN-I patients, but one study demonstrated that up to 60% of MEN-I patients will have pathologic evidence of a pituitary adenoma if an autopsy is performed.[51,52] The most common pituitary tumor found is prolactinoma. As compared with nonsyndromic patients, pituitary adenomas in MEN-I tend to be larger, more symptomatic, and have a higher recurrence rate after resection.[53] Pancreatic and gastrointestinal islet cell tumors are another significant component of MEN-I. Parathyroid and pituitary involvement with MEN-I can be effectively treated, which leaves the malignant potential of the gastrointestinal and pancreatic islet cell tumors as the major cause of mortality.[54–56] As with pituitary disease, there is a discrepancy between clinically apparent islet cell tumors (33% of MEN-I patients) and biochemical involvement (80%). Gastrinomas with Zollinger-Ellison syndrome are the most common clinical manifestation in this group. Insulinoma is the next most common clinically significant islet cell tumor, followed by rare tumors including vasoactive intestinal polypeptide-oma (VIPoma), somatostatinoma, and pancreatic polypeptide-oma. Aside from the classic parathyroid, pituitary, and pancreatic involvement, patients with MEN-I are at an increased risk of developing multiple other manifestations. For example, up to 5% of patients with MEN-I develop thymic carcinoids. Interestingly, these thymic carcinoids are found almost exclusively in male smokers with MEN-I.[57] Cutaneous tumors such as angiofibromas and collagenomas are more common in this group as are adrenocortical adenomas, thyroid adenomas, and spinal cord ependymomas.[58,59]

The MEN-I gene *MEN1* has been cloned and mapped to chromosome 11q13.[37,60] *MEN1* is a tumor suppressor gene that encodes for a protein named menin, and inactivation of this protein leads to tumorigenesis. Now that the gene is cloned, genetic testing is feasible. Prophylactic treatment is not performed in MEN-I, and therefore the knowledge that a patient had a MEN-I mutation prior to the onset of clinical symptoms is of little clinical utility. Furthermore, the sensitivity is low, and 30% of mutations go undetected by the current test.[61] It is for these reasons, along with the social concerns of diagnosing an otherwise asymptomatic patient with a congenital disorder, that universal acceptance of this test for first-degree relatives of MEN-I patients has not yet occurred.

Multiple Endocrine Neoplasia Type II

Multiple endocrine neoplasia type II (MEN-II) is divided into three subgroups: MEN-IIA; MEN-IIB; and familial medullary thyroid cancer (FMTC), which is a variant of MEN-IIA. As in MEN-I, these syndromes are inherited by an autosomal dominant mode of transmission. The three have medullary thyroid carcinoma as a common feature but differ in other clinical manifestations.

MEN-IIA is characterized by medullary thyroid carcinoma, pheochromocytoma, and hyperparathyroidism. Hyperparathyroidism affects 10 to 25% of these patients, and is more commonly asymptomatic and milder than the hyperparathyroidism found in MEN-I.[62,63] As in MEN-I, hyperparathyroidism in MEN-IIA is characterized by multiglandular hyperplasia, and treatment options for symptomatic patients are similar. However, because the symptom complex is milder and the recurrence rate after surgery is much less than that of MEN-I, bilateral neck exploration with removal of only grossly enlarged glands without cervical thymectomy is performed for most symptomatic patients.[64,65] If hypercalcemia is severe, more aggressive approaches such as subtotal or total parathyroidectomy with cervical thymectomy can be considered. The absence of hyperparathyroidism in MEN-IIB and FMTC makes the role of C-cell hyperplasia and elevated calcitonin as a causative factor of hyperparathyroidism in MEN-IIA less plausible. It has been found that the *ret* proto-oncogene is expressed in the parathyroid tumors of MEN-IIA, and, furthermore, specific *ret* mutations (codon 634) are found preferentially in families with MEN-IIA involving hyperparathyroidism. This leads to the conclusion that the parathyroid hyperplasia in MEN-IIA may be related to the expression of the mutant RET protein.[66] Medullary thyroid cancer is the most consistent finding of MEN-IIA and is found in 90 to 95% of patients. When MEN-IIA is confirmed by testing for the *ret* proto-oncogene, prophylactic thyroidectomy is recommended. The age at which this thyroidectomy should be performed is a controversial topic. For high-risk genetic alterations (e.g., codon 634), thyroidectomy is recommended by 5 years of age.[67] For intermediate-risk alterations, it is argued that thy-

Table 16.4 Clinical Presentation of Multiple Endocrine Neoplasia Type IIA (MEN-IIA)

Clinical Manifestation	Prevalence (MEN-IIA)
Medullary thyroid carcinoma	90–95%
Pheochromocytoma	40%
Hyperparathyroidism	10–25%

Less common features: cutaneous lichen amyloidosis, Hirschsprung disease

roidectomy can be performed later. Pheochromocytoma occurs in nearly 40% of patients with MEN-IIA. Biochemical screening by urinary or serum catecholamines is recommended for all patients with MEN-II or with medullary thyroid carcinoma. If patients are found to have pheochromocytoma, this should be surgically addressed prior to considering thyroidectomy or parathyroidectomy.[68] MEN-IIA is also associated with cutaneous lichen amyloidosis as well as Hirschsprung disease (**Table 16.4**).[69]

MEN-IIB also involves medullary thyroid carcinoma and pheochromocytoma but does not have an association with hyperparathyroidism. Medullary thyroid cancer is universal in these patients, is more aggressive than MTC found in MEN-IIA, and occurs at an earlier age. Timely diagnosis and early prophylactic thyroidectomy are imperative for the patient's ultimate prognosis. When MEN-IIB is diagnosed by *ret* testing, thyroidectomy is recommended by 6 months of age.[67] Pheochromocytomas occur in 40% of patients with MEN-IIB and should be evaluated and treated in the same manner as described for MEN-IIA. Marfanoid habitus, intestinal ganglioneuromas, and mucosal neuromas involving the lip and tongue are also common in MEN-IIB.[62]

Calciphylaxis

Calciphylaxis is a vascular and tissue manifestation of systemic disease. This primarily occurs in patients with secondary hyperparathyroidism and chronic renal failure, but isolated cases have been reported in patients with other underlying pathology such as alcoholic cirrhosis, vitamin D intoxication, primary hyperparathyroidism, multiple myeloma, and hypercalcemia of malignancy.[70,71] The term *calciphylaxis* is somewhat misleading because it implies an immunologic process. Other more specific terms are calcific uremic arteriolopathy, uremic small vessel disease, uremic gangrene syndrome, and uremic small-artery disease with medial calcification and intimal hyperplasia.[72–75] As these other more descriptive terms imply, calciphylaxis is characterized by systemic calcification of the tunica media of small vessels. This leads to the clinical manifestation of tissue ischemia and necrosis. Affected areas initially manifest as painful purpuric plaques with nodularity (**Fig. 16.4**) and typically progress to necrotic ulcers with eschar. The underlying muscle can be involved by the ischemic and necrotic

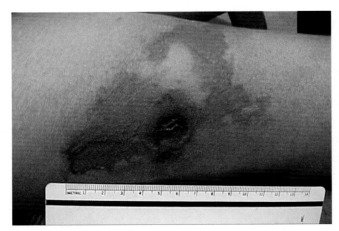

Fig. 16.4 Calciphylaxis lesion.

process. What ultimately leads to the poor prognosis associated with calciphylaxis is the superinfection that often ensues. The mortality rate remains between 60 and 87%, with patients usually succumbing to overwhelming infection and sepsis.[75]

Uremic small artery disease has been found to occur in 4% of patients on dialysis. Females are affected much more commonly than males and the mean age at presentation is between 48 and 57 years.[76] The pathogenesis is not well understood, but certain risk factors have been identified in animal models as well as patients. Elevated PTH, hyperphosphatemia, and elevated vitamin D levels seem to provide a milieu where calciphylaxis is more common. However, a superimposed event such as local tissue trauma, injection of medications, or elevation of other laboratory values often leads to the development of wounds in these sensitized patients. As previously discussed chronic renal failure leads to lower levels of vitamin D, which in turn decreases intestinal absorption of calcium leading to hypocalcemia and elevated parathormone levels. This secondary hyperparathyroidism ultimately leads to elevated calcium levels, and, with the addition of phosphate retention common in renal patients, elevated calcium-phosphate products lead to soft tissue and vascular calcification.[73] A calcium-phosphate product of 70 or greater increases the likelihood of developing calciphylaxis. Other factors felt to contribute to calciphylaxis are type 1 diabetes mellitus, protein C or protein S deficiency, calcium carbonate usage, prednisone, and administration of warfarin.[71,73,75]

With the lack of a specific test for calciphylaxis, the diagnosis remains a clinical one requiring a high degree of clinical suspicion. The development of a painful purpuric plaque in a dialysis patient should provoke close monitoring. Although laboratory abnormalities such as leukocytosis, hypercalcemia, hyperphosphatemia, and elevated PTH have been described, the confirmation of this diagnosis is with tissue biopsy showing medial calcification of small arteries and intimal hyperplasia.[73] There is no utility in imaging these patients for diagnostic purposes.

Once this diagnosis is suspected or confirmed, aggressive management is critical. The treatment involves attempting to correct the underlying hypercalcemia and hyperphosphatemia. This is accomplished by stopping vitamin D supplementation and prescribing a low-calcium dialysate and phosphate binders that are not calcium based (e.g., Renagel [sevelamer HCl]).[69,77] Dressing changes (with conventional or vacuum dressings) and surgical debridement of the necrotic wounds are important to prevent superinfection and ultimate sepsis.[78] The role of parathyroidectomy for calciphylaxis is controversial. Reports have advocated subtotal parathyroidectomy for improvement in wound healing, increased survival, and improvement of pain with the ulcers.[73,79] However, other reports have refuted these claims. Currently, there is no clear consensus on the role of, or extent of, parathyroidectomy in this patient population. Calciphylaxis carries such a grim prognosis that prevention is of the utmost importance. Meticulous management of the phosphate and calcium balance in renal patients can prevent the metabolic background, which has been shown to predispose these patients to calciphylaxis.

Hypoparathyroidism

Hypocalcemia can result from multiple factors including hypovitaminosis D, sepsis, hypoalbuminemia, hypomagnesemia, and fluoride poisoning. Hypoparathyroidism with decreased production of PTH or resistance to PTH can also cause significant hypocalcemia. Hypoparathyroidism is much less common than hyperparathyroidism, and is found in congenital as well as acquired forms. The most common cause is iatrogenic following thyroid or parathyroid surgery.[80]

Hypoparathyroidism occurring in children is most common in the neonatal period. The most common finding in the neonatal period is physiologic hypoparathyroidism with symptoms and biochemical evidence of hypoparathyroidism that is transient and warrants no treatment. The pathogenesis of this physiologic hypoparathyroidism is poorly understood, but known risk factors include maternal diabetes, birth asphyxia, and preterm delivery with low birth weight.[81] Other forms of hypoparathyroidism that occur early, in the first 24 hours of life, are caused by hypoplasia or agenesis of the parathyroid glands. DiGeorge anomaly is one example of parathyroid agenesis associated with other findings. DiGeorge is caused by failure of migration of neural crest cells into the 3rd and 4th pharyngeal pouches, which results in failure of appropriate development of the parathyroids and thymus. The clinical picture includes immune deficits secondary to the lack of T-cell function, hypoparathyroidism with hypocalcemia, cardiac defects including truncus arteriosus, and characteristic facies.[82,83] Microdeletions mapped to chromosome 22q11 have been described in up to 90% of DiGeorge patients.[84] Congenital hypoparathyroidism can occur in the face of normal-appearing parathyroid glands, and a collection of genetic defects has been described. There is an autosomal dominant form caused by a mutation in the CaSR. This mutation is an activating mutation that signals parathyroid cells and other cells in the body, indicating that there is adequate serum calcium, despite hypocalcemia. The clinical picture of hypocalcemia and hyperphosphatemia results in the presence of a normal intact PTH. This condition also has a paradoxical high or high normal urinary calcium due to activation of the calcium receptor in the renal tubule.[32] These patients are usually asymptomatic despite significant hypocalcemia, and attempts to treat the hypocalcemia should be reserved for symptomatic patients because treatment can result in elevated urinary calcium excretion, nephrolithiasis, nephrocalcinosis, and renal insufficiency.[32] There are two other forms of inherited hypoparathyroidism. One is a defect in the signal peptide of the PTH precursor preventing conversion to active PTH, and the other is inherited with sensorineural hearing loss and renal dysplasia, but the genetic defect is yet to be described.[85,86] Autosomal recessive and X-linked recessive forms of hypoparathyroidism have been reported, but specific genetic defects are not yet known. Late neonatal hypoparathyroidism occurs days after delivery. Two mitochondrial disorders, Kenny-Caffey syndrome and Kearns-Sayre syndrome, are associated with late neonatal hypoparathyroidism.[80]

Childhood hypoparathyroidism can also be seen as a part of an autoimmune complex. The most common example is seen with *h*ypoparathyroidism in conjunction with *a*drenal insufficiency and *m*ucocutaneous candidiasis, known as the HAM syndrome. Another syndrome with autoimmune destruction of the parathyroids is autoimmune polyglandular syndrome type I (also known as autoimmune polyendocrinopathy-candidiasis-ectodermal dystrophy [APECED] syndrome). Immunologic destruction of the hormone producing cells in the parathyroids is a common denominator in these two syndromes. Endocrinopathies in APECED, such as diabetes mellitus, hypogonadism, and hypothyroidism, must be excluded.[87]

Pseudohypoparathyroidism is a condition in which hypocalcemia and hyperphosphatemia are accompanied by elevated levels of PTH, indicating that the pathology is not absence of parathyroids or PTH but rather resistance of the end organs to the effects of PTH. There are two distinct forms of pseudohypoparathyroidism described. Type 1 is attributable to a blunted response of the cyclic adenosine monophosphate (cAMP) cascade to PTH, and is subdivided into type 1a, type 1b, and pseudopseudohypoparathy-

roidism, which is a related disorder. The gene coding for the stimulatory Gs-α1 protein in the adenylyl cyclase complex (GNAS1) has been shown to be involved in all of these disorders. The GNAS1 gene is known to be imprinted with the maternal allele expressed in the kidney. Therefore, maternal and paternal transmission differ in clinical presentations. Type 1a pseudohypoparathyroidism has a described mutation in GNAS1.[88] Manifestations of this disease include not only the above-mentioned metabolic findings but also short stature, round facies, and short metatarsal and metacarpal bones, which is also known as Albright hereditary osteodystrophy. The spectrum of disease in type 1a is the consequence of maternal transmission of a defective GNAS1, because the skeletal manifestations are seen in conjunction with renal manifestations.

In type 1b pseudohypoparathyroidism the defect in GNAS1 is felt to be limited to the kidney, because these patients have the characteristic hypocalcemia, hyperphosphatemia, and elevated PTH but do not have Albright hereditary osteodystrophy. This suggests that a maternal transmission is responsible in type 1b. There have been a few described defects in GNAS1 for type 1b that are different from the defect known to be responsible for type 1a and pseudopseudohypoparathyroidism. In type 2 pseudohypoparathyroidism the cAMP response to PTH is intact but the phosphate excretion in the kidney is altered, leading to the characteristic metabolic findings. It is felt that the downstream effects of cAMP are blunted due to resistance. The signal transduction defects seen in all of these disorders not only affect the response to PTH, but also can affect other hormonal responses in the patient. This can manifest as hypogonadism due to resistance to gonadotropins or hypothyroidism due to resistance to thyroid-stimulating hormone (TSH).[89] Pseudopseudohypoparathyroidism is the consequence of paternal transmission of the GNAS1 mutation described in type 1a, and includes Albright hereditary osteodystrophy but does not have hypocalcemia because the normal maternal allele expressed in the kidney preserves normal renal function.[90,91]

Although all of the above-mentioned syndromes and disease processes can cause hypoparathyroidism, the most common cause of hypoparathyroidism is iatrogenic following neck surgery. This can occur following thyroidectomy, parathyroidectomy, or central compartment neck dissections. It is estimated that 1 to 2% of patients undergoing total thyroidectomy for thyroid cancer develop hypoparathyroidism and hypocalcemia.[92,93]

References

1. Ahmad R, Hammond JM. Primary, secondary, and tertiary hyperparathyroidism. Otolaryngol Clin North Am 2004;37:701–713
2. AACE/AAES Task Force on Primary Hyperparathyroidism. The American Association of Clinical Endocrinologists and the American Association of Endocrine Surgeons position statement on the diagnosis and management of primary hyperparathyroidism. Endocr Pract 2005;11:49–54
3. Heath H, Hodgson SF, Kennedy MA. Primary hyperparathyroidism. Incidence, morbidity, and potential economic impact in a community. N Engl J Med 1980;302:189–193
4. Melton LJ. The epidemiology of primary hyperparathyroidism in North America. J Bone Miner Res 2002;17(suppl 2):N12–N17
5. Salti GI, Fedorak I, Yashiro T, et al. Continuing evolution in the

operative management of primary hyperparathyroidism. Arch Surg 1992;127:831–836

6. Bartsch D, Nies C, Hasse C, Willuhn J, Rothmund M. Clinical and surgical aspects of double adenoma in patients with primary hyperparathyroidism. Br J Surg 1995;82:926–929

7. Wynne AG, van Heerden J, Carney JA, Fitzpatrick LA. Parathyroid carcinoma: clinical and pathologic features in 43 patients. Medicine 1992;71:197–205

8. Ruda JM, Hollenbeak CS, Stack BC Jr. A systematic review of the diagnosis and treatment of primary hyperparathyroidism from 1995 to 2003. Otolaryngol Head Neck Surg 2005;132:359–372

9. Arnold A, Shattuck TM, Mallya SM, et al. Molecular pathogenesis of primary hyperparathyroidism. J Bone Miner Res 2002;17(suppl 2):N30–N36

10. Brown EM. The pathophysiology of primary hyperparathyroidism. J Bone Miner Res 2002;17(suppl 2):N24–N29

11. Clark OH, Wilkes W, Siperstein AE, Duh QY. Diagnosis and management of asymptomatic hyperparathyroidism: safety, efficacy, and deficiencies in our knowledge. J Bone Miner Res 1991;6:S135–S142

12. Talpos GB, Bone HG, Kleerekoper M, et al. Randomized trial of parathyroidectomy in mild asymptomatic primary hyperparathyroidism: patient description and effects on the SF-36 health survey. Surgery 2000;128:1013–1020

13. Rao DS. Parathyroidectomy for asymptomatic primary hyperparathyroidism (PHPT): is it worth the risk? J Endocrinol Invest 2001;24:131–134

14. Silverberg SJ, Bilezikian JP. Evaluation and management of primary hyperparathyroidism. J Clin Endocrinol Metab 1996;81:2036–2040

15. Summers GW. Surgical management of parathyroid disorders. In Cumming CW (ed.), Otolaryngology Head and Neck Surgery, 3rd ed. 1998:2519–2532

16. Khan AA, Bilezikian JP, Kung AW, et al. Alendronate in primary hyperparathyroidism: a double-blind, randomized, placebo-controlled trial. J Clin Endocrinol Metab 2004;89:3319–3325

17. Marcus R. The role of estrogens and related compounds in the management of primary hyperparathyroidism. J Bone Miner Res 2002;17(suppl 2):N146–N149

18. Shoback DM, Bilezikian JP, Turner SA, McCary LC, Guo MD, Peacock M. The calcimimetic cinacalcet normalizes serum calcium in subjects with primary hyperparathyroidism. J Clin Endocrinol Metab 2003;88:5644–5649

19. Heath DA, Heath EM. Conservative management of primary hyperparathyroidism. J Bone Miner Res 1991;6:S117–S120

20. Robert JH, Trombetti A, Garcia A, et al. Primary hyperparathyroidism: can parathyroid carcinoma be anticipated on clinical and biochemical grounds? Report of nine cases and review of the literature. Ann Surg Oncol 2005;12:526–532

21. Beus KS, Stack BC Jr. Parathyroid carcinoma. Otolaryngol Clin North Am 2004;37:845–854

22. Fraker DL. Update on the management of parathyroid tumors. Curr Opin Oncol 2000;12:41–48

23. Llach F, Velasquez Forero F. Secondary hyperparathyroidism in chronic renal failure: pathogenic and clinical aspects. Am J Kidney Dis 2001;38(suppl 5):S20–S33

24. Slatopolsky E, Robson AM, Elkan I, Bricker NS. Control of phosphate excretion in uremic man. J Clin Invest 1968;47:1865–1874

25. Canadillas S, Canalejo A, Santamaria R, et al. Calcium-sensing receptor expression and parathyroid hormone secretion in hyperplastic parathyroid glands from humans. J Am Soc Nephrol 2005;16:2190–2197

26. Gogusev J, Duchambon P, Hory B, et al. Depressed expression of calcium receptor in parathyroid gland tissue of patients with hyperparathyroidism. Kidney Int 1997;51:328–336

27. Yano S, Sugimoto T, Tsukamoto T, et al. Association of decreased calcium-sensing receptor expression with proliferation of parathyroid cells in secondary hyperparathyroidism. Kidney Int 2000;58:1980–1986

28. Goodman WG, Goldin J, Kuizon BD, et al. Coronary-artery calcification in young adults with end-stage renal disease who are undergoing dialysis. N Engl J Med 2000;342:1478–1483

29. Manns B, Stevens L, Miskulin D, Owen WF Jr, Winkelmayer WC, Tonelli M. A systematic review of sevelamer in ESRD and an analysis of its potential economic impact in Canada and the United States. Kidney Int 2004;66:1239–1247

30. Teng M, Wolf M, Lowrie E, Ofsthun N, Lazarus JM, Thadhani R. Survival of patients undergoing hemodialysis with paricalcitol or calcitriol therapy. N Engl J Med 2003;349:446–456

31. Ferris RL, Simental AA Jr. Molecular biology of primary hyperparathyroidism. Otolaryngol Clin North Am 2004;37:819–831

32. Pearce SH, Bai M, Quinn SJ, Kifor O, Brown EM, Thakker RV. Functional characterization of calcium-sensing receptor mutations expressed in human embryonic kidney cells. J Clin Invest 1996;98:1860–1866

33. Bai M, Pearce SH, Kifor O, et al. In vivo and in vitro characterization of neonatal hyperparathyroidism resulting from a de novo, heterozygous mutation in the Ca2+-sensing receptor gene: normal maternal calcium homeostasis as a cause of secondary hyperparathyroidism in familial benign hypocalciuric hypercalcemia. J Clin Invest 1997;99:88–96

34. Marx SJ, Stock JL, Attie MF, et al. Familial hypocalciuric hypercalcemia: recognition among patients referred after unsuccessful parathyroid exploration. Ann Intern Med 1980;92:351–356

35. Heath H III. The familial benign hypocalciuric syndromes. In: Bilezikian JP, Raisz LG, Rodan GA, eds. Principles of Bone Biology. SanDiego: Academic Press, 1996:769

36. Fitzpatrick LA. Hypercalcemia in the multiple endocrine neoplasia syndromes. Endocrinol Metab Clin North Am 1989;18:741–752

37. Malone JP, Srivastava A, Khardori R. Hyperparathyroidism and multiple endocrine neoplasia. Otolaryngol Clin North Am 2004;37:715–736

38. Schussheim DH, Skarulis MC, Agarwal SK, et al. Multiple endocrine neoplasia type 1: new clinical and basic findings. Trends Endocrinol Metab 2001;12:173–178

39. Arnold A. Clinical Manifestations and diagnosis of multiple endocrine neoplasia type 1. www.uptodate.com, 2005

40. Trump D, Farren B, Wooding C, et al. Clinical studies of multiple endocrine neoplasia type 1 (MEN1). Q J Med 1996;89:653–669

41. Rizzoli R, Green J 3rd, Marx SJ. Primary hyperparathyroidism in familial multiple endocrine neoplasia type I. Long-term follow-up of serum calcium levels after parathyroidectomy. Am J Med 1985;78:467–474

42. Hellman P, Skogseid B, Juhlin C, Akerstrom G, Rastad J. Findings and long-term results of parathyroid surgery in multiple endocrine neoplasia type 1. World J Surg 1992;16:718–722

43. Samaan NA, Ouais S, Ordonez NG, Choksi UA, Sellin RV, Hickey RC. Multiple endocrine syndrome type I. Clinical, laboratory findings, and management in five families. Cancer 1989;64:741–752

44. Wells SA, Farndon JR, Dale JK, Leight GS, Dilley WG. Long-term evaluation of patients with primary parathyroid hyperplasia managed by total parathyroidectomy and heterotopic autotransplantation. Ann Surg 1980;192:451–458

45. Malmaeus J, Benson L, Johansson H, et al. Parathyroid surgery in the multiple endocrine neoplasia type I syndrome: choice of surgical procedure. World J Surg 1986;10:668–672

46. Burgess JR, David R, Parameswaran V, Greenaway TM, Shepherd JJ.

The outcome of subtotal parathyroidectomy for the treatment of hyperparathyroidism in multiple endocrine neoplasia type 1. Arch Surg 1998;133:126–129

47. Shepherd JJ, Burgess JR, Greenaway TM, Ware R. Preoperative sestamibi scanning and surgical findings at bilateral, unilateral, or minimal reoperation for recurrent hyperparathyroidism after subtotal parathyroidectomy in patients with multiple endocrine neoplasiatype 1. Arch Surg 2000;135:844–84810896380

48. Hellman P, Ahlstrom H, Bergstrom M, et al. Positron emission tomography with 11C-methionine in hyperparathyroidism. Surgery 1994;116:974–981

49. Kivlen MH, Bartlett DL, Libutti SK, et al. Reoperation for hyperparathyroidism in multiple endocrine neoplasia type 1. Surgery 2001;130:991–998

50. Tonelli F, Spini S, Tommasi M, et al. Intraoperative parathyroid hormone measurement in patients with multiple endocrine neoplasia type 1 syndrome and hyperparathyroidism. World J Surg 2000;24:556–563

51. Burgess JR, Shepherd JJ, Parameswaran V, Hoffman L, Greenaway TM. Spectrum of pituitary disease in multiple endocrine neoplasia type 1 (MEN 1): clinical, biochemical, and radiological features of pituitary disease in a large MEN 1 kindred. J Clin Endocrinol Metab 1996;81:2642–2646

52. Padberg B, Schroder S, Capella C, et al. Multiple endocrine neoplasia type (MEN1) revisited. Virchows Arch 1995;426:541–548

53. Verges B, Boureille F, Goudet P, et al. Pituitary disease in MEN type 1 (MEN1): data from the France-Belgium MEN1 multicenter study. J Clin Endocrinol Metab 2002;87:457–465

54. Marx SJ, Vinik AI, Santen RJ, Floyd JC Jr, Mills JL, Green J 3rd. Multiple endocrine neoplasia type I: assessment of laboratory tests to screen for the gene in a large kindred. Medicine 1986;65:226–241

55. Skogseid B, Eriksson B, Lundqvist G, et al. Multiple endocrine neoplasia type 1: a 10-year prospective screening study in four kindreds. J Clin Endocrinol Metab 1991;73:281–287

56. Wamsteker EJ, Gauger PG, Thompson NW, Scheiman JM. EUS detection of pancreatic endocrine tumors in asymptomatic patients with type 1 multiple endocrine neoplasia. Gastrointest Endosc 2003;58:531–535

57. Teh BT, McArdle J, Chan SP, et al. Clinicopathologic studies of thymic carcinoids in multiple endocrine neoplasia type 1. Medicine 1997;76:21–29

58. Gibril F, Schumann M, Pace A, Jensen RT. Multiple endocrine neoplasia type 1 and Zollinger-Ellison syndrome: a prospective study of 107 cases and comparison with 1009 cases from the literature. Medicine 2004;83:43–83

59. Burgess JR, Harle RA, Tucker P, et al. Adrenal lesions in a large kindred with multiple endocrine neoplasia type 1. Arch Surg 1996;131:699–702

60. Larsson C, Skogseid B, Oberg K, Nakamura Y, Nordenskjold M. Multiple endocrine neoplasia type 1 gene maps to chromosome 11 and is lost in insulinoma. Nature 1988;332:85–87

61. Brandi ML, Gagel RF, Angeli A, et al. Consensus guidelines for diagnosis and therapy of MEN type 1 and type 2. J Clin Endocrinol Metab 2001;86:5658–5671

62. Raue F, Frank-Raue K, Grauer A. Multiple endocrine neoplasia type 2. Clinical features and screening. Endocrinol Metab Clin North Am 1994;23:137–156

63. Schuffenecker I, Virally-Monod M, Brohet R, et al. Risk and penetrance of primary hyperparathyroidism in multiple endocrine neoplasia type 2A families with mutations at codon 634 of the RET proto-oncogene. J Clin Endocrinol Metab 1998;83:487–491

64. Dotzenrath C, Cupisti K, Goretzki PE, et al. Long-term biochemical results after operative treatment of primary hyperparathyroidism associated with multiple endocrine neoplasia types I and IIa: is a more or less extended operation essential? Eur J Surg 2001;167:173–178

65. O'Riordain DS, O'Brien T, Grant CS, et al. Surgical management of primary hyperparathyroidism in multiple endocrine neoplasia types 1 and 2. Surgery 1993;114:1031–1037

66. Heath H, Sizemore GW, Carney JA. Preoperative diagnosis of occult parathyroid hyperplasia by calcium infusion in patients with multiple endocrine neoplasia, type 2a. J Clin Endocrinol Metab 1976;43:428–435

67. Machens A, Niccoli-Sire P, Hoegel J, et al. Early malignant progression of hereditary medullary thyroid cancer. N Engl J Med 2003;349:1517–1525

68. Wells SA, Dilley WG, Farndon JA, Leight GS, Baylin SB. Early diagnosis and treatment of medullary thyroid carcinoma. Arch Intern Med 1985;145:1248–1252

69. Verdy M, Weber AM, Roy CC, Morin CL, Cadotte M, Brochu P. Hirschsprung's disease in a family with multiple endocrine neoplasia type 2. J Pediatr Gastroenterol Nutr 1982;1:603–607

70. Beus KS, Stack BC Jr. Calciphylaxis. Otolaryngol Clin North Am 2004;37:941–948

71. Kent RB, Lyerly RT. Systemic calciphylaxis. South Med J 1994;87:278–281

72. Santos PW, Hartle JE, Quarles LD. Calciphylaxis. www.uptodate.com, 2005

73. Janigan DT, Hirsch DJ, Klassen GA, MacDonald AS. Calcified subcutaneous arterioles with infarcts of the subcutis and skin ("calciphylaxis") in chronic renal failure. Am J Kidney Dis 2000;35:588–597

74. Hafner J, Keusch G, Wahl C, et al. Uremic small-artery disease with medial calcification and intimal hyperplasia (so-called calciphylaxis): a complication of chronic renal failure and benefit from parathyroidectomy. J Am Acad Dermatol 1995;33:954–962

75. Coates T, Kirkland GS, Dymock RB, et al. Cutaneous necrosis from calcific uremic arteriolopathy. Am J Kidney Dis 1998;32:384–391

76. Angelis M, Wong LL, Myers SA, Wong LM. Calciphylaxis in patients on hemodialysis: a prevalence study. Surgery 1997;122:1083–1089

77. Don BR, Chin AI. A strategy for the treatment of calcific uremic arteriolopathy (calciphylaxis) employing a combination of therapies. Clin Nephrol 2003;59:463–470

78. Pliquett RU, Schwock J, Paschke R, Achenbach H. Calciphylaxis in chronic, non-dialysis-dependent renal disease. BMC Nephrol 2003;4:8

79. Kang AS, McCarthy JT, Rowland C, Farley DR, van Heerden JA. Is calciphylaxis best treated surgically or medically? Surgery 2000;128:967–971

80. Sutters M, Gaboury CL, Bennett WM. Severe hyperphosphatemia and hypocalcemia: a dilemma in patient management. J Am Soc Nephrol 1996;7:2056–2061

81. Mimouni F, Tsang RC. Neonatal hypocalcemia: to treat or not to treat? (A review). J Am Coll Nutr 1994;13:408–415

82. Muller W, Peter HH, Wilken M, et al. The DiGeorge syndrome. I. Clinical evaluation and course of partial and complete forms of the syndrome. Eur J Pediatr 1988;147:496–502

83. Muller W, Peter HH, Kallfelz HC, Franz A, Rieger CH. The DiGeorge sequence. II. Immunologic findings in partial and complete forms of the disorder. Eur J Pediatr 1989;149:96–103

84. Wilson DI, Burn J, Scambler P, Goodship J. DiGeorge syndrome: part of Catch 22. J Med Genet 1993;30:852–856

85. Arnold A, Horst SA, Gardella TJ, et al. Mutation of the signal peptide-encoding region of the preproparathyroid hormone gene in familial isolated hypoparathyroidism. J Clin Invest 1990;86:1084–1087

86. Bilous RW, Murty G, Parkinson DB, et al. Brief report: autosomal dominant familial hypoparathyroidism, sensorineural deafness, and renal dysplasia. N Engl J Med 1992;327:1069–1074

87. Finnish-German APECED Consortium. An autoimmune disease, APECED, caused by mutations in a novel gene featuring two PHD-type zinc-finger domains. Nat Genet 1997;17:399–403

88. Shapira H, Mouallem M, Shapiro MS, Weisman Y, Farfel Z. Pseudohypoparathyroidism type Ia: two new heterozygous frameshift mutations in exons 5 and 10 of the Gs alpha gene. Hum Genet 1996;97:73–75

89. Shapiro MS, Bernheim J, Gutman A, et al. Multiple abnormalities of anterior pituitary hormone secretion in association with pseudohypoparathyroidism. J Clin Endocrinol Metab 1980;51:483–487

90. Liu J, Litman D, Rosenberg MJ, et al. A GNAS1 imprinting defect in pseudohypoparathyroidism type IB. J Clin Invest 2000;106:1167–1174

91. Yu D, Yu S, Schuster V, et al. Identification of two novel deletion mutations within the Gs alpha gene (GNAS1) in Albright hereditary osteodystrophy. J Clin Endocrinol Metab 1999;84:3254–3259

92. Fitzpatrick LA, Arnold A. Hypoparathyroidism. In: DeGroot LJ, ed. Endocrinology, 3rd ed. Philadelphia: WB Saunders, 1995:1123

93. Scurry WC, Beus KS, Hollenbeak CS, Stack BC Jr. Perioperative parathyroid hormone assay for diagnosis and management of postthyroidectomy hypocalcemia. Laryngoscope 2005;115:1362–1366

17 Surgical Management of Hyperparathyroidism

Phillip K. Pellitteri

The recorded history of hyperparathyroidism in modern medicine is relatively short; nevertheless, several landmark events have contributed to the rapid evolution in the management of this disorder. Sir Richard Owen, a renowned British anatomist and curator, is generally acknowledged as being the first to describe the existence of the parathyroid glands in 1852.[1] In 1877, the Swedish medical student Ivar Sandstrom, reported the existence of small distinct glands adjacent to the thyroid gland in a dog.[2] Over the next 2 years, similar findings noted by Sandstrom in other small mammals led to the search for, and ultimate discovery of, a similar organ in humans (glandulae parathyroideae), which he reported on in 1880.

Early reports of clinical hyperparathyroidism involving the bone disease osteitis fibrosis cystica were noted by von Recklinghausen.[3] Askanazy[4] in 1904 associated the presence of osteomalacia with a potential parathyroid tumor following performance of an autopsy on a patient with nonfusing long bone fractures in whom a large (greater than 4 cm) mass was seen adjacent to the thyroid gland. An association between osteomalacia and parathyroid gland function was not linked until Jacob Erdheim,[5] a Viennese pathologist, discovered parathyroid gland morphologic and histologic abnormalities in patients with bone disease.

The noted American surgeon William Halsted, together with Herbert Evans,[6] a medical student at Johns Hopkins, characterized the blood supply to the parathyroid glands by the use of a vascular casting technique and emphasized that tetany after thyroidectomy was caused more by interruption of the vascular supply to the parathyroid glands than by their inadvertent removal. The work of Viennese surgeon Felix Mandl heralded the surgical treatment of parathyroid disease when he performed a series of neck explorations on Albert Gahne, a tram conductor crippled by parathyroid-induced bone disease.[7] This experience illustrated several important issues that would come to influence future work with surgical parathyroid disease, including clinical use of parathyroid transplantation in humans and the treatment of recurrent disease by reexploration. The association of elevated blood calcium levels and parathyroid dysfunction was well acknowledged when Charles Martell, a sea captain, was evaluated at the Massachusetts General Hospital (MGH) in 1927 and found to have hypercalcemia and generalized demineralization of the skeleton believed to be caused by hyperparathyroidism. The first two of a total of six operations performed on Captain Martell was by Dr. E. Richardson, chief of surgery at MGH. These first two neck explorations yielded only a single normal parathyroid gland on each side without identification of abnormal tissue.[8] A third neck exploration was performed in New York in 1929 by Dr. Russell Patterson without success. As renal function began to deteriorate with increasing symptoms of hyperparathyroidism, the patient returned to MGH under the care of Fuller Albright and Oliver Cope. Cope had experience in several parathyroid explorations under the supervision of Edward Churchill and began cadaver dissection preparation for reexploration of Martell, which he did on three occasions in 1932 without success. At the urging of Martell, who had read extensively about his own disease and the potential locations of ectopic parathyroid tissue, a mediastinal exploration, the seventh surgical procedure on Martell, was planned by Churchill. With Cope assisting, Churchill identified and removed most of a 3-cm tumor from the mediastinum, leaving an attached remnant portion with its vascular pedicle intact to avoid profound hypocalcemia. Several weeks following surgery, Martell experienced renal colic from an impacted ureteral stone, which required surgery; regrettably, this remarkable patient died from laryngospasm following this final operation.[9]

The Nobel Prize–winning work of Berson and Yallow in 1963 paved the way for accurate identification of parathyroid hormone levels in serum and heralded a new era in the presentation of patients with hyperparathyroidism. Instead of renal stones and bone abnormalities, patients are now minimally symptomatic or asymptomatic, without significant subjective complaints and very few (if any) clinical signs. In most instances, an elevated serum calcium and parathyroid hormone level represents the only abnormalities facing the surgeon.

This chapter discusses the surgical treatment of hyperparathyroidism relative to the current clinical profile of patients with a focus on contemporary surgical approaches. Elements that are critical to the success of surgical management, such as physiologic and localization studies, are highlighted as necessary, reserving a more thorough discussion for the reader in other areas of this text.

Indications for Surgery

The indications for performing surgery in patients with hyperparathyroidism may be categorized as those occurring in patients with primary hyperparathyroidism and those occurring in patients with renal-induced parathyroid disease. In patients with primary hyperparathyroidism the distinction between symptomatic patients and those with asymptomatic or minimally symptomatic disease is less relevant currently, as most patients present with minimally symptomatic disease. The accepted symptomatic clinical indications for operation include the presence of bone disease, kidney stones, or muscle weakness or fatigue of a degree that limits the patient's function. The finding of a total serum calcium level above 12 mg/dL in a patient who has either minimal or no symptoms also represents an indication for operative intervention. Patients in whom hyperparathyroidism has resulted in deterioration in mental function, such as altered memory or cognitive function, or frank psychosis, also warrant neck exploration.

The decision to perform surgical exploration in the medically stable, asymptomatic or minimally symptomatic patient with primary hyperparathyroidism is predicated on the potential for the development of complications from prolonged exposure to hypercalcemia and on the long-term benefit of surgery. In general, patients should be assessed for the risk of complications developing on the basis of disease severity at the time of diagnosis. Patients who were previously diagnosed and in whom complications have arisen over a short interval since diagnosis are at significant risk of developing further problems.

The age of the patient is not a contraindication to surgery; rather, the general medical condition and the potential for active quality of life should play a more prominent role in determining the recommendation for treatment.

Surgery in postmenopausal women should be given special consideration independent of the severity of hypercalcemia or the absence of symptoms. Women in this population are at greater risk for development of long-term skeletal complications from generalized demineralization and osteopenia (e.g., hip and vertebral fractures).[10] In a study by Silverberg and associates[11] examining 121 patients with primary hyperparathyroidism (101 of whom were asymptomatic), 61 had parathyroidectomy and 60 were followed expectantly. Whether patients were symptomatic or asymptomatic, the surgery resulted in correction of the hypercalcemia and an increase in bone mineral density of the lumbar spine and the femoral neck, but not of the radius. Of the 52 asymptomatic patients not having neck exploration, the serum calcium levels and the bone densitometry values did not change; however, 23% of them developed other indications for parathyroidectomy. A controlled prospective randomized clinical trial examining surgery versus no surgery in patients with mild asymptomatic primary hyperparathyroidism was conducted by Rao and colleagues.[12] In this investigation 53 patients with primary hyperparathyroidism were randomly assigned to either parathyroidectomy or observation and follow-up. Bone mineral density, biochemical characteristics, quality of life, and psychological function were measured at 6- or 12-month intervals for at least 24 months following treatment or observation. Significant improvement in bone marrow density was noted at the spine, femoral neck, hip, and forearm together with normalization of biochemical characteristics in patients undergoing parathyroidectomy. This was in contrast to patients undergoing follow-up observation without surgery who demonstrated reductions in bone mineral density at the femoral neck and total hip without significant changes in biochemical characteristics of the disease.

Major factors to be considered in determining the need for surgery are the potential for long-term benefit and the prospects for cure. In 85 to 90% of patients, hyperparathyroidism occurs as a result of a single adenoma. Exploration and removal of the adenoma is curative in greater than 95% of patients, and the long-term benefit and potential for cure is high. Primary sporadic hyperplasia occurs in approximately 10 to 12% of patients with hyperparathyroidism. Surgery in these patients involves subtotal parathyroidectomy, with the amount of tissue left ultimately determining the long-term effectiveness of the surgery. Because of the variable amount of parathyroid tissue left in the neck and thus the potential for variable activity, the prospect for cure is less reliable than for patients with adenoma. These patients have rates of cure that are reduced from those in whom an adenoma is removed.[13]

Given these considerations, the decision to perform surgery on patients who seem asymptomatic and who have no obvious metabolic complications is somewhat problematic. Although early surgical intervention seems to be favored, stringent criteria as to whether these patients should undergo surgery have not been clearly defined. About 50% of asymptomatic patients develop metabolic complications from hyperparathyroidism within 5 years of the onset of hypercalcemia.[14] To distinguish patients who might be suitable candidates for surgical treatment, a consensus conference held by the National Institutes of Health (NIH) in 1990 addressed the question of management in asymptomatic hyperparathyroidism.[15] Recommendations for surgical management or surveillance for patients with primary hyperparathyroidism derived from that conference predated much of what has evolved over the course of the past decade with respect to clinical experience with asymptomatic primary hyperparathyroidism, the evolution of contemporary surgical technique, and the development of newer technologies in preoperative localization. Accordingly, this conference was reconvened in early 2002 in an effort to reevaluate the original recommendations from the 1990 symposium and contemporize recommendations on the management of asymptomatic primary hyperparathyroidism.[16] The following is a review of the indications for surgery as suggested by the 2002 conference:

1 Serum calcium is greater than 1.0 mg/dL above the upper limit of normal.
2 Creatinine clearance is reduced greater than 30% for age in the absence of another cause.
3 A 24-hour urinary calcium is greater than 400 mg/dL.

4 Patients are younger than 50 years of age.
5 Bone mineral density measurement at the lumbar spine, hip, or distal radius is reduced greater than 2.5 standard deviations (by T score).
6 Patients request surgery, or patients are unsuitable for long-term surveillance.

These recommended indications are conservative; they provide a framework for surgical decision making but are not absolute or universal. The decision to perform surgery on a patient with primary hyperparathyroidism and metabolic complications is straightforward. The decision is less clear in asymptomatic patients or in those with minimal symptoms, and must be guided by the potential benefit of surgery, the patient's risk of complications developing from disease, the wishes of the patient, and, importantly, the experience of the surgeon. The success rate of surgery and the incidence of complications after parathyroidectomy have been documented to vary greatly, depending on the surgeon's experience. In one study, experienced Swedish surgeons achieved normal calcium in greater than 90% of patients, with recurrent laryngeal nerve complications realized in less than 1%. However, surgeons who perform fewer than 10 parathyroidectomies per year had a success rate of 70%, with 15% of patient remaining hypercalcemic and 14% becoming permanently hypocalcemic.[17] Therefore, in weighing potential benefit of surgery against risks for patients with asymptomatic hyperparathyroidism, the experience of the surgeon should be a primary consideration.

Although patients with mild to moderate hypercalcemia seldom experience rapid elevation in serum calcium level, the risk of symptoms developing and risks for potential end-organ damage increase with time. As a result, patients with untreated primary hyperparathyroidism appear to be at increased risk for major morbidity and mortality from cardiovascular disease.[18,19] In addition, parathyroidectomy appears to offer a distinct and measurable advantage in patients with mild asymptomatic primary hyperparathyroidism as indicated by the results of a randomized trial in which patients were subjectively surveyed by use of a standardized health survey instrument.[20] In this investigation, patients with mild symptomatic hyperparathyroidism were randomly assigned to surgery or observation and then assessed every 6 months following randomization for 2 years with the SF-36 Health Survey, an instrument that measures wellness.[21] Function was significantly improved in patients after parathyroidectomy as compared with patients who were observed. Further evidence for improvement in both function and quality of life following parathyroidectomy was noted in a follow-up study conducted by Edwards and associates,[22] in which 61 patients underwent a quality of life assessment before and at intervals up to 5 years following parathyroidectomy. When analyzing postoperative evaluations, the investigators noted that patients' perception of general health, muscle strength, energy level, and mood significantly improved following surgery.

In contrast to patients with primary hyperparathyroidism, the indications for parathyroid exploration in patients with renal failure–induced hyperparathyroidism are somewhat subjective and may be characterized as those manifested predating and following renal transplantation. Surgery is generally indicated when medical therapy fails to control progressive secondary hyperparathyroidism.[23–25] The clinical manifestations occurring in this disorder include persistent or worsening skeletal symptoms, intractable pruritus, and soft tissue calcifications.[26] The presence of biopsy-proven high turnover bone disease or calciphylaxis in a patient with chronic renal failure with secondary hyperparathyroidism is an additional indication for parathyroidectomy.[27–29] Parathyroidectomy may be indicated in some patients after successful renal transplantation because of the development of clinical manifestation similar to those of primary hyperparathyroidism, including hypercalcemia with nephrolithiasis, pancreatitis, central nervous system manifestations, and overt bone demineralization.[30] The presence of mild hypercalcemia in and of itself does not seem to be a serious threat to the patient after renal transplantation, but impaired kidney function in the presence of high parathyroid hormone levels and hypercalcemia represents an indication for parathyroidectomy, as is the association of kidney stones and long-standing hypercalcemia.[31–33]

Histopathologic Characteristics Influencing Surgical Approach

Single Gland Disease

Single glandular enlargement, or parathyroid adenoma, is the most common cause of hyperparathyroidism. In larger series of patients, where more uniformly accepted pathologic criteria are followed, approximately 80 to 85% of patients with primary hyperparathyroidism were found to have solitary parathyroid adenoma.[34–36] Parathyroid adenomata may occur in any of the four parathyroid glands but have been noted to involve inferior glands more commonly than superior glands.[37]

The gross appearance of parathyroid adenomas is variable but generally they are oval or bean-shaped, red-brown in color, and soft in consistency.[38,39] Adenomas may be bilobed or multilobulated in conformation. In up to 70% of adenomas, a rim of normal parathyroid tissue may be found around the hypercellular portion of the replaced normal gland (**Fig. 17.1**). However, the absence of this characteristic does not exclude the presence of a parathyroid adenoma. Under light microscopy, adenomas appear similar to normal parathyroid glands, exhibiting a thin fibrous capsule with a cellular framework arranged in nests and cords invested by a rich capillary network. Other growth patterns that may be found include acinar, follicular, and pseudopapillary patterns. Chief cells represent the dominant cell type in most parathyroid adenomas with oxyphil and transitional

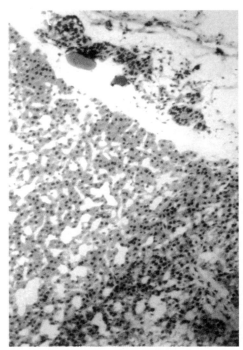

Fig. 17.1 Oil red "O" fat stain showing fat-suppressed rim of normal parathyroid tissue surrounding hypercellular area of parathyroid adenoma.

oxyphil cells, in varying proportions, interspersed within the parenchyma.[38–40] The chief cells in adenomas may be larger than found in normal glands and also exhibit a greater degree of nuclear pleomorphism and giant cell formation.[41,42] Variations in single glandular enlargement representative of parathyroid adenoma may occur and include the subtypes oncocytic adenoma, lipoadenoma, and atypical adenoma.

Oncocytic adenoma is a rare subtype of parathyroid adenoma (4.4–8.4% of adenomas) that is composed predominantly (greater than 80–90%) or exclusively of oxyphil cells.[43,44] Grossly, these tumors tend to be large and have been reported to range in size from 0.2 to 61 g; they are soft, spherical, ellipsoid, lobulated, or nodular, and range in color from light tan to dark orange-brown or mahogany.[45,46] Microscopically, the adenomas are composed predominantly of polygonal cells with abundant brightly eosinophilic granular cytoplasm and small round central hyperchromatic nuclei. Fat staining shows reduced cytoplasmic fat as per typical adenomas. Numerous mitochondria are densely packed throughout the cytoplasm on ultrastructural examination.

Lipoadenoma is another rare subtype of adenoma that was first described in 1958 as a parathyroid hamartoma.[47] The initial description was that of a nonfunctioning mass; subsequent reports documented that these lesions can be responsible for hyperparathyroidism.[48–50] The tumor is a lobulated yellow-tan mass composed of nests, acini, and cords of chief cells and occasional oxyphil and clear cells, intimately associated with large areas of adipose tissue or myxoid stroma.

A rim of normal parathyroid tissue may be present at the periphery.

Water-clear cell adenomas have been described, although their existence was initially doubted.[51] In contrast to the *large clear cell adenomas* that accumulate glycogen, true water-clear cell adenomas demonstrate a glycogen-free cytoplasm that is filled with membrane-bound vesicles.[52]

Atypical adenoma is the term that is used to describe parathyroid adenomas that exhibit atypical cytologic features without definite evidence of malignancy; that is, vascular or soft tissue invasion or metastases.[53] Nuclear atypia in these lesions is of limited value in distinguishing between parathyroid adenoma and carcinoma. Mitotic figures are common in adenomas; however, they may be seen in a small percentage of cases.[54] The malignant potential of atypical adenomas in terms of recurrent or metastatic behavior is uncertain. These lesions may exhibit conspicuous mitoses, adherence to surrounding tissues, trabecular cellular arrangements, capsular invasion, or broad fibrous bands.[55]

Multiple Gland Disease

In the absence of a known stimulus for parathyroid hormone secretion, the proliferation of parenchymal parathyroid cells leading to an increase in gland weight in multiple parathyroid glands is termed primary parathyroid hyperplasia. Two types of parathyroid hyperplasia exist: the common chief cell hyperplasia and the rare water-cell or clear cell hyperplasia.[56,57]

Chief Cell Hyperplasia

Chief cell hyperplasia was first demonstrated as a cause of primary hyperparathyroidism by Oliver Cope et al[58] in 1958. This accounts for approximately 15% of hyperparathyroidism in reported series; however, some reports have indicated that about half of primary hyperparathyroidism may be produced by hyperplasia. The stimulus for this disorder is not known; some studies have indicated the role of a possible circulating factor that can induce proliferation of parathyroid cells in culture. Approximately 30% of patients with chief cell hyperplasia have some type of familial hyperparathyroidism or one of the syndromes of multiple endocrine neoplasia (MEN).[56,57,59,60] Molecular studies have demonstrated that hyperplasias are ultimately associated with monoclonal proliferations.[61,62]

Grossly, there is enlargement of all four glands. The glands may be of variable size, or they may be uniformly enlarged. The dominant cell types are chief cells; however, one may also observe intermixed oxyphil cells and transitional oxyphil cells. Asymmetric gland enlargement due to cellular proliferations resulting in nodular formation may also be noted.[56,57]

The cytoplasmic fat in the chief cells is either reduced or absent.[56,57] The chief cell in nodular areas of cellular proliferation may be totally absent of any fat, whereas chief cells noted between the nodules may demonstrate abundant fat. Abnormal nuclei or mitoses are distinctly rare.[57]

Water-Clear Cell Hyperplasia

A proliferation of vacuolated water-clear cells in multiple parathyroid glands characterizes this rare form of hyperplasia. This pathology demonstrates a female predilection and leads to pronounced hypercalcemia and severe clinical disease. It represents the only parathyroid disorder in which the superior glands are definitively larger than the inferior parathyroid glands. Histologically the glands demonstrate diffuse proliferations of clear cells characterized by clear cytoplasm and small dense nuclei. Cytoplasmic lipid is generally not present; however, moderate amounts of glycogen may be identified. Histologically, water-clear cell hyperplasia bears a resemblance to renal cell carcinoma.[63]

Parathyroid Carcinoma

Parathyroid carcinoma has been reported to be responsible for 0.1 to 5% of cases of primary hyperparathyroidism.[64–68] It remains uncertain as to whether parathyroid carcinoma actually transforms from preexisting benign parathyroid lesions.[65,69] Carcinoma has been postulated to arise in the setting of primary parathyroid hyperplasia, notably familial hyperplasia.[70–72] Prior neck irradiation is not felt to be influential in the development of parathyroid carcinoma.[64,65]

Morphologic features diagnostic of parathyroid malignancy are problematic when applied to surgical decision making. In one series of 40 patients with metastatic parathyroid cancer, as many as 50% were thought to have benign disease by the operating surgeon and consulting pathologist during the time of initial exploration.[73] Metastases are the only certain sign of malignancy; however, metastatic behavior at the time of presentation is distinctly rare.[67]

Parathyroid carcinomas are characteristically large tumors, with as many as 30 to 50% being palpable at the time of presentation.[67,74] Although the average weights of carcinomas are reported to be greater than those of adenomas, there seems to be great overlap, indicating that weight alone may not be a major differentiating characteristic between benign and malignant lesions. Although parathyroid carcinomas generally arise in the usual parathyroid locations, they have uncommonly been described in ectopic supernumerary glands within the mediastinum.[75] Grossly, most parathyroid carcinomas are firm or hard in consistency and demonstrate a gray to white surface color, in contrast to adenomas, which tend to be soft and brown-tan in appearance. Malignant glands may demonstrate adherence to surrounding tissues and may be noted to extend to involve the soft tissues around the thyroid gland or the thyroid parenchyma itself. This morphologic characteristic alone is generally not enough to provide differentiation between benign and malignant disease since previous hemorrhage into a benign adenoma may be associated with fibrosis and adherence to adjacent structures.[65]

In contrast to regional lymphatic metastases, parathyroid carcinoma is more often associated with widespread local infiltration, with invasion into contiguous structures such as thyroid gland, strap muscles, trachea, and recurrent laryngeal nerve. Advanced distant metastasis has been demonstrated to occur in lung, bone, cervical and mediastinal lymph nodes, liver, and occasionally kidney and adrenal glands.[73,76] Pulmonary metastases are the most common distant metastatic site noted.[73]

The histologic diagnosis of parathyroid carcinoma remains problematic. Characteristically the entire gland is traversed by broad fibrous bands that seem to originate from the capsule and extend into the substance of tumor, leading to a nodular or lobulated appearance. Individual cells may be clear or rarely oxyphilic and are arranged in nests and trabeculae.[64] The cell itself may be uniformly bland or may demonstrate metaplasia, but the cases with minimal atypical findings may be difficult to distinguish from an adenoma.[68,77,78]

The presence of mitoses, which can be seen in most instances, has been suggested as a primary factor in definitively diagnosing parathyroid carcinoma.[79] However, mitotic figures may also be seen in parathyroid adenoma and hyperplasia, and their absence does not rule out a diagnosis of carcinoma.[80,81] Increased mitotic activity in unequivocal parathyroid carcinoma is an indicator of poor prognosis.[82] In the absence of an infiltrative growth pattern, the parathyroid lesion demonstrating some other feature of malignancy, including mitoses, may be designated as "atypical" adenoma.[83] Nonfunctioning parathyroid carcinomas have been rarely described, tending to be large and consisting of clear or oxyphil cells.[84,85]

Parathyroid carcinoma typically grows slowly and may demonstrate indolent clinical behavior. Patients with parathyroid carcinoma often die as a result of the effects of excessive parathyroid hormone (PTH) secretion and uncontrolled hypercalcemia rather than growth of the tumor mass itself. Surgical excision of recurrence or metastases may provide excellent palliation by reducing tumor burden and, consequently, hormone production.[86,87]

Surgical Approaches

Surgical Strategy: Determining the Approach

The optimal surgical approach in managing primary hyperparathyroidism is one in which normocalcemia is achieved while minimizing potential surgical morbidity, including recurrent laryngeal nerve injury, postexploration hypocalcemia, and persistent/recurrent hyperparathyroidism requiring reoperation. The approach selected should be individualized to the patient and disease entity (suspected single versus multiple gland disease) and should be time and cost efficient. The development of a surgical strategy in managing patients with primary hyperparathyroidism has in recent years evolved from the routine performance of a comprehensive bilateral neck exploration to a more focused unilateral approach. In theory, because most patients with primary hyperparathyroidism have a single hyperfunctioning adenoma as the offending lesion, it follows that the ideal surgical strategy would involve direct removal of the solitary abnormal gland in the least invasive and atraumatic manner. Incorporating this theoretical ideal into a practical and reliable surgical approach had previously been limited by two constraints: accurate preoperative localization of the abnormal gland, and an inability to intraoperatively confirm removal of all hyperfunctioning parathyroid tissue without performing a bilateral cervical exploration and identification of all four parathyroid glands.

Traditionally, the argument for performing a bilateral neck exploration in patients with suspected adenoma includes the demonstrated high success rate in achieving normocalcemia with a conventional bilateral approach in experienced hands (greater than 95% cure), the inability to accurately predict which side to selectively explore, and the potential risk of missing unsuspected multiple gland disease such as double adenoma or unsuspected sporadic diffuse hyperplasia.[88–93] Recent technologic advances have helped address these concerns, and there is now growing consensus shifting toward a less extensive, directed exploration in the approach to primary hyperparathyroidism. The first impetus to this paradigm shift was provided by improvements in preoperative imaging for the accurate localization of hyperfunctioning solitary adenomas through the use of technetium-99m-sestamibi imaging. The details of this technique as well as other localization modalities for identification of hyperfunctional parathyroid glands are discussed in Chapter 15. The second major advance involved the quest for a more precise and timely means of judging surgical success, which led to the development of assays to measure the intact parathyroid hormone (iPTH) molecule. With the ability to biochemically confirm removal of all hyperfunctional parathyroid tissue intraoperatively, the theoretic advantages of a directed unilateral cervical approach have increasingly become reality.[94–96]

Technique of Parathyroidectomy

Patient Preparation

Surgical exploration is generally performed with the patient under general anesthesia with endotracheal intubation. In patients who are medically unfit for general anesthesia, parathyroid exploration for removal of solitary adenoma localized preoperatively may be performed under local anesthesia supplemented by intravenous sedation.[97,98]

The patient should be positioned on the operating table with the neck hyperextended dorsally to provide optimal access to the cervicothoracic junction, particularly in those patients with a short wide neck. The arms of the patient should lie alongside the body to allow the surgeon and the assistant to stand adjacent to both sides of the neck comfortably. Long ventilation tubes are helpful in facilitating place-

ment of the ventilator at some distance from the operating table, which allows for rotation of the operating table away from the anesthesia equipment and personnel. Patients in whom directed or minimally invasive exploration is being performed should have an accessible intravascular site, intravenous or intraarterial, from which a peripheral sample of blood may be drawn to assess intact parathyroid hormone levels intraoperatively. Following the appropriate positioning and preparation of the patient on the operating table, the table may be adjusted in the reverse Trendelenburg position to decrease venous congestion in the central compartment of the neck.

Cervical Exploration

A low transverse cervical incision (Kocher) is designed two fingerbreadths above the suprasternal notch, usually over a natural skin crease and is carried down through the platysma. The incision may be designed according to the surgeon's preference with respect to the type of exploration being performed (**Fig. 17.2**). Focused procedures require a shorter incision than a traditional bilateral four-gland exploration. In any event, the incision should not extend beyond the anterior borders of the sternocleidomastoid muscles. After incising the platysma, the cranial skin–platysma flap is

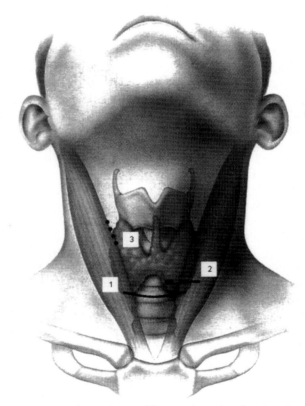

Fig. 17.2 Cervical incisions used for parathyroid exploration: 1, traditional Kocher incision; 2, directed unilateral (inferior gland); 3, directed unilateral (superior gland).

dissected upward to the notch of the thyroid cartilage and the caudal skin–platysma flap is dissected inferiorly to the suprasternal notch (the extent of subplatysmal dissection being dependent on the type of exploration being conducted, e.g., bilateral versus focused exploration). A self-retaining retractor is useful in spreading the cranial and caudal flaps to expose the midline strap muscles in the region of the thyroid bed and central neck structures. The midline raphe of the strap muscles is identified and separated from the thyroid notch to the suprasternal notch, thus allowing the sternohyoid muscles to be retracted laterally. It is generally unnecessary to divide the sternohyoid muscles. The sternothyroid muscle is then separated over the thyroid lobe on the side of the neck to be explored first, carefully elevating the muscle away from the thyroid capsule. Unlike the plane between the strap muscles, which is predominantly avascular, the plane separating the sternothyroid muscle from the true thyroid capsule may be quite vascular, and particular attention to hemostasis is important in carrying out this maneuver. Hemostasis during parathyroid exploration cannot be overemphasized, because blood-stained tissues hinder the ability of the surgeon to identify both abnormal and normal parathyroid glands within the fatty tissue of the central neck. The thyroid lobe on the side being explored is then retracted anteromedially to access the potential space posterior to the thyroid lobe. This is facilitated by exposing the dominant middle thyroid venous tributaries and dividing and ligating them to access this region, referred to as the viscerovertebral angle (VVA) (**Fig. 17.3**). Ligation of the superior thyroid artery is not necessary for adequate rotation of the thyroid anteromedially during this maneuver.

Once the VVA has been accessed, blunt dissection of fibroareolar tissue facilitates evaluation of the area where both normal and abnormal parathyroid glands generally reside. This permits visualization or palpation of enlarged parathyroid tissue with minimal dissection so as to prevent staining the tissues with blood. It is essential to maintain anteromedial retraction of the thyroid gland to expose the angle of visualization and subsequent exploration (**Fig. 17.4**). This is further facilitated by opening the fascial sheath (pretracheal fascia) connecting the carotid sheath and the thyroid gland. This maneuver provides access to the paraesophageal and retroesophageal spaces. Although identification of the recurrent laryngeal nerve is not generally mandatory, dissection in either the retroesophageal or paraesophageal space requires visualization of the nerve to prevent injury.

A systematic approach to the surgical identification of the parathyroid glands is essential to ensure a high success rate and to avoid missing abnormal glands. It is important to develop a methodical and disciplined sequence of exploration so as to minimize the potential for missing either normal or abnormal glands. The ability to palpate abnormal glands cannot be overemphasized. Often glands within the paraesophageal space just dorsal to the juxtaposition of the recurrent laryngeal nerve and the inferior thyroid artery may be quite readily palpated before they are seen. Palpation in the deep viscerovertebral angle generally directs the surgeon to the paraesophageal location, so that focal areas of meticulous dissection may be performed, thus minimizing the potential for significant tissue staining by blood and inadvertent devascularization of normal parathyroid glands. Initial palpation along the posterior aspect of the thyroid capsule, especially adjacent to the superior pole above the inferior thyroid artery entrance to the gland, at times demonstrates the presence of an enlarged superior parathyroid gland closely situated against the true thyroid capsule underneath a covering of pretracheal fascia (**Fig. 17.4**).

Depending on surgical preference, the usual trend is to identify the inferior glands initially. They tend to be larger and located more anteriorly; however, their location may also be less predictable and constant. Typically, they are found adjacent to the inferior pole of the thyroid gland or

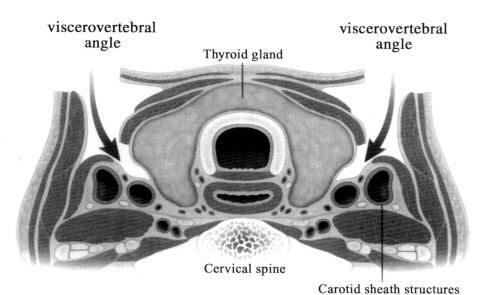

Fig. 17.3 The viscerovertebral angle (VVA).

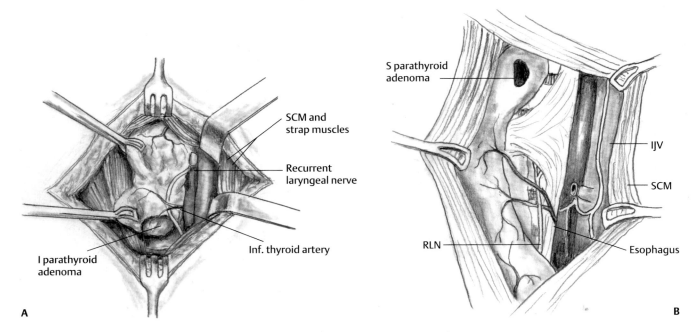

Fig. 17.4 (A) Anteromedial thyroid lobe retraction demonstrating structures within the viscerovertebral angle and inferior parathyroid adenoma. **(B)** Viscerovertebral angle exposure with superior parathy-roid adenoma adjacent to thyroid capsule. *Abbreviations:* IJV, internal jugular vein; RLN, recurrent laryngeal nerve; SCM, sternocleidomastoid.

within a tongue of thymic tissue inferior to the thyroid, the so-called thyrothymic ligament (**Fig. 17.5**). Commonly, they may be located anterior and slightly medial to the juxtaposition of the inferior thyroid artery and recurrent laryngeal nerve. The superior parathyroid glands are most commonly found along the posterior capsule of the thyroid gland at a point slightly lateral and posterior to the juxtaposition between the recurrent nerve and inferior thyroid artery. Blunt dissection along the posterior capsule often reveals the superior gland to be suspended in a teardrop fashion within a centimeter of the entrance of the recurrent laryngeal nerve traversing under the cricothyroid muscle. A helpful

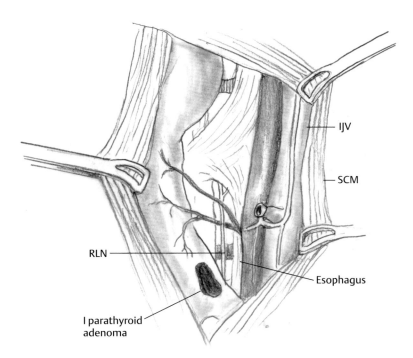

Fig. 17.5 Inferior parathyroid adenoma adjacent to the inferior thyroid pole.

maneuver in exposing the superior location is to divide the sternothyroid muscle close to the superior thyroid pole to maximize medial mobilization without devascularizing the superior pole of the thyroid gland.

Parathyroid glands are often (partially) surrounded by fat. Accordingly, any lobule of fat that is noted at sites that may harbor parathyroid glands should be carefully inspected. Thin fascia that covers the fat lobule may be opened and pressure applied, allowing the parathyroid gland to extrude or "blossom" out of the fat. Most normal parathyroid glands have a light brown or tobacco color, which is important in differentiating parathyroid glands from fat, which is generally more yellow, and from thyroid nodules, which are more rust red in color. Parathyroid glands surrounded by fat lobules also demonstrate a degree of freedom of mobility along the true thyroid capsule relative to the thyroid gland. It is helpful to bluntly dissect along the thyroid capsule with a Kitner (peanut) dissector to visualize moving structures within fat and adjacent to the true thyroid capsule. The close relationship of the pretracheal fascia overlying these pseudosubcapsular parathyroid glands allows this freedom of movement on blunt dissection. In contrast, a thyroid nodule mimicking a parathyroid gland does not enjoy this degree of freedom of movement and is more firmly attached to the central thyroid lobe without a plane of cleavage between it and the thyroid gland and without a vascular pedicle. Perithyroidal lymph nodes, particularly those within the thyrothymic ligament, may be confused with parathyroid glands. However, the consistency of lymph nodes is more firm than that of parathyroid glands, and lymph nodes are also noted to be more of a translucent white-gray than parathyroid glands.

During exploration, the vascular anatomy of both normal and abnormal parathyroid glands should be noted. Dissection of the superior parathyroid gland should be initiated at the outermost tip of this gland to prevent injury to the parathyroid vessels, which usually ascend from arterial anastomoses originating from the inferior thyroid artery. The dissection of the inferior parathyroid gland should begin at the caudal end of the gland, because the vascular pedicle generally enters on the upper or cranial side of the inferior parathyroid. Suspected devitalization of a normal parathyroid gland during dissection generally requires that it be reimplanted within cervical muscle.

Once the abnormal gland is identified, it is removed and sent to the laboratory for pathologic analysis. A thorough search is conducted to locate the second gland on the same side; if found, it, too, is biopsied and sent for pathologic determination. The performance of a frozen section on abnormal glands and identification of a second gland on the same side is not always required, depending on the type of exploration being performed. If the enlarged gland is reported as hypercellular and the second gland is normal or suppressed, the operation proceeds by accessing the VVA of the opposite side. Surgical preference and the type of procedure advocated (focused unilateral versus traditional bilateral) determine the extent of exploration at this point. In the event

that the second gland biopsied on the side explored first is found to be abnormal or if it appears enlarged, all four glands should be identified and histologically examined. In this instance, the presumptive diagnosis is sporadic hyperplasia, which requires subtotal (three-and-a-half-gland) parathyroidectomy. The distinction between adenoma and hyperplastic parathyroid tissue is at best difficult on frozen section analysis; therefore, the surgeon cannot rely on single-gland histologic analysis for definitive therapy.

The appearance of parathyroid tissue, both normal and hyperfunctional, is generally readily recognizable, provided the fibroareolar tissues remain free of excessive bloodstaining. In contrast to normal parathyroid tissue, parathyroid adenomata appear rust or beefy red in situ. They may be mottled or variegated in their coloring and they usually lighten on resection. In contrast, hyperplastic glands generally appear darker than adenoma, usually a dark rust, brown, or chocolate color resembling the color of thyroid tissue.

The failure to identify a missing gland suspected of being an adenoma, or, in the case of hyperplasia, failing to locate all glands, mandates a thorough dissection in an effort to locate abnormally located or ectopic parathyroid tissue. A systematic approach is undertaken to examine all areas potentially harboring an ectopic gland. It is imperative that the surgeon knows which gland is missing, with the understanding that a search is predicated on the likely variable or ectopic sites. Surgical dissection should address all areas accessible through a cervical approach, including the removal of thymic tissue within the superior mediastinum, examination of the retroesophageal space and carotid sheath to the hyoid bone, and thyroid lobectomy (lobotomy), if necessary (**Figs. 17.6** and **17.7**). Approximately 90% of all missed parathyroid adenomas are resectable through a transcervical

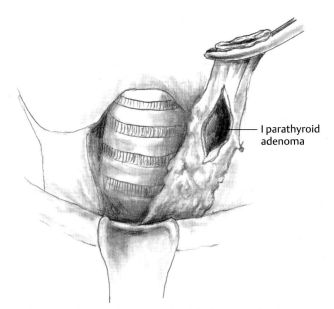

I parathyroid adenoma

Fig. 17.6 Intrathymic inferior parathyroid adenoma extracted from superior mediastinum.

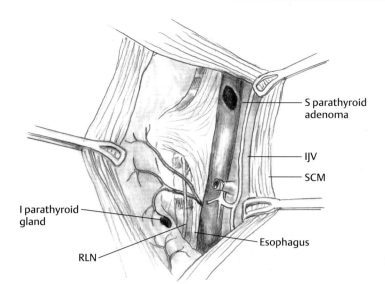

Fig. 17.7 Superior parathyroid adenoma within carotid sheath.

approach, and thus a missing gland is usually harbored in an ectopic location accessible to the surgeon at the initial operation.

Completing the Operation

After completion of the exploration, the operative field is irrigated with warm saline solution and inspected for adequate hemostasis. Particular attention to any normal parathyroid glands that were isolated and dissected is important to document apparent viability. Parathyroid glands judged to be poorly vascularized or of compromised viability should be reimplanted as discussed previously. Depending on the extent of operation, on the body habitus of the patient with respect to depth of dissection within the cervicothoracic junction, and on the degree of bleeding encountered, a drain may or may not be used. In most cases, drainage of the wound is not required because most dissections are limited and hemostatic. Depending on surgical preference, the skin may be closed in either a cuticular or subcuticular fashion after reapproximation of the strap muscles in the midline and closure of the platysma. An occlusive dressing is placed to prevent fluid collection under the incision.

Directed Exploration

Over the past decade, improved preoperative parathyroid localization has allowed alternative approaches to the conventional bilateral neck exploration, using smaller skin incisions, so-called minimally invasive parathyroidectomy (MIP). This terminology can be less than clear, because just how minimally invasive the procedure should be to qualify as such has previously lacked definition, and many of the terms and acronyms adopted during the developmental stages of these techniques have not been updated. Nevertheless, a minimally invasive approach to parathyroidectomy has become the procedure of choice in many endocrine centers and has been shown to be associated with an increase in the number of parathyroid explorations performed.[99] A potential reason for this increase may well reside in the perception that minimally invasive procedures are indeed less extensive, and so physicians are more prepared to refer patients for surgery. In a recent survey of referring endocrinologists, it was stated that 80% would refer more patients if MIP were readily available.[100]

The initial move away from a traditional bilateral approach to neck exploration in the mid-1980s was based on the principle that it would be sufficient to remove a single abnormal gland and visualize a normal second ipsilateral gland to avoid the need for a contralateral exploration.[101] Potentially this would reduce the theoretical higher incidence of complications associated with bilateral exploration. The choice of which neck side to initially approach was at first arbitrary, but was subsequently followed by the development of techniques such as esophagography, venography, and angiography. The general reservations noted at that time regarding the performance of a unilateral approach centered predominantly on the unreliability of the preoperative imaging, the presence of possible contralateral double adenomas, or diffuse asymmetric hyperplasia. As a result, the unilateral approach failed to gain universal support.

The development of improved modalities for preoperative localization significantly aided the evolution of a reliable unilateral approach. Thus, if one could accurately identify a single abnormal parathyroid gland preoperatively, the potential for directing a less invasive surgical approach to that gland and removing it became more realistic. This concept has led to the development of focused or directed unilateral cervical exploration which has, in turn, given rise to variations in the basic unilateral technique, some of which are discussed in greater detail in Chapter 19.

The directed approach to neck exploration utilizes preoperative localization together with the implementation of the intraoperative assay for parathyroid hormone determination (IOPTH) for the surgical management of primary

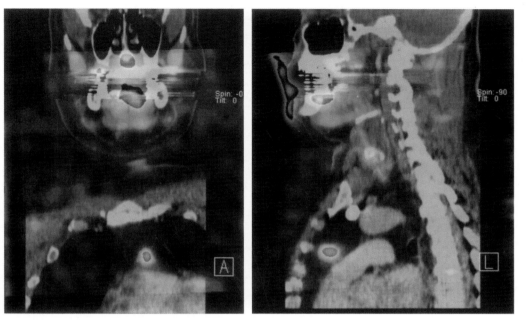

Fig. 17.8 Sagittal (**A**) and coronal (**B**) projections of fused technetium-99m (Tc-99m)-sestamibi and computed tomography images demonstrating ectopic mediastinal parathyroid adenoma.

hyperparathyroidism secondary to anticipated parathyroid adenoma. In the initial preoperative evaluation, all patients with disease entities exhibiting multiple gland hyperplasia, such as those with familial hyperparathyroidism and MEN types I or IIA, are determined to be candidates for standard bilateral cervical exploration and do not have localizing studies performed before the initial operation. A preoperative localizing study is obtained on all other patients with primary hyperparathyroidism, and, depending on surgical preference, may be combined with additional other localizing modalities. Examples of such include initial evaluation with a technetium-99m-sestamibi nuclear uptake scan combined with an anatomic localizing modality such as high-resolution ultrasound or computed tomography (CT) (**Fig. 17.8**). In this manner, the capabilities of both a physiologic and an anatomic localizing modality may be combined to enhance one's ability to localize hyperfunctional and morphologically enlarged parathyroid tissue. A thorough discussion of parathyroid localization modalities is more comprehensively covered in Chapter 15.

If the initial scan is inconclusive or equivocal, as judged by both the surgeon and nuclear medicine specialist, a standard bilateral cervical exploration is planned and performed, whether an enlarged gland is found on the side explored first or not. Failure to localize with an optimally performed technetium-99m-sestamibi scan, in the absence of significant thyroid disease, is strongly suggestive of sporadic diffuse hyperplasia.[102,103] If the nuclear scan identifies a discrete focus of nuclear activity on delayed imaging, suggestive of adenoma, a directed exploration to the side localized is performed, and biochemical confirmation of removal of all hyperfunctioning parathyroid tissue is obtained through the

use of IOPTH. It has been previously demonstrated that the most precipitous decrease in iPTH levels occurs 5 minutes after removal of all hyperfunctioning parathyroid tissue.[103] The short half-life of iPTH (roughly 2 to 5 minutes) allows peripheral blood samples to be obtained intraoperatively for rapid PTH testing anywhere from 7 to 10 minutes after excision of all suspected hyperfunctioning parathyroid tissue.[104] Accordingly, a peripheral blood sample for rapid iPTH assay is drawn at the time of abnormal gland identification (baseline) and subsequently 10 minutes after removal of all suspected hyperfunctioning parathyroid tissue. Degradation in the serum iPTH level exceeding 50%, noted in the postexcision intact PTH level compared with the preexcision or baseline level, provides biochemical confirmation of removal of all hyperfunctioning parathyroid tissue, allowing the procedure to be concluded without identification or biopsy of any other parathyroid glands. If the postexcision iPTH level degrades less than 50% of the baseline preexcision level, suggesting the presence of residual hyperfunctioning parathyroid tissue, a standard bilateral cervical exploration is performed.

Intraoperative PTH determination may be performed by several methods, one of which uses a radioimmunoassay developed through a simple, previously described modification of an intact PTH overnight assay method.[105] The intact PTH assay is a two-antibody sandwich system. One antibody (the capture antibody) is fixed to a plastic bead; the second is conjugated with a measurable marker. The amount of intact PTH present in a plasma sample can be determined by measuring the amount of the marker material remaining after all unbound solutions have been removed. Results of this rapid PTH assay are generally available within 8 to 10 minutes after submission to the radioimmunoassay laboratory. To overcome problems associated with sensitivity of the rapid immunoradiometric assay, researchers began conjugating the labeling antibody with chemiluminescent tracers to avoid the handling issues of their radioactive predecessors.[94,95,103] Since the introduction of the immunochemiluminometric assay (ICMA) in 1993, researchers have experimented with several different variations on this theme, and some manufacturers now offer so-called quick kits. Experience with this assay is consistent among the investigators in that a decrease of 50% or greater between the postexcision and baseline pre-excision PTH values is indicative of removal of all hyperfunctioning parathyroid tissue.[102,103,105–111] The major drawback of these kits is their high cost. However, because the assay negates the need for frozen section analysis in most cases, the overall cost is only slightly more expensive than the traditional unilateral approach.[94] These modifications can provide a cost-effective alternative to preformed kits, especially when weighed against the potential cost of a missed ectopic adenoma.[37]

The kinetics of postadenoma resection are important to understand if logical management strategies are based on these objective data. Libutti et al[112] demonstrated that the half-life of intact PTH varies within a short, brief window of 0.42 to 3.81 minutes. Randolph[113] demonstrated that the lowest values occur within 1 to 3 days. In up to 38% of patients with successful resection of a single parathyroid adenoma and return to normocalcemia, intact PTH levels may remain elevated at 1 month. Suggested mechanisms are cortical bone demineralization, increase in calcium receptor set point, and the development of a relative secondary hyperparathyroidism.[114,115]

Directed Mediastinal Exploration

Initial or reoperative exploration for parathyroid disease may require exploration of the mediastinum. Ectopic parathyroid glands located within the mediastinum and below the level of the thymus account for a small percentage (0.2%) of all abnormally located glands.[116] In contrast, in the reoperative setting, both Norton[117] and Wang[118] have shown that a more substantial proportion, 20% and 18%, respectively, of ectopically located adenomas reside in the mediastinum accessible only through a mediastinal approach. These inferior parathyroid glands are associated in almost all circumstances with the thymus with which they descend during embryonic development, having arisen within the thymus as a third pharyngeal pouch derivative. Several approaches to the mediastinum are available for exploration. The choice of approach used depends on the location of the putative adenoma within the mediastinal compartment. Localization studies that, in combination, corroborate and specify the mediastinal location are required before undertaking exploration. It has been the experience of most investigators that technetium-99m-sestamibi imaging together with an anatomic study such as CT or magnetic

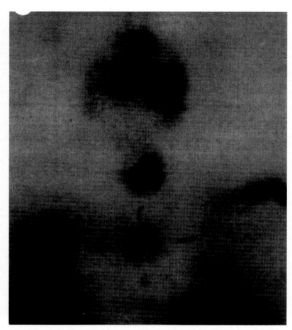

Fig. 17.9 Planar projection of Tc-99m-sestamibi image demonstrating mediastinal parathyroid adenoma.

resonance imaging (MRI) represents the optimal combination of physiologic- and anatomic-based imaging for localization (**Figs. 17.9** and **17.10**). The techniques available for approaching the mediastinum include transcervical and substernal with thymectomy with anterior retraction of the sternum for superior mediastinal glands; mediastinotomy with direct approach to the anterior middle and caudal mediastinal compartments; posterolateral thoracotomy for selective posteriorly located glands in the lower mediastinal compartment; and endoscopic, minimally invasive thoracoscopic mediastinal dissection for selectively focused exploration within the mediastinum.[119–121] In the contemporary setting, most mediastinal glands are approached through either a mediastinotomy or a video-assisted endoscopic

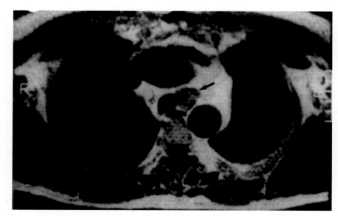

Fig. 17.10 Coronal magnetic resonance (MR) projection of patient in Fig. 17.9 exhibiting mediastinal adenoma (arrow) in the aortopulmonary window.

mediastinal exploration performed transcervically, owing to the capability of these techniques to safely address several areas within the mediastinal compartment and the lower cervical region immediately posterior to the clavicular heads and manubrium. Both these techniques also allow uninterrupted visualization of both recurrent laryngeal nerves, thus preventing inadvertent injury to these structures within the mediastinum.

Bilateral Neck Exploration

Situations in which localization studies are inconclusive or equivocal, or in which clinical circumstances suggest multiple gland disease preoperatively (MEN, familial hyperparathyroidism), mandate the performance of a traditional bilateral cervical exploration. Specifically, both sides of the neck are explored in an attempt to identify at least four parathyroid glands independent of whether the first side explored yields an enlarged gland or not. Routine biopsy of all normal-appearing glands is not recommended. Instead, incisional biopsy of glands is performed selectively. Intraoperative iPTH determination remains an important adjunct in the bilateral approach in that this modality serves to biochemically confirm removal of all hyperfunctioning parathyroid tissue and thus reduces the chance of missing ectopic multiglandular disease, whether as a result of "double adenoma" or ectopic supernumerary parathyroid glands.

Double Adenoma

The incidence of double parathyroid adenoma seems to increase with age. Synchronous double adenomas have been variably reported at rates ranging from 1 to 2% to as high as 10% in patients older than 60 years of age.[122,123] Approximately 50% of true double adenomas image accurately to each of the two locations (**Fig. 17.11**). Bilateral exploration is required despite the high suspicion of only two foci on localization because of the possibility of asymmetric hyperplasia. Intraoperative intact PTH assay provides biochemical confirmation that all hyperfunctional parathyroid tissue has been removed, in that a sequential drop in PTH levels will be noted after successive excision of the first and then second enlarged gland (**Fig. 17.12**). At least one other normal gland should be identified, but surgical biopsy and histologic anal-

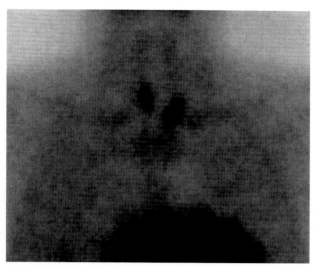

Fig. 17.11 Planar projection of Tc-99m-sestamibi image demonstrating bilateral parathyroid adenomata.

ysis of additional glands are not necessary, provided the final postexcision iPTH level ultimately decreases beyond 50% of the preexcision baseline level intraoperatively to within a normal range.

Sporadic Diffuse Hyperplasia

Ten to 15% of cases of primary hyperparathyroidism may occur as a result of multiglandular disease secondary to sporadic diffuse hyperplasia of the parathyroid glands. Depending on the surgeon's management philosophy, the initial approach to these patients generally includes performance of a nuclear imaging study using technetium-99m-sestamibi preoperatively unless the patient is known to have an endocrine or renal disorder involving multiglandular disease.

A scan that does not indicate an unequivocal area of nuclear uptake on delayed imaging raises the surgeon's suspicion of diffuse hyperplasia, thus mandating the need to comprehensively explore the neck bilaterally with histologic identification of at least one abnormal and one normal gland with the assurance that no additional grossly enlarged glands exist on either side. Forty percent of equivocal scans

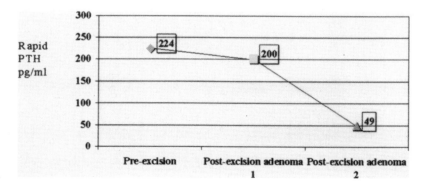

Fig. 17.12 Intact parathyroid hormone (iPTH) decay profile for double parathyroid adenoma resection.

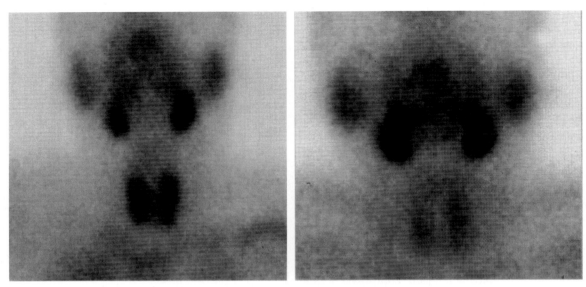

Fig. 17.13 Planar projection of Tc99m sestamibi image demonstrating no clear evidence of discrete nuclear uptake.

were associated with the ultimate finding of multiglandular disease at exploration in a series performed by the author (**Fig. 17.13**).

During comprehensive bilateral exploration, the surgeon endeavors to remove all enlarged glands (either single or multiple) and demonstrate the presence of a histologically normal gland in the event of less than four-gland disease. Rapid intraoperative iPTH assessment (**Fig. 17.14**) is performed to confirm the removal of all hyperfunctional parathyroid tissue, as per the same protocol used in the directed cervical exploration strategy. Failure to achieve this degree of parathyroid hormone degradation to a level that is within the normal laboratory range mandates further exploration, either for an ectopically located gland or, uncommonly, a supernumerary gland.

Following the identification of all enlarged hyperplastic glands in situ, the three largest glands are removed and histologically confirmed. Subtotal excision of the remaining gland follows, leaving at least one third to one half of the gland as a viable vascularized remnant. The titration of iPTH levels is

useful (utilizing IOPTH), in the preservation of a functional parathyroid remnant. Should the postexcision level fall below 10 pg/mL, consideration should be given to the cryopreservation of parathyroid tissue excised from the fourth gland. Although rarely necessary, this approach is favored over routine forearm autotransplantation of parathyroid tissue in that additional surgery is avoided and because a measurable iPTH level detected intraoperatively is generally predictive of euparathyroid function and normocalcemia.[37,124]

Familial Hyperparathyroidism

Familial hyperparathyroidism accounts for less than 5% of all cases of primary hyperparathyroidism.[125] This entity comprises a spectrum of autosomal-dominant inherited diseases that include MEN-I, MEN-IIA, non-MEN, and familial neonatal hyperparathyroidism. In contrast to sporadic primary hyperparathyroidism, patients with familial disease generally present at a younger age and are more likely to have multiglandular disease and persistent or recur-

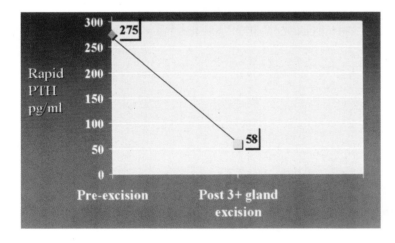

Fig. 17.14 iPTH decay profile for subtotal ($3\frac{1}{2}$ gland) parathyroidectomy.

rent hyperparathyroidism after parathyroidectomy. Subtotal or total parathyroidectomy in combination with bilateral transcervical thymectomy is more frequently necessary for definitive treatment, in contrast to the simple excision of a single adenoma, which is all that is generally required for approximately 80% of patients with sporadic primary hyperparathyroidism. Long-term follow-up of patients with familial disease is performed for early detection and treatment of other endocrine neoplasms associated with these disorders and for the detection of recurrent hyperparathyroidism. Because of the genetic implications of a heritable disease process, the screening of family members represents an important aspect of the overall management of familial hyperparathyroidism. As a result of the identification of causative genetic components in these disorders, the ability for genetic screening of family members and allowing for a global treatment plan for those individuals identified as gene carriers has become possible.

Multiple Endocrine Neoplasia Type I Multiple endocrine neoplasia type I represents an autosomal-dominant inherited syndrome characterized by the presence of neoplastic lesions involving the parathyroid glands, the anterior pituitary gland, the pancreas, and the duodenum. In addition to these affected organs, patients with this disorder may demonstrate carcinoid tumors of the bronchus or thymus, tumors of the ovaries, thyroid gland, adrenal glands, and multiple lipomas. MEN-I is an uncommon disorder occurring in 2 to 20 of every 100,000 persons.[29] A variable degree of penetrance characterizes the disorder, in that not all patients with MEN-I evolve to develop the complete syndrome. The appearance of primary hyperparathyroidism is the most consistent and common manifestation of MEN-I, occurring in greater than 95% of patients, usually before the age of 30, and represents the heralding manifestation of the syndrome.[126–128] Pancreatic endocrine tumors are most often multiple, characterized by islet cell tumors such as gastrinoma and insulinoma. A pituitary tumor is diagnosed in 30 to 40% of patients and is most commonly a prolactinoma. Hyperparathyroidism may occur up to 10 years before the onset of other endocrine disorders, and, as such, MEN-I should be considered in any patient diagnosed with primary hyperparathyroidism at an early age or with multiglandular disease.[128] MEN-I–induced hyperparathyroidism occurs as a result of diffuse four-gland parathyroid hyperplasia.[128–133] In general, the clinical manifestations and biochemical findings in patients with MEN-I are similar to those found in patients with sporadic primary hyperparathyroidism, and, as such, the diagnosis is made by documenting hypercalcemia associated with an elevated or inappropriately high iPTH level.[134] Some of the symptoms in patients with hyperparathyroidism associated with MEN-I may be masked by the Zollinger-Ellison syndrome or insulinoma.[128] Alternatively, MEN-I–induced hyperparathyroidism may also aggravate the clinical manifestations of the Zollinger-Ellison syndrome as a result of calcium stimulation

of gastrin secretion.[128] In considering the diagnosis of MEN-I, a screening biochemical analysis including levels of serum prolactin, glucose, basal gastrin, and pancreatic polypeptide should be obtained.

Wermer,[135] in 1954, noted that 50% of the offspring of individuals affected with the MEN-I syndrome inherited the disorder (without gender differentiation) and that this inheritance did not skip generations. This pattern of inheritance is characteristic of an autosomal dominant trait with a high degree of penetrance.[129,136]

The *MEN1* gene locus has been mapped to a section of chromosome 11 that was further shown to involve a mutation at the 11q13 locus.[137] Subsequently, the *MEN1* gene has been characterized as a tumor suppressor gene that encodes the protein menin.[138] Greater than 90% of patients with MEN-I have known germline menin gene mutations, and most MEN-I families have their own unique mutation that is predisposed to be heterozygous.[134,139]

Patients with MEN-I–induced hyperparathyroidism commonly demonstrate supernumerary parathyroid glands, which present a formidable management dilemma. The inability to recognize a supernumerary gland at the time of initial exploration for this disorder is a well-documented cause of recalcitrant disease.[128,140–142] The surgical approach in patients with this disorder should consist of a routine bilateral neck exploration with identification of all four parathyroid glands. The extensiveness of surgical resection of the parathyroid glands, once identified, is controversial, with advocates of both subtotal and total parathyroidectomy. Several investigators have reported their experience with subtotal parathyroidectomy in patients with MEN-I and hyperparathyroidism with varying degrees of surgical effectiveness.[128,132,133,142] Edis et al[141] reported that 82% of patients with chief cell hyperplasia had normal parathyroid function at least 1 year after subtotal parathyroidectomy. Of these, however, only six of 55 actually had hyperparathyroidism secondary to the MEN-I syndrome. In 12 patients undergoing subtotal parathyroidectomy for MEN-I–induced hyperparathyroidism as reported by Prinz et al,[142] only five ultimately achieved normocalcemia. The presence of a trophic factor has been theorized to represent the causative agent, resulting in a difference in success rates between patients treated for the hyperparathyroidism attributable to sporadic four-gland hyperplasia and that associated with the MEN-I syndrome. A potential parathyroid mitogenic humoral factor was identified by Brandi et al[143] in 1986 from the serum of patients with familial MEN-I syndrome. The mitogenic activity of this humoral factor persisted in the patient's plasma for up to 4 years following total parathyroidectomy. As a consequence, the chance of recurrence in these patients is potentially increased due to the exposure of the parathyroid remnant to this trophic factor. This theory was supported by Prinz et al,[142] who reported a patient with persistent hypoparathyroidism who required calcium supplementation for 10 years after subtotal parathyroidectomy before recurrent disease developed. The reexploration of this patient demonstrated that remnant parathyroid hyperplasia was the etiology of recurrence.

Other investigators have advocated total parathyroidectomy with autotransplantation as the procedure of choice for the initial operation in patients with MEN-I–induced primary hyperparathyoidism.[144,145] In this approach, four parathyroid glands are identified and removed with sectioning of the most morphologically normal-appearing gland into cubic centimeter fragments. The fragments are subsequently implanted into the brachioradialis muscle of the nondominant forearm. Sections from this gland may also be cryopreserved and successfully autotransplanted if the primary autograft does not function. Wells et al[145] pioneered this approach, and reported that 30% of the patients developed recurrent, graft-dependent hyperparathyroidism. It should be noted that only 50% of patients undergoing autotransplantation of cryopreserved parathyroid autografts develop permanent parathyroid function and normocalcemia.[146] Further evidence indicating the possible presence of a humoral factor initiating remnant growth is supplied by the findings of Mallette et al,[131] who reported a higher incidence of graft-dependent recurrence in patients with MEN-I treated with total parathyroidectomy and autotransplantation than in patients with sporadic hyperplasia undergoing the same operation. In patients undergoing total parathyroidectomy for MEN-I–induced hyperparathyroidism, the risk of missing ectopic or supernumerary parathyroid glands at the time of initial operation may be reduced by the utilization of intraoperative iPTH determination.[37]

Initial surgical exploration in patients with MEN-I and hyperparathyroidism may result in cure rates greater than 90%. The requisite for identifying all four parathyroid glands in these patients is emphasized by O'Riordain et al.[132] In this series, immediate cure was noted in 94% of patients; however, hypercalcemia was noted to be persistent in 19% of patients in whom fewer than four glands were visualized at initial operation, compared with 3% of patients in whom four glands or more were noted at initial surgery. In general, both persistent and recurrent disease rates are higher in patients who have less than total parathyroidectomy performed and in whom fewer than four glands are found at the time of initial operation.[129,132]

Multiple Endocrine Neoplasia Type IIA Multiple endocrine neoplasia type IIA is a syndrome characterized by medullary thyroid carcinoma, hyperparathyroidism, pheochromocytoma, Hirschsprung disease, and lichen planus amyloidosis. Eisenberg and Wallerstein,[147] in 1932, first reported a pheochromocytoma and concurrent thyroid carcinoma in a patient at autopsy. In 1961, Sipple[148] estimated that the incidence of thyroid cancer in patients with pheochromocytoma was 14 times higher than that of the normal population, and Cushman[149] subsequently reported a family with hereditary thyroid carcinoma and pheochromocytoma in which one affected member had a parathyroid tumor. The description and characterization of this syndrome, formerly known as Sipple syndrome, came to be known as multiple endocrine neoplasia type IIA (MEN-IIA).[150] The clinical entities associated with the MEN-IIA syndrome demonstrate a variable penetrance in patients, with the exception of medullary thyroid carcinoma, which is seen in essentially all affected individuals. Pheochromocytoma occurs in 70% of individuals affected, and hyperparathyroidism is reported least commonly, in approximately 20 to 35% of affected patients.[151–155]

The hyperparathyroidism associated with this disorder is usually diagnosed as a consequence of screening patients or family members with MEN-IIA or incidentally during thyroidectomy for C-cell hyperplasia or medullary thyroid carcinoma. In a review conducted by Raue et al,[154] 75% of patients with hyperparathyroidism associated with the MEN-IIA syndrome were diagnosed at the time of thyroidectomy with either C-cell hyperplasia or medullary thyroid carcinoma. These patients demonstrated normal serum calcium and parathyroid hormone levels preoperatively, and thus the diagnosis was made on the basis of intraoperative morphology or histology. Less commonly, a diagnosis of hyperparathyroidism is made as a result of the development of clinical symptoms that are similar to those encountered in sporadic primary hyperparathyroidism.[155] The hyperparathyroidism associated with MEN-IIA syndrome usually presents after the third decade of life in the form of mild asymptomatic hypercalcemia, and is generally acknowledged to be less aggressive than its counterpart noted for MEN-I or non-MEN syndromes.[132,153–155] Patients with hyperparathyroidism associated with MEN-IIA present with lower serum calcium levels, fewer symptoms or complications of hypercalcemia, less frequent multiple gland involvement, and a lower incidence of persistent or recurrent disease after surgical treatment, than patients with the MEN-I or non-MEN variety of hyperparathyroidism.

As is the case with MEN-I, MEN-IIA appears to be a genetic disease that is transmitted in an autosomal dominant fashion and with a high degree of penetrance but with variable expression. The heritable defect of the MEN-II syndrome has been mapped to the pericentromeric region of chromosome 10.[156,157] Subsequent work identified the *ret* protooncogene as a segment on chromosome 10 that encodes for a specific cell surface receptor complex, the exact function of which is poorly characterized. Mutations in the segment of the *ret* proto-oncogene coding for the extracellular domain of the tyrosine kinase receptor protein are responsible for producing the MEN-IIA phenotype.[158] This mutation is well characterized for its association with medullary thyroid carcinoma; however, its relationship to MEN-IIA–induced hyperparathyroidism is unknown.

In the event that parathyroid exploration for hyperparathyroidism associated with MEN-IIA is required, the presence of a pheochromocytoma must be excluded in patients prior to surgery. Unrecognized pheochromocytoma in a patient undergoing surgery under general anesthesia may result in a hypertensive crisis intraoperatively with potential catastrophic sequelae. Accordingly, these patients should be screened for the presence of a catecholamine-producing neoplasm of the adrenal gland, and thus a plasma collection for catecholamines, metanephrine, and non-metanephrine levels should be performed before surgery. Once the absence of this neoplasm is confirmed, the surgical approach in these patients is generally more conservative than in patients with MEN-I–associated hyperparathyroidism. A bilateral neck exploration is performed with identification of all four parathyroid glands. Although the hyperparathyroidism associated with patients affected with MEN-IIA demonstrates a higher incidence of multiglandular disease than patients with sporadic primary hyperparathyroidism, it is not as high as found in patients with MEN-I syndrome. Subtotal parathyroidectomy with removal of only the obviously morphologically enlarged parathyroid glands is the approach of choice in patients with MEN-II–associated hyperparathyroidism. Transcervical thymectomy is generally unwarranted, because supernumerary gland involvement is uncommon in these patients. In the event that all four glands are involved, transcervical thymectomy may be performed concurrent with subtotal parathyroidectomy. In surgery for medullary thyroid carcinoma, normal parathyroid glands in the superior position are generally preserved with resection of the inferior parathyroid glands and subsequent reimplantation, if necessary, so that lymph nodes in the central neck compartment and the anterior superior mediastinum are not excluded.

Exploration for patients with MEN-I– or –IIA–associated hyperparathyroidism is usually quite successful. Cance and Wells[151] have reported a 100% surgical success rate and 3% recurrence rate in treating patients with primary hyperparathyroidism associated with MEN-IIA. Unlike the hyperparathyroidism associated with MEN-I, where the extensiveness of parathyroid gland resection is important in defining operative success, the degree of resection does not seem to significantly influence the success rate in patients operated for parathyroid disease associated with MEN-IIA syndrome. O'Riordain et al[132] reported a 100% cure rate without recurrence whether total parathyroidectomy, subtotal parathyroidectomy, or excision of enlarged glands independently was performed.

Non–Multiple Endocrine Neoplasia Familial Hyperparathyroidism Hyperparathyroidism that occurs in the absence of other endocrinopathies in patients with at least one first-degree relative with surgically proven hyperparathyroidism and no personal or family history of multiple endocrine neoplasia has been termed non-MEN familial hyperparathyroidism (NMFH). It occurs in young patients with a mean age at diagnosis of approximately 36 years. Some of these patients experience the disorder as children, although presentation is uncommon before 10 years of age.[159] NMFH seems to be more aggressive than sporadic or MEN-IIA–related hyperparathyroidism; frequently, patients with this disorder manifest profound hypercalcemia and more frequently are seen in hypercalcemic crisis.[159,160] One third to one half of patients with NMFH present with renal stones and also commonly manifest other nonspecific signs and symptoms of hyperparathyroidism such as fatigue, weakness, hypertension, and peptic ulcer disease.[159] A high incidence of recalcitrant disease following treatment seems to be a characteristic feature of the clinical profile of patients with NMFH. Persistent or recurrent disease has been noted to occur at a rate of 33% in the 97 patients reported in the literature. This degree of recalcitrance contrasts markedly with a very low rate of recurrent disease following surgical treatment in patients with sporadic hyperparathyroidism.

Prior to initiating surgical treatment for this disorder it is important to exclude all other familial sources of hyperparathyroidism, as well as the entity known as benign familial hypocalciuric hypercalcemia (FHH). Once other clinical disorders have been excluded, patients with NMFH should be considered for parathyroid exploration because of the aggressive biologic behavior of this disorder. There is a high incidence of both multiglandular and supernumerary gland disease accounting for the high rate of recalcitrance following initial exploration. Similar to the other familial hyperparathyroidism disorders, a bilateral neck exploration with identification of all four parathyroid glands is performed. Either subtotal or total parathyroidectomy together with bilateral cervical thymectomy is generally performed with reimplantation of parathyroid tissue as necessary, depending on the extent of parathyroid gland resection. If only one or two parathyroid glands are morphologically enlarged, the goal of treatment is to resect all abnormal parathyroid tissue from one side of the neck, leaving existing remnant parathyroid tissue in the remaining side.[159] Intraoperative iPTH determination is helpful in determining the degree of hyperfunctional parathyroid tissue remaining after subtotal parathyroidectomy in these patients and may serve as an indicator of remnant parathyroid function once abnormally enlarged glands have been resected. Both the visualization and subsequent removal of abnormally enlarged glands and the intraoperative parathyroid hormone findings serve to guide the extensiveness of surgery in patients who manifest this disorder and have less than four glands appearing abnormal. It is important that these patients be followed long term to recognize if and when recalcitrant disease occurs.

Neonatal Hyperparathyroidism This is a rare condition that is characterized by severe hypercalcemia occurring in association with severe hypotonia, poor feeding, constipation, failure to thrive, and respiratory distress. The manifestations of this disorder often become evident during the first week of life; however, it may not become manifest until the age of 3 months or older.[159] Most instances of familial neonatal hyperparathyroidism have occurred in patients in whom a family history of benign familial hypocalciuric hypercalcemia has been present. The disease locus for FHH has been identified on the long arm of chromosome 3, and patients with FHH are heterozygous for the mutation, with one affected allele.[161,162] The presence of two defective alleles is believed to cause severe neonatal hyperparathyroidism.[163] Patients with this disorder require urgent parathyroid exploration and resection of all four glands. Total parathyroidectomy is advocated together with parathyroid reimplantation, bilateral transcervical thymectomy, and cryopreservation of parathyroid tissue because of a high recalcitrance rate for this disorder.

Hyperparathyroidism Associated with Renal Failure In contrast to the directed or focused exploration protocols for minimally invasive operations performed for solitary adenoma, the operation of choice for patients with renal-induced hyperparathyroidism at initial surgery is traditional four-gland bilateral exploration. The surgical principle of "not removing anything before seeing everything" is aptly applied in this situation. The two most widely used initial surgical procedures for the management of renal failure–induced hyperparathyroidism are subtotal parathyroidectomy and total parathyroidectomy with parathyroid autotransplantation with or without cryopreservation of parathyroid tissue. If subtotal parathyroidectomy is the procedure of choice, the smallest most morphologically normal-appearing parathyroid gland is selected to represent the remnant gland left in situ. The pole opposite the vascular pedicle is excised, leaving approximately one third to one half of the entire gland as a vascularized remnant. It is important that all parathyroid glands be in situ when this is accomplished so that, should the remnant prove to be nonviable after its sectioning, the next most normal-appearing gland is selected for the remnant, and the initial remnant is completely removed. It is generally easier to leave a superior remnant with a viable pedicle than an inferior one because of the proximity of the vascular pedicle to the normal position of the gland. The remnant is marked with a nonabsorbable suture or metal surgical clip. In the event that only three parathyroid glands are found after a comprehensive exploration, all three are removed. This circumstance has been noted to result in approximately 30% of patients remaining with the hyperparathyroid state.[164] If total parathyroidectomy and autotransplantation with or without cryopreservation is planned, all four parathyroid glands are removed after discovery, with the most normal-appearing gland selected as the autograft.[165] Ten to 15 cubic-millimeter fragments of the selected autotransplant gland are placed into several intramuscular pockets in the brachial radialis muscle of the nondominant forearm in a hemostatic fashion, preventing hemorrhage into the implant bed, which may result in poor "take" of the grafts.[145] Cryopreservation of the remaining portion of this autotransplant gland should be performed in the event that sufficient parathyroid function does not develop after revascularization of the implants.[166]

Advocates supporting one procedure versus the other are noted in the literature, but objective controlled trials dealing specifically with renal failure–induced hyperparathy-roidism are few. Of the trials conducted, the only prospective randomized series was reported by Rothmund et al,[167] who found that total parathyroidectomy with autotransplantation was superior to subtotal parathyroidectomy in controlling symptoms in a group of 40 patients with renal failure–induced hyperparathyroidism. In this series, in which patients were followed over a mean of 4 years postoperatively, four patients who were randomly assigned to the subtotal parathyroidectomy cohort experienced recurrent disease. The elimination of bone pain was significantly improved proportionately in patients who underwent total parathyroidectomy with autotransplantation. Three other independent reports compared both techniques in a retrospective analysis and found that both procedures resulted in similar outcomes.[168–170]

The success of subtotal parathyroidectomy is dependent on the size and viability of the remnant parathyroid gland left in situ. Nodular remnants are more likely to grow and result in recurrent hyperparathyroidism. This procedure has the theoretical advantage of producing less postoperative hypocalcemia because the remnant continues to function. The main disadvantage is that in the event that these remnants become hyperfunctional, the reoperations on many occasions are tedious, technically difficult, and carry increased risk of complications such as injury to the recurrent laryngeal nerve. In general, successful subtotal parathyroidectomy alleviated bone pain to a lesser degree than total parathyroidectomy with autotransplantation but carried less risk of postoperative low turnover bone disease.[170]

The effectiveness of total parathyroidectomy with autotransplantation depends on the nodularity of the gland from which the graft is obtained, and the number and weight of the fragments that are reimplanted. As in recurrent disease within a nodular remnant after subtotal parathyroidectomy, graft-dependent recurrence is three times greater when implanting a nodular gland instead of a diffusely hyperplastic one.[171] The advantage of autotransplantation is that should hyperparathyroidism recur in the graft remnant, partial resection of the remnant under local anesthesia with minimal morbidity may be accomplished.

Parathyroid Carcinoma

Primary hyperparathyroidism resulting from parathyroid carcinoma accounts for only 0.1 to 4% of patients affected.[67,172–175] Parathyroid carcinoma occurs with equal frequency in male and female patients; in contrast, parathyroid adenomas occur more frequently in women.[79] The epidemiology of parathyroid carcinoma offers few clues about its etiology and pathogenesis. The development of cancer of the parathyroid glands has been linked to chronic renal failure and dialysis[176–178] and to familial hyperparathyroidism syndromes including MEN-I and -IIA and the hereditary hyperparathyroidism-jaw tumor syndrome.[179] This syndrome is characterized by recurrent parathyroid adenomas, fibro-osseous tumors of the mandible, and Wilms tumors.[179]

In general, patients with parathyroid cancer have higher serum calcium levels, higher levels of intact parathyroid hormone, and more profound metabolic abnormalities than do patients with parathyroid adenoma or hyperplasia. A comprehensive and detailed discussion regarding the etiology and clinical characteristics of parathyroid carcinoma may be found in Chapter 16.

The definitive treatment of parathyroid cancer is en bloc resection of the tumor and areas of potential local invasion or regional metastasis. Parathyroid cancer frequently recurs in the central neck compartment, and typically exhibits a natural history marked by recurrent hypercalcemia. Therefore, performance of the appropriate surgical procedure during the initial operation is critical and is one of the most important prognostic factors associated with the management of parathyroid cancer.[180] The integrity of the parathyroid capsule should be maintained during dissection by use of an en bloc resection of the ipsilateral central neck contents including the thyroid lobe and tracheoesophageal soft tissues and lymphatics.[181] Structures such as the recurrent laryngeal nerve, esophageal wall, or strap muscles may require sacrifice if the tumor adheres to them; this reduces the risk of tumor spillage and local recurrence. The increased local control achieved with resection of the recurrent laryngeal nerve outweighs the complication of vocal cord paralysis, which may be managed by phonosurgical rehabilitative procedures.

A central compartment neck dissection (level VI), together with resection of soft tissues within the superior mediastinum, is important to appropriately stage any lymph node involvement that is not directly palpable during the initial surgery. Lymph node metastasis lateral to the jugular vein is rare in parathyroid cancer during the initial presentation.[182] Accordingly, prophylactic modified radical or selective dissection of levels I to V is not generally recommended. Neck dissection is reserved for patients with lymph node metastasis detected radiographically or by clinical examination in the jugular distribution or for patients with massive soft tissue invasion of lateral neck structures.

Although cure after resection of recurrent parathyroid carcinoma is rare, aggressive resection of local recurrence is recommended to control severe hypercalcemia. Selected patients achieve prolong disease-free intervals after one or more surgical procedures for recurrence in the neck or anterior superior mediastinum.[183]

In addition to the approach for both initial surgery of parathyroid carcinoma and local recurrence, an aggressive surgical approach to metastatic parathyroid cancer has been advocated to control marked hypercalcemia. Obara et al[184] reported on lung resection for metastasis from parathyroid cancer in which 32% of patients resected achieved a significant reduction in total serum calcium levels and 14% achieved long-term survival ranging from 9 to 30 years. Surgery for locally recurrent parathyroid cancer may be guided by preoperative localization studies to better define the extent and location of recurrent parathyroid cancer (**Fig. 17.15**). Nuclear localization studies must be interpreted with caution, however, because not all tumor foci may be detected, and in patients with very high intact parathyroid

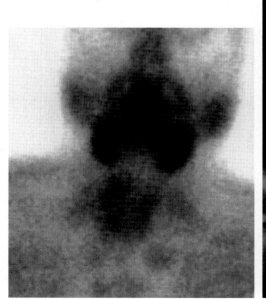

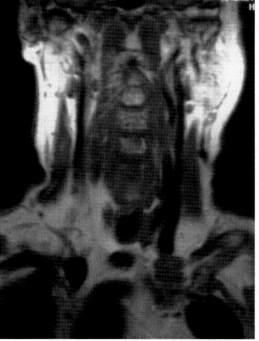

Fig. 17.15 Tc-99m-sestamibi planar image (**A**) and coronal MR projection (**B**) indicating hyperfunctional parathyroid tissue deep to the clavicular head in a patient with parathyroid carcinoma.

hormone levels, benign lesions of bone (brown tumors) may mimic metastases.[185–187]

It has been difficult to analyze the adjuvant roles of radiation and chemotherapy in the management of parathyroid cancer because of its low incidence. A National Cancer Database report describes the use of radiation therapy in combination with surgery in less than 7% of the 286 patients analyzed.[79]

Other reports have advocated the importance of complete en bloc resection followed by radiation therapy to increase local control.[188,189]

One must interpret these reports with care as patients in these series may not have had advanced resectable disease, a finding that characterized investigations where radiation therapy was thought to be a factor that worsened prognosis for parathyroid cancer.

Chemotherapy has proven to offer little in the management of parathyroid cancer. Minimal therapeutic response has been noted with a combination of 5-fluorouracil, cyclophosphamide, and dacarbazine, as well as the combination of methotrexate, doxorubicin, cyclophosphamide, and lomustine. Investigations reporting on the therapeutic results of these combinations were not conducted in a controlled environment and patient enrollment was small.[190,191]

Failed Exploration

A missed single adenoma represents the most common finding yielded on parathyroid reexploration conducted by the experienced parathyroid surgeon. Akerström et al[192] reported on 84 parathyroid reexplorations in 69 patients with primary hyperparathyroidism. Thirty-seven of these patients had missed adenomas and four had "double" adenomas, and only one adenoma was resected on the initial exploration.[192] The majority of the remaining patients had persistent hyperparathyroidism secondary to inadequate resection of parathyroid hyperplasia, with only four patients demonstrating recurrent "single" adenomas. Rotstein et al[193] summarized their experience with 28 reoperations for primary hyperparathyroidism. Solitary adenoma was identified in 24 patients, with two patients each having hyperplasia and carcinoma. Norman and Denham[194] used the technique of minimally invasive radio-guided parathyroidectomy for reoperative disease and resected 23 solitary adenomas from 24 patients. Jaskowiak et al[195] reviewed the NIH experience with 288 patients with persistent/recurrent hyperparathyroidism; 222 (77%) of these patients were ultimately demonstrated to have solitary adenomas.

In patients with renal failure–induced hyperparathyroidism, hyperplasia is the expected histopathology. Cattan et al[196] explored 89 patients for persistent or recurrent secondary hyperparathyroidism; 53 of these patients had undergone subtotal parathyroidectomy, whereas 36 had prior total parathyroidectomy with autotransplantation. Hypertrophy of the remnant was identified as the principal cause of recurrence in the subtotal group. In the group receiving total parathyroidectomy, recurrence was located in the autotransplant in one half; hyperplastic disease was identified in the neck or mediastinum in the remaining half.

When considering the possibility that failure to identify a single adenoma may be due to ectopic gland position, consideration of the surgical embryoanatomic relationships in the central neck is of primary importance. Parathyroid tissue originates from primordial pharyngeal endoderm formed in the third and fourth pharyngeal pouches during the fifth week of embryologic development (**Fig. 17.16**). The epithelial lining of the dorsal wing of the third pharyngeal pouch differentiates into primordial parathyroid glandular tissue, where the ventral portion of the pouch differentiates into the thymus. As the thymus migrates medially and inferiorly, it pulls the inferior parathyroid gland (parathymus) with it into the thymic tail. Eventually, the main portion of the thymus migrates to its final position in the upper thoracic

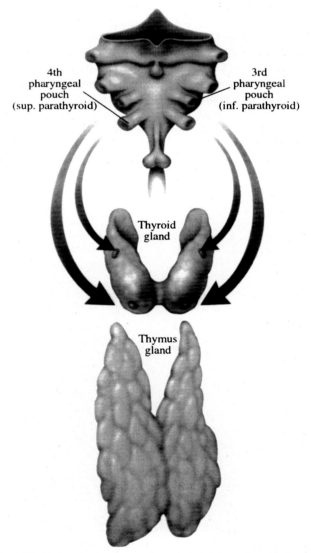

Fig. 17.16 Embryologic origin and descent of the parathyroid glands.

region, and its tail involutes, leaving the developing parathyroid gland to come to its position on the dorsal surface of the inferior pole of the thyroid gland. This glandular tissue eventully forms the inferior parathyroid gland. Simultaneously, the epithelium of the dorsal wing of the fourth pharyngeal pouch begins to differentiate into parathyroid glandular tissue. After separation from the regressing pouch, it becomes associated with the lateral portion of the caudally migrating thyroid and is carried a short distance medially and inferiorly until it resides posterior to the superior pole of the thyroid gland. This tissue eventually develops into the superior parathyroid gland. This embryologic pattern of development has significant implications for the identification of ectopic or normal glandular variance during the course of parathyroidectomy. The longer embryologic migration results in an extensive area of potential dispersal for the normal inferior parathyroid gland. In 61% of cases, the glands are situated at the level of the inferior poles of the thyroid lobes on the posterior, lateral, or anterior aspects. In 26% of cases, they are situated in the thyrothymic ligament or on the upper, cervical portion of the thymus. Less commonly, in 7% of cases, they are situated higher up at the level of the middle third of the posterior aspect of the thyroid lobes and may be confused with the superior parathyroid gland. Because of the embryonic descent of the thymus extending from the angle of the mandible to the pericardium, anomalies of migration of the parathymus are responsible for high or low ectopic locations of the inferior parathyroid gland. The incidence of higher ectopia along the carotid sheath, from the angle of the mandible to the lower pole of the thyroid, does not seem to exceed 1 to 2%.[197–199] Alternatively, if separation from the thymus is delayed, the inferior parathyroid gland may be pulled inferiorly into the anterior mediastinum to a varying degree. In this circumstance, the glands are usually within the thymus at the posterior aspect of its capsule, or still in contact with the great vessels of the mediastinum (**Fig. 17.17**). Lower ectopic regions such as these are noted in 3.9 to 5% of instances.[199,200]

The migration of the ultimobranchial bodies of the thyroid gland serve as a migratory tract for the superior parathyroid glands, which travel toward the lateral part of the main medial thyroid rudiment. In contrast to the inferior glands, the superior parathyroids have a relatively limited descent within the neck. They remain in contact with the posterior part of the middle third of the thyroid lobes. This limited embryonic migration explains why they remain relatively stable in their regional distribution when not pathologic. They are most commonly grouped at the posterior aspect of the thyroid lobes, in an area 2 cm in diameter, whose center is situated approximately 1 cm above the crossing of the inferior thyroid artery and the recurrent laryngeal nerve.[199,201] As a consequence of the extensive descent of the inferior parathyroid gland, the migration of the parathymus results in the inferior and superior glands crossing during development. The embryonic intersection of these glands explains why their grouping at the level of the inferior thyroid artery,

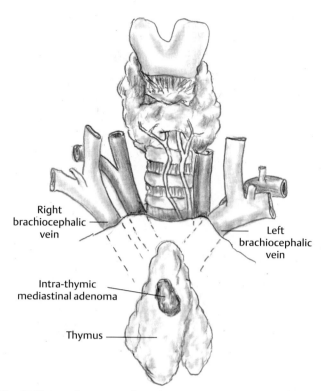

Fig. 17.17 Intrathymic parathyroid adenoma within the middle mediastinum.

Right brachiocephalic vein

Left brachiocephalic vein

Intra-thymic mediastinal adenoma

Thymus

at the junction of the middle and inferior thirds of the thyroid lobe, is in many respects quite close, depending on the degree of migration of the inferior parathyroid gland. Because of the limited migratory descent of the superior parathyroid gland, the area within which these glands disperse is limited, and thus congenital ectopic positions of the superior gland are unusual. In 13% of instances, the glands are located on the posterior aspect of the superior pole of the thyroid lobe in a laterocricoid, lateral pharyngeal, or cricothyroid position. In less than 1% of instances, they are located above the upper pole of the lobe. In 1 to 4% of instances, they are clearly posteriorly behind the pharynx or esophagus. Parathyroid glands that are found in the posterior superior mediastinum are usually neoplastic superior parathyroid glands that have migrated as a consequence of gravity and changes in intrathoracic pressure.[201] (**Fig. 17.18**).

In the NIH series, the most common ectopic site was within the thymus or mediastinum, accounting for 16.7% of ectopically located adenomas.[195] An intrathyroidal lesion was noted in 10% (22 patients) of the study population (**Fig. 17.19**). A similar percentage of patients had undescended parathyroid glands. These so-called parathymus lesions are located at the bifurcation of the carotid artery, high in the neck, and represent an inferior gland that is arrested in the descent from the third pharyngeal pouch (**Fig. 17.20**). Other typical ectopic locations included lesions within the carotid sheath and the retroesophageal space. Unusual ectopic locations include the aortopulmonary window in two patients,

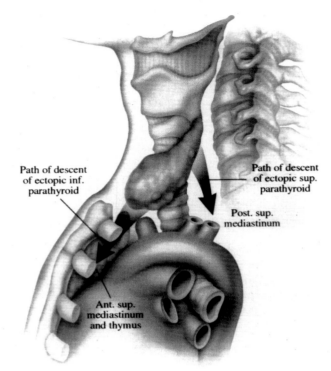

Fig. 17.18 Ectopic pathways for migration into the mediastinum.

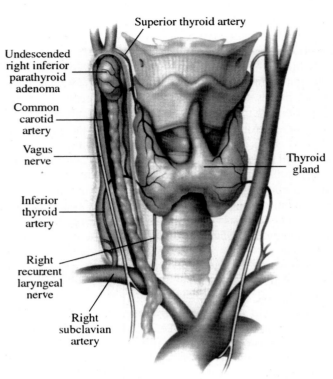

Fig. 17.20 Undescended inferior parathyroid adenoma associated with thymic tissue (parathymus).

the hypopharynx at the base of the tongue in one patient, the wall of the nasopharynx near the nasal septum in one patient, and within the vagus nerve high in the neck at the level of C1–C2 vertebra. Furthermore, three patients had lesions seated within the strap muscles, most likely occurring as a consequence of glandular effraction during the first exploration.[195] A comprehensive discussion detailing the management of recalcitrant hyperparathyroidism may be found in Chapter 18.

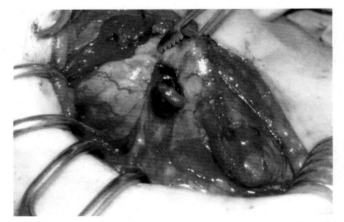

Fig. 17.19 Operative photograph demonstrating intrathyroidal parathyroid adenoma.

Cryopreservation of Parathyroid Tissue

William Halsted[202] was the first to describe parathyroid autotransplantation for the relief of postoperative tetany following thyroidectomy. In his 1907 paper, he described his experience with parathyroid autotransplantation in dogs, demonstrating successful autotransplantation following excision of the graft tissue, which subsequently resulted in the recurrence of symptomatic hypocalcemia. The first successful autotransplantation of parathyroid tissue in humans was performed by Lahey,[203] who reimplanted parathyroid tissue removed accidentally during thyroidectomy.

A period of quiescence in the interest in autotransplantation followed until Wells and colleagues[204] demonstrated synthesis and secretion of parathyroid hormone from autotransplanted parathyroid tissue in humans. In the 1975 report by Wells, postoperative function was confirmed clinically, histologically, and physiologically with a graft survival rate of 93%.

The indications for transplantation or reimplantation of parathyroid tissue include (1) total parathyroidectomy for the treatment of primary or secondary hyperparathyroidism due to diffuse parathyroid hyperplasia; (2) reimplantation of devascularized or accidentally resected normal parathyroid glands during extensive head and neck oncologic surgery, including thyroidectomy; and (3) parathyroid reexploration for recalcitrant hyperparathyroidism. The only absolute contraindication to parathyroid autotransplantation or reimplantation is in the setting of parathyroid carcinoma.

Although not strictly contraindicated, the autotransplantation of parathyroid tissue deriving from parathyroid adenoma is not recommended because of the greater potential for the development of recalcitrant hyperparathyroidism and the very slight potential for malignant degeneration.

An adjuvant technique that serves as an expansion of one's ability to reimplant parathyroid tissue is cryopreservation with delayed autotransplantation.

Technique of Autotransplantation and Cryopreservation

The technique of parathyroid autotransplantation has been classically described by Wells and colleagues.[204] Parathyroid tissue once excised is immediately placed in ice-cold 4% saline or tissue culture medium and chilled for 30 minutes. Devascularized normal parathyroid gland should be placed immediately upon recognition in the cold solution and may remain chilled until the completion of the operative procedure. A frozen section is typically obtained to confirm the presence of parathyroid tissue and avoid transplantation of adenomatous glands or nonparathyroid tissue sections.

Following tissue cooling, the parathyroid tissue may be conveniently diced into 1- to 2-mm cubes. In general, 15 to 20 cubics provide a satisfactory amount of parathyroid tissue for reimplantation or autotransplantation. In the event that tissue is being reimplanted because of inadvertent devascularization or removal, a choice of implantation site is usually the ipsilateral sternocleidomastoid muscle. The fascia of the muscle is generally incised, following which anywhere from one to three tissue cubes are inserted within the muscle pocket hemostatically and then subsequently closed and marked with a permanent suture.

In the event that abnormal parathyroid glands are being used following total parathyroidectomy for diffuse hyperplasia, and thus the possibility of required future excisions, the nondominant brachial radialis muscle is chosen as the preferred site for autotransplantation. This recipient site allows determination of graft function by sampling peripheral blood from the antecubital veins bilaterally and measuring the differential in parathyroid hormone levels. Future reexploration in this setting avoids the potential morbidity of a cervical reexploration while providing direct access to the graft with reduction of graft-implanted parathyroid tissue because of graft hyperfunction.

In the event that postoperative parathyroid function is uncertain, such as may occur in subtotal parathyroidectomy, cryopreservation of parathyroid tissue allowing for the potential for delayed autotransplantation represents a helpful adjuvant modality. With the improved capability of determining the level of parathyroid function intraoperatively using intraoperative parathyroid hormone assessment, the implementation of cryopreservation technique has become more refined and applied. Serum intact parathyroid hormone levels measured intraoperatively at a level less than 10 pg/mL following subtotal parathyroidectomy generally require cryopreservation of parathyroid tissue. In the setting of total parathyroidectomy for primary or secondary hyperparathyroidism, it is prudent to cryopreserve parathyroid tissue for delayed reimplantation in the event that initially autotransplanted parathyroid tissue does not result in normocalcemia postoperatively.

The technique of cryopreservation involves the placement of 1-mm cubes of parathyroid tissue in a cytoprotective solution of 10% dimethylsulfoxide (DMSO), 10% autologous serum, and 80% RPMI 1640, with glutamine and penicillin-streptomycin added.[205] Vials with the tissue in solution are then cooled to −80°C at a rate of 1°C per minute and maintained in the vapor phase of liquid nitrogen. Prior to autotransplantation, the preserved tissue is warmed to 37°C in a water bath and washed three times with 4% Waymouth's medium prior to transplantation.[206] Functionally, cryopreserved parathyroid tissue appears to incur a limited amount of physiologic derangement, potentially related to cellular processing or cellular expansion. In a report by Brennan and associates,[205] parathyroid hormone release was noted to decrease 10 to 60%, with only 50 to 60% of grafts achieving successful restoration of calcium homeostasis.

Autograft Revascularization The ability of parathyroid tissue to survive autotransplantation and restore calcium homeostasis indicates that the grafted tissue revascularizes to a sufficient extent to provide for physiologic demands as well as restoration of the calcium/parathyroid hormone axis. Evidence suggests that that parathyroid tissue induces angiogenesis, or the development of new blood vessels from existing blood vessels.[207] Carter and associates[207] have shown that parathyroid tissue upregulates production of vascular endothelial growth factor (VEGF), a potent endothelial cell mitogen. Although in vitro and in vivo studies have shown that VEGF can induce an angiogenic response, angiogenesis induced by parathyroid cells exceeds that induced by VEGF alone. This would suggest that other parathyroid produced factors may be involved in regulating angiogenesis together with VEGF. Carter and his group have shown that parathyroid tissue also upregulates angiopoietin-2, a peptide that mediates endothelial cell activity during angiogenesis and augments the stimulatory affects of VEGF.[207,208]

Autograft Recovery It may require several weeks to months for transplanted parathyroid tissue to become satisfactorily functional. During this recovery period, hypocalcemia is present and requires physiologic support. In the past it was believed that withholding calcium and moreover vitamin D supplementation would facilitate parathyroid graft recovery. This has been shown, in both human and animal studies, to be incorrect.[209,210] In addition, it has been shown that parathyroid-induced angiogenesis and graft revascularization occur independently of serum calcium and parathyroid hormone levels.[211] These findings would support the routine postoperative administration of calcium and vitamin D replacement during the graft recovery period. These supplements can then be progressively weaned over a time interval once intrinsic physiologic parathyroid and calcium homeostasis has been established.

Patients undergoing total parathyroidectomy and parathyroid transplantation receive supplementation that includes oral vitamin D_3 beginning 1 day postoperatively at a dose of 2 μg/day for 7 days. Oral calcium carbonate administration is initiated at 2 g/day once the total serum calcium level decreases to less than 8.0 mg/dL. A maintenance dose of approximately 0.5 to 1 μg of vitamin D_3 per day is initiated following the first week.

Hypocalcemic patients who become symptomatic postoperatively receive intravenous calcium gluconate; first a bolus of 2 g and then subsequently an IV infusion is established at 250 mg/day. Following the initiation of oral calcium supplementation and a stable or rising serum calcium level, the intravenous infusion is weaned rapidly. Following discharge, providing no symptoms recur, patients are monitored with total serum or ionized calcium levels every 2 to 4 weeks to determine the adequacy of replacement. Following establishment of stable parathyroid hormone levels or rising total serum calcium levels, vitamin D and oral calcium supplementation are discontinued.

Conclusion

The surgical management of hyperparathyroidism mandates a thorough, methodologic approach to diagnosis, patient evaluation, and the development of an appropriate surgical strategy. Advances in preoperative localization and the ability to rapidly assess the serum level of parathyroid hormone intraoperatively have allowed the fundamental surgical approach to become accurately directed, more refined, and less extensive, leading to improvements in outcome and reductions in treatment time, morbidity, and cost.

Although these technologic developments have effectively advanced the manner by which surgeons approach this disorder, they may not be universally applicable and thus should not serve as a substitute for a well-founded and traditional knowledge base in surgical embryology, anatomy, and meticulous technique. The majority of patients with hyperparathyroidism who undergo appropriate surgical therapy benefit symptomatically as well as metabolically.

References

1. Taylor S. Hyperparathyroidism: retrospect and prospect. Ann R Coll Surg Engl 1976;58:255–265
2. Seiple O. On a New Gland in Man and Several Mammals (Glandulae Parathyroideac). Sandstrom I, trans. Baltimore: Johns Hopkins Press, 1938
3. Von Recklinghausen F. Die fibrose oder deformlerende ostitis, die osteomalacie und die osteoplastiche Karzinosk in ihren gegenseltigen Beziehumgen. Excerpted from Taylor S. History of Hyperparathyroidism. Prog Surg 1968;18:1
4. Askanazy M. Uber ostitis deformans ohne osteldeo Genebe. Arb Pathol Inst Tubingen 1904;4:498
5. Erdheim J. Tetania parathyreopriva. Mitt Grenzgeb Med Chir 1906;16:632–744
6. Halsted WS, Evans HM. I. The parathyroid glandules: their blood supply and their preservation in operation upon the thyroid gland. Ann Surg 1907;46:489–506
7. McClellan WS, Hannon RR. A case of osteitis fibrosa cystica (osteomalacia?) with evidence of hyperactivity of the parathyroid bodies. Metabolic Study III. J Clin Invest 1930;8:249–258
8. Cope O, Keynes WM, Roth SI, Castleman B. Primary chief-cell hyperplasia of the parathyroid glands: a new entry in the surgery of hyperparathyroidism. Ann Surg 1958;148:375–388
9. Cope O. Surgery of hyperparathyroidism: the occurrence of parathyroids in the anterior mediastinum and the division of the operation into two stages. Ann Surg 1941;114:706–733
10. Kenny AM, MacGillivray DC, Pilbeam CC, Crombie HD, Raisz LG. Fracture incidence in postmenopausal women with primary hyperparathyroidism. Surgery 1995;118:109–114
11. Silverberg SJ, Shane E, Jacobs TP, Siris E, Bilizekian JP. A 10-year prospective study of primary hyperparathyroidism with or without parathyroid surgery. N Engl J Med 1999;341:1249–1255
12. Rao DS, Phillips ER, Divine GW, Talpos GB. Randomized controlled trial of surgery versus no surgery in patients with mild asymptomatic primary hyperparathyroidism. J Clin Endocrinol Metab 2004;89:5415–5422
13. Bruining HA, Birkenhager JC, Ong GL, Lamberts SW. Causes of failure in operation for hyperparathyroidism. Surgery 1987;101:562–565
14. Cristesson T. Primary hyperparathyroidism—pathogenesis, incidence and natural history. In: Rothmund M, Wells SA Jr, eds. Progress in Surgery, vol 18. Basel: Karger, 1986
15. National Institutes of Health conference. Diagnosis and management of asymptomatic primary hyperparathyroidism: consensus development conference statement. Ann Intern Med 1991;114:593–597
16. National Institutes of Health Conference. Asymptomatic primary hyperparathyroidism. Washington, DC: NIH, 2002
17. Malmaeus J, Granberg PO, Halvorsen J, et al. Parathyroid surgery in Scandinavia. Acta Chir Scand 1988;154:409–413
18. Nilsson IL, Aberg J, Rastad J, Lind L. Endothelial vasodilatory dysfunction in primary hyperparathyroidism is reversed after parathyroidectomy. Surgery 1999;126:1049–1055
19. Piovesan A, Molineri N, Casosso F, et al. Left ventricular hypertrophy in primary hyperparathyroidism: Effects of successful parathyroidectomy. Clin Endocrinol (Oxf) 1999;50:321–328
20. Talpos GB, Bone HG, Kleerekoper M, et al. Randomized trial of parathyroidectomy in mild asymptomatic primary hyperparathyroidism: patient description and effects on the SF-36 health survey. Surgery 2000;128:1013–1020
21. Wang C. Hyperfunctioning intrathyroid parathyroid gland: a potential cause failure in parathyroid surgery. J R Soc Med 1981;74:49–52
22. Edwards ME, Rotramel A, Beyer T, et al. Improvement in health-related quality of life symptoms of hyperparathyroidism is durable on long-term follow-up. Surgery 2006;140:655–663
23. Diethelm AG, Edwards RP, Whelchel JD. The natural history and surgical treatment of hypercalcemia before and after renal transplantation. Surg Gynecol Obstet 1982;154:481–490
24. Hognestad J, Flatmark A. Hyperparathyroidism in uremia and after kidney transplantation. Scand J Urol Nephrol Suppl 1977;42:137–139
25. Lundgren G, Asaba M, Magnusson G, Pieper R, Alveryd A. The role of parathyroidectomy in the treatment of secondary

hyperparathyroidism before and after renal transplantation. Scand J Urol Nephrol Suppl 1977;42:149–152

26. Demeure MJ, McGee DC, Wilkes W, Duh Q, Clark O. Results of surgical treatment for hyperparathyroidism associated with renal disease. Am J Surg 1990;160:337–340

27. DeVita MV, Rasenas LL, Bansal M, et al. Assessment of renal osteodystrophy in hemodialysis patients. Medicine (Baltimore) 1992;71:284–290

28. Duh QY, Lim RC, Clark OH. Calciphylaxis in secondary hyperparathyroidism: diagnosis and parathyroidectomy. Arch Surg 1991;126:1213–1218

29. Boey JH, Cooke TJC, Gilbert JM, et al. Occurrence of other endocrine tumors in primary hyperparathyroidism. Lancet 1975;2:781–784

30. D'Alessandro AM, Melzer JS, Pirsch JD, et al. Tertiary hyperparathyroidism after renal transplantation: operative indications. Surgery 1989;106:1049–1055

31. Chatterjee SN, Massry SG, Friedler RM, Singer FR, Berne TV. The high incidence of persistent secondary hyperparathyroidism after renal homotransplantation. Surg Gynecol Obstet 1976;143:440–442

32. Christensen MS, Nielsen HE. The clinical significance of hyperparathyroidism after renal transplantation. Scand J Urol Nephrol Suppl 1977;42:130–133

33. Pieper R, Alveryd A, Lundgren G, et al. Secondary hyperparathyroidism and its sequelae in renal transplant recipients. Scand J Urol Nephrol Suppl 1977;42:144–148

34. Coffey RJ, Lee TC, Canary JJ. The surgical treatment of primary hyperparathyroidism: a 20 year experience. Ann Surg 1977;185:518–523

35. DeLellis RA. Tumors of the Parathyroid Glands, Third Series, Fascicle 6. Washington, DC: Armed Forces Institute of Pathology, 1993:25

36. Ghandur-Mnaymneh L, Kimura N. The parathyroid adenoma. A histopathologic clarification with a study of 172 cases of primary hyperparathyroidism. Am J Pathol 1984;115:70–83

37. Pellitteri PK. Directed parathyroid exploration: evolution and evaluation of this approach in a single-institution review of 346 patients. Laryngoscope 2003;113:1857–1869

38. Fialkow PJ, Jackson CE, Block MA, Greenawald KA. Multicellular origin of parathyroid "adenomas." N Engl J Med 1977;297:696–698

39. Williams ED. Pathology of the parathyroid glands. Clin Endocrinol Metab 1974;3:285–303

40. van Heerden JA, Grant CS. Surgical treatment of primary hyperparathyroidism: an institutional perspective. World J Surg 1991;15:688–692

41. Lloyd HM, Jacobi JM, Cooke RA. Nuclear diameter in parathyroid adenomas. J Clin Pathol 1979;32:1278–1281

42. Rudberg C, Grimelius L, Johansson H, et al. Alteration in density, morphology, and parathyroid hormone release of dispersed parathyroid cells from patients with hyperparathyroidism. Acta Pathol Microbiol Immunol Scand [A] 1986;94:253–261

43. Bedetti CD, Dekker A, Watson CG. Functioning oxyphil cell adenoma of the parathyroid gland: a clinicopathologic study of ten patients with hyperparathyroidism. Hum Pathol 1984;15:1121–1126

44. Poole GV, Albertson DA, Marshall RB, Myers RT. Oxyphil cell adenoma and hyperparathyroidism. Surgery 1982;92:799–805

45. Christie AC. The parathyroid oxyphil cells. J Clin Pathol 1967;20:591–602

46. Ordonez NG, Ibanez ML, Mackay B, et al. Functioning oxyphil cell adenomas of parathyroid gland: Immunoperoxidase evidence of hormonal activity in oxyphil cells. Am J Clin Pathol 1982;78:681–689

47. Ober WB, Kaiser GA. Hamartoma of the parathyroid. Cancer 1958;11:601–606

48. Abul-Haj SK, Conklin H, Hewitt WC. Functioning lipoadenoma of the parathyroid gland: report of a unique case. N Engl J Med 1962;266:121–123

49. Daroca PJ, Landau RL, Reed RJ, Kappelman MD. Functioning lipoadenoma of the parathyroid gland. Arch Pathol Lab Med 1977;101:28–29

50. Hargreaves HK, Wright TC. A large functioning parathyroid lipoadenoma found in the posterior mediastinum. Am J Clin Pathol 1981;76:89–93

51. Castleman B, Mallory TB. Pathology of the parathyroid gland in hyperparathyroid gland in hyperparathyroidism: study of 25 cases. Am J Pathol 1935;11:1–69

52. Grenko RT, Anderson KM, Kauffman G, Abt AB. Water-clear cell adenoma of the parathyroid: a case report with immunohistochemistry and electron microscopy. Arch Pathol Lab Med 1995;119:1072–1074

53. Levin KE, Galante M, Clark OH. Parathyroid carcinoma versus parathyroid adenoma in patients with profound hypercalcemia. Surgery 1987;101:649–660

54. San-Juan J, et al. Significance of mitotic activity and other morphologic parameters in parathyroid adenomas and their correlation with clinical behavior [abstract]. Am J Clin Pathol 1989;92:523

55. DeLellis RA. Tumors of the Parathyroid Gland, Series 3, Fascicle 6. Washington, DC: Armed Forces Institute of Pathology, 1993:85

56. Grenko RT, Anderson KM, Kauffman G, et al. Water-clear cell adenoma of the parathyroid: a case report with immunohistochemistry and electronmicroscopy. Arch Pathol Lab Med 1995;119:1072–1074

57. Drueke TB. The pathogenesis of parathyroid gland hyperplasia in chronic renal failure. Kidney Int 1995;48:259–272

58. Cope O, Keynes WM, Roth SI, Castleman B. Primary chief-cell hyperplasia of the parathyroid glands: a new entity in the surgery of hyperparathyroidism. Ann Surg 1958;148:375–388

59. Adams PH, Chalmers T, Peters N, Rack JH, Truscott BM. Primary chief cell hyperplasia of the parathyroid glands. Ann Intern Med 1965;63:454–467

60. Wang CA, Castleman B, Cope O. Surgical management of hyperparathyroidism due to primary hyperplasia. Ann Surg 1982;195:384–392

61. Arnold A, Kim HG, Gaz RD, et al. Molecular cloning and chromosomal mapping of DNA rearranged with the parathyroid hormone gene in a parathyroid adenoma. J Clin Invest 1989;83:2034–2040

62. Friedman E, Bale AE, Marx SJ, et al. Genetic abnormalities in sporadic parathyroid adenoma. J Clin Endocrinol Metab 1990;71:293–297

63. LiVolgi VA, Asa SL. The Parathyroid Glands in Endocrine Pathology. Philadelphia: Churchill-Livingstone, 2002

64. Obara T, Fujimoto Y. Diagnosis and treatment of patients with parathyroid carcinoma: an update and review. World J Surg 1991;15:738–744

65. Smith JF, Coombs RRH. Histologic diagnosis of carcinoma of the parathyroid gland. J Clin Pathol 1984;37:1370–1378

66. van Heerden JA, Weiland LH, ReMine WH, Walls JT, Purnell DC. Cancer of the parathyroid glands. Arch Surg 1979;114:475–480

67. Wang CA, Gaz RD. Natural history of parathyroid carcinoma: diagnosis, treatment, and results. Am J Surg 1985;149:522–527

68. Wynne AG, van Heerden J, Carney JA, Fitzpatrick LA. Parathyroid carcinoma: clinical and pathologic features in 43 patients. Medicine (Baltimore) 1992;71:197–205

69. Kramer WM. Association of parathyroid hyperplasia with neoplasia. Am J Clin Pathol 1970;53:275–283

70. Dinnen JS, Greenwoood RH, Jones JH, Walker DA, Williams ED. Parathyroid carcinoma in familial hyperparathyroidism. J Clin Pathol 1977;30:966–975

71. Haghighi P, Astarita RW, Wepsic HT, Wolf PL. Concurrent primary parathyroid hyperplasia and parathyroid carcinoma. Arch Pathol Lab Med 1983;107:349–350

72. Kantarjian HM, Saad MF, Estey EH, Sellin RV, Samaan NA. Hypercalcemia in disseminated candidiasis. Am J Med 1983;74:721–724

73. Sandelin K, Tullgren O, Farnebo LO. Clinical course of metastatic parathyroid cancer. World J Surg 1994;18:594–598

74. Lumachi F, Basso SM, Basso U. Parathyroid cancer: etiology clinical presentation and treatment. Anticancer Res 2006;26:4803–4807

75. Kastan DJ, Kottamasu SR, Frame B, Greenwald KA. Carcinomas in a mediastinal fifth parathyroid gland. JAMA 1987;257:1218–1219

76. Schantz A, Castleman B. Parathyroid carcinoma. A study of 70 cases. Cancer 1973;31:600–605

77. Evans HL. Criteria for diagnosis of parathyroid carcinoma [abstract]. Lab Invest 1992;66:35A

78. Shane E, Bilezikian JP. Parathyroid carcinoma: a review of 62 patients. Endocr Rev 1982;3:218–226

79. Hundahl SA, Fleming ID, Fremgen AM, Menck HR. Two hundred eighty-six cases of parathyroid carcinoma treated in the U.S. between 1985–1995: a national cancer data base report. Cancer 1999;86:538–544

80. Chaitin BA, Goldman RL. Miotic activity in benign parathyroid disease. Am J Clin Pathol 1981;76:363–364

81. Snover DC, Foucar K. Miotic activity in benign parathyroid disease. Am J Clin Pathol 1981;75:345–347

82. Bondeson L, Sandelin K, Grimelius L. Histopathological variable and DNA cytometry in parathyroid carcinoma. Am J Surg Pathol 1993;17:820–829

83. Trigonis C, Cedermark B, Willems J, Hamberger B, Granberg PO. Parathyroid carcinoma—problems in diagnosis and treatment. Clin Oncol 1984;10:11–19

84. Merlano M, Conte P, Scarsi P, et al. Functioning parathyroid carcinoma. A case report. Tumori 1985;71:193–196

85. Yamashita H, Noguchi S, Nakayama I, et al. Light and electron microscopic study of nonfunctioning parathyroid carcinoma. Acta Pathol Jpn 1984;34:123–132

86. Shortell CK, Andrus CH, Phillips CE, Schwartz SI. Carcinoma of the parathyroid gland: a 30-year experience. Surgery 1991;110:704–708

87. Zisman E, Buckle RM, Deftos LJ, et al. Production of parathyroid hormone by metastatic parathyroid carcinoma. Am J Med 1968;45:619–623

88. Bonjer HJ, Bruining HA, Birkenhager JC, et al. Single and multigland disease in primary hyperparathyroidism: clinical followup, histopathology, and flow cytometric DNA analysis. World J Surg 1992;16:737–743

89. Howe JR. Minimally invasive parathyroid surgery. Surg Clin North Am 2000;80:1399–1426

90. Kaplan EL, Yashiro T, Salti G. Primary hyperparathyroidism in the 1990s. Choice of surgical procedures for this disease. Ann Surg 1992;215:300–317

91. Proye CA, Carnaille B, Bizard JP, et al. Single and multigland disease in seemingly sporadic primary hyperparathyroidism revisited: where are we in the 1990s? A plea against unilateral parathyroid exploration. Surgery 1992;112:1118–1122

92. Shaha AR, Jaffe BM. Cervical exploration for primary hyperparathyroidism. J Surg Oncol 1993;52:14–17

93. Weber CJ, Swell CW, McGarity WG. Persistent and recurrent sporadic primary hyperparathyroidism: histopathology, complications, and results of reoperation. Surgery 1994;116:991–998

94. Irvin GL, Derlso GT. A new, practical intraoperative parathyroid hormone assay. Am J Surg 1994;168:466–468

95. Irvin GL, Prudhomme DL, Deriso GT, Sfakianakis G, Chandarlapaty SK. A new approach to parathyroidectomy. Ann Surg 1994;219:574–579

96. Patel PC, Pellitteri PK, Patel NM, Fleetwood MK. Use of a rapid intraoperative parathyroid hormone assay in the surgical management of parathyroid disease. Arch Otolaryngol Head Neck Surg 1998;124:559–562

97. Chen H, Sokoll LJ, Udelsman R. Outpatient minimally invasive parathyroidectomy: a combination of sestamibi—SPECT localization, cervical block anesthesia and intraoperative parathyroid hormone assay. Surgery 1999;126:1016–1021

98. Inabnet WB, Fulla Y, Richard B, et al. Unilateral neck exploration under local anesthesia: the approach of choice for asymptomatic primary hyperparathyroidism. Surgery 1999;126:1004–1009

99. Delbridge L. Minimally invasive parathyroidectomy: the Australian experience. Asian J Surg 2003;26:76–81

100. Denham DW, Norman J. Bilateral neck exploration for all parathyroid patients is an operation for the history books. Surgery 2003;134:513

101. Tibblin S, Bondeson AG, Ljungberg O. Unilateral parathyroidectomy in hyperparathyroidism due to parathyroid adenoma. Ann Surg 1982;195:245–252

102. Carty SE, Worsey J, Virji MA, Brown ML, Watson CG. Concise parathyroidectomy: the impact of preoperative SPECT 99mTc sestamibi scanning and intraoperative quick parathormone assay. Surgery 1997;122:1107–1114

103. Kao PC, van Heerden JA, Taylor RL. Intraoperative monitoring of parathyroid procedures by a 15-minute parathyroid hormone immunochemiluminometric assay. Mayo Clin Proc 1994;69:532–537

104. Nussbaum SR, Thompson AR, Hutcheson KA, Gaz RD, Wang CA. Intraoperative measurement of parathyroid hormone in the surgical management of hyperparathyroidism. Surgery 1988;104:1221–1227

105. Fleetwood MK, Quinton L, Wolfe J, et al. Rapid PTH assay by simple modification of Nichols Intact PTH-parathyroid hormone assay kit. Clin Chem 1996;42:1498

106. Inabnet WB, Kim CK, Haber RS, Lopchinsky RA. Radio guidance is not necessary during parathyroidectomy. Arch Surg 2002;137:967–970

107. Irvin GL, Dembrow VD, Prudhomme DL. Clinical usefulness of an intraoperative "quick parathyroid hormone" assay. Surgery 1993;114:1019–1022

108. Monchik JM, Barellini L, Langer P, Kahya A. Minimally invasive parathyroid surgery in 103 patients with local/regional anesthesia without exclusion criteria. Surgery 2002;131:502–508

109. Nussbaum SR, Thompson AR, Hutscheson KA, et al. Intraoperative measurement of PTH 1–84: A potential use of the clearance of PTH to assess surgical cure of hyperparathyroidism. Surgery 1988;104:1121–1127

110. Sofferman RA, Standage J, Tang ME. Minimal access parathyroid surgery using intraoperative parathyroid hormone assay. Laryngoscope 1998;108:1497–1503

111. Udelsman R, Donovan PI, Sokoll LJ. One hundred consecutive minimally invasive parathyroid explorations. Ann Surg 2000;232:331–339

112. Libutti SK, Alexander HR, Bartlett DL, et al. Kinetic analysis of the rapid intraoperative parathyroid hormone assay in patients

during operation for hyperparathyroidism. Surgery 1999;126: 1145–1150

113. Randolph GW. Surgery of the Thyroid and Parathyroid Glands. Philadelphia: WB Saunders, 2003

114. Wang TS, Ostrower ST, Heller KS. Persistently elevated parathyroid hormone levels after parathyroid surgery. Surgery 2005;138:1130–1135

115. Mandal AK, Udelsman R. Secondary hyperparathyroidism is an expected consequence of parathyroidectomy for primary hyperparathyroidism: a prospective study. Surgery 1998;124:1021–1026

116. Gilmour JR. The gross anatomy of the parathyroid glands. J Pathol Bacteriol 1938;46:133–149

117. Norton JA. Re-operation for missed parathyroid adenoma. Adv Surg 1997;31:273–297

118. Wang CA. Parathyroid re-exploration. A clinical and pathological study of 112 cases. Ann Surg 1977;186:140–145

119. Prinz RA, Lonchyna V, Carnaille B, Wurtz A, Proye C. Thoracoscopic excision of enlarged mediastinal parathyroid glands. Surgery 1994;116:999–1004

120. Miccoli P, Berti P, Materazzi G, Ambrosini CE, Fregoli L, Donatini G. Endoscopic bilateral neck exploration versus quick intraoperative parathyroid hormone assay (gPTHa) during endoscopic parathyroidectomy: a prospective randomized trial. Surg Endosc 2008;22:398–400

121. Inabnet WB, Chu CA. Transcervical endoscopy–assisted mediastinal parathyroidectomy with intraoperative hormone monitoring. Surg Endosc 2003;17:1678

122. Harness JK, Ramsburg SR, Nishiyama RH, Thompson NW. Multiple adenomas of the parathyroids: do they exist? Arch Surg 1979;114:468–474

123. Tezelman S, Shen W, Shaver JK. Double parathyroid adenomas: clinical and biochemical characteristics before and after parathyroidectomy. Ann Surg 1993;218:300–307

124. Tanaka Y, Seo H, Tominaga Y, et al. Factors related to the recurrent hyperfunction of autografts after total parathyroidectomy in patients with severe secondary hyperparathyroidism. Surg Today 1993;23:220–227

125. Evans DB, Rich TA, Cote GJ. Surgical management of familial hyperparathyroidism. Ann Surg Oncol 2007;14:1525–1527

126. Brandi ML, and et al. Familial multiple endocrine neoplasia type I: a new look at pathophysiology. Endocr Rev 1987;8:391–405

127. Deveney CW. Multiple endocrine neoplasia type 1. In: Clark OH, Dub QY, eds. Textbook of Endocrine Surgery. Philadelphia: WB Saunders, 1997:556

128. Kraimps JL, Duh QY, Demeure M, Clark OH. Hyperparathyroidism in multiple endocrine neoplasia syndrome. Surgery 1992;112:1080–1086

129. Lee CH, Tseng LM, Chen JY, Hsiao HY, Yang AH. Primary hyperparathyroidism in multiple endocrine neoplasia type 1: individualized management with low recurrence rates. Ann Surg Oncol 2006;13:103–109

130. Hellman P, Skogseid B, Juhlin C, Akerstrom G, Rastad J. Findings and long-term results of parathyroid surgery in multiple endocrine neoplasia type 1. World J Surg 1992;16:718–722

131. Mallette LE, Blevins T, Jordan PH, Noon GP. Autogenous parathyroid grafts for generalized primary hyperplasia: contrasting outcome in sporadic hyperplasia versus multiple endocrine neoplasia type I. Surgery 1987;101:738–745

132. O'Riordain DS, O'Brien T, Grant CS, et al. Surgical management of primary hyperparathyroidism in multiple endocrine neoplasia types 1 and 2. Surgery 1993;114:1031–1037

133. van Heerden JA, Kent RB, Sizemore GW, Grant CS, ReMine WH. Primary hyperparathyroidism in patients with multiple endocrine neoplasia syndromes. Arch Surg 1983;118:533–536

134. Kraimps JL, Barbler J. Familial hyperparathyroidism in multiple endocrine neoplasia syndromes. In: Clark OH, Duh QY, eds. Textbook of Endocrine Surgery. Philadelphia: WB Saunders, 1997:381

135. Wermer P. Genetic aspects of adenomatosis of endocrine glands. Am J Med 1954;16:363–371

136. Johnson GJ, Summerskill WH, Anderson VE, Keating FR. Clinical and generic investigation of a large kindred with multiple endocrine adenomatosis. N Engl J Med 1967;277:1379–1385

137. Larsson C, Skogseid B, Oberg K, Nakamura Y, Nordenskjold M. Multiple endocrine neoplasia type 1 gene maps to chromosome 11 and is lost in insulinoma. Nature 1988;332:85–87

138. Chandrasekharappa SC, Guru SC, Manickam P, et al. Positional cloning of the gene for multiple endocrine neoplasia–type 1. Science 1997;276:404–407

139. Sato F, Duh QY. Multiple endocrine neoplasia syndrome. In: Prinz RA, Scaren ED, eds. Endocrine Surgery. Georgetown, TX: Landes Bioscience, 2000:263

140. Cope O. Editorial: hyperparathyroidism—too little, too much surgery? N Engl J Med 1976;295:100–102

141. Edis AJ, van Heerden JA, Scholz DA. Results of subtotal parathyroidectomy for primary chief cell hyperplasia. Surgery 1979;86: 462–469

142. Prinz RA, Gamvros OI, Sellu D, Lynn JA. Subtotal parathyroidectomy for primary chief cell hyperplasia of the multiple endocrine neoplasia type I syndrome. Ann Surg 1981;193:26–29

143. Brandi ML, Aurbach GD, Fitzpatrick LA, et al. Parathyroid mitogenic activity in plasma from patients with familial multiple endocrine neoplasia type 1. N Engl J Med 1986;314:1287–1293

144. Wells SA, Ellis GJ, Gunnels JC, Schneider AB, Sherwood LM. Parathyroid autotransplantation in primary parathyroid hyperplasia. N Engl J Med 1976;295:57–62

145. Wells SA, Farndon JR, Dale JK, Leight GS, Dilley WG. Long-term evaluation of patients with primary parathyroid hyperplasia managed by total parathyroidectomy and heterotopic autotransplantation. Ann Surg 1980;192:451–458

146. McHenry CR, Senger DB, Calandro NK. The effect of cryopreservation on parathyroid cell viability and function. Am J Surg 1997;174:481–484

147. Eisenberg AS, Wallerstein H. Pheochromocytoma of the suprarenal medulla (paraganglioma): a clinicopathology study. Arch Pathol (Chic) 1932;14:818

148. Sipple JH. The association of pheochromocytoma with carcinoma of the thyroid gland. Am J Med 1961;31:163–166

149. Cushman P. Familial endocrine tumors: report of two unrelated kindreds affected with pheochromocytomas, one also with multiple thyroid carcinomas. Am J Med 1962;32:352–360

150. Steiner AL, Goodman AD, Powers SR. Study of a kindred with pheochromocytoma, medullary thyroid carcinoma, hypoparathyroidism and Cushing's disease: multiple endocrine neoplasia type 2. Medicine 1968;47:371–409

151. Cance WG, Wells SA. Multiple endocrine neoplasia type IIa. Curr Probl Surg 1985;22:1–56

152. Chong GC, Beahrs OH, Sizemore GW, Woolner LH. Medullary carcinoma of the thyroid gland. Cancer 1975;35:695–699

153. Howe JR, Norton JA, Wells SA. Prevalence of pheochromocytoma and hyperparathyroidism in multiple endocrine neoplasia type 2A: results of long-term follow-up. Surgery 1993;1114:1070–1077

154. Raue F, Frank-Raue K, Grauser A. Multiple endocrine neoplasia type 2. Clinical features and screening. Endocrinol Metab Clin North Am 1994;23:137–156

155. Raue F, Kraimps JL, Dralle H, et al. Primary hyperparathyroidism in multiple endocrine neoplasia type 2A. J Intern Med 1995;238:369–373

156. Mathew CG, Chin KS, Easton DF, et al. A linked genetic marker for multiple endocrine neoplasia type 2A on chromosome 10. Nature 1987;328:527–528

157. Simpson NE, Kidd KK, Goodfellow PJ, et al. Assignment of multiple endocrine neoplasia type 2A on chromosome 10 by linkage. Nature 1987;328:528–530

158. Mulligan LM, Kwok JB, Healey CS, et al. Germline mutation of the RET protooncogene in multiple endocrine neoplasia type 2A. Nature 1993;363:458–460

159. Huang SM. Familial hyperparathyroidism. In: Clark OH, Duh QY, eds. Textbook of Endocrine Surgery. Philadelphia: WB Saunders, 1997:385

160. Huang SM, Duh QY, Shaver J, et al. Familial hyperparathyroidism without multiple endocrine neoplasia. World J Surg 1997;21:22–28

161. Heath H. Familial benign hypercalcemia—from clinical description to molecular genetics. West J Med 1994;160:554–561

162. Heath H, Jackson CE, Otterud B, Leppert MF. Genetic linkage analysis in familial benign (hypocalciuric) hypercalcemia: evidence for locus heterogeneity. Am J Hum Genet 1993;53:193–200

163. Pollack MR, Brown EM, Chou YW, et al. Mutations in the human Ca^{2r} sensing receptor gene cause familial hypocalciuric hypercalcemia and neonatal severe hyperparathyroidism. Cell 1993;75:1297–1303

164. Llach F. Parathyroidectomy in chronic renal failure: indications, surgical approach and the use of calcitriol. Kidney Int Suppl 1990;29:S62–S68

165. Sitges-Serra A, Caralps-Riera A. Hyperparathyroidism associated with renal disease: pathogenesis, natural history, and surgical treatment. Surg Clin North Am 1987;67:359–377

166. Wells SA, Gunnells JC, Shelburne JD, Schneider AB, Sherwood LM. Transplantation of the parathyroid glands in man: clinical indications and results. Surgery 1975;78:34–44

167. Rothmund M, Wagner PK, Schark C. Subtotal parathyroidectomy versus total parathyroidectomy and autotransplantation in secondary hyperparathyroidism: a randomized trial. World J Surg 1991;15:745–750

168. Malmaeus J, Akerstrom G, Johansson H, et al. Parathyroid surgery in chronic renal insufficiency. Subtotal parathyroidectomy versus total parathyroidectomy with autotransplantation to the forearm. Acta Chir Scand 1982;148:229–238

169. Takagi H, Tominaga Y, Uchida K, et al. Subtotal versus total parathyroidectomy with forearm autograft for secondary hyperparathyroidism in chronic renal failure. Ann Surg 1984;200:18–23

170. Welsh CL, Taylor GW, Cattell WR, Baker LR. Parathyroid surgery in chronic renal failure: Subtotal parathyroidectomy or autotransplantation? Br J Surg 1984;71:591–592

171. Delmonico FL, Wang CA, Rubin NT, et al. Parathyroid surgery in patients with renal failure. Ann Surg 1984;200:644–647

172. Mittendorf EA, McHenry CR. Parathyroid carcinoma. J Surg Oncol 2005;89:136–142

173. Cohn K, Silverman M, Corrado J, Sedgewick C. Parathyroid carcinoma: the Lahey Clinic experience. Surgery 1985;98:1095–1110

174. Hakaim AG, Esselstyn CB. Parathyroid carcinoma: 50-year experience at The Cleveland Clinic Foundation. Cleve Clin J Med 1993;60:331–335

175. van Heerden JA, Weiland LH, ReMine WH, Walls JT, Purnell DC. Cancer of the parathyroid glands. Arch Surg 1979;114:475–480

176. Boyle NH, Ogg CS, Hartley RB, Owen WJ. Parathyroid carcinoma secondary to prolonged hyperplasia in chronic renal failure and in coeliac disease. Eur J Surg Oncol 1999;25:100–103

177. Miki H, Sumitomo M, Inoue H, Kita S, Monden Y. Parathyroid carcinoma in patients with chronic renal failure on maintenance hemodialysis. Surgery 1996;120:897–901

178. Takami H, Kameyama K, Nagakubo I. Parathyroid carcinoma in a patient receiving long-term hemodialysis. Surgery 1999;125:239–240

179. Yoshimoto K, Endo H, Tsuyuguchi M, et al. Familial isolated primary hyperparathyroidism with parathyroid carcinoma: clinical and molecular features. Clin Endocrinol (Oxf) 1998;48:67–72

180. Sandelin K, Auer G, Bondeson L, Grimelius L, Farnebo LO. Prognostic factors in parathyroid cancer: a review of 95 cases. World J Surg 1992;16:724–731

181. Shane E. Clinical review 122: parathyroid carcinoma. J Clin Endocrinol Metab 2001;86:485–493

182. Obara T, Fujimoto Y. Diagnosis and treatment of patients with parathyroid carcinoma: an update and review. World J Surg 1991;15:738–744

183. Favia G, Lumachi F, Polistina F, D'Amico DF. Parathyroid carcinoma: sixteen new cases and suggestions for correction management. World J Surg 1998;22:1225–1230

184. Obara T, Okamoto T, Ito Y, et al. Surgical and medical management of patients with pulmonary metastasis from parathyroid carcinoma. Surgery 1993;114:1040–1048

185. Lu G, Shih WJ, Xiu JY. Technetium-99m MIBI uptake in recurrent parathyroid carcinoma and brown tumors. J Nucl Med 1995;36:811–813

186. Sandelin K, Thompson NW, Bondeson L. Metastatic parathyroid carcinoma: dilemmas in management. Surgery 1991;110:978–986

187. Sarfati E, Desportes L, Gossot D, et al. Acute primary hyperparathyroidism. Br J Surg 1989;76:979–981

188. Chow E, Tsang RW, Brierley JD, Filice S. Parathyroid carcinoma—the Princess Margaret Hospital experience. Int J Radiat Oncol Biol Phys 1998;41:569–572

189. Lillemoe KD, Dudley NE. Parathyroid carcinoma: pointers to successful management. Ann R Coll Surg Engl 1985;67:222–224

190. Bukowski RM, Sheeler L, Cunningham J, Esselstyn C. Successful combination chemotherapy for metastatic parathyroid carcinoma. Arch Intern Med 1984;144:399–400

191. Chahinian AP, Holland JF, Nieburgs HE, et al. Metastatic nonfunctioning parathyroid carcinoma: ultrastructural evidence of secretory granules and response to chemotherapy. Am J Med Sci 1981;282:80–84

192. Akerström G, Rudberg C, Grimelius L, et al. Causes of failed primary exploration and technical aspects of re-operation in primary hyperparathyroidism. World J Surg 1992;16:562–568

193. Rotstein L, Irish J, Gullane P, Keller MA, Sniderman K. Re-operative parathyroidectomy in the era of localization technology. Head Neck 1998;20:535–539

194. Norman J, Denham D. Minimally invasive radioguided parathyroidectomy in the reoperative neck. Surgery 1998;124:1088–1092

195. Jaskowiak N, Norton JA, Alexander HR, et al. A prospective trial evaluating a standard approach to re-operation for missed parathyroid adenoma. Ann Surg 1996;224:308–322

196. Cattan P, Halimi B, Aidan K, et al. Re-operation for secondary uremic hyperparathyroidism: are technical difficulties influenced by initial surgical procedure? Surgery 2000;127:562–565

197. Akerström G, Malmaeus J, Bergstrom R. Surgical anatomy of human parathyroid glands. Surgery 1984;95:14–21

198. Fraker DL, Doppman JL, Shawker TH, et al. Undescended parathyroid adenoma: an important etiology for failed operations for primary hyperparathyroidism. World J Surg 1990;14:342–348

199. Linch DC, Watson LC, Cowie AG. Ectopic parathyroid adenomas. J R Soc Med 1980;73:638–640
200. Henry JF, Denizot A. Anatomic and embryologic aspects of primary hyperparathyroidism. In: Barbier J, Henry JF, eds. Primary Hyperparathyroidism. Paris: Springer-Verlag, 1992:5
201. Thompson NW. Surgical anatomy of hyperparathyroidism. In: Rothmund M, Wells SA Jr, eds. Parathyroid Surgery. Basel, Karger, 1986:59
202. Halsted WS. Auto- and isotransplantation in dogs, of parathyroid glandules. J Exp Med 1909;11:175–199
203. Lahey FH. The transplantation of parathyroids in partial thyroidectomy. Surg Gynecol Obstet 1926;42:508–509
204. Wells SA, Grunnels J, Caulie S, Schneider JD, Arthur B, Sherwood L. Transplantation of the parathyroid glands in man: clinical indications and results. Surgery 1975;78:34–44
205. Brennan MF, Brown EM, Sears HF, Aurbach GD. Human parathyroid cryopreservation in vitro testing of function by parathyroid hormone release. Ann Surg 1978;187:87–90
206. Wells SA, Grunnels JC, Gutman RA, Shelborne JD, Schneider AB, Sherwood LM. The successful transplantation of frozen parathyroid tissue in man. Surgery 1977;81:86–90
207. Carter WB, Uy K, Ward MD, Hoying JB. Parathyroid-induced angiogenesis is VEGF-dependent. Surgery 2000;128:458–464
208. Holash J, Maisonpierre PC, Compton D, et al. Vessel cooption, regression, and growth in tumors mediated by angiopoietins and VEGF. Science 1999;284:1994–1998
209. Funahashi H, Tanaka Y, Imal T, et al. Parathyroid hormone suppression by 22-oxacalcitrol in the severe parathyroid hyperplasia. J Endocrinol Invest 1998;21:43–47
210. Imai T, Tanaka Y, Kikumori T, Ohiwa M, Matsuura N, Funahashi H. Surgical management of preclinical medullary thyroid carcinoma in MEN2A. Thyroidol Clin Exp. 1998;10:143–147
211. Carter WB, Crowell SL, Boswell CA, Williams SK. Stimulation of angiogenesis by canine parathyroid tissue. Surgery 1996;120:1089–1094

18 Reoperation for Hyperparathyroidism

Tzeela Cohen and Ashok R. Shaha

The history of reoperation for hyperparathyroidism is as old as the history of parathyroid surgery itself. In 1925, Felix Mandel from Vienna described the first parathyroidectomy for hyperparathyroidism (HPT). Soon thereafter, in 1926, Oliver Cope from Massachusetts General Hospital published his experience in the field. One of Dr. Cope's first patients was Captain Charles Martel, whose unfortunate story demonstrates the great challenge of treating persistent HPT. Captain Martel's neck was explored six times in vain, while the adenoma responsible for his debilitating disease was hidden in his mediastinum, lateral to the superior vena cava. Without the opportunity to use a Google search, it was the patient himself who urged his physicians to explore the mediastinum, based on his personal knowledge of anatomy.[1]

Great advances have been made over the past two decades in the treatment of primary hyperparathyroidism. Introduction of noninvasive and highly sensitive localization studies, combined with an efficient means for intraoperative prediction of cure, have made these operations seem easy.

The problem of surgical failure does persist, however, and is even seen in highly selective groups of patients,[2,3] demonstrating that surgical judgment and skill is still a crucial component for a successful outcome despite technologic innovation. John Doppman, a radiologist working in the field, warned in 1986, "The only localization study needed for initial surgery for hyperparathyroidism is to localize an experienced endocrine surgeon," a sentiment still not outdated. The lesson Dr. Oliver Cope, the American pioneer of parathyroid surgery, learned from his mentor, Dr. Edward Churchill at Massachusetts General Hospital, is still applicable: "Success of parathyroid surgery must lie in the ability of the surgeon to know a parathyroid gland when he [sees] it, to know the distribution of the glands when they hide, and also to be delicate enough in the technique to be able to make use of this knowledge."[4]

Causes of Recurrent or Persistent Hypercalcemia/Hyperparathyroidism

The reasons for recurrent or persistent hypercalcemia after initial surgery can be divided into three major categories (**Table 18.1**):

1 The wrong diagnosis leads to a nonindicated operation.
2 Surgery was indicated, but was inadequate for the disease process.
3 The surgical technique failed.

Misdiagnosis

Only a small percentage of patients with recurrent hypercalcemia fall into the category of nonindicated surgery or incorrect diagnosis. Even though the most common cause of hypercalcemia in the outpatient setting is primary HPT, the differential diagnosis is broad.[5,6] In most cases, a thorough physical examination, a carefully recorded medical and family history, and a few simple laboratory tests (such as serum calcium and phosphorus, serum PTH, and 24-hour urinary calcium) are sufficient for the diagnosis. Still, even in high-volume specialized centers, some patients may undergo surgery in vain.[7]

Benign familial hypocalciuric hypercalcemia (BFHH) is a commonly reported reason for persistent hypercalcemia after parathyroidectomy. This is a hereditary disease transmitted in an autosomal dominant fashion with 80% penetrance, caused by an inactivating mutation in the calcium-sensing receptor (CaSR) gene.[8]

Benign familial hypocalciuric hypercalcemia should be suspected in a patient with mild, persistent hypercalcemia starting at young age that was not corrected by previous surgery. Upon questioning, a family history of hypercalcemia and failed surgery may be obtained. The key for correct diagnosis in these patients is measurement of 24-hour collection of urinary calcium, which typically should be under 50 mg/24 hours. Unfortunately, occasionally measured

Table 18.1 Causes of Recurrent or Persistent Hyperparathyroidism

Misdiagnosis
Nonindicated surgery
Benign familial hypocalciuric hypercalcemia
Hypercalcemia with adequate parathyroid function
Inadequate surgery
Multiple-gland hyperplasia
Multiple adenomas
Parathyroid carcinoma
Local recurrence of benign disease and parathyromatosis
Failed surgery
Missed adenoma
Missed ectopic adenoma
Supernumerary glands

values are significantly higher, leading to the wrong diagnosis and an unnecessary operation.[7]

Inadequate Surgery

Many patients fall into this category, primarily due to the following four undetected conditions.

Multiple-Gland Hyperplasia

Failure to diagnose multiple-gland disease is not uncommon. In several different studies, multiple-gland hyperplasia was diagnosed in up to 17% of patients who underwent surgery for primary hyperparathyroidism.[4,7,9] The figures are higher in reoperation studies from specialized centers, reaching 20 to 37%.[6,10] The key to success in these patients is making the right diagnosis preoperatively and thereby ensuring the appropriate surgical treatment. Family history is essential for both parathyroid related problems and other malignancies associated with the multiple endocrine neoplasia (MEN) syndrome. Accurate diagnosis is the cornerstone for delivering appropriate treatment to the patient and other family members.

Multiple Adenomas

The exact incidence of multiple adenomas is unknown, but has been found to range from 2 to 14% in different studies.[4,7,9,11] Multiple adenomas can cause either persistent disease, with hypercalcemia developing within 6 months after the primary operation, or recurrent disease with hypercalcemia developing more than 6 months after the initial operation. In the era of minimally invasive parathyroid surgery and unilateral neck exploration guided by preoperative localization with sestamibi scan, failure to localize the additional adenoma preoperatively leads to a failed operation.[12] Even the addition of a rapid PTH test to a unilateral exploration may not be sufficient in these cases.[9]

In some cases it may be impossible to preoperatively predict whether the disease is caused by a single or multiple adenomas versus multiglandular hyperplasia, such as with lithium-associated hyperparathyroidism (LAHPT).

Patients treated with lithium for more than 10 years are prone to developing primary hyperparathyroidism secondary to either a single adenoma or multiple-gland disease.[13] Failure to explore all four glands may lead to disease persistence after removal of a single adenoma. The use of a rapid PTH test during the operation may help in differentiating hyperplasia from single or multiple adenomas in these patients.[14]

Parathyroid Carcinoma

Parathyroid carcinoma is a rare tumor; according to the National Cancer Database, about 30 new cases of parathyroid carcinoma are diagnosed annually in the United States, with a 10-year survival rate of 49%.[15] In studies of patients undergoing initial surgery for hyperparathyroidism, the incidence of parathyroid carcinoma ranges from less than 1%[7,16] to 5%.[11] The importance of correctly diagnosing these patients cannot be overstressed.

Preoperatively, a family history of parathyroid carcinoma, excessively high serum calcium levels, or the presence of a very large adenoma should raise suspicion and encourage discussion with the patient regarding a wide resection.

Intraoperatively, recognition of the locally invasive character and abnormal appearance of the lesion compared with a typical adenoma mandates an en-bloc resection of the lesion. If the tumor is adherent to the thyroid lobe and cannot be separated easily, an ipsilateral thyroid lobectomy should be performed along with excision of the parathyroid tumor. Local recurrence is common and often the patient requires multiple operations.[17] The use of a rapid PTH test in these operations can help achieve maximal tumor resection.[18]

Postoperatively, testing for molecular markers is warranted. Germline mutations in *HRPT2* are responsible for the hyperparathyroidism–jaw tumor (HPT-JT) syndrome. Family members carrying this gene have a high risk of developing parathyroid carcinoma. In some of the seemingly sporadic tumors, a germline mutation may be found, necessitating family testing.[19,20]

Local Recurrence of Benign Disease and Parathyromatosis

Recurrent or persistent hyperparathyroidism can be secondary to local recurrence of a benign adenoma at the site of resection. The term *parathyromatosis* describes small nodules of benign, hyperplastic parathyroid tissue found in the former operation site, either in the neck or the mediastinum, causing hyperparathyroidism and hypercalcemia. Overall, this phenomenon is rare but may be seen, most often, in the setting of chronic renal failure and secondary hyperparathyroidism.[21]

Jaskowiak et al[10] described the National Institutes of Health (NIH) experience with this entity. In 17 patients with recurrent hyperparathyroidism, adenoma was discovered at the site of previous excision, situated in dense scar tissue with evidence of old suture material. The combination of the anatomic finding, the pathologic characteristics of the tissue, and the benign course of disease in these patients are the keys to distinguishing this entity from parathyroid carcinoma.

Failed Surgery

By far, the most common cause of persistent and recurrent hyperparathyroidism is failure to locate and excise the diseased or enlarged gland.

Failure to Locate a Normally Positioned Adenoma

In most studies with a large series of reoperations for hyperparathyroidism, the vast majority of adenomas are found in their native location or along the route of expected migration of an enlarged gland in the tracheoesophageal groove.[6,10,22] In a series from Tampa, Florida,[23] 17 patients underwent surgery after a previous operation failed to identify an adenoma seen on a preoperative sestamibi scan. The adenomas in all patients were found as expected from the scans, proving both the accuracy of the localization and the failure of surgical technique.

Failure to Locate an Ectopic Adenoma

Studies of reoperations for HPT report that in 24 to 44% of cases, the adenoma is eventually found in an ectopic location.[10,22] The most common ectopic location is the mediastinum and thymus, which occurs in 18% of cases.[10] The next most common location is within the thyroid capsule, a so-called intrathyroidal adenoma, in 7 to 10% of cases.[10,22] Other ectopic locations include retroesophageal adenomas, situated between the esophagus and the spine in the pharyngeal wall and the pterygopalatine fossa, and within the epineurium of the vagus nerve.[24] An undescended parathyroid gland situated at or superior to the carotid bifurcation was found in 7% of reoperated patients.[25] Other locations described are anterior to the trachea, at the aortopulmonary window, behind the ventricle,[26] at the base of the tongue,[10] and in the wall of the nasopharynx.[10]

Failure to Treat Supernumerary Glands

The problem of supernumerary glands is of crucial importance in the treatment of patients with HPT secondary to hyperplasia. When following a presumably successful operation with removal of most parathyroid tissue, if hypercalcemia persists or recurs, one needs to suspect the existence of an additional enlarged gland that, most often, will be situated at an ectopic location.[27]

Diagnosis and Treatment of Recurrent or Persistent Hypercalcemia/Hyperparathyroidism (Table 18.2)

Name the Disease

The combination of a thorough history and physical exam, review of the family history, and performing simple laboratory tests (serum calcium, phosphorus, and PTH, and 24-hour urine calcium) should be sufficient for a diagnosis in most patients.

Name the Reason for Failure

Based on the correct diagnosis, by reviewing previous blood tests, localization studies, operative notes, and pathology, one can name the reason for failure: whether the operation was not indicated in the first place, was inade-

Table 18.2 The "Ten Commandments" of Reoperative Parathyroid Surgery

1. Name the disease.
2. Name the reason for failure.
3. Define the indication for surgery: advantages versus disadvantages.
4. Define the goal of surgery.
5. Use preoperative localization studies.
6. Strive to achieve at least two concurrent localization studies.
7. Plan the operative approach, and have a backup plan as well.
8. Ensure intraoperative localization studies are available in case needed.
9. Use intraoperative quality-control studies.
10. Think of the future.

quate to the disease process, or failed due to poor surgical technique.

Define the Indication for Surgery: Advantages Versus Disadvantages

The indications for reoperation are similar to those for primary operation. Symptomatic patients and selected asymptomatic patients should meet the criteria according to the new NIH consensus guidelines:[28] t-score less than –2.5 on bone density assessment, unexplained decreased creatinine clearance by 30% of expected levels, serum calcium 1 mg/dL above the upper normal limit, urinary calcium >400 mg/24 hours and age >50. For asymptomatic patients with suspicious laboratory findings, it is wise to weigh the anticipated benefit of a repeated operation against the risks of complication from reoperation. Careful follow-up is reasonable in these patients, because many of them remain asymptomatic for many years without additional surgery.[29,30] One of the main indications for surgery in this group, however, is progressive osteoporosis.

Define the Goal of Surgery

Before embarking upon surgery, the goals of the procedure should be set. When dealing with reoperative surgery, the goal should be the identification of an enlarged parathyroid gland situated in the area marked by preoperative studies, the removal of which will cause sufficient decrease in PTH levels drawn during the operation.

When the diagnosis is multiple-gland hyperplasia, the goal should be to systematically expose all parathyroid tissue, excise it, and plan ahead to determine whether cryopreservation or autotransplantation may be needed. If the previous operation resulted in excision of four or more glands, the possibility of supernumerary glands should be entertained, and every effort for localization should be made. In the rare case of parathyroid carcinoma, the goal of the operation must be maximal disease debulking, which can be monitored with serial measurements of PTH during the operation.

Use Preoperative Localization Studies, and Strive to Achieve at Least Two Concurrent Localization Studies

The surgeon's aim is to achieve reliable localization using noninvasive techniques, but it is wiser to judiciously use invasive tests when indicated rather than attempting surgery in an operated neck after previous surgical failure.

Noninvasive Studies

Sestamibi Scan   Today, the sestamibi scan is by far the most reliable localization study for parathyroid adenomas. First introduced in 1989 by Coakley et al,[31] it has gained wide popularity. In a meta-analysis of 6331 patients, published by Denham et al[32] in 1998, the sestamibi scan was shown to be a cost-effective localization study, with 90% sensitivity and 98.85% specificity. The addition of single photon emission computed tomography (SPECT) can increase sensitivity.[33,34]

Still, the sestamibi scan is not infallible because false-negative rates may reach 22%. False-negative results are more common in patients with normocalcemia, small adenomas, multigland disease, and ectopic adenomas.[35] Failure to identify an adenoma despite a positive test was attributed at times to an inherent false-positive rate for this scan. Some authors suggested that reactive lymph nodes and thyroid adenomas or carcinomas may mimic parathyroid adenomas.[31,36]

With a properly performed scan and thorough exploration of the neck, the incidence of false-positive scans is very low. Norman et al[23] performed reoperations for primary HPT in 17 patients after previous negative neck exploration that failed to identify a sestamibi-proven parathyroid adenoma. All patients underwent a repeat scan that was similar to their original scan. At repeat exploration, adenomas were found in all as predicted by the scan. Axelrod et al[37] reviewed scans in patients with undescended inferior adenomas found during reoperation for persistent hyperparathyroidism. In the three patients studied, the adenoma was seen on the preoperative scan but was misread as an ipsilateral submandibular gland. The addition of lateral views and the use of wide-field scans help discriminate between intrathyroid lesions and adenomas, and allows evaluation of the mediastinum, which is the most common site for an ectopic parathyroid gland in the setting of reoperation. However, the sestamibi scan has its limitations. Sensitivity seems to decline with a multinodular goiter, and it is a poor tool for localization of hyperplastic glands.

Ultrasound of the Neck   In a large study of patients who underwent surgery for HPT, a neck ultrasound (US) had a reasonable sensitivity of 61% and a positive predictive value of 87%.[38] In a series of 62 patients undergoing reoperation at the NIH, preoperative US had a 90% sensitivity and 87% specificity with an overall accuracy of 84%.[39] In this study, concordance between the US and sestamibi scan findings was a good predictor of successful operation. US can be of great help for evaluation of intrathyroidal adenoma; on the other hand, the presence of multinodular goiter can greatly reduce the accuracy of this test.[40]

Computed Tomography and Magnetic Resonance Imaging   Computed tomography (CT) and magnetic resonance imaging (MRI) are not as sensitive as the previously presented modalities, but still can be of great value in the setting of reoperation. It is most useful for ectopic adenomas, mediastinal adenomas, and recurrent carcinomas.[41] Jaskowiak et al[10] routinely performed CT scan of the neck and chest in patients with recurrent or persistent HPT after prior exploration. The true-positive rate was 52%, with a 16% false-positive result. MRI was used less commonly in this series, but showed similar results, with 48% true positive and 14% false positive. Similar results have also been shown in other studies.[42] A CT-guided fine-needle aspiration (FNA) of a suspicious lesion can increase the specificity of this study. When biopsy is impossible due to location or was attempted and failed, including the area of the lesion in an "extended field," a sestamibi scan can help verify the physiologic nature of the radiologic finding.

Invasive Studies

Fine-Needle Aspiration   A US- or CT-guided FNA of a suspected parathyroid adenoma with analysis of the aspirate for PTH is a highly sensitive technique for localization before reoperation.[10,43,44] The drawback is low specificity and the theoretical threat of causing tissue seeding along the needle track.

Angiography   Superselective digital subtraction angiography (DSA) is a sensitive method for localization of ectopic parathyroid tissue.[45] This invasive procedure is indicated for patients with recurrent or persistent HPT in whom previous noninvasive testing failed to identify the adenoma. The procedure involves catheterization of six different arteries: internal mammary arteries bilaterally, both inferior thyroid arteries, and either both superior thyroid arteries or the common carotid arteries.

Selective Venous Sampling   Similar to DSA, this procedure is reserved for selected patients. Selective venous sampling is performed by catheterization of veins draining the neck and mediastinum.[46] By comparing PTH levels taken from iliac veins with those obtained from thyroid veins (superior, middle and inferior), vertebral veins, and the thymic vein, the anticipated localization of the adenoma will be at the area with venous PTH levels that are at least twice as high as the systemic levels. A 75 to 88% true-positive rate and a 0 to 12% false-positive rate are reported in published studies.[10,47,48]

Plan the Operative Approach, and Have a Backup Plan as Well

Most reoperations in the neck can be performed through the original lower neck transverse incision. After entering the neck, it is useful to approach the tracheoesophageal groove by entering medial to the medial border of the sternocleidomastoid muscle and proceeding from lateral to medial, thus avoiding the midline scarring. This is also called the lateral trapdoor approach. Plan the systemic neck exploration based on localization studies and knowledge of parathyroid gland anatomy and embryology. The superior parathyroid gland is commonly located behind the upper pole of the thyroid; its absence should initiate a search along the tracheoesophageal groove, lateral to the esophageal wall and behind it. The lower gland is classically located at the junction of the inferior thyroid artery and the recurrent laryngeal nerve, lying anterior to the nerve. In its absence one should dissect caudally toward the lowest edge of the thyroid gland and the mediastinum. Following the vessels feeding the adenoma may help localization even when it is embedded within the thymic fat. In the case of an undescended parathyroid adenoma diagnosed preoperatively, the best approach is via a high oblique neck incision as opposed to using the old transverse scar.[25]

Unilateral Versus Bilateral Neck Exploration

The use of localization studies has led to a trend toward limited explorations, but at the price of a significant recurrence rate.[12] Even after so-called confirmation of a successful excision with the use of a rapid PTH test, an additional adenoma may be found in a significant number of patients upon completion of the neck exploration.[9] For this reason, it seems prudent to perform a full four-gland exploration in patients who failed a previous operation.

Minimally Invasive Radio-Guided Parathyroidectomy

Minimally invasive radio-guided parathyroidectomy (MIRP) is optional only in patients with a well-defined adenoma localized preoperatively with a technetium (Tc)-sestamibi scan, and was found to be quite reliable in the setting of primary operations.[49] One to 3 hours before the operation, the patient is injected with the radioactive isotope. The neck is explored through a small incision using a hand-held gamma probe. Removal of hyperactive tissue that leads to marked count decrease in the parathyroid bed and equalization of radioactive counts in all neck fields, which by itself shows radioactivity of at least 20% of the initial value, are indicative of a successful operation. The same technique was tested and found useful in the reoperative setting.[50] Because this technique is limited to simple cases of well-localized adenoma, it is unclear to what degree this offers an advantage over exploration by a skilled surgeon.

Mediastinal Adenomas

Approximately 20% of reoperative parathyroid adenomas are located in the mediastinum. The vast majority of these are amenable to resection via a low transverse cervical incision.[51] These glands most likely represent cervical parathyroid glands descending into the chest. Their blood supply, originating in the neck, can be followed, thus helping in their discovery. The deeper mediastinal adenomas may represent lower adenomas that migrated further into the chest in the embryonic period; others are believed to develop primarily in the chest and are fed by mediastinal vessels. Although the first group is more common and is treated with a conventional cervical approach, the second group is challenging, and treatment often requires mediastinal exploration.

In 1981, Russell et al[52] published the Mayo clinic experience with mediastinotomies for parathyroid tumors. In a series of 38 patients operated on between 1942 and 1980, 37 patients had previous neck exploration and two had previous mediastinal exploration. The operation was successful in 37 patients, but with a significant morbidity rate. In 47% of patients the tumor was located in the thymus; in 21% it was found in the anterior mediastinum adjacent to the thymus; in 24% it was found in intimate relation to the ascending aorta, aortic arch, and great vessels; and in 5% the tumor was found adherent to the pericardium.

During the last decade with the increasing practice of video-assisted thoracoscopies (VAT) in thoracic surgery, this technique has been tested for the retrieval of mediastinal parathyroid tumors. Kumar et al[53] reported their experience in one patient with a 2 × 2 cm adenoma embedded in thymic tissue. They performed a three-trocar thoracoscopy and excised the gland en-bloc with the thymic tissue. The authors summarized a total of 26 patients described in the English-language literature who underwent such a procedure and conclude that this procedure is safe for well-localized adenomas.

In rare cases angiographic ablation can be used for treatment of ectopic adenomas, mostly mediastinal. In this technique a large dose of contrast is injected into the perfusing artery. Long-term success rates up to 67% were reported.[54] The advantage of this approach is an early convalescence without jeopardizing the feasibility of performing salvage surgery if needed. This treatment method is not suitable in cases where the only functioning parathyroid tissue is the adenoma; for these patients an operation with either immediate autotransplantation or cryopreservation of parathyroid tissue is more desirable.

Ensure Intraoperative Localization Studies Are Available in Case Needed

Intraoperative ultrasound can identify adenomas in up to 71% of patients with a sensitivity rate of 85%.[10] Intraoperative US can help confirm localization of adenoma seen on preoperative ultrasound or other localization studies.

This is especially useful in the case of intrathyroid adenoma, where FNA can be done from the suspected lesion and the aspirate analyzed for PTH in a rapid fashion prior to thyroidectomy.

As stated before, nuclear-guided surgery is limited to patients with a positive sestamibi scan. It is reasonable to suggest that in complicated reoperative cases with extensive scarring, availability of this tool may facilitate the operation.

Use of Intraoperative Quality-Control Studies

For many years, surgeons hoped for a simple, reliable, and quick technique to predict successful operation, particularly in the reoperative setting.[55] The best available tool today to predict cure rate after parathyroidectomy is the rapid PTH test. Introduced by Irvin et al[56] in the 1990s, it gained popularity rapidly. PTH levels should be drawn before the operation commences and again 10 minutes after removal of the suspected hyperfunctioning parathyroid tissue. A decrease in PTH level of 50% and above is compatible with removal of the adenoma and predicts a cure with a sensitivity of 96%, a specificity of 100%, and overall accuracy of 97% in the setting of primary operation.[38,57] Weber et al[58] published their experience with this assay. It was proven highly accurate for prediction of cure after resection of a single adenoma, but was inaccurate in patients with multiple adenomas or hyperplasia. A similar experience was published by Sebag et al.[42] Intraoperative PTH successfully predicted cure in 44 of 49 patients with a 90% sensitivity rate and 90% positive predictive value. In cases with multiple-gland hyperplasia, the false-negative rate was 17% compared with 0% for single adenoma patients.

In the reoperative setting, PTH levels can help guide the extent of exploration and resection. Its use in patients with parathyroid carcinoma can potentially assist in accomplishing complete debulking of localized and metastatic disease. Frozen section of the excised lesion is recommended if a PTH test is not available or when the aim of the operation is removal of all parathyroid tissue, and is mandatory before immediate autotransplantation. Another proposed means of tissue verification is by aspirating the tissue for a rapid PTH test.[59]

Think of the Future

The two most important complications of parathyroid surgeries are hypocalcemia and recurrent laryngeal nerve injury. Hypocalcemia after reoperation can be very distressing and may require long-term treatment with calcium and vitamin D, starting just a few hours after the operation. Some patients sustain permanent hypocalcemia. Because the remaining functioning parathyroid tissue left after previous operations cannot be assessed accurately before surgery, it is hard to predict who will develop postoperative hypocalcemia. Elaraj et al[60] proposed that a drop of PTH levels greater than 84% compared with the pre-resection value is a predictor of hypocalcemia in patients undergoing surgery for multiglandular disease.

The need for immediate autotransplantation or delayed transplantation of parathyroid tissue has to be evaluated preoperatively. Multiple previous operations and operations for hyperplastic glands are more likely to lead to long-term hypoparathyroidism. In these cases it is wise to preserve viable, pathologically confirmed parathyroid tissue on the operating field for autotransplantation at the end of the procedure. If the risk for postoperative hypoparathyroidism seems high, cryopreservation of parathyroid tissue allows repeat transplantation if the initial effort failed or for delayed transplantation in patients in whom the risk of persistent postoperative hypoparathyroidism is considered moderate.[61] Graft function can be proved in 60% of patients undergoing delayed cryopreserved parathyroid autograft. In more than two-thirds of them, normocalcemia can be established without the use of medications. Long periods of cryopreservation have been associated with graft failure.[62]

Some authors advocate the use of recurrent laryngeal nerve (RLN) monitoring in these difficult cases. Yarbrough et al[63] from the Mayo Clinic showed that the use of RLN monitoring did not decrease the complication rate. Their conclusion was that routine careful nerve exposure is the best way to avoid such complications.

References

1. Bauer W, Federman DD. Hyperparathyroidism epitomized: the case of Captain Charles E. Martell. Metabolism 1962;11:21–29

2. Henry JF, Sebag F, Tamagnini P, Forman C, Silaghi H. Endoscopic parathyroid surgery: results of 365 consecutive procedures. World J Surg 2004;28:1219–1223

3. Rubello D, Pelizzo MR, Boni G, et al. Radioguided surgery of primary hyperparathyroidism using the low-dose 99mTc-sestamibi protocol: multiinstitutional experience from the Italian Study Group on Radioguided Surgery and Immunoscintigraphy (GISCRIS). J Nucl Med 2005;46:220–226

4. Cope O. The study of hyperparathyroidism at the Massachusetts General Hospital. N Engl J Med 1966;274:1174–1182

5. Schwartz SR, Futran ND. Hypercalcemic hypocalciuria: a critical differential diagnosis for hyperparathyroidism. Otolaryngol Clin North Am 2004;37:887–896 xi.

6. Bruining HA, Birkenhager JC, Ong GL, Lamberts SW. Causes of failure in operations for hyperparathyroidism. Surgery 1987;101:562–565

7. van Heerden JA, Grant CS. Surgical treatment of primary hyperparathyroidism: an institutional perspective. World J Surg 1991;15:688–692

8. Hendy GN, D'Souza-Li L, Yang B, Canaff L, Cole DE. Mutations of the calcium-sensing receptor (CASR) in familial hypocalciuric hypercalcemia, neonatal severe hyperparathyroidism, and autosomal dominant hypocalcemia. Hum Mutat 2000;16:281–296

9. Siperstein A, Berber E, Mackey R, Alghoul M, Wagner K, Milas M. Prospective evaluation of sestamibi scan, ultrasonography, and

rapid PTH to predict the success of limited exploration for sporadic primary hyperparathyroidism. Surgery 2004;136:872–880

10. Jaskowiak N, Norton JA, Alexander HR, et al. A prospective trial evaluating a standard approach to reoperation for missed parathyroid adenoma. Ann Surg 1996;224:308–320 discussion 320–321

11. Lumachi F, Ermani M, Basso S, Zucchetta P, Borsato N, Favia G. Localization of parathyroid tumours in the minimally invasive era: which technique should be chosen? Population-based analysis of 253 patients undergoing parathyroidectomy and factors affecting parathyroid gland detection. Endocr Relat Cancer 2001;8:63–69

12. Baliski CR, Stewart JK, Anderson DW, Wiseman SM, Bugis SP. Selective unilateral parathyroid exploration: an effective treatment for primary hyperparathyroidism. Am J Surg 2005;189:596–600 discussion 600

13. Awad SS, Miskulin J, Thompson N. Parathyroid adenomas versus four-gland hyperplasia as the cause of primary hyperparathyroidism in patients with prolonged lithium therapy. World J Surg 2003;27:486–488

14. Hundley JC, Woodrum DT, Saunders BD, Doherty GM, Gauger PG. Revisiting lithium-associated hyperparathyroidism in the era of intraoperative parathyroid hormone monitoring. Surgery 2005;138:1027–1031 discussion 1031–1032

15. Hundahl SA, Fleming ID, Fremgen AM, Menck HR. Two hundred eighty-six cases of parathyroid carcinoma treated in the U.S. between 1985–1995: a National Cancer Data Base Report. The American College of Surgeons Commission on Cancer and the American Cancer Society. Cancer 1999;86:538–544

16. Sandelin K, Thompson NW, Bondeson L. Metastatic parathyroid carcinoma: dilemmas in management. Surgery 1991;110:978–986 discussion 986–988

17. Kebebew E, Arici C, Duh QY, Clark OH. Localization and reoperation results for persistent and recurrent parathyroid carcinoma. Arch Surg 2001;136:878–885

18. Clayman GL, Gonzalez HE, El-Naggar A, Vassilopoulou-Sellin R. Parathyroid carcinoma: evaluation and interdisciplinary management. Cancer 2004;100:900–905

19. Weinstein LS, Simonds WF. HRPT2, a marker of parathyroid cancer. N Engl J Med 2003;349:1691–1692

20. Shattuck TM, Valimaki S, Obara T, et al. Somatic and germ-line mutations of the HRPT2 gene in sporadic parathyroid carcinoma. N Engl J Med 2003;349:1722–1729

21. Kollmorgen CF, Aust MR, Ferreiro JA, McCarthy JT, van Heerden JA. Parathyromatosis: a rare yet important cause of persistent or recurrent hyperparathyroidism. Surgery 1994;116:111–115

22. Thompson GB, Grant CS, Perrier ND, et al. Reoperative parathyroid surgery in the era of sestamibi scanning and intraoperative parathyroid hormone monitoring. Arch Surg 1999;134:699–704 discussion 704–705

23. Norman JG, Jaffray CE, Chheda H. The false-positive parathyroid sestamibi: a real or perceived problem and a case for radioguided parathyroidectomy. Ann Surg 2000;231:31–37

24. Chan TJ, Libutti SK, McCart JA, et al. Persistent primary hyperparathyroidism caused by adenomas identified in pharyngeal or adjacent structures. World J Surg 2003;27:675–679 Epub 2003 May 13

25. Billingsley KG, Fraker DL, Doppman JL, et al. Localization and operative management of undescended parathyroid adenomas in patients with persistent primary hyperparathyroidism. Surgery 1994;116:982–989 discussion 989–990

26. Corvera CU, Jablons D, Morita E, Clark OH. Retrocardiac parathyroid tumor: a rare mediastinal site. Surgery 2004;135:104–107

27. Wang CA. Parathyroid re-exploration. A clinical and pathological study of 112 cases. Ann Surg 1977;186:140–145

28. Bilezikian JP, Potts JT Fuleihan Gel-H, et al. Summary statement from a workshop on asymptomatic primary hyperparathyroidism: a perspective for the 21st century. J Clin Endocrinol Metab 2002;87:5353–5361

29. Silverberg SJ, Shane E, Jacobs TP, Siris E, Bilezikian JP. A 10-year prospective study of primary hyperparathyroidism with or without parathyroid surgery. N Engl J Med 1999;341:1249–1255

30. Wermers RA, Khosla S, Atkinson EJ, et al. Survival after the diagnosis of hyperparathyroidism: a population-based study. Am J Med 1998;104:115–122

31. Coakley AJ, Kettle AG, Wells CP, O'Doherty MJ, Collins RE. 99Tcm sestamibi–a new agent for parathyroid imaging. Nucl Med Commun 1989;10:791–794

32. Denham DW, Norman J. Cost-effectiveness of preoperative sestamibi scan for primary hyperparathyroidism is dependent solely upon the surgeon's choice of operative procedure. J Am Coll Surg 1998;186:293–305

33. Moka D, Voth E, Dietlein M, Larena-Avellaneda A, Schicha H. Technetium 99m-MIBI-SPECT: A highly sensitive diagnostic tool for localization of parathyroid adenomas. Surgery 2000;128:29–35

34. Sfakianakis GN, Irvin GL, Foss J, et al. Efficient parathyroidectomy guided by SPECT-MIBI and hormonal measurements. J Nucl Med 1996;37:798–804

35. Merlino JI, Ko K, Minotti A, McHenry CR. The false negative technetium-99m-sestamibi scan in patients with primary hyperparathyroidism: correlation with clinical factors and operative findings. Am Surg 2003;69:225–229 discussion 229–230

36. Liu Y, Chun KJ, Freeman LM. "Shine through" on dual tracer parathyroid scintigraphy: a potential pitfall in interpretation. Clin Nucl Med 2005;30:145–149

37. Axelrod D, Sisson JC, Cho K, Miskulin J, Gauger PG. Appearance of ectopic undescended inferior parathyroid adenomas on technetium Tc 99m sestamibi scintigraphy: a lesson from reoperative parathyroidectomy. Arch Surg 2003;138:1214–1218

38. Grant CS, Thompson G, Farley D, van Heerden J. Primary hyperparathyroidism surgical management since the introduction of minimally invasive parathyroidectomy: Mayo Clinic experience. Arch Surg 2005;140:472–478 discussion 478–479

39. Feingold DL, Alexander HR, Chen CC, et al. Ultrasound and sestamibi scan as the only preoperative imaging tests in reoperation for parathyroid adenomas. Surgery 2000;128:1103–1109 discussion 1109–1110

40. Klingler PJ, Strolz S, Profanter C, et al. Management of hyperparathyroidism in an endemic goiter area. World J Surg 1998;22:301–307 discussion 307–308

41. Clark P, Wooldridge T, Kleinpeter K, Perrier N, Lovato J, Morton K. Providing optimal preoperative localization for recurrent parathyroid carcinoma: a combined parathyroid scintigraphy and computed tomography approach. Clin Nucl Med 2004;29:681–684

42. Sebag F, Shen W, Brunaud L, Kebebew E, Duh QY, Clark OH. Intraoperative parathyroid hormone assay and parathyroid reoperations. Surgery 2003;134:1049–1055 discussion 1056

43. MacFarlane MP, Fraker DL, Shawker TH, et al. Use of preoperative fine-needle aspiration in patients undergoing reoperation for primary hyperparathyroidism. Surgery 1994;116:959–964 discussion 964–5

44. Sacks BA, Pallotta JA, Cole A, Hurwitz J. Diagnosis of parathyroid adenomas: efficacy of measuring parathormone levels in needle aspirates of cervical masses. AJR Am J Roentgenol 1994;163:1223–1226

45. Miller DL, Chang R, Doppman JL, Norton JA. Localization of parathyroid adenomas: superselective arterial DSA versus superselective conventional angiography. Radiology 1989;170(3 pt 2):1003–1006

46. Sugg SL, Fraker DL, Alexander R, et al. Prospective evaluation of selective venous sampling for parathyroid hormone concentration in patients undergoing reoperations for primary hyperparathyroidism. Surgery 1993;114:1004–1009

47. Jones JJ, Brunaud L, Dowd CF, Duh QY, Morita E, Clark OH. Accuracy of selective venous sampling for intact parathyroid hormone in difficult patients with recurrent or persistent hyperparathyroidism. Surgery 2002;132:944–950 discussion 950–951

48. Estella E, Leong MS, Bennett I, et al. Parathyroid hormone venous sampling prior to reoperation for primary hyperparathyroidism. ANZ J Surg 2003;73:800–805

49. Norman J, Chheda H. Minimally invasive parathyroidectomy facilitated by intraoperative nuclear mapping. Surgery 1997;122:998–1003 discussion 1003–1004

50. Norman J, Denham D. Minimally invasive radioguided parathyroidectomy in the reoperative neck. Surgery 1998;124:1088–1092 discussion 1092–1093

51. Clark OH. Mediastinal parathyroid tumors. Arch Surg 1988;123:1096–1100

52. Russell CF, Edis AJ, Scholz DA, Sheedy PF, van Heerden JA. Mediastinal parathyroid tumors: experience with 38 tumors requiring mediastinotomy for removal. Ann Surg 1981;193:805–809

53. Kumar A, Kumar S, Aggarwal S, Kumar R, Tandon N. Thoracoscopy: the preferred method for excision of mediastinal parathyroids. Surg Laparosc Endosc Percutan Tech 2002;12:295–300

54. Doherty GM, Doppman JL, Miller DL, et al. Results of a multidisciplinary strategy for management of mediastinal parathyroid adenoma as a cause of persistent primary hyperparathyroidism. Ann Surg 1992;215:101–106

55. Spiegel AM, Eastman ST, Attie MF, et al. Intraoperative measurements of urinary cyclic AMP to guide surgery for primary hyperparathyroidism. N Engl J Med 1980;303:1457–1460

56. Irvin GL, Dembrow VD, Prudhomme DL. Operative monitoring of parathyroid gland hyperfunction. Am J Surg 1991;162:299–302

57. Irvin GL, Dembrow VD, Prudhomme DL. Clinical usefulness of an intraoperative "quick parathyroid hormone" assay. Surgery 1993;114:1019–1022 discussion 1022–1023

58. Weber CJ, Ritchie JC. Retrospective analysis of sequential changes in serum intact parathyroid hormone levels during conventional parathyroid exploration. Surgery 1999;126:1139–1143 discussion 1143–1144

59. Perrier ND, Ituarte P, Kikuchi S, et al. Intraoperative parathyroid aspiration and parathyroid hormone assay as an alternative to frozen section for tissue identification. World J Surg 2000;24:1319–1322

60. Elaraj DM, Remaley AT, Simonds WF, et al. Utility of rapid intraoperative parathyroid hormone assay to predict severe postoperative hypocalcemia after reoperation for hyperparathyroidism. Surgery 2002;132:1028–1033 discussion 1033–1034

61. Brennan MF, Brown EM, Spiegel AM, et al. Autotransplantation of cryopreserved parathyroid tissue in man. Ann Surg 1979;189:139–142

62. Cohen MS, Dilley WG, Wells SA, et al. Long-term functionality of cryopreserved parathyroid autografts: a 13-year prospective analysis. Surgery 2005;138:1033–1040 discussion 1040–1041

63. Yarbrough DE, Thompson GB, Kasperbauer JL, Harper CM, Grant CS. Intraoperative electromyographic monitoring of the recurrent laryngeal nerve in reoperative thyroid and parathyroid surgery. Surgery 2004;136:1107–1115

19 Advanced Techniques in Parathyroid Surgery

Robert A. Sofferman

The anatomic studies by Gilmour[1] have determined that most individuals have four parathyroid glands. However, in the surgical investigation required in patients with primary hyperparathyroidism, the 5% of patients with only three or more than four parathyroids gland may pose a special quandary during surgery. A thorough knowledge of parathyroid embryology should direct the surgeon to inspect specific ectopic sites or regions. However, after this somewhat tedious exploration is accomplished, the surgeon will complete the procedure without knowing if the hyperparathyroid process has been corrected. Certainly with an identified large single gland and one adjacent ipsilateral or contralateral normal parathyroid, the procedure terminates with a greater than 96% chance of success. In fact, this approach was performed by Dr. C. A. Wang,[2] a highly experienced and respected surgeon of his day. Because preoperative imaging studies were not reliable, and thus not employed in his practice of parathyroid surgery, a correct side of entry was a chance event, permitting the unilateral approach in less than 50% of his patients. In addition, if a unilateral procedure was accomplished by an initial entry to the correct side, the potential of missing a second adenoma in the opposite neck still existed. Wang accepted this potential failure as an inherent risk of the technique with the understanding that a revision procedure would involve entry into a previously unoperated side.

An often-quoted phrase from Doppman[3] at the 1991 National Institutes of Health (NIH) Consensus Conference on Parathyroid Surgery, "The only required localization study is identification of an experienced parathyroid surgeon" is worthy of retrospective study. Prior to 1992 when technetium-sestamibi became a practical reality, the technetium thallium scans and ultrasound yielded unpredictable results. Based on these studies, the possibility of focused or uniglandular surgery would have been limited and likely have required conversion to traditional bilateral four-site inspection. In addition, the experienced surgeon recognizes first the location and appearance of the normal parathyroid gland and the sometimes subtle size difference of the pathologic gland and where to look for the aberrant gland when it is not in its cardinal position. Inherent in this experience is the need for accurate decision making, such as which glands to remove and which to retain, judicious use of frozen section, when to consider thyroidectomy, and when to consider autotransplantation or cryopreservation. These among many other intraoperative considerations are the elements that mandate careful thinking and action if patients with hyperparathyroidism are to be well served.

Localization studies, most specifically technetium-sestamibi with or without single photon emission computed tomography (SPECT), are extremely helpful surgical adjuncts but taken alone have some inherent risks. The reliance on this scan alone as a roadmap to targeted surgery creates a false sense of confidence and perhaps an attitude that parathyroid surgery is easy. In reality, most cases with definitively positive scans are straightforward and uncomplicated. Occasionally the enlarged parathyroid is not precisely found where it is imaged and may be retroesophageal, intrathyroidal, or lateral in the carotid sheath. In these circumstances, other preoperative and intraoperative maneuvers are helpful. When the positively imaged gland cannot be identified visually, palpation is the most important tool in proper identification of the enlarged gland. This maneuver, performed in a careful and systematic manner, is critical to finding the target and may save the patient many ancillary localization studies and revision surgery. Thus it is clear that planned bilateral exploration is the most basic parathyroid procedure and should be in the knowledge base of any surgeon who becomes involved in this surgery.

With the advent of excellent preoperative imaging (technetium-99m-sestamibi and high-resolution ultrasound), surgical intervention has changed from bilateral inspection of all parathyroid glands to a more focused approach to the single adenoma. There are several reasons for this technique, most of which are medically logical and some of which are driven by the desire of the patient for more limited surgery. In reality, there are even some marketing considerations from the surgical community, which is oriented to convince endocrinologists and referring physicians that the focused surgery is safer, simpler, and worthy of consideration for nearly every patient with any degree of primary hyperparathyroidism. In addition, the Internet has now become a competitive arena for advertising the limited procedure directed primarily at patients who might choose to travel to a distant surgery center, believing that the smallest incision is the ideal surgery.

Minimal access parathyroidectomy (MAP) is a specific procedure reported from the Mayo Clinic.[4] However, all of the procedures described in this chapter utilize minimal access techniques. These procedures begin with preoperative imaging such as the technetium-99m-sestamibi scan with or without SPECT and high-resolution ultrasound. The ultrasound may seem superfluous when the sestamibi is positive, but may be pivotal in circumstances when the adenoma is actually intrathyroidal. In addition, concurrent thyroid pathology may be detected in the process of assessing the position and number of enlarged parathyroid glands. I have identified several thyroid malignancies in this way that might have otherwise remained undetected for an indeterminant period of time. Concurrent thyroid and parathyroid surgery can then be accomplished to the benefit of the patient. Additionally, preoperative ultrasound may detect enlargement of more than one parathyroid gland, which would suggest the possibility of four-gland hyperplasia or even a double adenoma circumstance. There are instances in which only one of two enlarged glands are positive on sestamibi, and ultrasound may lead the surgeon to suspect ipsilateral or bilateral dual adenomas.

If the scans clearly identify a discrete single adenoma, several choices exist for surgical intervention, including the following:

1   Bilateral four-site inspection
2   Direct resection through a midline conventional collar incision
3   Minimally invasive parathyroidectomy through a 2.5-cm midline incision
4   Direct incision over the adenoma site based on gamma probe direction
5   Video-assisted endoscopic parathyroidectomy

Virtually all of the limited approaches are based on the premise that a small incision is preferable. This concept certainly can be challenged. The aesthetic comparison of a small unilateral incision or trocar entry incisions versus a larger carefully positioned and repaired midline transverse incision of about 5 cm has not been formally debated, but the question has authentic value. The critical features of any of the limited procedures are adequate exposure and identification of important neurovascular structures, proper hemostasis, and a guarantee that the hyperparathyroid state has been corrected. If resection alone based on a sestamibi scan is the chosen technique, a success rate of approximately 90% can be expected. This is well below the accepted standard of 96%, and there are other considerations in failure. A revision procedure places the recurrent laryngeal nerves at accelerated risk, and frequently the revision parathyroidectomy occurs in a field where previously normal parathyroids have either been removed or devascularized.

Intraoperative Parathyroid Hormone Assessment

Parathyroid hormone is a polypeptide composed of 84 amino acids with the active amino terminal at one end and inactive carboxyl unit at the other. Originally assays measured midrange or terminal fragments but were not representative of true parathyroid hormone (PTH) levels. With fragmentation of the polypeptide, falsely elevated parathyroid levels would be indirectly interpreted by these older measurements. Measurement of the full intact molecule became the desired reality with the immunoradiometric assay (IRMA) in the late 1980s. Although this assay represented a major advance in the accurate delineation of PTH levels, and modification in the 24-hour turnaround time allowed its practical intraoperative use, there were several disadvantages that invited a search for an alternative measurement tool. The short isotope half-life reduced its shelf life, and there were cumbersome personnel and disposal issues with the intraoperative use of radioactive materials. Additionally, 15% of intraoperative studies were significantly inaccurate. In the early 1990s the two-site chemiluminescent antibody assay was introduced, which offered a solution to the aforementioned problems.[5] The assay utilizes a goat polyclonal antibody to one end of the PTH molecule attached to a polystyrene bead, which immobilizes and fixes the molecule. A second goat antibody labeled with an acridinium ester attaches to the opposite free end, effectively trapping the intact PTH polypeptide as a "sandwich" (**Fig. 19.1**). Free-labeled antibody and fragments are separated and discarded by special reagents and repeated washes. The tubes containing the washed beads with trapped PTH molecules are then exposed to trigger solutions in a luminometer. A specific amount of blue light is then emitted through these chemical interactions as relative light units (RLUs) and the emission is compared with standard curves (**Fig. 19.2**). The linear relationship between light emission and peptide concentration is very accurate, but the routine assay time of 2 hours is impractical for operative use. By modifying the incubation temperature to 45°C, essentially heating it from room temperature, only 7 minutes are required to render an accurate analysis.

This single step in the assay allows the tool to be useful for intraoperative measurements. Several companies manufacture this technology (e.g., Nichols Institute Diagnostics, San Clemente, CA, and Diagnostics Products Corporation, Los Angeles, CA), which can also be used for other diagnostic purposes such as thyroid and endocrine assessment, cardiac markers, toxic screens, allergy testing, and certain infectious disease measurements. This multipurpose feature creates an opportunity for hospital laboratories to purchase this expensive equipment. PTH measurement represents only a small portion of the menu of uses, which makes the purchase argument stronger even for the community hospital. When the central chemistry laboratory is employed for intraoperative PTH measurement, a few practical modifications are required to optimize efficiency. This system must be readied and standardized in advance, and a courier must be present on standby in the operating room to deliver the pre- and post-removal samples as efficiently as possible. This small practical maneuver represents a reasonable alternative to the Quick Kit (60-4257 Nichols Institute Diagnostics), which is positioned in or adjacent to the operating room and run by a technician. These assay kits are expensive, requiring a

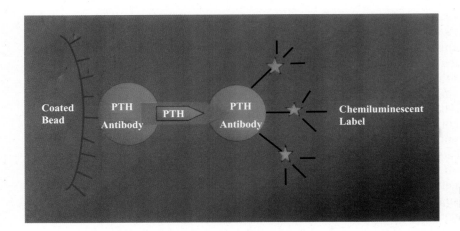

Fig. 19.1 Diagrammatic representation of chemiluminescent "sandwich" parathyroid hormone (PTH) assay.

pooled sequence of patients to reduce costs for each patient analysis.

The first reported use of intraoperative PTH was essentially a pilot study by Nussbaum and coworkers[6] at Massachusetts General Hospital in 1998. Thirteen patients were reported from that study, each of whom had pre- and post-removal immunoradiometric and PTH assays with normalization of PTH levels after single-gland resection. Libutti et al,[7] who did kinetic studies at the NIH, demonstrated that PTH has a short half-life, which can vary between 0.42

and 3.81 minutes. This singular fact allows for the utility of intraoperative measurements in predicting success of the single-gland excision without the requirement to inspect other parathyroid glands.

Dr. George Irvin is perhaps the most vocal and published proponent for the use of intraoperative PTH in the surgical management of primary hyperparathyroidism. The impetus for his interest was a 1990 failed exploration. After 4 months a revision procedure that involved a contralateral thyroid lobectomy was performed, and success was confirmed by

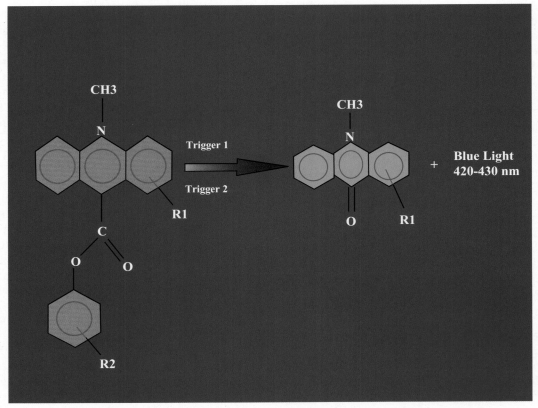

Fig. 19.2 Chemical reaction of acridinium ester with trigger 1 (alkaline solution) and trigger 2 (hydrogen peroxide) to produce light emission representative of precise intact parathyroid hormone levels.

intraoperative PTH. His 133-case experience with intraoperative PTH from 1993 to 1999 resulted in a reduction of operative failure with initial parathyroidectomy from 6% to 1.5%.[8] Perhaps of greater note was an improvement in successful reoperative parathyroidectomy from 76 to 94% after intraoperative PTH was employed. In 1992, Chapuis et al[9] reported a series of 45 patients undergoing uniglandular parathyroidectomy with local anesthesia and concurrent intraoperative IRMA PTH assessment. The authors' criterion for success was normalization of PTH, which can be a misleading end point. Of 320 cases performed with intraoperative PTH at the University of Vermont, three early failures were due to acceptance of this concept without appreciation of the importance of the 50% or greater reduction in levels from baseline. This 50% requirement was initially reported in 1994 by Irvin and Deriso in a series of 16 patients whose levels diminished by more than 50% at the 5-minute post-removal interval.[10] The hope that a shorter interval of sampling might reduce operative time has some inherent risks.

Randolph et al[11] found that 11% of cured patients have a delayed decrement beyond the 5-minute interval. In addition, there may be artifactual elevations in parathyroid hormone levels subsequent to surgical manipulation. Kao et al[12] at the Mayo Clinic reported a patient with PTH increase to 146% above baseline at the 5-minute interval, presumably due to excessive release of hormone early in the dissection. Kao et al favored a 15-minute interval during their initial clinical experience to counteract this issue. Currently it appears as if a 10-minute interval between pathologic gland removal and blood sampling is adequate. In addition, if the intraoperative PTH falls by a 50% decrement from baseline and is also determined to fall into the normal range, the patient's predicative postoperative calcium will be normal.[13] If these criteria are not met and the surgeon is certain that uniglandular disease is the clinical problem, it is reasonable to obtain a second post-removal sample when the inadequate report has been received in the operating room. When the second sample has then been procured and transferred to laboratory analysis, it is reasonable to proceed with inspection of the remaining parathyroid sites. Not infrequently the second sample will have decreased appropriately, allowing the procedure to terminate, and further exploration and manipulation of possible parathyroid tissues will not have affected the second result. If the second sample remains elevated, continued exploration is required until a second adenoma or hyperplastic glands have all been identified. In our experience an additional sample has been required in 10% of cases.

Irvin et al[14] report that 14% of cases did not meet satisfactory requirements for terminating surgery based on the previously described PTH criteria. Occasionally intraoperative PTH levels fall below the lowest level of normal (10–65 pg/mL) after subtotal parathyroidectomy or even resection of a single adenoma. This should not be cause for alarm or for consideration of parathyroid autotransplantation. The remaining parathyroid glands may be physiologically suppressed as a result of the hypersecreting state from the enlarged autonomously functioning parathyroid and require several hours to develop proper activity. In contrast, after total thyroidectomy the parathyroid hormone level should fall within the normal range as long as one or more of the parathyroid glands are viable. If intraoperative PTH is utilized and determined to be below normal, previously dissected parathyroid glands should be examined for viability. Any glands that are venous engorged or suspect should be considered for autotransplantation. In this circumstance, without autotransplantation, there is a significant potential for permanent hypocalcemia.

Following parathyroidectomy, the PTH level changes over the subsequent days to weeks. These changes may not be apparent because sequential parathormone levels are not generally obtained as long as the patient reverts to eucalcemia. Not uncommonly, PTH levels may remain elevated for 10 days to 3 months in spite of normalization of calcium levels, and this circumstance should not be misinterpreted as a persistence or recurrence of hyperparathyroidism.[15] Potential explanations for this seeming biochemical paradox are bone remineralization and transient secondary hyperparathyroidism, an increase in calcium set point, and changes in calcium receptors.

Patients with diffuse four-gland hyperplasia represent 10 to 15% of the pool of those with primary hyperparathyroidism. Depending on the individual biologic activity of each enlarged gland, there is a sequential PTH decrement as each gland is removed.[16] After the remaining gland has been addressed (likely leaving half of one viable enlarged parathyroid gland) the PTH levels should fall into the normal range and certainly should have receded by more than 50% of baseline. If the level falls below the lower limit of normal, autotransplantation of some of the previously removed parathyroid tissue should be seriously considered. This differs from the management of uniglandular parathyroid disease, where the remaining glands can be functionally suppressed.

Intraoperative PTH analysis is especially helpful in revision surgery where the functional status of parathyroid tissue other than the targeted enlarged gland is unknown. In addition, surgical reexploration may be difficult and lead to iatrogenic devascularization of remaining parathyroid glands in the exploratory process. Here is an illustrative case of the utility of intraoperative PTH in assisting in the determination of the extent of revision surgery: A patient with symptomatic recurrent nephrolithiasis presented for a surgical parathyroidectomy. The past medical history was marked by a total thyroidectomy, bilateral radical neck dissection, and orthovoltage external radiation therapy for a presumed aggressive thyroid cancer 30 years previously. Surgical records were no longer available. The surgical field was severely scarred and extensive collateral venous circulation was expected and encountered during parathyroid exploration. Fortunately, the technetium-99m-sestamibi scan was positive and localizing. In conjunction with recurrent laryngeal nerve monitoring, the side of entry and the ability to locate the recurrent laryngeal nerve allowed safe, successful parathyroidectomy. However, without intraoperative PTH analysis, there would not have been any way of determining the status of the remaining parathyroid glands. With a unilateral sestamibi-delayed washout, the exploration of the opposite side was probably not necessary or a risk worth taking. Fortunately, the PTH value receded by more than 50%, and the procedure was able to be terminated without any consideration of autotransplantation.

Occasionally, persistent unresolved hyperparathyroidism requires reexploration without the assistance of positive imaging. Reexploration always requires inspection of previous operative reports but they may not be helpful in considering which side to enter first. Irvin et al[17] utilized sequential massage of the neck with matched PTH analysis to assist in exploration of the proper side. They reported the utility of massage and diagnostic spike in three of 14 reoperative ectopic cases. Taylor et al[18] compared internal jugular vein and venous sample from the arm to predict a correct side of entry in 76% of routine parathyroid procedures and two cases of failed prior exploration. Similarly, Irvin et al employed this differential venous sampling technique in reoperative surgery. They entered the correct side based on these samples in a series of nine of 10 patients. Sugg et al[19] published a large series of 86 reoperative patients who did not localize on ultrasound, computed tomography (CT) scan with contrast, technetium-thallium scan, or contrast magnetic resonance imaging (MRI). Selective angiography of the neck and mediastinum was then performed. If the occult enlarged parathyroid could not be demonstrated, selective venous sampling via the Seldinger technique was performed analyzing samples from the superior, middle, and inferior thyroid veins, thymic veins, and occasional vertebral veins. Rapid PTH was performed on all samples, and 28 patients demonstrated a diagnostic gradient.

Patients with renal failure and secondary hyperparathyroidism may not demonstrate a reduction in PTH level for a prolonged period of time even after total parathyroidectomy. The half-life of PTH in patients with significant renal disease is nearly three times as long as in normal individuals. Lokey et al[20] reported a series of 80 patients requiring total parathyroidectomy in chronic renal failure and utilized a 20-minute interval after removal of the last enlarged gland as a surgical end point. The PTH results of total parathyroidectomy and thymectomy are still more variable in renal patients, but all patients must demonstrate at least a 50% gradient and finalize near the upper limit of normal.

In summary, intraoperative PTH is a major advance in the surgical management of hyperparathyroidism. It is well integrated into more limited surgical procedures and has substantially reduced the risk of failed exploration. Patients with double adenomas, one of which may not image with sestamibi, are discovered intraoperatively as a direct result of this technology. Diffuse hyperplasia can now be better managed, and decisions for reimplantation and a host of surgical scenarios have a refined and logical foundation.

Minimal Access Parathyroidectomy

Minimal access parathyroidectomy (MAP) is a term coined by Clive Grant[4] at the Mayo Clinic; the procedure was first performed in June 1998. A nearly similar term, *minimally invasive parathyroidectomy* (MIP), implies that conventional open parathyroidectomy is an invasive technique. The MAP procedure depends on accurate preoperative localization and is characterized by a small skin incision usually 2.5 to 3 cm. In fact, MAP differs little from most contemporary parathyroid surgery with the exception of the size of the incision. With the aid of accurate preoperative localization, a directed approach to a single adenoma is the goal of nearly all current surgery for primary hyperparathyroidism. With the aid of magnification and careful soft tissue technique, conventional parathyroid exploration should not be considered at all invasive. Rather, without the need to incise muscle and the fact that blood supply to the adenoma is discrete and independent of the thyroid gland, parathyroid adenoma resection is usually devoid of significant bleeding or hematoma risk. Most inferior adenomas do not displace or involve the recurrent laryngeal nerve, and approaches to the superior parathyroid gland usually require careful identification of the nerve itself.

In my experience, no patient undergoing parathyroidectomy has ever demonstrated paresis or paralysis of recurrent laryngeal nerve function. MAP demands accurate preoperative localization and technetium-sestamibi with or without SPECT is the foundation of imaging. However, even with a positive focal scan, multiple gland hyperplasia or double adenoma may be present, with the additional enlarged parathyroid failing to demonstrate uptake. High-resolution ultrasound has traditionally occupied a second tier of identification, probably due to the fact that it evolved in an era when high-resolution transducers and ideal image processing were not available. The complementary addition of high-resolution ultrasound allows more precise determination of the existence of multiple gland disease. In this circumstance, a more conventional open procedure with an expanded size of incision would be more likely.

Minimal access parathyroidectomy is a technique developed by surgeons. Udelsman[21] and Grant[4] in separate reports indicate a cure rate of 97 to 100%. This procedure is identical in concept to the conventional uniglandular approach, with the exception of the size of the incision, which measures approximately 3 cm. At the Mayo Clinic, 30 to 50% of patients with surgical hyperparathyroidism are selected for a MAP. Approximately half of the patients required or requested general anesthesia, and localization is based on sestamibi scans. Intraoperative PTH failed to decrease in 8.5% of patients, requiring further conventional exploration with conversion of a small midline incision to a more conventional size and inspection of the four cardinal sites.

Because this technique has specific requirements for an identifiable imaged gland, there are expected limitations to its application. Failure to image with sestamibi, multiple endocrine neoplasia (MEN) syndrome and concomitant hyperparathyroidism, revision procedures, familial hyperparathyroidism, multiple gland imaging, and concurrent need for thyroidectomy are reported contraindications for this technique. Other realistic limitations may preclude the obese patient and those with a low-lying larynx where exposure problems are anticipated.

This procedure is likely to have been developed through a combination of factors. Although some have compared its evolution to the transition from open cholecystectomy to the laparoscopic technique, there are flaws in this analogy. Although it is true that the cosmetic benefits are obvious and a genuine advance, one important advantage of the laparoscopic cholecystectomy is the avoidance of the morbidity of muscle division. Along with less invasive retraction and all of the associated comfort benefits, this procedure has revolutionized abdominal surgery. In contradistinction, modern conventional parathyroidectomy is remarkably noninvasive. Dissection planes involve principally adipose and fascial tissues, and bleeding is limited and easily controlled. Muscle division is usually unnecessary, and postoperative pain is generally minor and easily controlled. For all of these reasons, patients undergoing conventional parathyroidectomy can usually be discharged to home care within a few hours of surgery. Thus the only realistic advantage may seem to be the smaller incision, which does have a down side. The exposure is more limited and retraction requirements are greater. Although this does not seem to translate into an increase in complications, this procedure has been reported by a limited number of experienced surgeons. It would seem that MAP is somewhat patient driven as a procedure, which idealizes a technique that offers little cosmetic advantage over modern open parathyroidectomy. Perhaps it has in part become a counterpoint to the radio-guided procedure that Internet advertising has placed in a competitive marketing position.

Methylene Blue

In 1966 Klopper and Moe[22] demonstrated the efficiency of toluidine blue in differentially staining normal parathyroid glands in dogs. However, toxic side effects of arrhythmia and cardiac arrest eliminated its clinical use in humans. In 1971, Dudley[23] reported the use of a related thiazin dye, tetramethylthionine (methylene blue) in the selective identification of parathyroid tissue. His initial recommendation of an intravenous infusion of 5 mg per kilogram 1 hour prior to neck exploration proved to be safe and effective. The mechanism of action is incompletely understood but may be explained in the same way preferential uptake of technetium-sestamibi by parathyroid adenoma occurs. Both substances are lipophilic cations and readily diffuse through the mitochondrial cell membrane. Parathyroid adenomas demonstrate increased oxyphil cells, which are highly laden with mitochondria. Orloff[24] reported a 96% anatomic correlation between positive sestamibi imaging and methylene blue staining. Sherlock and Holl-Allen[25] demonstrated that a more concentrated infusion of 7.5 mg per kilogram produces better differential staining, and there may be timing

issues as well. Some authors suggest a divided dosage 1 hour prior to induction and the remainder a half-hour later. Others have recommended a constant infusion during induction with completion over a 15-minute interval.

Kuriloff and Sanborn[26] report an experience in 35 patients with primary hyperparathyroidism receiving methylene blue infusion at induction for surgery. The anesthesiologist and surgeon were aware of expected pseudocyanosis and possible oximetry demonstrating pseudohypoxia. In this series all but one of the adenomas stained with methylene blue, with most demonstrating a dark blue to purple color. Most importantly, three ectopic adenomas were readily identified because of the staining characteristics. Normal glands and diffuse hyperplasia stained to a lesser degree. Normal parathyroid glands may stain lightly, and in this series only 46% demonstrated any visible blue hue. In patients undergoing thyroidectomy, 87% of normal parathyroids concentrated methylene blue with 50% staining intensely. Suppressed nonadenoma glands in primary hyperparathyroidism do concentrate methylene blue but the stain is very light. This differential staining may assist the surgeon in distinguishing hyperplastic from normal glands.

Skin pseudocyanosis is usually mild and disappears within 24 hours, and greenish-blue urine color may persist for 10 days; patients should be warned of these anticipated issues. Methylene blue is used in these low doses to treat methemoglobulinemia and for the initial management of cyanide poison, as the reduced hemoglobin binds free cyanide ions pending more definitive treatment. During surgery, PO_2 of arterial blood gas determination during the use of methylene blue is usually normal in spite of low pulse oximetry of 60 to 65%, with an average recovery to the normal range occurring within 15 minutes after infusion.

Schell and Dudley[27] report a series of 688 patients in which only methylene blue infusion was used without any preoperative localization or intraoperative PTH. A cure rate of 99.7% was achieved. This procedure may be used effectively in reoperation after failed initial neck exploration, and in one series of 24 revision cases where the patients were eventually cured on reexploration, all demonstrated blue stain in the identified enlarged parathyroid gland. The safety of this technique has been confirmed in most large series, but the anesthesia literature does register some cautions. A few sporadic reports suggest prolonged postoperative disorientation, and one patient with a malignant hyperthermia profile developed secondary hyperparathyroidism and renal failure,[28] which would suggest that methylene blue should not be employed in patients with poor renal clearance.

Video-Assisted Parathyroidectomy

The first endoscopic parathyroidectomy was performed in 1996 by Gagner.[29] His midline approach has been adopted by others, with and without CO_2 insufflation. The midline approach allows access to the lower pole of the thyroid and inferior glands, but the superior glands are more problematic due to required anteromedial retraction of the thyroid gland. Jean-François Henry et al[30] developed a more direct lateral approach that enters on the line of the anterior border of the sternocleidomastoid muscle. Because this is a lateral-unilateral approach, preoperative imaging with ultrasound and sestamibi is required. The criteria for this and other limited endoscopic procedures are as follows:

1   Absence of significant goiter
2   No prior neck surgery
3   No familial hyperparathyroidism or suspect multiglandular disease
4   No marked hypercalcemia or excessive PTH values
5   Not applicable for secondary hyperparathyroidism

This lateral approach through a 15-mm skin incision allows exploration from the superior pole to the thymus and potentially into the anterior and posterior mediastinum. In Henry et al's first 44 cases, 91% of adenomas were correctly identified by endoscopic exploration. A conversion to an open procedure was required in 16% of these cases because of identification failure or a suspicion of multigland disease.

Paolo Miccoli et al[31] reported the single-institution experience of the University of Pisa from 1997 to 2003 of 370 patients managed with minimally invasive video-assisted parathyroidectomy (MIVAP). This midline technique is similar to that of Gagner without insufflation, employing external retraction for exposure. A 30-degree 5-mm endoscope and a variety of 2-mm complementary instruments are fundamental to the procedure; 98.3% of these patients were cured, and video-assisted exploration was successful in 94% of cases. The mean operative time was 36 minutes, and 5.6% of cases required a concomitant thyroidectomy. Complications were uncommon, consisting of 10 cases of hypoparathyroidism, one hematoma, and three recurrent laryngeal nerve palsies.

Video-assisted parathyroidectomy appears to be a logical progression from standard bilateral open exploration with the advent of reliable preoperative imaging and confinement to a directed regional exploration with the support of intraoperative PTH. The incision is small but may be offset by the cosmetic limitations of trocar entry points. Perhaps its greatest obstacle is the technology. These procedures are destined to be performed by a few surgeons who can develop an endoscopic case load, thus reducing operative time and complication rate. In spite of the improving experience and results achieved with MIVAP, a recurrent laryngeal palsy rate of 1% is disturbing and must be addressed if these procedures are to be recommended instead of open surgery. Its time may have come, and the future will determine whether the more occasional surgeon practicing parathyroid and thyroid surgery can easily master these techniques safely.

Radio-Guided Parathyroidectomy

The gamma probe has been effectively employed in the identification of sentinel nodes in melanoma and other malignant primary head and neck tumors. In 1999, Murphy and Norman[32] reported their experience with 12,090 tissue specimens from 345 patients with primary hyperparathyroidism. Parathyroid and other tissues from the head and neck were evaluated within $3\frac{1}{2}$ hours after sestamibi injection, and radioactive counts were determined with the gamma probe and compared with the background. Lymph nodes, normal parathyroid glands, and fat were equal or less than 2.2% of background. Normal thyroid tissues and diffuse hyperplasia of the parathyroid gland never exceeded values greater than 16%. In contrast, parathyroid adenomas exceeded background by more than 20% in all cases, and most averaged 59% ± 9% above the background. Norman reported a subsequent experience with this technique performing about 900 cases per year (unpublished data presented at the 6th International Conference on Head and Neck Cancer, Washington, DC, 2004). Eighty percent of his cases are performed with the gamma probe and limited dissection, and he claims a cure rate of 99% without frozen section or intraoperative PTH. He emphasizes that the probe is not utilized to find the enlarged parathyroid glands but rather to use the 20% rule in ex vivo evaluation of the removed parathyroid tissue. Murphy and Norman's extensive described experience subsequent to the original report in 1999 has continued to confirm that removed parathyroids with greater than 20% ex vivo counts are always single adenomas, allowing termination of surgery.

A study by Caudle et al[33] reviews minimally invasive radio-guided parathyroidectomy (MIRP), preoperative sestamibi localization, and selective frozen section without the use of intraoperative PTH in 140 acute patients; 96% of these patients were cured. A study by Chen et al[34] compared the projected success of gamma probe values with intraoperative PTH in 254 patients undergoing MIP from 2001 to 2004. The positive predictive value for resection based on sestamibi alone was 81%, radio-guided resection 88%, and resection with intraoperative PTH 99.5%. The authors conclude that intraoperative PTH has the highest sensitivity, positive predictive value, and accuracy of all perioperative adjunctive modalities.

Finally, Orlo Clark[35] employed the gamma probe in 75 consecutive cases to determine whether the technique provided any advantage beyond his conventional surgical management. His conclusion and the published opinion of Shaha et al[36] conclude that the use of radio-guided surgery does not confer any surgical or curative advantage. In spite of this, patients are often influenced by new technology and marketing. It is clear that radio-guided parathyroidectomy and the seeming limited incision capability have combined appeal for the patient anticipating parathyroid surgery. However, the use of high-resolution ultrasound and technetium scan with or without SPECT are the true advances that allow minimal access surgery. The relative confirmatory benefits of either gamma probe ex vivo measurements or intraoperative PTH have their proponents, and both offer intraoperative opportunities to determine single versus multigland disease.

Mediastinal Parathyroid

Ectopic parathyroid glands in the anterior mediastinum may be retrieved through cervical thymectomy unless they are so inferior in location that the innominate vessels are at risk of injury. Preoperative cervicoplanar or SPECT sestamibi gives significant information about this question, but precise localization is usually required to allow the best surgical decision to evolve. MRI and CT with contrast and now possibly positron emission tomography (PET)-CT are complementary to the sestamibi scan and determine ideal localization. A full or upper median sternotomy is direct and safe, with some limited associated morbidity as a result of the chondro-osseous split. Thoracoscopic approaches have been developed, and the accrued experience of 38 patients between 1994 and 2002 has been summarized by Bodner et al[37] in their review of 19 publications on the subject. Of these 38 cases, three required conversion to open sternotomy. In seven patients, supplementary radio-guidance was required for localization during thoracoscopy. Video-assisted thyroid surgery (VATS) is hampered by poor vision control and limited exploration ability.

Although this chapter discusses surgically related advances in parathyroidectomy, a novel and exciting option now exists for the management of ectopic parathyroid adenomas in the anterior and posterior mediastinum. Sacks and Palotta[38] have described an arteriographic ablation for mediastinal adenomas using intraarterial absolute alcohol in preference to Gelfoam obliteration for cervical adenomas. The safety of alcohol in the mediastinum is a result of an "end organ" vascular supply. Five of six patients with mediasti-

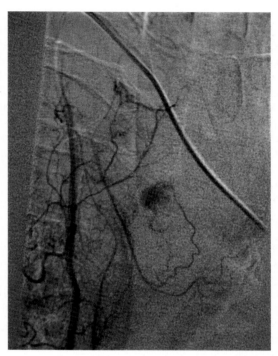

Fig. 19.3 Superselective internal mammary angiogram demonstrating the blush of mediastinal parathyroid adenoma. Courtesy of Barry Sachs, MD.

nal adenomas have been successfully cured of their hyperparathyroidism with arteriographic ablation. The technique (**Figs. 19.3** and **19.4**) requires a diagnostic selective internal mammary artery angiogram and subselective catheterization with five 10-cc boluses of 60 to 70% regular ionic

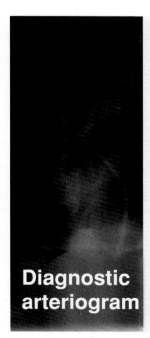
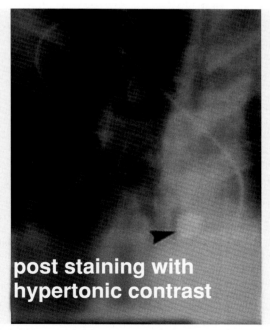
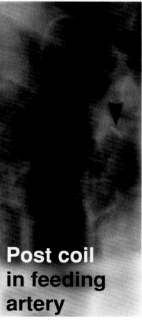

Diagnostic arteriogram

post staining with hypertonic contrast

Post coil in feeding artery

Fig. 19.4 Sequence of angiogram, alcohol ablation, and coil occlusion of discrete vessels to parathyroid adenoma. Arrows designate location of tumor. Courtesy of Barry Sachs, MD.

contrast infusion. The contrast has two destructive effects: it is directly cytotoxic to the adenoma, and the contrast is hyperosmolar and produces cellular dehydration and destruction. In circumstances where the vascular supply to the adenoma persists after contrast infusion, alcohol destruction can then be utilized. Occasionally, Gelfoam or coil obliteration of the end artery may be required. Although this procedure is uncommon, it may offer the least invasive option for managing the mediastinal parathyroid adenoma. Only time and greater numbers of cases managed in this way will determine the safety and efficacy of angiographic ablation.

Conclusion

Since the 1989 report by Coakley et al[39] on the applicability of technetium-sestamibi for identification of parathyroid adenoma, the surgical landscape has changed dramatically. The combination of high-resolution ultrasound, technetium-sestamibi, and intraoperative PTH has allowed focused uni-

lateral exploration through small incisions. Interestingly, this surgical change has produced better patient acceptance of a recommendation for surgery and a more liberal attitude by endocrinologists about referring patients for curative parathyroidectomy. Although there are many new tools that parallel the improvements in preoperative imaging, every surgeon performing parathyroidectomy must be fully comfortable with conventional bilateral exploration. It is critical for the surgeon to understand the embryology of parathyroid migration and potential sites of ectopic location. This knowledge is complementary to preoperative imaging. Although these aforementioned advances allow more focused targeted surgery, the principal objective must still be the proper identification of the pathologic state and its correction with a single procedure. Revision surgery is difficult for the patient and surgeon, with a higher complication rate and risk of permanent hypoparathyroidism. For the first time in the history of parathyroid surgery, it is now possible for surgeons to have intraoperative confirmation of the completion of objectives.

References

1. Gilmour JR. The gross anatomy of the parathyroid glands. J Pathol 1938;46:133–149
2. Wang CA. Surgical management of primary hyperparathyroidism. Curr Probl Surg 1990;125:985
3. Doppman JL. NIH Consensus Conference on Primary Hyperparathyroidism, 1991
4. Grant CS. Minimal access parathyroidectomy. In: Randolph GW, ed. Surgery of the Thyroid and Parathyroid Glands. Philadelphia: WB Saunders, 2003:549–556
5. Sofferman RA, Standage J, Tang ME. Minimal access parathyroid surgery using intraoperative parathyroid hormone assay. Laryngoscope 1998;108:1497–1503
6. Nussbaum SR, Thompson AP, Hutchinson KA, Gaz RD, Wang CA. Intraoperative measurement of parathyroid hormone in the surgical management of hyperparathyroidism. Surgery 1988;104:1121–1127
7. Libutti SK, Alexander HR, Bartlett HR, et al. Kinetic analysis of the rapid intraoperative parathyroid hormone assay in patients during aspiration for hyperparathyroidism. Surgery 1999;126:1145–1151
8. Boggs JE, Irvin GL, Carneiro DM, Madinari AS. The evolution of parathyroidectomy failures. Surgery 1999;126:998–1002
9. Chapuis Y, Icard P, Fulla Y, et al. Parathyroid adenomectomy under local anesthesia with intra-operative monitoring of UcAMP and/or 1-84 PTH. World J Surg 1992;16:570
10. Irvin GL, Deriso GT. A new, practical intraoperative parathyroid hormone assay. Am J Surg 1994;168:466–468
11. Sofferman RA, Randolph GW. Intraoperative parathyroid hormone assessment during parathyroidectomy. In: Randolph GW. Surgery of the thyroid and parathyroid glands. Philadelphia: WB Sanders, 2003, p.559
12. Kao PC, van Heerden JA, Taylor RL. Intraoperative monitoring of parathyroid procedures by a 15 minute parathormone immuno-chemiluminectric assay. Mayo Clin Proc 1994;69:532–537
13. Proctor MD, Sofferman RA. Intraoperative hormone testing: what have we learned? Laryngoscope 2003;113:706–714
14. Irvin GL, Dembrow VD, Prudhomme DL. Clinical usefulness of in-

traoperative "quick parathyroid hormone" assay. Surgery 1993;114:1019–1022
15. Starr FL, DeCresce R, Prinz RA. Normalization of intraoperative parathyroid hormone does not predict normal postoperative parathyroid hormone levels. Surgery 2000;128:930–935
16. Clary BM, Garner SC, Leight GS. Intraoperative parathyroid hormone monitoring during parathyroidectomy for secondary hyperparathyroidism. Surgery 1997;122:1034–1038
17. Irvin GL, Molinari AS, Figueroa C, Carneiro DM. Improved success rate in reoperative parathyroidectomy with intraoperative PTH assay. Ann Surg 1999;229:874–878
18. Taylor J, Fraser W, Banaszkiewicz P, Drury P, Atkins P. Lateralization of parathyroid adenomas by intraoperative PTH estimation. J R Coll Surg Edinb 1996;41:174–177
19. Sugg SL, Fraker DL, Alexander R, et al. Prospective evaluation of selective venous sampling for parathyroid hormone concentration in patients undergoing reoperations for primary hyperparathyroidism. Surgery 1993;114:1004–1009
20. Lokey J, Pattou F, Mondragon-Sanchez A, et al. Intraoperative decay profile of intact (1-84) parathyroid hormone in surgery for secondary hyperparathyroidism–a consecutive series of 80 patients. Surgery 2000;128:1029–1034
21. Udelsman R, Donovan PI, Sokoll LJ. One hundred consecutive minimally invasive parathyroid explorations. Ann Surgery 2000;232:331
22. Klopper PJ, Moe RE. Demonstration of the parathyroids during surgery in dogs, with preliminary report of results in some clinical cases. Surgery 1966;59:1101–1107
23. Dudley NE. Methylene blue for rapid identification of the parathyroids. BMJ 1971;3:680–681
24. Orloff LA. Methylene blue and sestamibi: complimentary tools for localizing parathyroids. Laryngoscope 2001;111:1901–1904
25. Sherlock DJ, Holl-Allen RT. Intravital methylene blue staining of parathyroid glands and tumors. Ann R Coll Surg Engl 1984;66:396–398
26. Kuriloff DB, Sanborn KV. Rapid intraoperative localization of parathyroid glands utilizing methylene blue infusion. Otolaryngol Head Neck Surg 2004;131:616–622

27. Schell SR, Dudley NE. Clinical outcomes and fiscal consequences of bilateral neck exploration without preoperative radionuclide imaging or minimally invasive techniques. Surgery 2003;133:32–39

28. Mathew S, Linhartova L, Raghuraman G. Hyperpyrexia and prolonged postoperative disorientation following methylene blue infusion during parathyroidectomy. Anaesthesia 2006;61:580–583

29. Gagner M. Endoscopic subtotal parathyroidectomy in patients with primary hyperparathyroidism. Br J Surg 1996;83:875

30. Henry JF, Defechereux T, Gramatica L, de Boissezon C. Minimally invasive videoscopic parathyroidectomy by lateral approach. Langenbecks Arch Surg 1999;384:298–301

31. Miccoli P, Berti P, Materazzi G, et al. Results of video-assisted parathyroidectomy: single institution's six year experience. World J Surg 2004;28:1216–1218

32. Murphy C, Norman J. The 20 percent rule: a simple instantaneous radioactivity measurement defines cured and allows elimination of frozen sections and hormone assays during parathyroidectomy. Surgery 1999;126:1023–1029

33. Caudle AS, Brier SE, Calvo BF, Kim HJ, Meyers MO, Ollila DN. Experienced radio-guided surgery teams can successfully perform minimally invasive radio-guided parathyroidectomy without intraoperative parathyroid hormone assays. Am Surg 2006;72:785–790

34. Chen H, Mack E, Starling JR. A comprehensive evaluation of perioperative adjuncts during minimally invasive parathyroidectomy: which is most reliable? Ann Surg 2005;242:375–380

35. Clark O. Presentation at the conference on surgery of the thyroid and parathyroid glands, November 9–10, 2001, Boston, Massachusetts Eye & Ear Infirmary

36. Shaha AR, Patel SG, Singh B. Minimally invasive parathyroidectomy: the role of radio-guided surgery. Laryngoscope 2002;112:2166–2169

37. Bodner J, Prommegger R, Profanter C, Schmid T. Thoracoscopic resection of mediastinal parathyroids: current status and future perspectives. Minim Invasive Ther Allied Technol 2004;13:199–204

38. Sachs BA, Pollotta J. Angiographic ablation of parathyroid adenomas. In: Kadir S, ed. Current Practice of Interventional Radiology. Philadelphia: BC Decker, 1991

39. Coakley AJ, Kettle AG, Wells CP, O'Doherty MJ, Collins RE. 99Tcm sestamibi-a new agent for parathyroid imaging. Nucl Med Commun 1989;10:791–794

V Special Topics

20 Complications of Thyroid Surgery

Mark J. Jameson and Paul A. Levine

Thyroid surgery is extremely safe, and serious postoperative morbidity is quite uncommon. The most concerning complications are recurrent laryngeal nerve (RLN) injury and permanent hypoparathyroidism resulting in persistent hypocalcemia. Thyroid surgeons must be well versed in these as well as other complications and their management.

Wound Complications

Wound complications such as infection, hematoma, seroma, skin flap necrosis, and hypertrophic scarring/keloid formation are uncommon after thyroid surgery. The risk of these complications is increased when the patient has had prior radiation therapy or when a neck dissection is performed concomitantly.[1]

Postoperative bleeding after thyroidectomy is either immediate or delayed, but is most often arterial. Immediate bleeds typically occur at the time of extubation; the neck rapidly expands, or frank blood is noted filling the drains.[1] In this situation, the airway is quickly secured and the neck is explored. Because of this possibility, which is often related to aggressive coughing or straining, Reeve and Thompson[2] recommend routinely applying pressure to the neck as the patient is extubated. Alternatively, this can be achieved with a pressure dressing. Delayed hematomas develop more slowly and generally occur within the first 24 hours postoperatively, with most significant hematomas becoming obvious within 8 hours. These bleeds may be noticed only when breathing is subjectively more difficult, and in this situation, the airway status must be rapidly assessed. If urgent decompression is necessary, the wound must be opened and evacuated, and an emergency airway obtained, if necessary.

Abbas et al[3] studied 918 thyroid and 350 parathyroid surgeries of which six (0.7%) and four (1.1%), respectively, required reoperation for postoperative bleeding. Of these, two wounds were opened emergently at the bedside, and one patient required emergent tracheotomy. With the exception of one bleed, which occurred 5 days postoperatively, all the bleeds occurred between 2 and 48 hours after the operation.[3] Other large series have noted the incidence of hemorrhage to be approximately 1%.[2,4,5]

Seromas occur infrequently and are usually easily treated with pressure dressing after needle aspiration or passive drain placement. Although it is common practice to place a drain for prevention of hematoma or seroma after thyroidectomy, Shaha and Jaffe[6] noted no difference in outcome whether or not a drain was used. They recommended selective use of drains for large dead space, large substernal goiter, or subtotal thyroidectomy for large multinodular goiter or Graves disease.

Wound infections are noted in 0.1 to 0.3% of cases[2,4,5] and can generally be treated with oral antibiotics after drainage of any purulent collection. Hypertrophic scars can be treated with injected steroids or other scar reduction techniques. In known keloid formers, prophylactic steroid injections in the early postoperative period should be considered.

Laryngeal Nerve Injury

Recurrent Laryngeal Nerve

The published incidence of RLN injury varies widely (0.3 to 17%[1]). This variation is likely the result of multiple confounding factors. First is the definition of "nerve injury." RLN neuropraxia resulting in temporary true vocal cord (TVC) paresis can occur even with minimal manipulation of the nerve. Permanent paralysis occurs when the nerve is transected. In some cases, these injuries go unnoticed or are not documented in the medical record, making retrospective analysis difficult. Second, the physiologic effect of RLN injury is variable. Depending on the degree of injury, damage to the RLN may cause hoarseness, mild dysphagia, or airway compromise of variable magnitude. In some patients, vocal cord paresis and even total paralysis is nearly imperceptible by simply listening to the voice and does not generate any complaints from the patient, particularly if the paralyzed vocal cord has stabilized in the midline rather than in the paramedian position. Many patients who undergo thyroidectomy do not have detailed sequential laryngeal examinations after surgery, and even fewer have this type of evaluation preoperatively. Third, the incidence of RLN injury is so low that very large studies are required to accurately assess the problem. In general, permanent injury to the RLN is anticipated in approximately 1% of thyroid lobectomies; the rate increases slightly in total thyroidectomy because both nerves are at risk, and the average degree of disease tends to be somewhat higher. The rate of injury also increases in the reoperative setting. Bilateral RLN injury is quite rare.

Operator experience and operative technique play a large role in RLN injury. Accordingly, loupe magnification and microsurgical technique have been shown in a randomized trial of 97 patients to significantly reduce operative time and overall morbidity.[7] Although not statistically significant, the rates of transient and permanent RLN palsy were reduced in the microsurgical group, as were the rates of hematoma and transient and permanent hypoparathyroidism.[7] Herranz-Gonzalez et al[8] found that the three most significant factors contributing to RLN injury, after operator experience, are histology, second operation, and failure to identify the nerve. When the RLN is injured, it is likely to happen in one of three sites: at the thoracic inlet, crossing inferior thyroid vessels, or at the Berry ligament.[1] On the right, the nerve tends to be more lateral and superficial than on the left, where it ascends vertically in the tracheoesophageal groove. On either side, the surgeon must be aware of the variable relationship to the inferior thyroid artery and the possibility of single or multiple branch points before entry into the larynx. For these reasons, the safest approach is to identify the RLN low in the neck and trace it superiorly to its laryngeal entry. It is also important to remember that, in somewhat less than 1% of cases, a nonrecurrent nerve is reported on the right. This can occur as a direct branch from the vagus nerve at the level of the cricothyroid membrane or a partially recurrent nerve looping around inferior thyroid vessels. Both aberrancies are due to anomalous development of the subclavian artery from the aortic arch rather than brachiocephalic artery.[1] Nonrecurrent laryngeal nerve on the left has been reported only in rare cases of situs inversus.

In recent years, there has been significant interest in neurophysiologic monitoring in an effort to avoid RLN injury. This is typically performed using an endotracheal tube with electrodes that allow monitoring of TVC activity, similar to facial nerve integrity monitoring. Studies have demonstrated conflicting results. In a retrospective study of 116 monitored nerves versus 120 control nerves, Robertson et al[9] noted RLN paralysis in 2.5% of nerves in the control group and 0.86% of nerves in the monitored group. However, the difference was not statistically significant due to the extremely low rate of this complication. The authors also noted a slightly increased risk of paresis in advanced T-stage malignancy (T3/T4), and recommended consideration of RLN monitoring in this setting. They also noted the additional benefits of monitoring, including continuous feedback during nerve dissection, which may be particularly useful in the teaching setting, and the ability to stimulate the nerve at the end of the procedure to confirm integrity.[9] In a study of 20 patients undergoing reoperative central compartment neck dissection with recurrent laryngeal nerve monitoring using hook wire electrodes, Kim et al[10] noted that no patient with normal preoperative vocal cord function suffered postoperative paresis or paralysis.

Superior Laryngeal Nerve

The external branch of the superior laryngeal nerve (EBSLN) innervates the cricothyroid muscle, which controls the timbre of the voice by regulating the amount of tension on the TVCs when they are approximated. Injury to the EBSLN results in impaired pitch control, particularly at higher pitches.

Early vocal fatigue may also be noted, but these changes often go unnoticed except by vocal professionals.

The EBSLN travels with the superior thyroid vessels until it separates to enter the cricothyroid muscle. Thus, if superior thyroid vessels are clamped and divided as a group, approximately 20% of patients will be at risk for nerve injury.[2] There is some debate about whether or not the nerve should be identified in every case. Although some authors have advocated making this identification, it is generally accepted that individual ligation of the superior thyroid vessels immediately adjacent to the thyroid capsule avoids injury to the EBSLN. In a prospective randomized study with 449 superior pole ligations, Bellantone et al[11] demonstrated that the group in which the superior thyroid artery branches were ligated separately at the capsule had no EBSLN injuries and took significantly less operative time. Interestingly, in the group where every effort was made to identify the nerve, it could not be found in 11.6% of cases.

Combined Nerve Injury

Combined loss of the RLN and the EBSLN on the same side results in significantly more dramatic symptoms compared with isolated RLN injury; patients exhibit breathier voice, intermittent cough, and occasional aspiration with liquids. The TVC appears lateral and inferior to the normal cord with no adduction during phonation.[1]

Treatment

Although of questionable value, most surgeons prefer to attempt primary repair if the RLN is transected intraoperatively. Although normal function will not be restored, there may be some beneficial tone and reduced atrophy of the vocalis muscle, leading to improved voice quality.[12] Results are generally disappointing, and many patients require additional intervention. Although some authors have had significant success with reinnervation techniques,[13] they tend, in general, to yield unpredictable results with a prolonged delay from surgery to benefit. Thus most surgeons currently choose static medialization for paralyzed TVCs.[14] This approach moves the paralyzed cord toward midline to narrow or close the glottic gap during phonation. The drawback is reduction of the airway; candidates must be free of airway difficulty preoperatively. TVC injection has been performed with various materials and the typical drawback for paralyzed patients is loss of benefit over time.[14] The transient nature, however, can be beneficial for patients who are severely paretic but still have the chance of some recovery of function. Medialization laryngoplasty (type 1 thyroplasty) is permanent but reversible and is generally the procedure of choice; it can be performed under local anesthesia so that vocal quality can be tested intraoperatively.[14,15] Arytenoid adduction, cricothyroid subluxation, or adduction arytenopexy may be useful adjunct procedures to further improve vocal performance in selected patients.[14,15]

Hypothyroidism

Hypothyroidism is expected with total thyroidectomy. It can sometimes be seen with hemithyroidectomy as well, particularly in patients in whom hypothyroidism is predicted as a result of their underlying disease (e.g., long-standing Graves disease or Hashimoto thyroiditis). In their retrospective analysis of 90 patients, Miller et al[16] demonstrated an overall incidence of hypothyroidism of 27% after hemithyroidectomy. The rate was higher in patients with Hashimoto thyroiditis and multinodular goiter, and the majority of cases developed in the first 6 to 12 months after surgery. The patients who ultimately became hypothyroid tended to have a higher preoperative thyroid-stimulating hormone (TSH). It is important to note that curative radiation to the neck is associated with hypothyroidism in 20 to 30% of patients; half of these occur within 5 years of therapy.[17] Thus patients undergoing hemithyroidectomy after neck irradiation may be at a much greater risk for permanent hypothyroidism.

Hypocalcemia (Hypoparathyroidism)

Incidence

Temporary hypocalcemia has been reported to occur in 6 to 35% of cases,[5,18-23] whereas permanent hypocalcemia is much less frequent, in 0.7 to 8% of cases.[5,8,18-22] Rates of hypocalcemia vary significantly based on criteria (e.g., laboratory cutoff selected, symptomatic complaints), distribution of operations in the study (e.g., percent total thyroidectomies, which are higher risk versus thyroid lobectomy), length of follow-up, amount of anticipatory treatment, and so on.

Etiology

The etiology of postoperative hypoparathyroidism after thyroidectomy has not been definitively identified and is likely multifactorial. It is possible that hemodilution resulting from intraoperative fluid administration plays a role.[24] It has also been demonstrated that calcitonin release after thyroid gland manipulation may result in peripheral insensitivity to parathyroid hormone (PTH).[25] Additionally, injury to, devascularization of, or removal of parathyroid glands are likely causative mechanisms.[26] One would anticipate that inadvertent parathyroidectomy would contribute. However, Sasson et al[21] demonstrated that, although postoperative hypocalcemia increased with total thyroidectomy compared with less extensive thyroid surgery, unintentional parathyroidectomy is not associated with increased risk of postoperative hypocalcemia. In this study of 69 total thyroidectomies and 72 thyroid lobectomies, incidental parathyroidectomy occurred in 15% of cases. These parathyroids were noted to be intrathyroidal (50%), extracapsular (31%), and in the central compartment (19%). The risk of incidental parathyroidectomy increased with associated modified radical neck dissection.

Factors that contribute to postoperative hypocalcemia include extent of surgery, experience of the operator, and the number of glands left behind.[27] Most surgeons strive to preserve at least two functional parathyroids; if the remaining glands are thought to have sustained significant injury, appear nonviable, or are found on inspection of the specimen before sending it to pathology, autotransplantation is recommended. Zedenius et al[28] reported no permanent hypoparathyroidism in 100 consecutive cases where autotransplantation was performed. Lo and Lam[29] had similar results with 98 patients, but 21.4% were still noted to develop transient hypocalcemia.

Management

Postoperative hypocalcemia is the most significant practical problem related to thyroid surgery. In this age of cost control and minimization of hospital stays, predicting which patients will exhibit hypocalcemia and require treatment is a major focus of current clinical research. Although many surgeons argue for overnight postoperative inpatient observation for thyroidectomy patients because of the risk of hematoma, there are proponents of same-day discharge after thyroidectomy in selected cases. The biggest impediment to same-day discharge is predicting who will develop hypocalcemia and to what extent (i.e., amount of treatment required). Even setting aside the possibility of performing thyroidectomy as outpatient surgery, cost savings would likely be substantial if patients could confidently be discharged within 24 hours of their surgery. Both PTH and calcium levels have become candidates to predict postoperative hypocalcemia.

In a group of 40 thyroidectomy patients studied by Lam and Kerr,[30] 12 patients developed postoperative hypocalcemia. PTH levels drawn at 1 hour postoperatively were less than or equal to 8 pg/mL (0.8 pmol/L) in all 12 cases. Vescan et al[31] further refined this concept in a study of 199 patients undergoing total thyroidectomy in which the rate of transient hypocalcemia was 22%. PTH levels were drawn at 1 hour postoperatively. A PTH level of less than 10.4 pg/mL (1.1 pmol/L) predicted hypocalcemia with 99% specificity; only one of 155 normocalcemic patients had a PTH level in this range. A PTH level greater than 15.1 pg/mL (1.6 pmol/L) predicted normocalcemia with a sensitivity of 95%; two of 44 hypocalcemic patients had a PTH level in this range. The authors also noted that, in this cohort, the average hospital stay was 2.1 and 3.6 days for normocalcemic and hypocalcemic patients, respectively, and they recommended that, for patients with a PTH below 10.4 pg/mL at 1 hour postoperatively, calcium and vitamin D supplementation should be started immediately to perhaps reduce the length of hospital stay for these patients.

Lombardi et al[32] noted that 15 of 16 patients who developed postoperative hypocalcemia in their study had 4- and 6-hour postoperative PTH levels less than 10 pg/mL. They also noted that PTH levels continued to decrease for as long as 4 hours after total thyroidectomy, which may make assessment of intraoperative or immediate postoperative PTH a poor predictor of postoperative hypocalcemia. Chia et al[23] prospectively studied PTH levels in 103 patients who underwent thyroid and parathyroid surgery. They noted that no patients who underwent thyroid lobectomy or parathyroid adenoma excision developed postoperative hypocalcemia, whereas 22% of total thyroid patients exhibited clinically significant hypocalcemia. In their study, all of the patients who required calcium supplementation had PTH levels of less than 15 pg/mL (1.6 pmol/L) at 8 hours after surgery, and 75% of the patients in this group ultimately required calcium supplementation, yielding a sensitivity and specificity of 100% and 90.5%, respectively, for this test. The authors recommended that patients with a PTH level of less than 15 pg/mL at 8 hours postoperatively should be considered for early supplementation and observed for hypocalcemia. On average, total thyroidectomy patients did not achieve a stable calcium level until 25 hours postoperatively.

Other investigators have pursued the early postoperative trend in calcium level as a predictor of hypocalcemia. Gulluoglu et al[33] drew serum calcium levels at 8, 14, 24, and 48 hours postoperatively and noted that the slope of change in calcium level between 8 and 14 hours independently predicted calcium status. Luu et al[34] used ionized calcium levels drawn preoperatively and at 2 and 8 hours postoperatively. All patients with a positive slope between the preoperative calcium level and either postoperative level or between the two postoperative levels maintained normocalcemia. The slopes between the preoperative calcium level and the 8-hour postoperative level and between the two postoperative levels were significantly different when normocalcemic patients were compared with hypocalcemic patients. However, no clear cutoff value could be established.

Payne et al[35] pursued the combined use of PTH and calcium levels. They initially validated the role of 1- and 6-hour postoperative PTH and corrected calcium levels in predicting hypocalcemia. They showed that patients with PTH levels of 28 pg/mL or greater and calcium levels of 8.56 mg/dL or greater at 6 hours postoperatively were not at risk for developing hypocalcemia. In a subsequent study, patients who met these criteria were discharged, whereas patients

with PTH levels at or below 8 pg/mL at 1 hour postoperatively were empirically started on calcium and vitamin D supplementation.[36] The result was a decrease in the rate of transient hypocalcemia from 28% to 9% and a reduction in average hospital stay by 10 hours. Patient satisfaction level increased and costs were reduced by an average of $766 per patient.

Further refinement of predictive criteria for hypocalcemia will be required before early discharge will be widely accepted. In addition, many centers do not have access to rapid PTH assessment or, if they do, it is quite expensive. However, widespread use of the test will likely lower its cost, and, if use of the test allows many patients to be discharged early, it will likely be cost-effective. Certainly further studies are warranted. Because of these limitations on PTH assessment, many centers have algorithms in place to aggressively manage postoperative calcium and thus minimize the postoperative hospital stay. Reeve and Thompson[2] recommend that asymptomatic patients with calcium below 8.0 mg/dL (normal range, 8.6–10.2) be started on 2 to 3 g of calcium carbonate, educated regarding the symptoms of hypocalcemia, and discharged. In patients with calcium levels below 7.5 mg/dL or who are symptomatic, treatment with 2 to 3 g of calcium carbonate plus 0.25 to 0.5 μg of rapid-acting vitamin D (calcitriol; Rocaltrol) is begun. These patients stay in the hospital for an additional day and are then discharged if they remain asymptomatic. Most can be quickly weaned off supplemental calcium, although a small percentage require 3 months or more of treatment. Particularly when calcium levels do not respond as expected to supplementation, magnesium levels should be checked and repleted if necessary.

We have adopted an aggressive calcium replacement protocol in an effort to shorten the hospital stay for postthyroidectomy patients. **Table 20.1** describes our typical treatment regimen based on serum calcium level, which is drawn on the evening of the operation (6 to 8 hours postoperatively) and the following morning. If necessary, repeated samples are drawn on a daily basis or twice daily if intravenous (IV) replacement is required, until the level is greater than 8.0. All patients are discharged with education regarding the symptoms of hypocalcemia and its management. Patients

Table 20.1 Postthyroidectomy Calcium Management

Serum Ca²⁺	IV Ca²⁺ Replacement	Oral Ca²⁺ Replacement	Vitamin D	Disposition
>8.0	–	–	–	Educate patient and discharge postoperative day 1
7.5–8.0	–	1 g elemental Ca t.i.d.	–	Educate patient and discharge when serum Ca²⁺ >8.0 and no IV replacement in previous 24 hours; check serum Ca²⁺ in 3–5 days
7.0–7.5	–	1.5 g elemental Ca t.i.d.	0.5 μg calcitriol b.i.d.	(see note above)
<7.0 or symptomatic	2 g calcium gluconate	1.5 g elemental Ca q.i.d.	1 μg calcitriol b.i.d.	(see note above)

are not discharged if IV replacement was required within the previous 24 hours. For patients requiring calcium supplementation, a serum level is drawn 3 to 5 days after discharge, and the replacement doses are adjusted accordingly. Magnesium levels are checked with each calcium measurement (at least daily) and aggressively repleted as necessary. Although numbers at present are not adequate for statistical analysis, we anticipate that instituting very early calcium replacement in patients who may develop postoperative hypoparathyroidism will slightly reduce the average length of stay for postthyroidectomy patients. Although hypercalcemia is occasionally noted at the postdischarge calcium check, we have had no cases of symptomatic hypercalcemia with the regimen described.

Thyrotoxic Storm

Thyrotoxic storm can be triggered by thyroid surgery on hyperthyroid patients. Because of better medical control of thyroid function, this is now a rare complication. In potentially hyperthyroid patients, preoperative thyroid function tests should be performed. When it is necessary to operate on hyperthyroid patients, euthyroid status can be achieved rapidly using inhibitors of peripheral deiodination, antithyroid agents, and beta-blockade. Panzer et al[37] achieved excellent success using a regimen including iopanoic acid (500 mg b.i.d.), dexamethasone (1 mg b.i.d.), propylthiouracil or methimazole, and a beta-blocker. This regimen achieved euthyroid status in 17 severely hyperthyroid patients requiring surgery, and no surgery-related thyroid storm was encountered. It is important to continue beta-blockade for an appropriate period postoperatively.[2]

Thyrotoxic storm should be treated with high-dose thioureas (e.g., propylthiouracil 200 mg q6h) with subsequent administration of iodide several hours later. The heart rate must be monitored and controlled with beta-blockade. Prednisone may aid in inhibiting peripheral conversion of thyroxine to triiodothyronine.[1]

Airway Obstruction

Airway obstruction after thyroid surgery is rare and is related to either hematoma or bilateral vocal cord paralysis. When bilateral RLN injury occurs, patients may demonstrate stridor and dyspnea immediately on extubation or soon thereafter. Although unusual, bilateral RLN injury may not be immediately obvious, but these patients develop airway obstruction over time as the vocal cords move to a more paramedian position.

Laryngotracheal/Esophageal Injury

Injury to the larynx, trachea, or esophagus is rare in thyroid surgery. These structures can be at risk when aggressive retraction is used, resulting in distortion of normal anatomy, or when there is significant deviation of the midline structures. Because of its anatomic location, cervical sympathetic trunk injury is rare, but can occur when extirpation of a goiter or cancer requires retroesophageal dissection. In a large Australian series, Horner syndrome was noted in two of 10,201 cases.[2]

Conclusion

Pneumothorax is rare but can occur when extensive subclavicular dissection is necessary. Nonspecific perioperative morbidity is rare with thyroidectomy and includes myocardial infarction (0.2%), stroke (0.6%), and pneumonia (0.6%).[4] In several moderate to very large series, mortality was 0 to 0.8%.[4,5,8]

References

1. Kennedy TL. Surgical complications of thyroidectomy. Oper Tech Otolaryngol Head Neck Surg 2003;14:74–79
2. Reeve T, Thompson NW. Complications of thyroid surgery: how to avoid them, how to manage them, and observations on their possible effect on the whole patient. World J Surg 2000;24:971–975
3. Abbas G, Dubner S, Heller KS. Re-operation for bleeding after thyroidectomy and parathyroidectomy. Head Neck 2001;23:544–546
4. Bhattacharyya N, Fried MP. Assessment of the morbidity and complications of total thyroidectomy. Arch Otolaryngol Head Neck Surg 2002;128:389–392
5. Rosato L, Avenia N, Bernante P, et al. Complications of thyroid surgery: analysis of a multicentric study of 14,934 patients operated on in Italy over 5 years. World J Surg 2004;28:271–276
6. Shaha AR, Jaffe BM. Selective use of drains in thyroid surgery. J Surg Oncol 1993;52:241–243
7. Testini M, Nacchiero M, Piccinni G, et al. Total thyroidectomy is improved by loupe magnification. Microsurgery 2004;24:39–42
8. Herranz-Gonzalez J, Gavilan J, Matinez-Vidal J, Gavilan C. Complications following thyroid surgery. Arch Otolaryngol Head Neck Surg 1991;117:516–518
9. Robertson ML, Steward DL, Gluckman JL, Welge J. Continuous laryngeal nerve integrity monitoring during thyroidectomy: does it reduce risk of injury? Otolaryngol Head Neck Surg 2004;131:596–600
10. Kim MK, Mandel SH, Baloch Z, et al. Morbidity following central compartment reoperation for recurrent or persistent thyroid cancer. Arch Otolaryngol Head Neck Surg 2004;130:1214–1216
11. Bellantone R, Boscherini M, Lombardi CP, et al. Is the identification of the external branch of the superior laryngeal nerve mandatory in thyroid operation? Results of a prospective randomized study. Surgery 2001;130:1055–1059
12. Chou FF, Su CY, Jeng SF, Hsu KL, Ly KY. Neurorrhaphy of the recurrent laryngeal nerve. J Am Coll Surg 2003;197:52–57
13. Crumley RL. Unilateral recurrent laryngeal nerve paralysis. J Voice 1994;8:79–83
14. Hartl DM, Travagli JP, Leboulleux S, Baudin E, Brasnu DF, Schlumberger M. Clinical review: current concepts in the management of unilateral recurrent laryngeal nerve paralysis after thyroid surgery. J Clin Endocrinol Metab 2005;90:3084–3088
15. Zeitels SM. New procedures for paralytic dysphonia: adduction

arytenopexy, Goretex medialization laryngoplasty, and cricothyroid subluxation. Otolaryngol Clin North Am 2000;33:841–854

16. Miller FR, Paulson D, Prihoda TJ, Otto RA. Risk factors for the development of hypothyroidism after hemithyroidectomy. Arch Otolaryngol Head Neck Surg 2006;132:36–38

17. Jereczek-Fossa BA, Alterio D, Jassem J, Gibelli B, Tradati N, Orecchia R. Radiotherapy-induced thyroid disorders. Cancer Treat Rev 2004;30:369–384

18. Bergamaschi R, Becouarn G, Roncerary J, Arnaud JP. Morbidity of thyroid surgery. Am J Surg 1998;176:71–75

19. Pappalardo G, Guadalaxara A, Frattaroli FM, Illomei G, Falaschi P. Total compared with subtotal thyroidectomy in benign nodular disease: personal series and review of published reports. Eur J Surg 1998;164:501–506

20. Mishra A, Agarwal G, Agarwal A, Mishra SK. Safety and efficacy of total thyroidectomy in hands of endocrine surgery trainees. Am J Surg 1999;178:377–380

21. Sasson AR, Pingpank JF, Wetherington RW, Hanlon AL, Ridge JA. Incidental parathyroidectomy during thyroid surgery does not cause transient symptomatic hypocalcemia. Arch Otolaryngol Head Neck Surg 2001;127:304–308

22. Higgins KM, Mandell DL, Govindaraj S, et al. The role of intraoperative rapid parathyroid hormone monitoring for predicting thyroidectomy-related hypocalcemia. Arch Otolaryngol Head Neck Surg 2004;130:63–67

23. Chia SH, Weisman RA, Tieu D, Kelly C, Dillmann WH, Orloff LA. Prospective study of perioperative factors predicting hypocalcemia after thyroid and parathyroid surgery. Arch Otolaryngol Head Neck Surg 2006;132:41–45

24. Demeester-Mirkine N, Hooghe L, Van Geertruyden J, De Maertelaer V. Hypocalcemia after thyroidectomy. Arch Surg 1992;127:854–858

25. Watson CG, Steed DL, Robinson AG, Deftos LJ. The role of calcitonin and parathyroid hormone in the pathogenesis of post-thyroidectomy hypocalcemia. Metabolism 1981;30:588–589

26. Wingert DJ, Friesen SR, Iliopoulos JI, Pierce GE, Thomas JH, Hermreck AS. Post-thyroidectomy hypocalcemia: incidence and risk factors. Am J Surg 1986;152:606–610

27. Pattou F, Combemale F, Fabre S, et al. Hypocalcemia following thyroid surgery: incidence and prediction of outcome. World J Surg 1998;22:718–724

28. Zedenius J, Wadstrom C, Delbridge L. Routine autotransplantation of at least one parathyroid gland during total thyroidectomy may reduce permanent hypoparathyroidism. Aust N Z J Surg 1999;69:794–797

29. Lo CY, Lam KY. Postoperative hypocalcemia in patients who did or did not undergo parathyroid autotransplantation during thyroidectomy: a comparison study. Surgery 1998;124:1081–1086

30. Lam A, Kerr PD. Parathyroid hormone: an early predictor of postthyroidectomy hypocalcemia. Laryngoscope 2003;113:2196–2200

31. Vescan A, Witterick I, Freeman J. Parathyroid hormone as a predictor of hypocalcemia after thyroidectomy. Laryngoscope 2005;115:2105–2108

32. Lombardi CP, Raffaelli M, Princi P, et al. Early prediction of postthyroidectomy hypocalcemia by one single iPTH measurement. Surgery 2004;136:1236–1241

33. Gulluoglu BM, Manukyan MN, Cingi A, Yegen C, Yalın R, Aktan AO. Early prediction of normocalcemia after thyroid surgery. World J Surg 2005;29:1288–1293

34. Luu Q, Andersen PE, Adams J, Wax MK, Cohen JI. The predictive value of perioperative calcium levels after thyroid/parathyroid surgery. Head Neck 2002;24:63–67

35. Payne RJ, Hier MP, Tamilia M, Mac Namara E, Young J, Black MJ. Same-day discharge after total thyroidectomy: the value of 6-hour serum parathyroid hormone and calcium levels. Head Neck 2005;27:1–7

36. Payne RJ, Tewfik MA, Hier MP, et al. Benefits resulting from 1- and 6-hour parathyroid hormone and calcium levels after thyroidectomy. Otolaryngol Head Neck Surg 2005;133:386–390

37. Panzer C, Beazley R, Braverman L. Rapid preoperative preparation for severe hyperthyroid Graves' disease. J Clin Endocrinol Metab 2004;89:2142–2144

21 Radio-Guided Thyroid Surgery

James Ragland and Brendan C. Stack Jr.

The use of radio-guided surgery has evolved from the experiences in sentinel lymph node mapping in breast cancer and melanoma to include parathyroid, thyroid, prostate, pulmonary, and gastric cancers.[1-7] Early reports from these new experiences of radio-guided surgery are mostly positive. The use of radio-guided surgical approaches for thyroid carcinoma is one of the newest uses of this technology. This method is most promising for helping surgeons better manage local recurrence and regional metastatic spread in the neck, but has the possibility of applications at any location. This chapter describes how using readily available radioisotopes can precisely identify thyroid tissue and make reoperation safer and more effective.

Background

The management of the neck in thyroid carcinoma has long been debated. The propensity for local recurrence for well-differentiated thyroid cancer (WDTC) can be high even after total thyroidectomy and postoperative treatment with iodine 131 (I-131). Simon et al[8] reported on 252 patients with differentiated thyroid carcinoma treated with total thyroidectomy and postoperative I-131 for tumors higher than stage I, and found 31% required reoperation for regional recurrence. A significant increase in recurrence was found in patients who did not have an initial neck dissection. Performance of lymph node dissection was an independent predictor of survival.[9,10] Using a focused surgical approach to cervical lymphatics is proving to be a valuable technique to localize and excise recurrent metastatic thyroid carcinoma.[7] Traditional radiographic imaging techniques, such as ultrasound, computed tomography (CT), and magnetic resonance imaging (MRI), are sensitive at defining anatomic abnormalities but lack the specificity of radioactive uptake studies at identifying thyroid tissue versus postoperative scar or other anatomic changes.[11] Due to the relatively good prognosis for patients with recurrent thyroid carcinoma, it will be difficult to assess an increase in overall survival with radio-guided surgery for many years. This should not, however, discourage the use of this approach as well as its prospective study. A detailed discussion of the pathophysiology of metastatic thyroid disease is beyond the scope of this chapter. Instead, we focus on the techniques, methods, and future plans for radio-guided thyroid operations and how this technique can be incorporated into the practice of thyroid surgeons.

Radio-guided surgery enhances the surgeon's ability to quickly identify and remove thyroid tissue that otherwise might not be grossly identifiable intraoperatively or identifiable by preoperative imaging, and confirms that no residual tissue remains at the end of the procedure. To work with probes that are easily handled and sensitive to a radionuclide in tissues, two technologies using either diodes or scintillating crystals can be employed, depending on the energy of the radioisotope to be used.[12] It should be noted that there is a difference between radio-guided surgery and traditional sentinel lymphoscintigraphy. When using lymphoscintigraphy for identification of a sentinel node or pathway of drainage from a tumor bed, vital blue dye or radioactive marker is injected into the tumor bed and the first-echelon lymph nodes are found and removed either by following the dye or by gamma-probe localization. This nodal level is presumed to have the highest likelihood of containing occult tumor (an indirect localization).[13] If the nodes are positive for tumor spread, a formal unguided dissection of regional lymph nodes is often performed. Radio-guided surgery is able to directly identify tissue of interest in any location or distance from primary tumor by using systemic administration of radiotracer specifically taken up by thyroid cells and thus allowing the intraoperative localization with a gamma probe.[4,14-16] This ability to localize is independent of lymphatic flow.

Littmann et al[17] first reported using I-131 and intraoperative probe-guided neck dissection in thyroid carcinoma in 1980. Waddington et al[18] reported using the technique to localize a persistent recurrence of medullary thyroid carcinoma in 1994 with the somatostatin analogue indium-111 pentetreotide. Beginning in the late 1990s many of the radioisotopes used in thyroid diagnostic imaging, including technetium-99m-sestamibi, 18-fluoro-2-deoxyglucose positron emission tomography (^{18}F-FDG-PET), and iodines 131 and 123, have been used in localization surgeries.[11,18-25] The decision to use one isotope over another from a surgical standpoint is usually made based on which radioisotope was used for the original diagnosis of recurrence/persistence. A positive uptake scan is dependent on the affinity of the tumor cells for a certain radioisotope. This in itself is a major area of study in the imaging of thyroid carcinoma. Because there are many isotopes available for clinical thyroid imaging, we discuss them individually.

Iodine

Total thyroidectomy, followed by I-131 treatment and thyroid hormone replacement therapy, represents the standard of care for most patients with differentiated thyroid

Table 21.1 Properties of Iodine Isotopes

	Energy	Half-life	Emission	Surgical Timing
I-123	159 keV	13 hours	Gamma	12–24 hours
I-131	364 keV	8 days	Gamma and Beta	5 days to 3 weeks

Data from Gulec SA, Eckert M, Woltering EA. Gamma probe-guided lymph node dissection ("gamma picking") in differentiated thyroid carcinoma. Clin Nucl Med 2002;27:859–861.

cancer.[26] Management of locoregional recurrence after the initial treatment is somewhat controversial, as some authors recommend repeated I-131 treatments and others recommend surgical resection.[27,28] Indeed, I-131 uptake was still detectable after three I-131 treatment doses in 24% of patients in a large series by Pacini et al,[29] indicating persistent disease.[30] Even a negative high dose I-131 scan with negative thyroglobulin levels may not be adequate in predicting cure.[29] This issue is further confounded by a proliferation of patients with measurable thyroglobulin without clinically demonstrable disease.

Radio-guided thyroid surgery (RGTS) using both I-131 and I-123 have been described[7,25,31,32] (**Table 21.1**). I-123, which is exclusively a gamma emitter, is about six times more detectable than I-131, a mixed gamma and beta emitter, on imaging scans for the same administered activity.[33] This makes I-123 a better choice for diagnostic and follow-up imaging.[33] I-131 is still commonly used for imaging, due to its lower cost, availability, and use as the therapeutic workhorse of medical thyroid ablation. Its ablative properties come from its β-emissions, which can be present even in low imaging doses of 2 to 10 mCi. This has led to the description of the *stunning* phenomenon, which is another disadvantage of using I-131 for imaging. Stunning occurs when a low imaging dose (2 to 10 mCi) of I-131 is given, which causes a later therapeutic dose (100 to 150 mCi) to have less therapeutic effect due to a blunted uptake by previously stunned thyroid cells.[33,34] To avoid stunning and to increase sensitivity to more lesions on imaging, low diagnostic doses of 2 to 5 mCi are not recommended prior to RGTS, only full therapeutic doses of 100 mCi or more.[33,35] In fact, early in RGTS descriptions, Travagli et al[11] described 18 patients in their study who had an I-131 total body scan (TBS) with both 2 to 5 mCi and 100 mCi. In 10 patients (56%), the high-dose I-131 TBS depicted foci of uptake that were not suspected with 2 to 5 mCi, thus stopping the low-dose arm of the study altogether. Only one report has recently recommended low diagnostic doses of 2 to 5 mCi of I-131 in a series of only four patients.[36]

Although various authors have described I-131 RGTS on a case report basis, the intraoperative protocol for recurrent WDTC first proposed by Travagli et al,[11] and followed up by Salvatori et al[35] takes place over 1 week. It begins on day 0 when the patient receives 100 mCi of I-131 in a hypothyroid state (thyroid-stimulating hormone [TSH] >30 μU/mL). An I-131 TBS and spot neck images are obtained on day 4. On day 5, a complete neck dissection of neoplastic areas is performed using an intraoperative handheld gamma probe. After resection is completed, the tissues of the dissected neck are rescanned with the handheld gamma probe to verify complete resection. The protocol finishes after 7 days (day 7) when an image is obtained using the residual radioactivity from the initial dose to confirm the completeness of surgery.[11,25,35] The patient inclusion criteria for both series was the presence of persistent or recurrent radioiodine-positive lymph node metastases after at least two radioiodine treatments. Other criteria were clinical evidence of lymph node metastases, positive neck ultrasonography (US) or neck and chest CT studies, and detectable serum Tg values.[11,35]

Both authors demonstrated the benefit of the radioguided method by identifying tumor intraoperatively that was either not seen on imaging or would have been missed due to its presence in scar, behind carotid sheath vessels, or within the mediastinum. In fact, Travagli's series of 54 patients and Salvatori's 10 patients showed that 15% and 53%, respectively, of lesions found histologically were only picked up by gamma-probe guidance. Because the authors were also performing complete neck dissections, both studies were able to give false-negative rates of 25% and 5%, respectively, based on histologic lesions not found by either I-131 imaging or gamma probe. This was taken as evidence that complete nodal dissection with probe guidance in cases of recurrence is superior to gamma-probe "picking" of lesions. The lesion to background (L/B) ratio found by Travagli to indicate tumor was as low as 1.5:1. Of note, even though a high dose of I-131 was given only 4 days prior to surgery, no significant amount of radiation exposure was detected on the surgeon or the instruments in either study.[11,35]

The above protocol is not the only method of I-131 RGTS. Spieth et al[37] in 2003 described the use of recombinant human TSH (Thyrogen®, thyrotropin α, Genzyme Corp., Cambridge, MA) given prior to a therapeutic 151-mCi dose of I-131 and radio-guided surgery for papillary carcinoma. This not only allowed the suspected recurrence to be localized by scintigraphy and subsequently with the gamma probe, but also kept the patient from having to be hypothyroid through the perioperative period. Scurry et al[7] recently reported using RGTS to identify nonpalpable papillary carcinoma 3 weeks after the original ablative/treatment dose of I-131 (**Fig. 21.1**). Indeed, further progress may lie in the use of prototype portable gamma cameras that can theoretically perform postoperative imaging while still in the operating room.[38]

I-123-metaiodobenzylguanidine (I-123-MIBG) has also been used in RGTS.[24,31,33,39] Its advantage over I-131 as an imaging modality has allowed it to be used to identify WDTC that was negative on I-131 scans. It has been described for use in papillary and multiple endocrine neoplasia type II (MEN-II)-associated medullary thyroid carcinoma. Technical differences in RGTS between the two radioisotopes are substantial as described by Gulec et al.[24] I-123 emits a 159-keV gamma photon, compared with the high-energy 364 keV of I-131. This necessitates using a different gamma-probe setting for localization, specifically 152 keV. This is close to the energy of technetium-99m (Tc-99m), and the preprogrammed setting for technetium can be used. Uptake of I-123 by the thyroid gland is almost immediate compared with I-131. Any thyroid tissue present retains the radioiodine for several days and allows for washout of normal iodine-avid salivary tissues over a short time. This provides the optimal L/B ratio and places surgical timing at around 12 to 24 hours. The half-life of I-123 is 13 hours compared with 8 days for I-131. Oral forms of Na–I-123 are available in capsules and have been used for RGTS in as low as 1-mCi oral doses.

The clinical descriptions of I-123 in RGTS are limited to case reports. Shimotake et al[39] in Japan described focal resection of hot spots of recurrent medullary thyroid carcinoma in the neck. In a promising report, Gulec et al[24] used RGTS with I-123 to perform the neck exploration during the initial thyroidectomy in one patient. Foci of tumor were found in two lymph nodes less than 0.5 cm with an L/B ratio of 10:1. These nodes were otherwise nonidentifiable, and this patient would not have had lymph node resection without this localization.[24]

I-125 is another radioactive iodine isotope. However, due to its low-energy photons, it is poorly seen on preoperative imaging. Therefore, it requires another imaging modality for recurrence to be diagnosed. The low energy may also inhibit it from being localized behind other structures such as the sternum or clavicles and is thus not beneficial in RGTS.[37] Its long half-life of almost 60 days is not practical with other isotopes being readily available.[24]

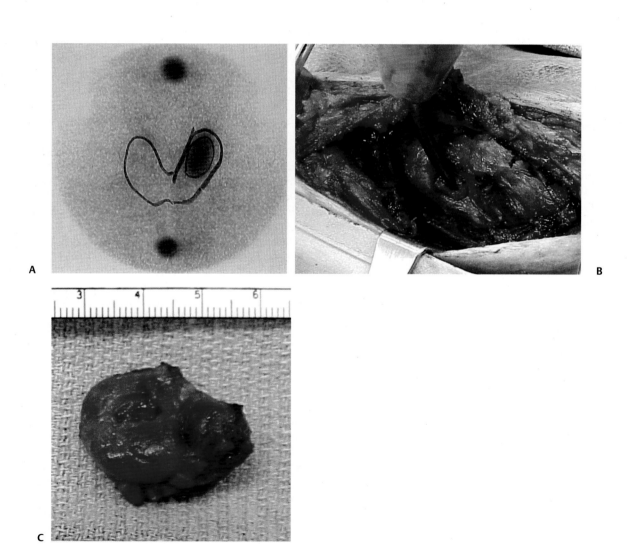

Fig. 21.1 **(A)** A postsurgical scan from a patient referred for postoperative I-131 ablation. Significant uptake was noted in the left upper lobe. Superior and inferior uptake is seen at the chin and sternal markers by nuclear medicine. **(B)** The left thyroid bed was explored and residual thyroid tissue was identified. **(C)** The excised thyroid tissue was identified as radioactive in vivo and ex vivo. There was a drop of the operative bed down to background after the lesion was removed.

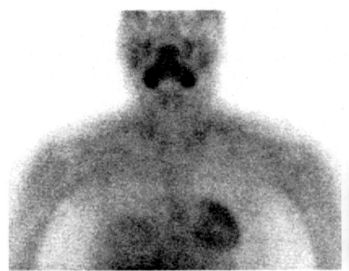
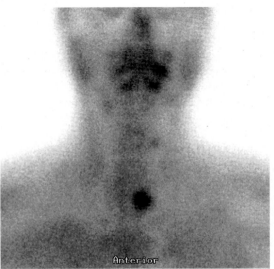

Fig. 21.2 **(A)** A patient with a regional recurrence of thyroid cancer that is not iodine avid. **(B)** The same patient as in **A** with a focus of technetium-99m uptake in the left lower neck. This uptake was used on a separate occasion to effect a successful radio-guided surgical excision of this lesion.

Technetium-99 Guided Surgery

Technetium-99m and Tc-99m–labeled agents such as sestamibi (Tc-99m-MIBI) have been used for thyroid imaging for many years. It is one of the many radioisotopes whose benefit comes to bear when the tumor is no longer iodine-avid, or is considered a nonfunctioning WDTC. Using Tc-99m is also described for use with medullary thyroid carcinoma or non–follicle-derived thyroid carcinoma.[22]

Despite their inability to take up radio-labeled iodine agents, nonfunctioning WDTC metastases generally maintain the capability to secrete thyroglobulin (Tg). Elevated Tg combined with negative iodine uptake scans is the basis for use of other isotopes, such as 18-FDG and Tc-99m, in the search for recurrent thyroid disease. Tc-99m-MIBI imaging was found to have a 94% sensitivity in localizing iodine-negative lesions in the neck. When Tc-99m was compared head to head with I-131 in patients with known iodine-avid tumors, however, the two agents were equally sensitive.[19,40] So far, reports of the use of Tc-99m-MIBI in RGTS for recurrent well-differentiated thyroid cancer (WDTC) have been in patients with extensive scarring from previous surgeries, and the use of the guided technique facilitated the resections.[23,41]

Technical aspects of using Tc-99m for RGTS were first described by Boz et al[23] and later by Rubello et al.[41] It has a half-life of only 6 hours and emits gamma energy at 140 keV. Its use is similar to that of other RGTS methods described. Boz et al described a patient case report using Tc-99m given at a dose of 20 mCi 2 hours prior to surgery and found a tumor-to-background ratio of 4:1 as compared to the lesion detected on scintigraphy, which showed the tumor bed equal to background after resection and normal postoperative Tg levels.[23] Rubello et al modified the method for 46 patients using 1 mCi low-dose Tc-99m and administering it in the operating room immediately prior to surgery to reduce overall radioactive exposure. They found a tumor-to-background ratio of 2.44:1 ± 0.93. Rubello et al also reported that Tc-99m delivers a lower radiation dose to operative personnel than I-131[25,41] (**Fig. 21.2**).

Recently, a Tc-99m–labeled somatostatin analogue, Tc-99m-depreotide (NeoTect, Berlex, Montvale, NJ), was described and may hold promise in future RGTS protocols in medullary thyroid carcinoma (MTC). MTC is of neuroendocrine origin and contains high levels of somatostatin receptors, making its detection amenable to radio-labeled somatostatin analogues.[18,42]

Indium-111 Pentetreotide

Indium-111-pentetreotide, Octreoscan, is a radio-labeled somatostatin analogue that has been used for the detection of somatostatin receptor positive tumors, which are predominantly of neuroendocrine origin such as medullary thyroid carcinoma.[18,22,42–49] It was the isotope used in the first description of radio-guided thyroid surgery for recurrence by Waddington et al[18] in 1994. Method descriptions for using indium-111-pentetreotide in RGTS are limited. Adams et al[22] described the optimal timing of surgical resection after dose administration to be within 24 hours. They also recommended a tumor-to-background ratio of 2:1. Overall, however, their limited series showed indium-111-pentetreotide to be inferior to Tc-99m(V)-DMSA for RGTS in medullary thyroid carcinoma.

As would be expected, indium-111-pentetreotide is not an effective agent for WDTCs such as papillary and follicular carcinoma.[50] It has been shown to be useful for the detection of primary and metastatic neuroendocrine tumors of the head and neck that are larger than 1.5 cm.[44] Technetium-99m-depreotide (NeoTect), a somatostatin receptor analogue tagged with Tc-99m, could have wider impact in the future for medullary thyroid carcinoma due to Tc-99m being more widely used and less expensive.[42,43]

Thallium 201

Thallium 201 is a nonspecific tumor localizing radioisotope for use in patients who may have thyroid cancer recurrence despite having negative iodine uptake scans. The usefulness of this agent, however, is uncertain due to sensitivities found in the literature ranging from 45 to 94%, but this agent overall is similar to Tc-99m in iodine-negative patients.[19,51–54] Though RGTS using thallium 201 has not been described to date, it is reasonable to assume that given a patient with an elevated Tg, and positive thallium-201 scan, indicating a site of recurrence, that a radio-guided approach could be taken.

Thallium emits gamma rays of 167 keV, making it close to Tc-99m for probes with fixed isotope settings; otherwise, an adjustable probe offers better fine-tuning into a 20% detection window. The physical half-life of thallium 201 is 73 hours, but it has relatively rapid uptake into tissues, allowing the possibility of either same-day surgical procedures or delayed procedures to allow for scheduling after a positive scan. The usual intravenously administered dose for clinical imaging in adults is 2.0 to 3.0 mCi. Estimated total body radiation exposure dose for thallium 201 is 0.72 rad/3 mCi.[55] Thallium also does not require a hypothyroid state for uptake. These are technical details to be considered if a radio-guided approach is considered after a positive thallium-201 uptake scan and the need for surgery is determined.

Positron Emission Tomography–Guided Surgery

With positron emission tomography (PET) imaging becoming more frequently used in thyroid metastatic follow-up, being able to harness the radioactive output of ^{18}F-FDG-PET in RGTS was the logical next step. The basis for the emerging use of ^{18}F-FDG-PET is centered around the consistent finding of a "flip-flop" between radioiodine positive and ^{18}F-FDG-PET–positive tumors.[47,56–58] This means that in patients with elevated Tg and positive radioiodine scans, the ^{18}F-FDG-PET scan is usually negative, whereas in patients with elevated Tg and negative radioiodine scans, the ^{18}F-FDG-PET scan is usually positive and indicates a more aggressive tumor with a higher mortality rate.[56,59] Based on these findings, and the results by Wang et al[60] that showed I-131 had little or no treatment effect on tumors that were

^{18}F-FDG-PET positive, surgical resection is a more imperative option.

Kraeber-Bodere et al[21] described the feasibility of RGTS with ^{18}F-FDG as an agent for radio-guided surgery in the first published report of this technique. In their protocol, patients with positive PET scans and elevated Tg were given a mean dose of 265 MBq (range, 165 to 526) of ^{18}F-FDG 30 minutes prior to surgery. Six of these patients were given recombinant TSH (rTSH) stimulation with 0.9 mg 24 to 48 hours prior to surgery based on reports of increased ^{18}F-FDG uptake compared with nonstimulation patients.[61] A hand-held gamma probe with a BgO scintillator (Modelo 2 Localization Monitor; Oris/Damri, Gif-sur-Yvette, France) was used intraoperatively. ^{18}F-FDG emits a high-energy radiation of 511 keV, requiring a probe with a range capable of that level. (This probe is currently not Food and Drug Administration [FDA] approved, and is therefore labeled as experimental for this purpose). Due to the rapid washout and short half-life of 110 minutes for FDG, a decay constant K is used to compare counts obtained at different times (K = $2^{(\text{time}/108\text{minute})}$, corrected counts = counts $\times$ 1/K) (K = time since the injection divided by the ^{18}F half life). All lesions detected by preoperative ^{18}F-FDG-PET were also detected with the probe. The tumor-to-background ratios were relatively close to one another, but by using tumor-to-shoulder rather than tumor-to-neck, the difference was increased from 1.40 to 1.73. Mean radioactivity at the tumor site was decreased by 22% after resection of the identified lesion. The ex vivo mean tumor-to-normal tissue ratio was higher than prior to removal (in vivo readings) at 2.4 (**Fig. 21.3**). The surgeon's hands were exposed to 90 to 270 μSv of radiation, which is considered to be minor. Patients need to be as inactive as possible prior to this procedure, similar to during a PET scanning, secondary to the increased uptake of FDG into metabolically active normal tissues. In fact, tension in neck muscles has been interpreted as nodal metastasis on routine PET imaging.[62]

Overall, PET imaging and the use of ^{18}F-FDG have many advantages over thyroid radio-isotopes. ^{18}F-FDG does not require any thyroid function to be present in highly dedifferentiated tumors because its uptake is based on metabolic activity. Increased metabolic activity is associated with a more aggressive tumor in most instances including thyroid carcinoma. It is able to identify tumor even when the ability to make Tg is lost from dedifferentiation. PET has superior resolution to single photon emission computed tomography (SPECT) imaging used with other radioisotopes; PET resolution is on the order of 5 mm or less compared with 1 to 1.5 cm for SPECT. Better imaging results are obtained by rTSH stimulation and a euthyroid state, which precludes the need for a hypothyroid state.

Conclusion

Although radio-guided thyroid surgery is still very early in its development, it is offering promise for the future

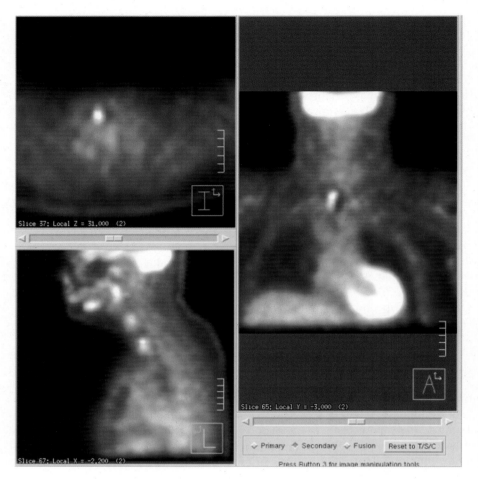

Fig. 21.3 A patient with iodine negative, 18-FDG-PET–positive thyroid cancer recurrence in the central neck. Images are shown from the upper left in a clockwise order: axial, coronal, and sagittal. The sagittal image demonstrates physiologic uptake in Waldeyer ring, and the mylohyoid and intrinsic laryngeal muscles. This patient was given an FDG dose on the morning of surgery to guide the exploration and successful excision of recurrent cancer.

of recurrent and metastatic thyroid cancer surgery. It may not be long before RGTS will be part of the initial thyroidectomy rather than an adjunct to treatment of recurrent disease. Even though it appears to make surgical excisions of recurrences easier, it should be remembered that it is still a localization and adjunctive method, and a fo-

cused lymph node level(s) dissection is still the recommendation for most recurrent metastatic thyroid disease. Radio-guided "berry picking" of radioactive lesions is essentially the same approach as has been done for clinically evident cervical nodal disease in the past and should be discouraged.

References

1. Kitagawa Y, Fujii H, Mukai M, Kubota T, Otani Y, Kitajima M. Radio-guided sentinel node detection for gastric cancer. Br J Surg 2002;89:604–608
2. Sortini D, Feo CV, Carcoforo P, et al. Thoracoscopic localization techniques for patients with solitary pulmonary nodule and history of malignancy. Ann Thorac Surg 2005;79:258–262
3. Wawroschek F, Vogt H, Wengenmair H, et al. Prostate lymphoscintigraphy and radio-guided surgery for sentinel lymph node identification in prostate cancer. Technique and results of the first 350 cases. Urol Int 2003;70:303–310
4. Albertini JJ, Cruse CW, Rapaport D, et al. Intraoperative radio-lympho-scintigraphy improves sentinel lymph node identification for patients with melanoma. Ann Surg 1996;223:217–224
5. Cuntz MC, Levine EA, O'Dorisio TM, et al. Intraoperative gamma detection of 125I-lanreotide in women with primary breast cancer. Ann Surg Oncol 1999;6:367–372
6. Ruda JM, Hollenbeak CS, Stack BC. A systematic review of the diag-

nosis and treatment of primary hyperparathyroidism from 1995 to 2003. Otolaryngol Head Neck Surg 2005;132:359–372
7. Scurry WC, Lamarre E, Stack B. Radioguided neck dissection in recurrent metastatic papillary thyroid carcinoma. Am J Otolaryngol 2006;27:61–63
8. Simon D, Goretzki PE, Witte J, Roher HD. Incidence of regional recurrence guiding radicality in differentiated thyroid carcinoma. World J Surg 1996;20:860–866 discussion 866
9. Rosa Pelizzo M, Toniato A, Boschin IM, et al. Locally advanced differentiated thyroid carcinoma: a 35-year mono-institutional experience in 280 patients. Nucl Med Commun 2005;26:965–968
10. Hay ID, Bergstralh EJ, Goellner JR, Ebersold JR, Grant CS. Predicting outcome in papillary thyroid carcinoma: development of a reliable prognostic scoring system in a cohort of 1779 patients surgically treated at one institution during 1940 through 1989. Surgery 1993;114:1050–1057, discussion 1057–1058

11. Travagli JP, Cailleux AF, Ricard M, et al. Combination of radioiodine (131I) and probe-guided surgery for persistent or recurrent thyroid carcinoma. J Clin Endocrinol Metab 1998;83:2675–2680

12. Tenenbaum F, Ricard M. [Perioperative detection probes. Evaluation and perspectives in endocrinology.] Ann Endocrinol (Paris) 1997;58:39–46

13. Stack BC Jr. Lymphoscintigraphy and Sentinel Lymph Node Biopsy Techniques in Cutaneous Melanoma. Facial Plastic Surgery Clinics of North America 2003:61–67

14. Wong JH, Cagle LA, Morton DL. Lymphatic drainage of skin to a sentinel lymph node in a feline model. Ann Surg 1991;214:637–641

15. Morton DL, Wen DR, Wong JH, et al. Technical details of intraoperative lymphatic mapping for early stage melanoma. Arch Surg 1992;127:392–399

16. Stack BC, Lowe VJ, Hardeman S. Radioguided surgical advancements for head and neck oncology. South Med J 2000;93:360–363

17. Littmann K, Magdsick G, Strotges MW, Eigler FW. [Intraoperative localization measurement following preoperative radioiodine marking to facilitate the treatment of differentiated thyroid carcinoma.] Chirurg 1980;51:389–394

18. Waddington WA, Kettle AG, Heddle RM, Coakley AJ. Intraoperative localization of recurrent medullary carcinoma of the thyroid using indium-111 pentetreotide and a nuclear surgical probe. Eur J Nucl Med 1994;21:363–364

19. Seabold JE, Gurll N, Schurrer ME, Aktay R, Kirchner PT. Comparison of 99mTc-methoxyisobutyl isonitrile and 201Tl scintigraphy for detection of residual thyroid cancer after 131I ablative therapy. J Nucl Med 1999;40:1434–1440

20. Carril JM, Quirce R, Serrano J, et al. Total-body scintigraphy with thallium-201 and iodine-131 in the follow-up of differentiated thyroid cancer. J Nucl Med 1997;38:686–692

21. Kraeber-Bodere F, Cariou B, Curtet C, et al. Feasibility and benefit of fluorine 18-fluoro-2-deoxyglucose-guided surgery in the management of radioiodine-negative differentiated thyroid carcinoma metastases. Surgery 2005;138:1176–1182

22. Adams S, Acker P, Lorenz M, Staib-Sebler E, Hor G. Radioisotope-guided surgery in patients with pheochromocytoma and recurrent medullary thyroid carcinoma: a comparison of preoperative and intraoperative tumor localization with histopathologic findings. Cancer 2001;92:263–270

23. Boz A, Arici C, Gungor F, Yildiz A, Colak T, Karayalcin B. Gamma probe-guided resection and scanning with TC-99m MIBI of a local recurrence of follicular thyroid carcinoma. Clin Nucl Med 2001;26:820–822

24. Gulec SA, Eckert M, Woltering EA. Gamma probe-guided lymph node dissection ("gamma picking") in differentiated thyroid carcinoma. Clin Nucl Med 2002;27:859–861

25. Rubello D, Salvatori M, Pelizzo MR, et al. Radio-guided surgery of differentiated thyroid cancer using (131)I or 99mTc-Sestamibi. Nucl Med Commun 2006;27:1–4

26. Shaha AR. Management of the neck in thyroid cancer. Otolaryngol Clin North Am 1998;31:823–831

27. Grebe SK, Hay ID. Thyroid cancer nodal metastases: biologic significance and therapeutic considerations. Surg Oncol Clin North Am 1996;5:43–63

28. Coburn M, Teates D, Wanebo HJ. Recurrent thyroid cancer. Role of surgery versus radioactive iodine (I131). Ann Surg 1994;219:587–593, discussion 593–585

29. Pacini F, Cetani F, Miccoli P, et al. Outcome of 309 patients with metastatic differentiated thyroid carcinoma treated with radioiodine. World J Surg 1994;18:600–604

30. Bachelot A, Leboulleux S, Baudin E, et al. Neck recurrence from thyroid carcinoma: serum thyroglobulin and high-dose total body scan are not reliable criteria for cure after radioiodine treatment. Clin Endocrinol (Oxf) 2005;62:376–379

31. Mansberg R, Crawford B, Uren RF, Thompson JF. Minimally invasive radio-guided surgery for recurrent thyroid cancer using iodine-123. Clin Nucl Med 2005;30:43–44

32. Schachter P, Shimonov M, Lorberboim M. [Combined radioiodine (I-131) treatment and radio-guided surgery for recurrent cervical well-differentiated thyroid cancer.] Harefuah 2005;144:168–172

33. Ali N, Sebastian C, Foley RR, et al. The management of differentiated thyroid cancer using 123I for imaging to assess the need for 131I therapy. Nucl Med Commun 2006;27:165–169

34. Robbins RJ, Schlumberger MJ. The evolving role of (131)I for the treatment of differentiated thyroid carcinoma. J Nucl Med 2005;46(suppl 1):28S–37S

35. Salvatori M, Rufini V, Reale F, et al. Radio-guided surgery for lymph node recurrences of differentiated thyroid cancer. World J Surg 2003;27:770–775

36. Negele T, Meisetschlager G, Bruckner T, Scheidhauer K, Schwaiger M, Vogelsang H. Radio-guided surgery for persistent differentiated papillary thyroid cancer: case presentations and review of the literature. Langenbecks Arch Surg 2006;391:178–186, Epub 2006 Feb 21

37. Spieth ME, Standiford SB, Starkman ME, Gough J. Recombinant TSH-stimulated, radioguided differentiated thyroid carcinoma surgery. Clin Med Res 2003;1:53–56

38. Sanchez F, Benlloch JM, Escat B, et al. Design and tests of a portable mini gamma camera. Med Phys 2004;31:1384–1397

39. Shimotake T, Tsuda T, Aoi S, Fumino S, Iwai N. Iodine 123 metaiodobenzylguanidine radio-guided navigation surgery for recurrent medullary thyroid carcinoma in a girl with multiple endocrine neoplasia type 2B. J Pediatr Surg 2005;40:1643–1646

40. Casara D, Rubello D, Saladini G, et al. Clinical approach in patients with metastatic differentiated thyroid carcinoma and negative 131I whole body scintigraphy: importance of 99mTc MIBI scan combined with high resolution neck ultrasonography. Tumori 1999;85:122–127

41. Rubello D, Piotto A, Pagetta C, Pelizzo MR, Casara D. (99m)Tc-MIBI radio-guided surgery for recurrent thyroid carcinoma: technical feasibility and procedure, and preliminary clinical results. Eur J Nucl Med Mol Imaging 2002;29:1201–1205

42. Weiner RE, Thakur ML. Radiolabeled peptides in oncology: role in diagnosis and treatment. BioDrugs 2005;19:145–163

43. Bangard M, Behe M, Guhlke S, et al. Detection of somatostatin receptor-positive tumours using the new 99mTc-tricine-HYNIC-D-Phe1-Tyr3-octreotide: first results in patients and comparison with 111In-DTPA-D-Phe1-octreotide. Eur J Nucl Med 2000;27:628–637

44. Whiteman ML, Serafini AN, Telischi FF, Civantos FJ, Falcone S. 111In octreotide scintigraphy in the evaluation of head and neck lesions. AJNR Am J Neuroradiol 1997;18:1073–1080

45. Valli N, Catargi B, Ronci N, et al. Evaluation of indium-111 pentetreotide somatostatin receptor scintigraphy to detect recurrent thyroid carcinoma in patients with negative radioiodine scintigraphy. Thyroid 1999;9:583–589

46. Schirmer WJ, Melvin WS, Rush RM, et al. Indium-111-pentetreotide scanning versus conventional imaging techniques for the localization of gastrinoma. Surgery 1995;118:1105–1113

47. Gotthardt M, Battmann A, Hoffken H, et al. 18F-FDG PET, somatostatin receptor scintigraphy, and CT in metastatic medullary thyroid carcinoma: a clinical study and an analysis of the literature. Nucl Med Commun 2004;25:439–443

48. Tisell LE, Ahlman H, Wangberg B, et al. Somatostatin receptor scintigraphy in medullary thyroid carcinoma. Br J Surg 1997;84:543–547

49. Berna L, Chico A, Matias-Guiu X, et al. Use of somatostatin analogue scintigraphy in the localization of recurrent medullary thyroid carcinoma. Eur J Nucl Med 1998;25:1482–1488

50. Garin E, Devillers A, Le Cloirec J, et al. Use of indium-111 pentetreotide somatostatin receptor scintigraphy to detect recurrent thyroid carcinoma in patients without detectable iodine uptake. Eur J Nucl Med 1998;25:687–694

51. Brendel AJ, Guyot M, Jeandot R, Lefort G, Manciet G. Thallium-201 imaging in the follow-up of differentiated thyroid carcinoma. J Nucl Med 1988;29:1515–1520

52. Dadparvar S, Krishna L, Brady LW, et al. The role of iodine-131 and thallium-201 imaging and serum thyroglobulin in the management of differentiated thyroid carcinoma. Cancer 1993;71:3767–3773

53. Hoefnagel CA, Delprat CC, Marcuse HR, de Vijlder JJ. Role of thallium-201 total-body scintigraphy in follow-up of thyroid carcinoma. J Nucl Med 1986;27:1854–1857

54. Unal S, Menda Y, Adalet I, et al. Thallium-201, technetium-99m-tetrofosmin and iodine-131 in detecting differentiated thyroid carcinoma metastases. J Nucl Med 1998;39:1897–1902

55. Okudan B, Smitherman TC. The value and throughput of rest thallium-201/stress technetium-99m sestamibi dual-isotope myocardial SPECT. Anadolu Kardiyol Derg 2004;4:161–168

56. Robbins RJ, Wan Q, Grewal RK, et al. Real-time prognosis for metastatic thyroid carcinoma based on FDG-PET scanning. J Clin Endocrinol Metab 2006;91:498–505

57. Brandt-Mainz K, Muller SP, Gorges R, Saller B, Bockisch A. The value of fluorine-18 fluorodeoxyglucose PET in patients with medullary thyroid cancer. Eur J Nucl Med 2000;27:490–496

58. Al-Nahhas A. Dedifferentiated thyroid carcinoma: the imaging role of 18F-FDG PET and non-iodine radiopharmaceuticals. Nucl Med Commun 2004;25:891–895

59. Feine U, Lietzenmayer R, Hanke JP, Held J, Wohrle H, Muller-Schauenburg W. Fluorine-18-FDG and iodine-131-iodide uptake in thyroid cancer. J Nucl Med 1996;37:1468–1472

60. Wang W, Larson SM, Tuttle RM, et al. Resistance of [18f]-fluorodeoxyglucose-avid metastatic thyroid cancer lesions to treatment with high-dose radioactive iodine. Thyroid 2001;11:1169–1175

61. Chin BB, Patel P, Cohade C, Ewertz M, Wahl R, Ladenson P. Recombinant human thyrotropin stimulation of fluoro-D-glucose positron emission tomography uptake in well-differentiated thyroid carcinoma. J Clin Endocrinol Metab 2004;89:91–95

62. Cook GJ, Maisey MN, Fogelman I. Normal variants, artefacts and interpretative pitfalls in PET imaging with 18-fluoro-2-deoxyglucose and carbon-11 methionine. Eur J Nucl Med 1999;26:1363–1378

22 Office-Based Ultrasound of the Thyroid and Parathyroid Glands

David L. Steward

Incorporation of neck ultrasound (US) into an office practice can improve patient care and satisfaction, build a thyroid and parathyroid surgical practice, and be fiscally sound. Office-based US machines are portable because they are about the size of a laptop computer, thus allowing easy transport to multiple practice locations, hospital floors, or operating rooms. Physicians, whether they are endocrinologists, surgeons, or radiologists, who perform their own US obtain exponentially more information through real-time imaging than can be obtained by viewing only static images. A great advantage of office-based US is that the physician who will be making the final diagnostic and therapeutic decisions has control over an inherently dynamic imaging study. When coupled with greater knowledge of patients' clinical history and disease pathophysiology, this invariably results in greater diagnostic yield.

Indications and Technique

Thyroid

Neck ultrasound is widely accepted as the optimal modality for evaluation of thyroid nodularity, and the thyroid is one of the easiest neck structures to image with US. The technique involves B mode (gray scale) scanning in the transverse/axial plane first on one side and then the other. One half of the trachea should be visible on the medial aspect of the screen and the great vessels visible laterally. A light touch minimizes compression of the jugular vein.

Longitudinal/sagittal imaging is used selectively, once pathology is identified, for confirmation and sizing in the cranial-caudal dimension. Holding the probe between the thumb and first two fingers near the skin interface allows the ring or little finger to brace on the patient to prevent sliding unintentionally. For subtle changes in position, the probe can be slightly tilted back and forth, which allows more precise movement than sliding the probe along the skin surface. Color power Doppler can be utilized to assess vascularity. Once an image is localized in real time, the image can be frozen, labeled, sized, and saved or printed for the patient's file.

The depth of penetration of the ultrasound waves depends on the frequency, with lower frequency probes penetrating more deeply than higher frequency. Most contemporary probes for office US of the neck include multiple frequencies ranging from 5 to 10 MHz or 7 to 12 MHz, providing the depth of the lower frequencies and higher resolution of the higher frequencies. The long axis of the ultrasound probe used predominately in the neck is approximately 3 cm and corresponds to the side-to-side span of the ultrasound waves. In contrast, the short axis is approximately 1 cm but the thickness of the ultrasound waves is smaller than 1 mm; hence the sound waves emanating and returning from the probe can be thought of as roughly shaped like a credit card.

The image created by ultrasound results from the piezo-electric effect of the transducer probe, which alternately sends and receives sound waves, converting them to electrical impulses. Gel is required to bridge the interface between the probe and skin surfaces. The thyroid gland should be homogeneous and of intermediate gray scale, and is considered the reference echogenicity for comparison to other structures. Abrupt interfaces between one type of tissue and another result in reflection of a greater proportion of sound waves than those that continue to penetrate, often resulting in a bright (hyperechoic) signal with a dark (hypo- or anechoic) shadow beyond. The trachea is a good example, with hyperechoic cartilage rings. Coarse calcifications within the thyroid are even more dramatic in this regard. Solid hyperfunctioning thyroid nodules tend to be mildly hyperechoic with respect to the surrounding gland. Fluid-filled or cystic nodules tend to be hypoechoic, similar to vascular structures. Cystic nodules can be differentiated from vessels as one scans from inferior to superior because nodules appear and then disappear, whereas vessels continue in one direction or another. Color Doppler can also be used but is rarely needed to differentiate nodules from vessels once sufficient experience is gained. Doppler can be used to assess the vascularity of the gland overall or a discrete nodule. Untreated Graves patients demonstrate increased vascularity throughout a relatively homogeneous thyroid gland. In contrast, Hashimoto's thyroiditis usually appears heterogeneous, with splotchy ill-defined hypoechoic areas and decreased vascularity, often associated with benign-appearing reactive lymph nodes especially inferior to the thyroid gland.

Ultrasound provides the most accurate sizing, and its sensitivity for thyroid malignancy approaches 90% in experienced hands.[1,2] Sonographic features suggestive of malignant thyroid nodules are shown in **Table 22.1**[1-3] and **Fig. 22.1**. Decisions regarding which thyroid nodules to biopsy

Table 22.1 Ultrasound Features Suggestive of Thyroid Nodule Malignancy

Irregular border
Hypoechoic
Spheroid shape
Microcalcifications
Increased intranodule vascularity

Table 22.2 Proportion of Sonographic Features in Benign Lymph Nodes Versus Papillary Carcinoma Nodal Metastasis

Ultrasound Appearance	% of Benign Nodes	% of Malignant Nodes
Size >0.6 cm	17%	93%
Absence of echogenic hilum	10%	88%
Hyperechoic relative to muscle	5%	86%
Round shape	30%	80%
Calcifications	0%	50%
Cystic component	0%	20%

in multinodular goiter should be made based not just on size but also on sonographic features suggestive of malignancy. Biopsy of the largest nodule is recommended even if sonographic features appear benign. Any nodule that appears suspicious by the criteria listed in **Table 22.1** should undergo biopsy, independent of size.

Lymph Nodes

Neck ultrasound with serum thyroglobulin is replacing radioiodine scanning for thyroid cancer surveillance with sensitivities of 96% versus 21% for recurrence.[4,5] Sonographic features of papillary carcinoma nodal metastasis are shown in **Table 22.2**[6] and **Fig. 22.2**. Lymphatic ultrasound is technically more challenging than for the thyroid gland, because most lateral lymph nodes are subcentimeter and sandwiched between the sternocleidomastoid (SCM) and prevertebral musculature. Head and neck surgeons usually have an advantage over their endocrine colleagues with their intimate knowledge of lymphatic drainage patterns and complex anatomy of the neck. The largest nodes almost always appear on the posterior aspect of the submandibular gland (level I) and are rarely involved in thyroid cancer. In contrast, lymph nodes identified in levels II, III, IV, and VI should be carefully evaluated for features of malignancy. Lymph nodes posterior to the great vessels

likely represent metastasis along the inferior thyroid artery. Lymph nodes indenting the jugular vein are also highly suspicious.

A systematic routine should be employed for thyroid cancer surveillance, imaging inferiorly from the innominate artery to the thyroid cartilage superiorly to encompass level VI, then scanning inferiorly from the subclavian along the great vessels superiorly to the tail of the parotid and submandibular gland to encompass levels II to IV. Level V is imaged last, and it is most difficult, but it rarely demonstrates nodal metastasis without involvement in level II, III, or IV. Neck US should be performed every 6 to 12 months for the first 3 years after initial treatment for thyroid cancer, and annually thereafter. However, in low-risk cases with an initial undetectable thyroid-stimulating hormone (TSH)-stimulated thyroglobulin, negative antithyroglobulin antibodies, and negative neck ultrasound, basal thyroglobulin and less frequent ultrasound surveillance may be sufficient.[7]

Neck ultrasound should be performed preoperatively to assess for nodal metastasis any time that fine-needle aspiration (FNA) suggests papillary or medullary carcinoma such that adequate nodal dissection can be performed at the time of thyroidectomy.[8–10] Neck US is more sensitive than

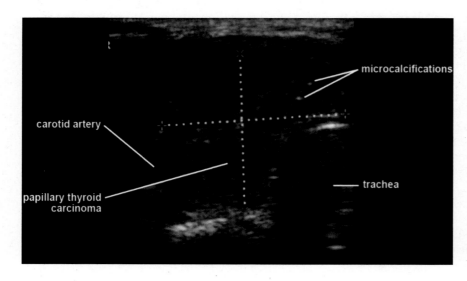

Fig. 22.1 Transverse axial image of large right papillary thyroid carcinoma with microcalcifications.

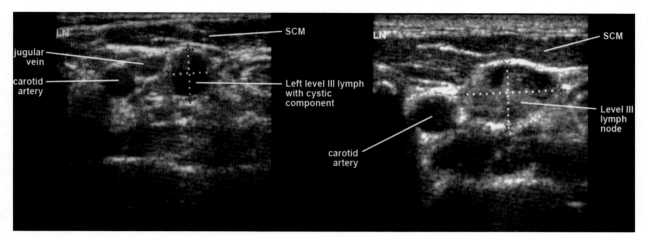

Fig. 22.2   (A,B) Transverse axial images of left level III nodal metastasis. *Abbreviation:* SCM, sternocleidomastoid.

computed tomography (CT) or magnetic resonance imaging (MRI) for nodal metastasis, often identifying subcentimeter nodal metastasis without difficulty.

Thyroid Fine-Needle Aspiration

When coupled with fine-needle biopsy, sensitivity and specificity for malignancy is further improved with lower rates of nondiagnostic specimens and reduced sample error problems when compared with fine-needle biopsy by palpation alone.

The preferred technique for US-guided FNA involves inserting the needle in the direction of the long axis of the probe to visualize the entire needle (**Fig. 22.3**) as opposed to the short axis, which visualizes only a tiny portion of the needle. Keeping the bevel of the needle tip up increases the echogenicity of the needle tip, allowing exact localization for sampling even subcentimeter lesions.

A $1\frac{1}{2}$-inch, 22-gauge needle is preferred for fine-needle biopsy, with a 25-gauge needle used for local anesthetic infiltration under the skin and anticipated needle track. A min-

imum of two separate needle samples per lesion is required but three or four are recommended. Needle biopsy performed via a fine capillary sampling technique (no syringe) is less painful, creates less bleeding, and provides better cellular architecture for the cytopathologist.[11] Proper fine-needle aspiration technique involves applying negative pressure to the syringe, only when the needle is within the lesion to be sampled. The negative pressure is then released prior to removal of the needle. The aspiration technique does increase the yield of the sample, and thus a combination of both techniques is optimal, with capillary sampling performed on the first pass. The exception is for cystic nodules, where the fluid should initially be aspirated into the syringe so as not to be lost. Subsequent needle passes should focus on more solid areas or the border of the cystic component, or preferably suspicious areas such as those demonstrating microcalcifications. Specimens should be placed on a glass slide or CytoLyt solution (Cytyc Corp., Marlborough, MA) should be used. If medullary carcinoma is suspected, specimen should be sent to the lab in CytoLyt, with instructions to perform calcitonin staining on the cell block.

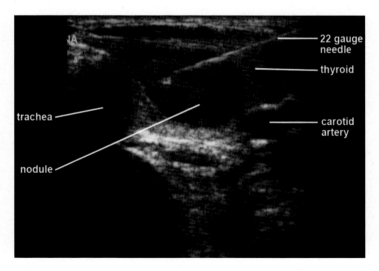

Fig. 22.3 Transverse axial image of ultrasound guided fine-needle biopsy using long axis technique.

Lymph Node Fine-Needle Aspiration

Fine-needle biopsy is often necessary to confirm nodal metastasis suspected on US, especially prior to consideration for revision surgery. However, US-guided FNA of lymph nodes is technically more challenging than for thyroid nodules due to their small size, proximity to great vessels, and tendency to bounce off the needle or, once "stuck," to move back and forth with the needle rather than allowing the needle to pass back and forth within them. Sending the needle wash for thyroglobulin measurement can aid in the diagnosis of metastatic lymph nodes but not thyroid nodules because thyroglobulin is produced by both benign and malignant thyroid tissue but should not be present in lymph nodes.[12] The aspirate should be rinsed in 1 cc of normal saline and sent in a red-topped tube to the chemistry laboratory for analysis. Simultaneous serum thyroglobulin testing is recommended to avoid false positive from blood aspirated during the biopsy.

Parathyroid

Preoperative parathyroid localization is effectively performed with office-based ultrasound but is technically more challenging than thyroid imaging. The sensitivity of US exceeds that of sestamibi for localization to the correct quadrant (87% vs. 58%) or side (91% vs. 74%).[13] Other surgeons have also demonstrated improved sensitivity of office-based US over sestamibi.[14,15] The typical sonographic appearance of parathyroid adenomas is a smooth ellipsoid- or crescent-shaped hypoechoic mass abutting the posterior surface of the thyroid if superior, and near the inferior pole of the thyroid if inferior. Examples of both are shown in **Figs. 22.4** and **22.5**.

Differentiating a superior from inferior parathyroid adenoma sonographically can at times be difficult, especially when the superior gland is located inferiorly. Using the posterior surface of the carotid artery as a surrogate marker for the plane of the recurrent laryngeal nerve on transverse

imaging can be helpful. Adenomas located deep/posterior to this plane are likely superior glands even if located near or below the inferior pole of the thyroid. This information can be very helpful intraoperatively, especially if performing a minimally invasive approach.

If an adenoma is not identified in the typical locations, search for ectopic locations should be performed to include the carotid sheath, the retroesophagus, the intrathymus, the anterior/superior mediastinum, and the intrathyroid. To improve superior mediastinal imaging, the patient should hyperextend the neck, and the probe should be used transversely at the clavicle while angling the probe to image inferiorly. This allows for easy imaging of the innominate and subclavian vasculature and can often identify superior mediastinal adenomas. To improve imaging posteriorly around the prevertebral fascia, turning up the far field gain can help, as can lowering the transducer frequency for greater depth of penetration.

Parathyroid Fine-Needle Aspiration

Parathyroid adenomas have such a characteristic appearance sonographically that tissue confirmation preoperatively is rarely necessary and cannot differentiate adenoma from carcinoma. However, when coupled with needle aspiration and measurement of parathyroid hormone (PTH) from the aspirate (diluted in 1 cc saline), intrathyroid parathyroid adenomas can be reliably differentiated from thyroid nodules.[15,16] Cytology should be performed to rule out thyroid malignancy, but it may be difficult to differentiate thyroid from parathyroid origin on cytology alone without the use of special stains (thyroglobulin, TTF1, parathormone). If special stains are desired, the aspirated specimen should be sent in CytoLyt solution rather than placed on glass slides so that a cell block can be set up. Parathyroid FNA with measurement of parathyroid hormone from the aspirate can be used to confirm suspected intrathyroidal parathyroid

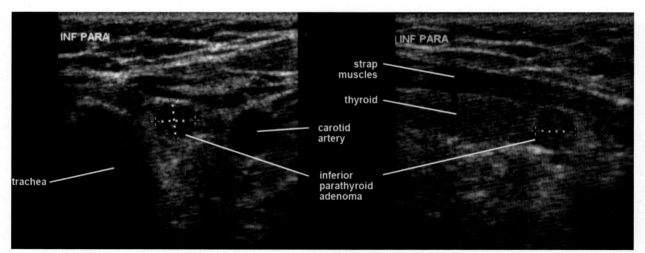

A　　**B**

Fig. 22.4 **(A,B)** Transverse axial and longitudinal/sagittal views of left inferior parathyroid adenoma. *Abbreviation:* INF PARA, inferior parathyroid.

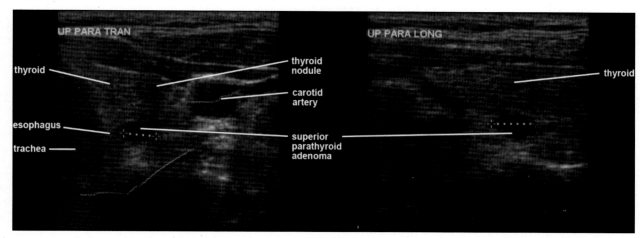

Fig. 22.5   (A,B) Transverse axial and longitudinal/sagittal views of left superior parathyroid adenoma. *Abbreviations:* UP PARA LONG, superior parathyroid, longitudinal image; UP PARA TRAN, superior parathyroid, transverse image.

adenomas either preoperatively or intraoperatively with rapid PTH measurement.

Thyroid Incidentalomas

Routine performance of neck ultrasound for preoperative parathyroid localization allows for identification of incidental thyroid pathology that can be biopsied preoperatively. This has been shown to reduce unnecessary thyroid surgery at the time of parathyroidectomy and to allow appropriate thyroidectomy and node dissection in cases of concomitant thyroid malignancy.[17] Thyroid pathology can be picked up incidentally during US for parathyroid localization. The latter case resulted in recognition of multiple endocrine neoplasia type IIa (MEN-IIa) syndrome and allowed biochemical screening to rule out pheochromocytoma prior to parathyroidectomy, thyroidectomy, and bilateral neck dissections.

Certification and Coding

Certification courses are available through the American College of Surgeons and the American Association of Clinical Endocrinologists and are strongly recommended. Verification of competency remains the responsibility of the physician.

Documentation requires at least a formal written report and digital or hardcopy image. It is recommended that diagnostic ultrasounds be performed for about 1 year prior to billing for them, while referring patients to radiology for a confirmatory scan, until the surgeon develops skill in scan performance and interpretation. During this period, however, FNA performed with US guidance was billed.

The correct Current Procedural Terminology (CPT) code for diagnostic neck US is 76536. When US-guided FNA is performed, two separate CPT codes should be used: 76942 and 10022. The first represents the use of US for needle placement and the second for FNA performed with US guidance. These codes are repeated for each nodule, node, or mass biopsied but not for each needle pass into the same specimen. For example, if a patient is seen for evaluation of a palpable thyroid nodule, a diagnostic US is performed (76536) confirming bilateral dominant nodules followed by US FNA of both nodules with four needle passes through each of the two nodules (76942 × 2, and 10022 × 2).

As a rough estimate of the procedure volume required to cover the cost of an office-based US machine, 100 US CPT procedure codes billed annually would cover a $30,000 machine in approximately 3 years. At the time of this writing Medicare reimbursement was about $78 for 76536 and $125 each for 76942 and 10022.

References

1. Shimura H, Haraguchi K, Hiejima Y, et al. Distinct diagnostic criteria for ultrasonographic examination of papillary thyroid carcinoma: a multicenter study. Thyroid 2005;15:251–258
2. Chammas MC, Gerhard R, de Oliveira IR, et al. Thyroid nodules: evaluation with power Doppler and duplex Doppler ultrasound. Otolaryngol Head Neck Surg 2005;132:874–882
3. Alexander EK, Marqusee E, Orcutt J, et al. Thyroid nodule shape and prediction of malignancy. Thyroid 2004;14:953–958
4. Pacini F, Molinaro E, Castagna MG, et al. Recombinant human thyrotropin-stimulated serum thyroglobulin combined with neck ultrasonography has the highest sensitivity in monitoring differen-

tiated thyroid carcinoma. J Clin Endocrinol Metab 2003;88:3668–3673
5. Torlontano M, Crocetti U, Augello G, et al. Comparative evaluation of recombinant human thyrotropin-stimulated thyroglobulin levels, 131I whole-body scintigraphy, and neck ultrasonography in the follow-up of patients with papillary thyroid micro carcinoma who have not undergone radioiodine therapy. J Clin Endocrinol Metab 2006;91:60–63 Epub 2005 Oct 11
6. Rosario PW, de Faria S, Bicalho L, et al. Ultrasonographic differentiation between metastatic and benign lymph nodes in patients with papillary thyroid carcinoma. J Ultrasound Med 2005;24:1385–1389

7. Torlontano M, Attard M, Crocetti U, et al. Follow-up of low risk patients with papillary thyroid cancer: role of neck ultrasonography in detecting lymph node metastases. J Clin Endocrinol Metab 2004;89:3402–3407

8. Solorzano CC, Carneiro DM, Ramirez M, et al. Surgeon-performed ultrasound in the management of thyroid malignancy. Am Surg 2004;70:576–580

9. Ito Y, Tomoda C, Uruno T, et al. Preoperative ultrasonographic examination for lymph node metastasis: usefulness when designing lymph node dissection for papillary microcarcinoma of the thyroid. World J Surg 2004;28:498–501 Epub 2004 Apr 19

10. Kouvaraki MA, Shapiro SE, Fornago BD, et al. Role of preoperative ultrasonography in the surgical management of patients with thyroid cancer. Surgery 2003;134:946–954, discussion 954–955

11. Ceresini G, Corcione L, Morganti S, et al. Ultrasound-guided fine-needle capillary biopsy of thyroid nodules, coupled with on-site cytologic review, improves results. Thyroid 2004;14:385–389

12. Baskin HJ. Detection of recurrent papillary thyroid carcinoma by thyroglobulin assessment in the needle washout after fine-needle aspiration of suspicious lymph nodes. Thyroid 2004;14:959–963

13. Steward DL, Danielson GP, Afman CE, Welge JA. Parathyroid adenoma localization: surgeon–performed ultrasound vs. sestamibi. Laryngoscope 2006 Aug; 116(8):1380–1384

14. Berri RN, Lloyd LR. Detection of parathyroid adenoma in patients with primary hyperparathyroidism: the use of office-based ultrasound in preoperative localization. Am J Surg 2006;191:311–314

15. Solorzano CC, Carneiro-Pla DM, Irvin GL. Surgeon-performed ultrasonography as the initial and only localizing study in sporadic primary hyperparathyroidism. J Am Coll Surg 2006;202:18–24

16. Stephen AE, Milas M, Garner CN, et al. Use of surgeon-performed office ultrasound and parathyroid fine needle aspiration for complex parathyroid localization. Surgery 2005;138:1143–1150, discussion 1150–1151

17. Milas M, Mensah A, Alghoul M, et al. The impact of office neck ultrasonography on reducing unnecessary thyroid surgery in patients undergoing parathyroidectomy. Thyroid 2005;15:1055–1059

Outpatient Thyroidectomy

Thyroid surgery has evolved significantly over the past century. Once a procedure that was considered "breathtaking heroics fraught with danger to the patient and almost certain bereavement for the family,"[1,2] currently more than 80,000 thyroidectomy procedures are performed each year in the United States.[1,2] Because of the proximity of the thyroid gland to vital structures, thyroidectomy has traditionally been performed as an inpatient procedure with a several-day hospitalization. Over the past decade, patient and industry-driven motivation to contain costs without compromising care has prompted a paradigm shift toward outpatient and short-stay surgery in virtually all surgical disciplines. Advances in technology and surgical techniques have allowed surgeons to expand the indications for outpatient surgery to include more invasive operations such as appendectomy, cholecystectomy, and more recently thyroid and parathyroid surgery.

The principal concerns following thyroidectomy include the development of a neck hematoma, acute airway compromise, recurrent laryngeal nerve palsy, and symptomatic hypocalcemia. Life-threatening hematoma, which occurs with an incidence of 0.3 to 1.2%, has led many endocrine surgeons to argue for a mandatory 23-hour postoperative observation period.[3,4] Some suggest that 23-hour observation may identify an additional 38 to 50% of complications that would be otherwise missed in outpatient procedures.[5,6]

Alternatively, McHenry[7] argues that a routine 24- to 48-hour hospital admission may not be justified because most significant neck hematomas manifest either immediately following endotracheal tube removal or early in the postoperative period. Furthermore, delayed neck hematomas or seromas, which may occur up to 2 to 3 days after surgery, are not usually of clinical significance. These issues are explored in depth in this chapter, and a logical algorithm for selected outpatient thyroidectomy is provided.

Drains in Thyroid Surgery

Although many endocrine surgeons continue to utilize drains in thyroidectomy wounds, their routine use has been challenged since 1986.[8] Corsten et al[9] and Pothier[10] independently conducted meta-analyses to evaluate the efficacy of suction drainage in the prevention of postoperative hematomas. Neither found evidence that routine drainage of thyroidectomy wounds prevented hematomas, and no difference in complication rates could be demonstrated. Evolutions in surgical practices have also led many to question the use of drains. For example, subtotal thyroidectomy, which carries an increased risk of bleeding from remnant thyroid tissue, has largely been replaced by total lobectomy and total thyroidectomy.[11] Advances in technology assist surgeons in achieving a better balance between hemostasis and tissue preservation. For instance, Harmonic technology (Ethicon Endosurgery, Cincinnati, OH) (**Fig. 23.1**) provides the ability

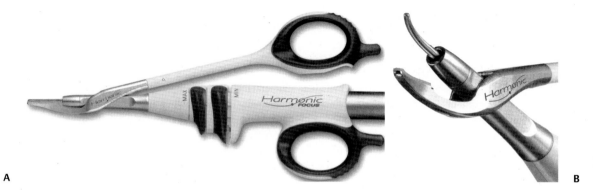

A   B

Fig. 23.1 The Harmonic Focus™ (Ethicon Endosurgery, OH) is a single-patient-use instrument. (**A**) The device is specifically designed for head and neck applications, and provides the ability to dissect as well as to coagulate and cut with hand-activation. (**B**) The working tip is curved and consists of an active blade (upper part), and an inactive blade (lower part). The active blade transmits frictional energy that has the ability to seal and divide vessels up to 5 mm in diameter.

Table 23.1 Criteria for Using Drains

- History of bleeding dyscrasia
- Extensive dissection for substernal goiter
- Concomitant neck dissection
- Large goiter with substantial remaining dead space

to cut and coagulate while reducing the amount of collateral tissue injury, whereas continuous nerve monitoring allows surgeons to closely gauge trauma to the recurrent laryngeal nerve. Our practice for using drains is presented in **Table 23.1**.

Management of Calcium

The most common complication following thyroid surgery is transient hypocalcemia, with an incidence ranging from 2 to 30%.[1,12–17] The etiology of hypocalcemia is multifactorial, with parathyroid insufficiency being the predominant cause. Other contributing factors include reduced stores of vitamin D, hemodilution, carcinoma, and thyrotoxic osteodystrophy.[18,19] In an effort to minimize hospital stays, many authors have attempted to identify risk factors for the development of postoperative hypocalcemia; however, invoking a reliable protocol remains difficult.[12,13,18–20]

Monitoring Serum Calcium Levels

In the absence of reliable preoperative predictors of hypocalcemia, investigators have relied on serum calcium measurements to direct early treatment.[12–14,20] Several authors have shown that an up-sloping curve derived from serum calcium levels obtained at several intervals postoperatively can predict normocalcemia.[15,21] These results, however, take nearly 24 hours to obtain. Adams et al[12] retrospectively reviewed postoperative calcium levels in 128 patients who underwent either parathyroid surgery or nonparathyroid operations including total thyroidectomy, completion thyroidectomy, and other operations thought to put the parathyroid glands at risk. They found that an initial positive slope was 100% predictive of normocalcemia in nonparathyroid patients, and 90% predictive in parathyroid patients. In the nonparathyroid group, a decline in ionized calcium less than 0.25% per hour carried an 85% chance of patients remaining normocalcemic. Their study is limited due to small numbers and a lack of standardized postoperative timing for blood draws. In a follow-up study,[20] the authors attempted to identify a routine that would predict patients at risk for hypocalcemia using a preoperative and 2-hour postoperative ionized calcium level. Although they were unable to find a statistically significant difference between these two levels, they found that patients who became hypocalcemic had an average percent decline in ionized calcium (iCa) of 1.671% per hour ($p = .006$).

In a similar approach, Husein et al[14] prospectively enrolled 68 patients who underwent total thyroidectomy. Corrected serum calcium levels were drawn at 6, 12, and 20 hours and twice daily. Transient hypocalcemia was seen in 21% of patients and permanent hypocalcemia in 6%. The authors found that patients who exhibited a positive slope between 6- and 12-hour calcium levels (defined as a change >0 mmol/L) remained normocalcemic with a positive predictive value of 85.7%. A slope of ≥0.02 between 6 and 12 hours was associated with normocalcemia 97% of the time. Using this algorithm, the authors were able to discharge patients 1 day earlier on average. Bentrem et al[13] obtained total and iCa levels at 8, 16, and 22 hours postoperatively. The iCa levels obtained at 16 hours allowed identification of patients who would eventually develop hypocalcemia 94.4% of the time. The authors also found that iCa levels more accurately correlated with symptomatic hypocalcemia than total calcium and allowed identification of more patients at risk for significant hypoparathyroidism.

In McHenry's[7] review of same-day thyroid surgery, all cases of hypocalcemia were treated successfully on an outpatient basis with no adverse sequelae. He advocates measurement of serum calcium on the morning after surgery in selected patients at risk for postthyroidectomy hypocalcemia. Lo Gerfo et al[16] reported a 6% rate of transient hypocalcemia, with all cases successfully treated on an outpatient basis.

Several issues complicate the utilization of calcium monitoring, however. Serum calcium levels may take 24 to 48 hours to decline. Furthermore, it has been shown that a fall in postoperative calcium within 24 hours is not specific to thyroid surgery. Demeester-Mirkine et al[22] showed that many patients undergoing operations outside the cervical area exhibit declines in serum calcium level similar to those after routine thyroidectomy. Parathyroid hormone (PTH) levels, however, did not fall after nonthyroid operations.

Monitoring Serum Parathyroid Hormone Levels

The poor reliability of serum calcium levels in the prediction of hypoparathyroidism in the immediate postoperative period has prompted several investigators to seek ways to utilize intact PTH (iPTH) for this purpose. Lo et al[23] reported that a $>75\%$ decline in iPTH 10 minutes following removal of the thyroid gland correlated with the development of postoperative hypocalcemia with a sensitivity of 100%, specificity of 72%, and an overall accuracy of 75%. In their series, all patients with normal iPTH after thyroidectomy remained normocalcemic during the postoperative period. They concluded that use of iPTH can avoid the costs of additional serum calcium monitoring and facilitate early discharge.

Lombardi et al[24] described 53 consecutive patients who underwent total or completion thyroidectomy. iPTH was measured at induction of anesthesia, at skin closure, and at 2, 4, 6, 24, and 48 hours after surgery. The authors found that postoperative iPTH levels were reduced (<10 pg/mL) in hypocalcemic patients at all times measured. All normocalcemic patients had perioperative iPTH levels in the normal range. iPTH levels <10 pg/mL at 4 and 6 hours predicted hypocalcemia with 100% specificity and 94% sensitivity, whereas iPTH measurements obtained earlier were less accurate in predicting hypocalcemia.

Scurry et al[25] reported similar findings in a study of 63 total or completion thyroidectomy patients. Additionally they found that an absolute PTH level of 7 pg/mL was most sensitive and specific for predicting hypocalcemia. In their series, patients undergoing completion thyroidectomy were at greater risk of developing hypocalcemia compared with patients undergoing total thyroidectomy.

Based on the findings of these authors, the evaluation of iPTH appears to represent a reasonable option in the prediction of postoperative hypocalcemia, but costs may prevent widespread adoption.

Prophylactic Calcium Supplementation

An alternative solution to the challenge of postoperative calcium management is to administer prophylactic calcium supplementation. Moore[26] was the first to describe this approach to avoid hypocalcemic crisis and promote earlier discharge after total thyroidectomy. More recently, Bellantone et al[27] reviewed their experience of 79 total thyroidectomy patients who were randomly assigned to one of three groups. Patients in group A received no treatment, whereas group B patients received oral calcium (1 g three times daily), and group C patients received the same dose of oral calcium combined with calcitriol (1 μg twice daily). Eleven patients in group A experienced symptomatic hypocalcemia requiring administration of oral calcium and vitamin D, compared with only two patients in group B and three in group C. Two of the patients in group A required IV calcium supplementation ($p <.01$) compared with none in groups B and C. Although it has been shown that vitamin D administration may inhibit PTH secretion by normally functioning parathyroid glands,[28] no difference in iPTH levels was encountered in this series. The authors conclude that administration of oral calcium with or without vitamin D can effectively prevent symptomatic hypocalcemia and allows for safe and early discharge.

Clinical Experience with Outpatient Thyroid Surgery

Several authors have described satisfactory experiences with outpatient or short-stay thyroidectomy. McHenry,[7] for example, retrospectively reviewed 80 patients with nodular thyroid disease who underwent thyroidectomy; 71 patients were discharged after 23 hours, and the remaining nine had planned hospital admissions due to medical conditions, concomitant neck dissection, median sternotomy, or soft tissue tumor resection. Complications included hematoma in one patient, recurrent laryngeal nerve paresis in two patients, and transient hypocalcemia in eight patients. The neck hematoma occurred following an episode of severe coughing and increased blood pressure in the operating room, immediately after extubation. All episodes of hypocalcemia were managed on an outpatient basis, with one patient requiring subsequent hospitalization for anxiety. There were no mortalities. Cost savings were 32% for unilateral thyroidectomy and 47 to 56% for total thyroidectomy.

Sahai et al[29] reviewed short-stay total thyroidectomies ($n = 75$) and hemithyroidectomies ($n = 36$). In their series all patients were discharged after 23-hour observation. Morbidity included transient hypocalcemia in nine patients, two of whom were symptomatic and required readmission and treatment with additional calcium and vitamin D. Both were discharged after overnight observation. The remaining hypocalcemic patients were asymptomatic and diagnosed on routine blood testing as outpatients. One patient required readmission for treatment of a wound infection.

Although reports of extended or short-stay thyroid surgery are prevalent in the literature, little data exist regarding true outpatient thyroidectomy. Steckler[30] initially reported on outpatient procedures, but limited his population to hemithyroidectomy in noncancer cases. Subsequently, Lo Gerfo et al[16] and then Mowschenson and Hodin[31] extended this indication by including total thyroidectomy in their series, again, hospitalizing patients for 4 to 8 hours after surgery.

Most recently, Terris et al[11] conducted a prospective, nonrandomized study of 52 patients undergoing true outpatient thyroidectomy. Patients were discharged directly from the ambulatory recovery unit (usually 2 to 2.5 hours after surgery) once they were able to ambulate, to tolerate a diet, and to manage pain with oral medications. There were no significant complications. One patient required readmission for anxiety. The authors observed significant cost savings in patients undergoing outpatient surgery compared with a similar group of patients who were admitted following surgery.

Protocol for Outpatient Thyroidectomy

Our protocol for performing outpatient thyroid surgery is presented in **Table 23.2**. Inpatient observation should be considered in patients requiring drains, in those with significant medical comorbidity, or in patients in whom there is a concern regarding stability of the airway.

Outpatient Parathyroidectomy

The conventional surgical approach for primary hyperparathyroidism is bilateral neck exploration. Although this modality is associated with high cure rates and few complications, technologic advances (including technetium-99m [Tc-99m]-sestamibi and ultrasound scanning) along with patient motivation factors have driven a trend toward minimally invasive techniques.[33,34] Although bilateral exploration remains the standard of care for four-gland hyperplasia, the advent of minimally invasive parathyroidectomy (MIP) has led to significant decreases in cost, recovery time, and hospital stay while maintaining the same high

Table 23.2 Protocol for Outpatient Thyroidectomy

Indications:

- Cooperative patient interested in outpatient surgery
- Availability of person to take patient home
- Medically fit caregiver
- No concomitant procedure requiring inpatient admission[32]

(Suspected or confirmed malignancy does not contraindicate outpatient surgery)

Discharge parameters:

- Stable wound and airway
- Normal vital signs
- Tolerating oral diet
- Pain controlled with oral medications
- Patients and families are counseled regarding signs and symptoms of hematoma (patients are instructed to return to the hospital immediately should these symptoms arise)

Calcium management (total or completion thyroidectomy):

- Oscal-D 1 gram t.i.d. for the first postoperative week, 1 gram b.i.d. for the second postoperative week, 1 gram daily for the third postoperative week
- Patients and families are counseled regarding the signs and symptoms of hypocalcemia and instructed to increase supplementation and notify their physician should symptoms arise

---

cure rates and low complication rates in selected patients with localized disease. It has been reported that minimally invasive parathyroidectomy is the procedure of choice used by 92% of the members of the International Association of Endocrine Surgeons in patients with localized, single-gland disease.[35–37] One review revealed that MIP has resulted in earlier referral for surgical intervention by endocrinologists.[38]

Minimally invasive parathyroidectomy was discussed at greater length in earlier chapters; however, it is worth mentioning that because of the reduced dissection required, drains are rarely used. Because only one of the four parathyroid glands is disturbed, postoperative hypocalcemia is rare. Therefore, this surgical technique particularly lends itself to an outpatient approach.

Clinical Experience with Outpatient Parathyroidectomy

In their review of MIP, Chen et al[39] showed that 79% of patients were discharged within 3 hours postoperatively. When compared with historical controls, the total hospital charges were approximately $3174 in patients who underwent MIP versus $6328 in patients who had bilateral neck

exploration. Cure rates and morbidity were similar in this series.

Similarly, Cohen et al[35] were able to discharge 86% of patients on the day of surgery. Postoperative cure was achieved in 98.6% of patients with a mean follow-up of about 15 months. No patient experienced significant morbidity. Despite their successful experience, Cohen et al caution that surgeons should remain hypervigilant about the development of any degree of neck swelling. They recommend that patients be observed in recovery for 2 to 3 hours after surgery with a low threshold for continued hospital observation if any concerns develop.

Norman et al[40] reviewed 17 cases of MIP in patients who had undergone at least one prior failed neck exploration. In all cases, a preoperative Tc-99m sestamibi had localized an adenoma and was subsequently deemed to be a false positive by the original surgeon. Prior to reoperation, a repeat Tc-99m sestamibi was obtained, and demonstrated the same focus of increased radio-uptake. Reexploration was undertaken utilizing a radio-guided technique with a handheld gamma probe. In 100% of cases, an adenoma was successfully located in the region indicated by the preoperative Tc-99m sestamibi, and removed; 88% of patients were discharged on the same day.

The classic teaching regarding serial monitoring of calcium levels following parathyroid surgery has been

Table 23.3 Protocol for Outpatient Parathyroidectomy

Indications:

- Localizing imaging study
- Cooperative patient interested in outpatient surgery
- Availability of person to take patient home
- Medically fit patient
- No concomitant procedure requiring inpatient admission[32]

Discharge parameters:

- Stable wound and airway
- Normal vital signs
- Tolerating oral diet
- Pain controlled with oral medications
- Patients and families are counseled regarding signs and symptoms of hematoma (patients are instructed to return to the hospital immediately should these symptoms arise)

Calcium management:

- Oscal-D 1 gram t.i.d. for the first postoperative week, 1 gram b.i.d. for the second postoperative week, 1 gram daily for the third postoperative week
- Patients and families are counseled regarding the signs and symptoms of hypocalcemia and instructed to increase supplementation and notify their physician should symptoms arise

challenged during this era of MIP. Although preexisting vitamin D deficiency can occasionally predispose to hypocalcemia, the only meaningful risk relates to the potential phenomenon of "bone hunger," in which the chronically calcium-depleted bones abruptly sequester serum calcium following the removal of the previously overproducing parathyroid adenoma before the remaining previously suppressed parathyroid glands are fully functional. This is a transient event when it occurs, however, and a large volume of experience suggests that it can be averted by prophylactic calcium supplementation.[26,35]

Protocol for Outpatient Parathyroidectomy

Our protocol for performing outpatient parathyroidectomy is presented in **Table 23.3**. Outpatient procedures are not yet advisable for patients undergoing subtotal parathyroidec-tomy or concomitant surgeries requiring inpatient observation. Admission should be considered for individuals with a diagnosis of parathyroid carcinoma.

Conclusion

Outpatient surgery of the thyroid and parathyroid glands offers significant benefits in regard to patient satisfaction and improved resource utilization. Additionally, this approach allows patients to recover in the comfort of their own home, thereby avoiding exposure to nosocomial infections and iatrogenic complications. With advances in surgical instrumentation and techniques and the addition of prophylactic calcium supplementation, the risk of complications is low. Therefore, outpatient thyroid and parathyroid surgery represents a viable alternative to conventional inpatient surgery.

References

1. Tapscott WJ. A brief history of thyroid surgery. Curr Surg 2001;58:464–466
2. Higgins KM, Mandell DL, Govindaraj S, et al. The role of intraoperative rapid parathyroid hormone monitoring for predicting thyroidectomy-related hypocalcemia. Arch Otolaryngol Head Neck Surg 2004;130:63–67
3. Abbas G, Dubner S, Heller KS. Re-operation for bleeding after thyroidectomy and parathyroidectomy. Head Neck 2001;23:544–546
4. Spanknebel K, Chabot JA, DiGiorgi M, et al. Thyroidectomy using monitored local or conventional general anesthesia: an analysis of outpatient surgery, outcome and cost in 1,194 consecutive cases. World J Surg 2006;30:813–824
5. Burkey SH, Van Heerden JA, Thompson GB, Grant CS, Schleck CD, Farley DR. Reexploration for symptomatic hematomas after cervical exploration. Surgery 2001;130:914–920
6. Schwartz AE, Clark OH, Ituarte P, LoGerfo P. Therapeutic controversy: thyroid surgery—the choice. J Clin Endocrinol Metab 1998;83:1097–1105
7. McHenry CR. "Same day" thyroid surgery: an analysis of safety, cost savings, and outcome. Am Surg 1997;63:586–589
8. Kristoffersson A, Sandzen B, Jarhult J. Drainage in uncomplicated thyroid and parathyroid surgery. Br J Surg 1986;73:121–122
9. Corsten M, Johnson S, Alherabi A. Is suction drainage an effective means of preventing hematoma in thyroid surgery? A meta-analysis. J Otolaryngol 2005;34:415–417
10. Pothier DD. The use of drains following thyroid and parathyroid surgery: a meta-analysis. J Laryngol Otol 2005;119:669–671
11. Terris DJ, Moister B, Seybt MW, Gourin CG, Chin E. Outpatient thyroid surgery is safe and desirable. Otolaryngol Head Neck Surg 2007;136:556–559
12. Adams J, Andersen P, Everts E, Cohen J. Early postoperative calcium levels as predictors of hypocalcemia. Laryngoscope 1998;108:1829–1831
13. Bentrem DJ, Rademaker A, Angelos P. Evaluation of serum calcium levels in predicting hypoparathyroidism after total/near-total thyroidectomy or parathyroidectomy. Am Surg 2001;67:249–251
14. Husein M, Hier MP, Al-Abdulhadi K, Black M. Predicting calcium status post thyroidectomy with early calcium levels. Otolaryngol Head Neck Surg 2002;127:289–293
15. Lam A, Kerr PD. Parathyroid hormone: an early predictor of post-thyroidectomy hypocalcemia. Laryngoscope 2003;113:2196–2200
16. Lo Gerfo P, Gates R, Gazetas P. Outpatient and short-stay thyroid surgery. Head Neck 1991;13:97–101
17. Warren FM, Andersen PE, Wax MK, Cohen JI. Intraoperative parathyroid hormone levels in thyroid and parathyroid surgery. Laryngoscope 2002;112:1866–1870
18. McHenry CR, Speroff T, Wentworth D, Murphy T. Risk factors for post-thyroidectomy hypocalcemia. Surgery 1994;116:641–648
19. Moore C, Lampe H, Agrawal S. Predictability of hypocalcemia using early postoperative serum calcium levels. J Otolaryngol 2001;30:266–270
20. Luu Q, Andersen PE, Adams J, Wax MK, Cohen JI. The predictive value of perioperative calcium levels after thyroid/parathyroid surgery. Head Neck 2002;24:63–67
21. Marohn MR, LaCivita KA. Evaluation of total/near-total thyroidectomy in a short stay hospitalization. Surgery 1995;118:943–947
22. Demeester-Mirkine N, Hooghe L, Van Geertruyden J, De Maertelaer V. Hypocalcemia after thyroidectomy. Arch Surg 1992;127:854–858
23. Lo CY, Luk JM, Tam SC. Applicability of intraoperative parathyroid hormone assay during thyroidectomy. Ann Surg 2002;236:564–569
24. Lombardi CP, Raffaelli M, Princi P, et al. Early prediction of postthyroidectomy hypocalcemia by one single iPTH measurement. Surgery 2004;136:1236–1241
25. Scurry WC, Beus KS, Hollenbeak CS, Stack BC. Perioperative parathyroid hormone assay for diagnosis and management of postthyroidectomy hypocalcemia. Laryngoscope 2005;115:1362–1366
26. Moore FD. Oral calcium supplements to enhance early hospital discharge after bilateral surgical treatment of the thyroid gland or exploration of the parathyroid glands. J Am Coll Surg 1994;178:11–16
27. Bellantone R, Lombardi CP, Raffaelli M, et al. Is routine supplementation therapy (calcium and vitamin D) useful after total thyroidectomy. Surgery 2002;132:1109–1113
28. Zisman AL, Ghantous W, Schinleber P, Roberts L, Sprague SM. Inhibition of parathyroid hormone: a dose equivalency study of paricalcitol and doxercalciferol. Am J Nephrol 2005;25:591–595
29. Sahai A, Symes A, Jeddy T. Short-stay thyroid surgery. Br J Surg 2005;92:58–59
30. Steckler RM. Outpatient thyroidectomy: a feasibility study. Am J Surg 1986;152:417–419

31. Mowschenson PM, Hodin RA. Outpatient thyroid and parathyroid surgery: a prospective study of feasibility, safety, and costs. Surgery 1995;118:1051–1053

32. Samson PS, Reyes FR, Saludares WN, Angeles RP, Francisco RA, Tagorda ER. Outpatient thyroidectomy. Am J Surg 1997;173:499–503

33. Chen H, Zeiger MA, Gordon TA, Udelsman R. Parathyroidectomy in Maryland: effects of an endocrine center. Surgery 1996;120:948–952

34. Van Heerden JA, Grant CS. Surgical treatment of primary hyperparathyroidism: an institutional perspective. World J Surg 1991;15:688–692

35. Cohen MS, Finkelstein SE, Brunt LM, et al. Outpatient minimally invasive parathyroidectomy using local/regional anesthesia: a safe and effective operative approach for selected patients. Surgery 2005;138:681–689

36. Udelsman R. Six hundred fifty-six consecutive explorations for primary hyperparathyroidism. Ann Surg 2002;235:665–670

37. Udelsman R, Donovan PI, Sokoll LJ. One hundred consecutive minimally invasive parathyroid explorations. Ann Surg 2000;232:331–339

38. Gallagher SF, Denham DW, Murr MM, Norman JG. The impact of minimally invasive parathyroidectomy on the way endocrinologists treat primary hyperparathyroidism. Surgery 2003;134:910–917

39. Chen H, Mack E, Starling JR. A comprehensive evaluation of perioperative adjuncts during minimally invasive parathyroidectomy. Which is most reliable? Ann Surg 2005;242:375–383

40. Norman JG, Jaffray CE, Chheda H. The false-positive parathyroid sestamibi: a real or perceived problem and a case for radioguided parathyroidectomy. Ann Surg 2000;231:31–37

Index